T0329683

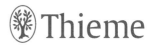

The Surgical Handbook

Michael Karsy, MD, PhD, MSc
Neurosurgical Resident
Department of Neurosurgery
University of Utah Medical Center
Salt Lake City, Utah

Hussam Abou-Al-Shaar, MD
Neurosurgical Resident
Department of Neurological Surgery
University of Pittsburgh Medical Center
Pittsburgh, Pennsylvania

Jian Guan, MD
Neurosurgeon
Department of Neurosurgery
Pacific Neuroscience Institute
Torrance, California

Rebecca Kim, MD, MPH
Instructor
Department of Surgery
Medical College of Wisconsin
Milwaukee, Wisconsin

Jeffrey B. Horn, MD
Assistant Clinical Professor
Department of Anesthesiology
University of Utah Medical Center
Salt Lake City, Utah

115 illustrations

Thieme
New York • Stuttgart • Delhi • Rio de Janeiro

Library of Congress Cataloging-in-Publication Data is available with the publisher.

Thieme Publishers New York
333 Seventh Avenue, New York, NY 10001 USA
+1 800 782 3488, customerservice@thieme.com

Georg Thieme Verlag KG
Rüdigerstrasse 14, 70469 Stuttgart, Germany
+49 [0]711 8931 421, customerservice@thieme.de

Thieme Publishers Delhi
A-12, Second Floor, Sector-2, Noida-201301
Uttar Pradesh, India
+91 120 45 566 00, customerservice@thieme.in

Thieme Publishers Rio de Janeiro,
Thieme Publicações Ltda.
Edifício Rodolpho de Paoli, 25º andar
Av. Nilo Peçanha, 50 – Sala 2508,
Rio de Janeiro 20020-906 Brasil
+55 21 3172-2297

Cover design: Thieme Publishing Group
Typesetting by TNQ Technologies, India

Printed in USA by King Printing Company, Inc.   5 4 3 2 1

ISBN 978-1-68420-128-0

Also available as an e-book:
eISBN 978-1-68420-129-7

Important note: Medicine is an ever-changing science undergoing continual development. Research and clinical experience are continually expanding our knowledge, in particular our knowledge of proper treatment and drug therapy. Insofar as this book mentions any dosage or application, readers may rest assured that the authors, editors, and publishers have made every effort to ensure that such references are in accordance with **the state of knowledge at the time of production of the book**.

Nevertheless, this does not involve, imply, or express any guarantee or responsibility on the part of the publishers in respect to any dosage instructions and forms of applications stated in the book. **Every user is requested to examine carefully** the manufacturers' leaflets accompanying each drug and to check, if necessary in consultation with a physician or specialist, whether the dosage schedules mentioned therein or the contraindications stated by the manufacturers differ from the statements made in the present book. Such examination is particularly important with drugs that are either rarely used or have been newly released on the market. Every dosage schedule or every form of application used is entirely at the user's own risk and responsibility. The authors and publishers request every user to report to the publishers any discrepancies or inaccuracies noticed. If errors in this work are found after publication, errata will be posted at www.thieme.com on the product description page.

Some of the product names, patents, and registered designs referred to in this book are in fact registered trademarks or proprietary names even though specific reference to this fact is not always made in the text. Therefore, the appearance of a name without designation as proprietary is not to be construed as a representation by the publisher that it is in the public domain.

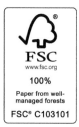

To my wife, Odessa, and children, Penelope and Philip, for their continued support. To all my mentors and patients who have continued to teach me every day.

– Michael Karsy

To my parents, Izzat and Lina, for their endless love and encouragement. To my brothers and my mentors for their continuous support and guidance.

– Hussam Abou-Al-Shaar

To my parents, without whom none of this would be possible.

– Jian Guan

To the students and residents who inspire us all to keep teaching, learning, and asking why.

– Rebecca Kim

To my beautiful wife, Melissa, and daughter, Charlotte, for their unwavering support and dedication to our family. Without their love and support, my life would be trivial. To Dr. Mark Harris, MD, MPH, for his mentorship and resolute collaboration on this personal and professional journey.

– Jeffrey B. Horn

Contents

Edited by Line Kemeyou and Milos Buhavac

Michael Karsy and Milos Buhavac

Michael Karsy and Milos Buhavac

Line Kemeyou and Josef Stehlik

Michael Karsy and Milos Buhavac

Michael Karsy and Milos Buhavac

Michael Karsy and Milos Buhavac

Contents

Contents

Preface

The increasing complexity and rapid transformation of modern surgical treatment has resulted in greater surgical subspecialization than ever before. A dizzying array of procedures exists for patients, which has undoubtedly improved outcomes for surgical patients. However, increasing specialization has led to limited communication between surgical teams and created challenges in training surgeons.

Greater difficulty exists in understanding much of the surgical nuances of decision-making. Providers may not always recognize pathology outside of their specialty or know how to initiate workup, which can delay patient care. Nowhere is this more evident than during training where providers have limited surgical knowledge, are just gaining surgical experience, and have multiple demands on their time. The heterogeneity of surgical exposure during training also results in variability in the knowledge and abilities of surgeons.

This book was designed to fill in some of these gaps. It aims to cover all the major surgical subspecialties, including information on disease recognition and anticipated treatment, classification of disease subtypes, highlighting of where controversies in management exist, and a starting point for additional individualized learning. It also strives to increase insight into surgical fields beyond one's own specialty. The sections can be read independently, or the book can be read cover to cover, depending on an individual's needs. The handbook has been geared to also be useful to residents and medical students on surgical rotations, as well as other providers managing surgical patients, such as advance practice providers, internists, emergency medicine physicians, and anesthesiologists. The goal of this book is not to replace expert consultation or more comprehensive sources but instead inform practitioners earlier to a patient condition and allow for more timely consultation with appropriate providers.

Michael Karsy, MD, PhD, MSc
Hussam Abou-Al-Shaar, MD
Jian Guan, MD
Rebecca Kim, MD, MPH
Jeffrey B. Horn, MD

Acknowledgments

We would like to thank Timothy Hiscock, Executive Editor, and Gaurav prabhuzantye, Project Manager from Thieme Medical Publishers, for their tireless efforts to make this idea become a reality. We also thank all the team members and editors from Thieme Medical Publishers who worked on this project.

We would like thank Kristin Kraus, MSc, Academic Editor from the University of Utah for her help with chapter editing and formatting.

Finally, we would like to thank all the contributing authors and section editors who took time from their busy practices to help impart some of their knowledge to others and improve surgical training.

Contributors

Hussam Abou-Al-Shaar, MD
Neurosurgical Resident
Department of Neurological Surgery
University of Pittsburgh Medical Center
Pittsburgh, Pennsylvania

Cigdem Akcabay, MD
Maternal-Fetal Medicine Fellow
Department of Obstetrics and Gynecology
University of Cukurova, School of Medicine
Adana, Turkey

Jeremiah Alt, MD, PhD
Associate Professor
Department of General Surgery
Division of Otolaryngology–Head & Neck Surgery
University of Utah
Salt Lake City, Utah

Erol Arslan, MD
Maternal-Fetal Medicine Specialist
Department of Obstetrics and Gynecology
University of Health Sciences
Van Training and Research Hospital
Van, Turkey;
Visitor Researcher
Division of Maternal–Fetal Medicine
University of Utah
Salt Lake City, Utah

Alana Aylward, MD
Otolaryngology Resident
Department of General Surgery
Division of Otolaryngology–Head & Neck Surgery
University of Utah
Salt Lake City, Utah

Eric Babajanian, MD
Otolaryngology Resident
Department of General Surgery
Division of Otolaryngology–Head & Neck Surgery
University of Utah
Salt Lake City, Utah

Bridger Battaglia, BS
Medical Student
Department of General Surgery
Division of Otolaryngology–Head & Neck Surgery
University of Utah
Salt Lake City, Utah

Erica F. Bisson, MD, MPH
Associate Professor
Department of Neurosurgery
University of Utah Medical Center
Salt Lake City, Utah

Landon Blumel, MD
Attending Anesthesiologist
Anesthesiology Consultants of
   Cheyenne LLC
Cheyenne, Wyoming

Emilee Borgmeier, MD
Visiting Instructor
Department of Anesthesiology
University of Utah
Salt Lake City, Utah

Nasreen Bowhan, MD
Attending Dermatologists
Department of Dermatology
SSM Health/Dean Medical Group
Madison, Wisconsin

Ronald Buczek, DO
Hand Fellow
Visiting Instructor
Department of General Surgery
University of Utah
Salt Lake City, Utah

Milos Buhavac, MBBS, MA
Critical Care Fellow
Visiting Instructor
Department of General Surgery
University of Utah
Salt Lake City, Utah

Michael Burrow, MD
Ophthalmology Resident
Department of Ophthalmology
University of Utah
Salt Lake City, Utah

Austin Cannon, MD
General Surgery Resident
Department of General Surgery
University of Utah
Salt Lake City, Utah

Richard Cannon, MD
Assistant Clinical Professor
Department of General Surgery
Division of Otolaryngology–Head & Neck Surgery
University of Utah
Salt Lake City, Utah

Adrienne Carey, MD
Assistant Professor
Division of Infectious Diseases
University of Utah
Salt Lake City, Utah

Eric W. Cerrati, MD
Assistant Clinical Professor
Department of General Surgery
Division of Otolaryngology–Head & Neck Surgery
University of Utah
Salt Lake City, Utah

Chad Condie, PharmD, BCCCP
Clinical Pharmacist
Pharmacy Services
U Health University of Utah
Salt Lake City, Utah

Jeffrey Dillon, MD
Assistant Clinical Professor
Department of Anesthesiology
University of Utah
Salt Lake City, Utah

David Dorsey, MD
Assistant Clinical Professor
Department of Anesthesiology
University of Utah
Salt Lake City, Utah

Stephen J. Fenton, MD, FACS, FAAP
Assistant Professor
Division of Pediatric Surgery
Department of Surgery
University of Utah
Primary Children's Hospital
Salt Lake City, Utah

Michelle D. Ford, BHS, CST
Instrument Coordinator
University of Utah
Salt Lake City, Utah

Brent Geffen, MD
Otolaryngology Resident
Department of General Surgery
Division of Otolaryngology–Head & Neck Surgery
University of Utah
Salt Lake City, Utah

Mohit Gilotra, MD
Assistant Professor
Department of Orthopedic Surgery
University of Maryland
Baltimore, Maryland

Fulya Gokdagli, MD
Obstetrics and Gynecology Specialist
Department of ART and Reproductive Genetics
Istanbul Memorial Hospital
Istanbul, Turkey

Jian Guan, MD
Attending Neurosurgeon
Department of Neurosurgery
Pacific Neuroscience Institute
Torrance, California

Mark Harris, MD, MPH
Associate Professor
Vice Chair for Education
Department of Anesthesiology
University of Utah
Salt Lake City, Utah

Gregory W.J. Hawryluk, MD, PhD, FRCSC
Assistant Clinical Professor
Section of Neurosurgery
University of Manitoba
Winnipeg, Manitoba

Jeffrey B. Horn, MD
Assistant Clinical Professor
Department of Anesthesiology
University of Utah Medical Center
Salt Lake City, Utah

Randy L. Jensen, MD, PhD
Professor
Department of Neurosurgery
University of Utah
Salt Lake City, Utah

Yashar Kalani, MD, PhD
Associate Professor
Department of Neurosurgery
University of Virginia
Charlottesville, Virginia

Michael Karsy, MD, PhD, MSc
Neurosurgical Resident
Department of Neurosurgery
University of Utah Medical Center
Salt Lake City, Utah

Logan Kelly, PharmD, BCPS
Clinical Pharmacist
Department of Pharmacy Services
University of Utah
Salt Lake City, Utah

Line Kemeyou, MD
Assistant Professor
Department of Internal Medicine
Division of Cardiovascular Disease
University of Utah
Salt Lake City, Utah

John R. Kestle, MD
Professor
Department of Neurosurgery
University of Utah
Primaries Children's Hospital
Salt Lake City, Utah

Rebecca Kim, MD, MPH
Instructor
Department of Surgery
Medical College of Wisconsin
Milwaukee, Wisconsin

Jeyan Kumar, MD
Neurosurgical Resident
Department of Neurosurgery
University of Virginia
Charlottesville, Virginia

Jim Lai, MD
Physical Medicine and Rehabilitation Resident
Department of Physical Medicine and Rehabilitation
Sinai Hospital
Baltimore, Maryland

Mark A. Mahan, MD
Assistant Professor
Department of Neurosurgery
University of Utah School of Medicine
Salt Lake City, Utah

Mansour Mathkour, MD, MSc
Neurosurgery Resident
Department of Neurosurgery
Tulane University
New Orleans, Louisiana

Erin McCormack, MD
Neurosurgery Resident
Department of Neurosurgery
Tulane University
New Orleans, Louisiana

Hilary McCrary, MD, MPH
Otolaryngology Resident
Department of General Surgery
Division of Otolaryngology–Head & Neck Surgery
University of Utah
Salt Lake City, Utah

Ryan McTish, PharmD
Clinical Pharmacist
Department of Pharmacy Services
University of Utah
Salt Lake City, Utah

Marcus M. Monroe, MD
Assistant Professor
Department of General Surgery
Division of Otolaryngology–Head & Neck Surgery
University of Utah
Salt Lake City, Utah

Christopher Ian Newberry, MD
Otolaryngology Resident
Department of General Surgery
Division of Otolaryngology–Head & Neck Surgery
University of Utah
Salt Lake City, Utah

Bao Nguyen, MD
General Surgery Resident
Department of Surgery
University of Utah
Salt Lake City, Utah

Antony Ocon, MD, PhD
Rheumatology Fellow
Department of Medicine
Division of Allergy, Immunology, and Rheumatology
University of Rochester Medical Center
Rochester, New York

Min Park, MD
Associate Professor
Department of Neurosurgery
University of Virginia
Charlottesville, Virginia

Dorothea Rosenberger, MD, PhD
Professor of Anesthesiology and Critical Care
    Medicine
Diplomate
European Society of Anesthesiology and Intensive
    Care (DESA)
Department of Anesthesiology
University of Utah Health
School of Medicine
Salt Lake City, Utah

Katie Russell, MD
Assistant Professor
Division of Pediatric Surgery
Department of Surgery
University of Utah
Primary Children's Hospital
Salt Lake City, Utah

Stephen Sams, MD
Assistant Professor
Department of Anesthesiology
University of Utah
Salt Lake City, Utah

Wayne Shipley, PharmD, BCCCP
Clinical Pharmacist
Department of Pharmacy Services
University of Utah
Salt Lake City, Utah

Faizi Siddiqi, MD
Professor
Department of Plastic Surgery
University of Utah
Salt Lake City, Utah

Emily Spivak, MD, MHS
Associate Professor
Department of Internal Medicine
Division of Infectious Diseases
University of Utah
Salt Lake City, Utah

Josef Stehlik, MD
Professor
Department of Internal Medicine
Division of Cardiovascular Disease
University of Utah
Salt Lake City, Utah

Fatma Betul Tuncer, MD
Craniofacial Surgery Fellow
Department of Surgery
Division of Plastic Surgery
University of Utah
Salt Lake City, Utah

Jacob Veith, MD
Plastic Surgery Resident
Department of Plastic Surgery
University of Utah
Salt Lake City, Utah

Rachel Elizabeth Ward, MD
Associate Staff Dermatologist
Department of Dermatology
Cleveland Clinic Foundation
Cleveland, Ohio

Andrea Weitz, MD
General Surgery Resident
Department of General Surgery
University of Utah
Salt Lake City, Utah

Cem Yalçinkaya, MD
Gynecologic Oncology Specialist
Department of Obstetrics and Gynecology
University of Health Sciences
Umraniye Training and Research Hospital
Istanbul, Turkey

Michael Yim, MD
Otolaryngology Fellow
Department of General Surgery
Division of Otolaryngology–Head & Neck Surgery
University of Utah
Salt Lake City, Utah

1 General Perioperative and Operative Management

Edited by Jeffrey B. Horn and Mark Harris

1.1 Perioperative Risk

Emilee Borgmeier and Jeffrey Dillon

1.1.1 Overview

- Predicting perioperative surgical risk is a challenging endeavor, which involves taking into account the patient's known past medical history, current surgical procedure, and patient status.
- Knowing which patients can proceed to surgery without further intervention versus those who may need further optimization is a skill that is paramount in physicians who practice medicine in the perioperative period.
- Fundamentals of this practice include understanding who is at increased risk for complications in the perioperative period and why, and understanding when intervention or further testing is indicated prior to proceeding with surgery.

1.1.2 Adverse Events

- Adverse events defined as Major Adverse Cardiac and Cerebrovascular Event (MACE) include the following[1]:
  - Sudden cardiac death.
  - Cerebrovascular death.
  - Myocardial infarction (MI).
  - New congestive heart failure (CHF).
  - Nonfatal cardiac arrest.
  - New arrhythmia.
  - Postoperative angina.
  - Postoperative nonfatal stroke.
- When attempting to study these types of events, articles and reviews may choose to incorporate only some of those events into their risk calculation.
- Definition of risk:
  - Low-risk procedure (MACE risk < 1%):
    - Examples: Superficial surgeries, cataract surgeries, plastic surgery, dental procedures, ambulatory surgery.
  - Elevated risk procedure (MACE risk ≥ 1%):
    - Examples: Intrathoracic procedures, intraperitoneal procedures, aortic, peripheral vascular, head and neck surgery.
- Impact of individual risk factors on perioperative risk:
  - Detailed information regarding other specific risk factors is summarized below from the 2014 ACC/AHA Guideline on Perioperative Cardiovascular Evaluation and Management of Patients Undergoing Noncardiac Surgery[2] unless otherwise referenced.
  - History of previous MI *without* revascularization procedure:
    - Elevated risk of perioperative MACE if operation performed within 60 days of MI.
    - Elective surgery performed < 6 months after MI puts patients at elevated risk for perioperative stroke.
  - History of previous MI *with* revascularization procedure (PCI)[3]:
    - Concern is for in-stent rethrombosis leading to repeat MI.
    - Drug-eluting stent (DES) placement precludes elective noncardiac surgery until 6 months after stent placement.
    - Bare metal stent placement precludes elective noncardiac surgery until at least 30 days poststent placement.

- Emergency surgery before the above time periods requires a discussion between the surgical team, anesthesia team, and patient regarding risks and benefits of bleeding vs. in-stent rethrombosis.
  ○ Age:
  - Age greater than 65 is associated with higher incidence of perioperative stroke.
  ○ Heart failure:
  - History of reduced or preserved ejection fraction heart failure (HF), or physical exam findings consistent with untreated HF are at elevated risk of perioperative MACE.
  - Those that are not optimized medically and who show signs of fluid overload are at highest risk, as well as those with left ventricular ejection fraction (LVEF) < 30% *regardless of optimization status.*[4]
  - Best evidence supports the following medications for decreased mortality in reduced ejection fraction HF (but should *not* be initiated perioperatively): Angiotensin-converting enzyme (ACE) inhibitor or angiotensin receptor blocker (ARB), beta blocker (carvedilol specifically), spironolactone.
  - In one large study, elective noncardiac surgeries in patients with known *optimized* HF did not have higher perioperative mortality rates, but did have significantly longer hospital stays, higher rates of readmission, and overall long-term mortality rates were higher.[5]
  - Diastolic dysfunction is also related to elevate risk of MACE, longer hospitalization, and higher rates of perioperative HF, according to a study of patients undergoing major vascular surgery.[6]
  ○ Cardiomyopathy:
  - Other types of cardiomyopathies include restrictive cardiomyopathy (such as amyloidosis), peripartum cardiomyopathy, and hypertrophic obstructive cardiomyopathy; management depends on knowledge of each specific disease process. All are at increased risk of MACE, but quantification and specific risk factors have not been elucidated.
  ○ Valvular heart disease:
  - In a patient with clinically suspected moderate or greater valvular disease, a perioperative echocardiogram is recommended if there has not been one performed in the past year, or there have been significant functional changes since the patient's last echocardiogram (Class IC).
  - In patients who meet indications for intervention of their valvular disease based on symptoms and severity, intervention on the valve prior to elective noncardiac surgery is effective in reducing the risk of perioperative MACE (Class IC).
  - In patients with *severe but asymptomatic aortic stenosis*, elevated risk elective noncardiac surgery is reasonable, given that there is appropriate intraoperative and postoperative hemodynamic monitoring (Class IIa).
  - In patients with *severe but asymptomatic mitral stenosis that is not favorable for percutaneous balloon commissurotomy*, elevated risk elective noncardiac surgery may be reasonable if there is appropriate intraoperative and postoperative hemodynamic monitoring (Class IIb).
  - In patients with asymptomatic severe mitral regurgitation *or* asymptomatic severe aortic insufficiency (with normal LVEF), elevated risk noncardiac surgery is reasonable with adequate intraoperative and postoperative hemodynamic monitoring (Class IIa).
  ○ Arrhythmia:
  - Many patients have a history of a known arrhythmia, most often atrial fibrillation or frequent preventricular contractions (PVCs).
  - History of PVCs does not confer elevated risk for MACE.
  - If atrial fibrillation is a new diagnosis, cardiac workup should occur prior to elective noncardiac surgery, along with discussion of management of anticoagulation.
  - In otherwise stable, preexisting atrial fibrillation, no further workup is needed; they are at higher risk for left atrial appendage clot formation, but not MACE.
  ○ Implanted cardiac devices[7,8,9]:
  - See Chapter 6.6 Implantable Cardiovert Defibrillators and Pacemakers.
  - Care team should have understanding of the implanted device, and the initial reasoning for placement (typically tachyarrhythmia, bradyarrhythmia, or low ejection fraction heart failure), and the current functional status of the device, and patient dependence on device for cardiac output.
  - Temporary, external pacemaker or defibrillator should be readily available in case of device failure or interference.

Table 1.1 Breakdown of basic pacemaker modes

Paced	Sensed	Response
O = None	O = None	O = None
A = Atrium	A = Atrium	I = Inhibited
V = Ventricle	V = Ventricle	T = Triggered
D = Dual (A + V)	D = Dual (A + V)	D = Dual (T + I)

- – "Cardiac implantable electronic device (CIED)" as a term includes both pacemakers and defibrillators.
- ○ Implantable cardioverter defibrillator (ICD) function:
  - – Electromagnetic interference caused by cautery (especially monopolar), nerve stimulators, radiofrequency ablation, and shock wave lithotripsy can cause inappropriate defibrillation.
  - – Place electrocautery dispersal pads such that the current is not directed in a path through the device, use bipolar cautery if possible, or monopolar cautery in short bursts.
  - – Surgery below umbilicus: Generally accepted that there is no need to turn off ICD.
  - – Surgery above umbilicus: ICD function is typically turned off by either interrogation of device or by placing magnet over device intraoperatively.
  - – Returning the device to its original functionality in either postanesthetic care unit (PACU) or ICU when appropriate and cannot be forgotten.
- ○ Pacemaker function:
  - – Electromagnetic interference can mimic intrinsic cardiac activity, and cause the device to inappropriately pace/sense/inhibit, potentially leading to decreased or no cardiac output depending on the underlying pathology.
  - – Place electrocautery dispersal pads such that the current is not directed in a path through the device, use bipolar cautery if possible, or monopolar cautery in short bursts.
  - – Mode of pacing should be discovered either from device interrogation, patient history or by electrocardiogram (ECG).
  - – Mode described typically as a series of three letters: XXX, describing codes for the three functions Paced, Sensed, Response in that order (▶ Table 1.1).
  - – Surgery below umbilicus: Reprogramming device not generally recommended.
  - – Surgery above umbilicus: Generally recommended that device be temporarily reprogrammed to an asynchronous mode, such as AOO or DOO as appropriate, which disables the sensing function of the device, minimizing the chance for electromagnetic interference.
  - – Most common set modes are VVI or DDD during the perioperative period.
- ○ Emergencies involving implanted cardiac devices:
  - – What if you don't know what type of device the patient has, and neither do they or the medical record? History and physical, including ECG. Chest X-ray can also differentiate between ICD and pacemaker (there is a thick, radiopaque line associated with an ICD, versus two thin leads in a pacemaker).

1.1.3 Perioperative Management: Who Do I Order Further Testing for?

- Preoperative testing is often a confusing aspect of preoperative care, as it is difficult to find definitive predictive data.
- It is known, however, that many tests are ordered reflexively; do not add to the patients care and therefore reflect a large cost burden on the healthcare system, estimated in the US alone to cost $18 billion annually.[10]
- The basic guideline is that preoperative testing should not be ordered routinely; rather, selective individual tests based on a specific patient's clinical situation whose results would likely change or allow optimization of surgical or anesthetic management should be considered.
- The following is a review of the current practice recommendations from the 2012 American Society of Anesthesiologists practice advisory,[11] the 2014 American College of Family Physician's Practice Guidelines,[12] and the 2014 American College of Cardiology/American Heart Association Practice Guidelines[2]:

○ ECG: Not indicated unless high-risk surgery is planned, or the patient has known cardiovascular disease or concern for new cardiovascular disease or arrhythmia. May also be considered if patient has strong risk factors for cardiovascular disease (i.e., smoking history, diabetes mellitus, etc.).

○ Echocardiogram: Not routinely recommended. It is reasonable to perform preoperative echocardiography to assess left ventricular (LV) function in patients with dyspnea of unknown origin or in patients with known systolic or diastolic heart failure or valvular pathology with worsening dyspnea or other significant change. It is also reasonable to obtain a repeat echocardiogram in patients with a history of systolic or diastolic heart failure who have been clinically stable and in whom there has been no assessment in the previous 12 months.

○ Noninvasive cardiac stress testing: Not routinely recommended. Need for preoperative cardiac stress testing can be determined by an evaluation of the patient's functional status or capacity. This can be measured using metabolic equivalents (METs), where 1 MET represents the resting oxygen consumption of the patient (▶ Table 1.2). Patients who have 4 METs or greater typically do not require preoperative stress testing, whereas those patients with < 4 METs functional capacity may benefit from preoperative noninvasive cardiac stress testing to assess for possible need of coronary revascularization prior to elective surgical procedures (▶ Fig. 1.1).

Table 1.2 Examples of activities consistent with different levels of functional activity expressed in metabolic equivalents (METs)

< 4 METs	4 METs	> 4 METs
Basic activities of daily living	Climb 1 flight of stairs	Climb > 1 flight of stairs
Light housework	Mopping floors	Heavy housework such as scrubbing floors or moving furniture
Pulling weeds	Raking leaves	Mowing the lawn (not a rider-mower)
Office work	Golfing with a cart	Golfing on foot
Walking on level ground at 2–3 mph	Walking uphill slowly or on level ground at 3–4 mph	Walking uphill or on level ground at > 4 mph

Abbreviation: mph, miles per hour.

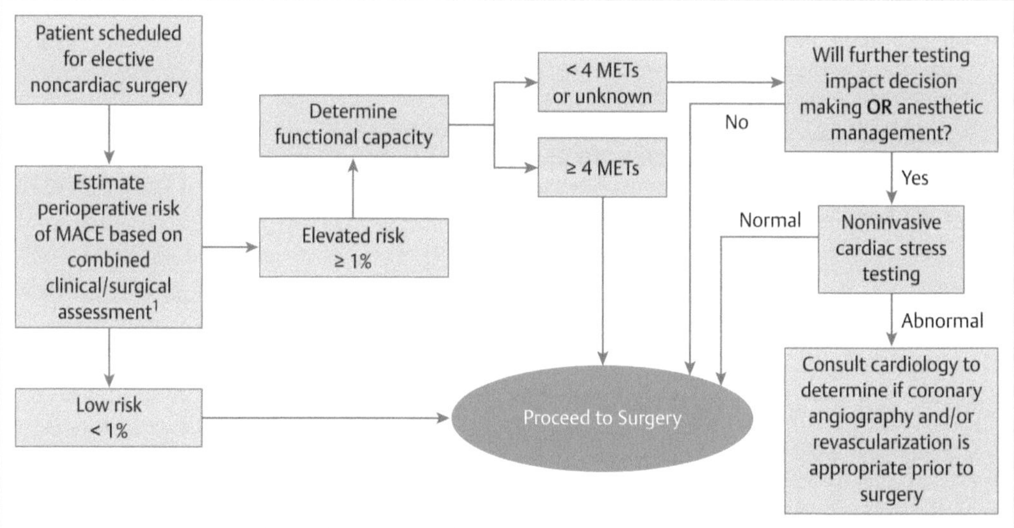

Fig. 1.1 Stepwise approach to perioperative cardiac assessment for CAD and determining need for preoperative noninvasive cardiac stress testing prior to elective surgery. Adapted from 2014 ACC/AHA Practice Guidelines,[2] 2012 ASA Practice Advisory,[11] and the 2014 ACFP Practice Guidelines.[12]

○ Chest X-ray: Not routinely recommended. Consider appropriateness if patient has significant pulmonary disease, new signs or symptoms of respiratory infection, or concerns for significant volume overload.

○ Pulmonary function tests/spirometry: Not routinely recommended. May consider if patient has significant pulmonary disease, and/or surgical interventions will significantly change pulmonary status (i.e., lobectomy or pneumonectomy).

○ Coagulation studies: Not routinely recommended. Reasonable in patients with known liver, renal dysfunction or known coagulation disorder prior to certain surgical interventions and neuraxial anesthesia.

○ Serum chemistry: Not routinely recommended. May be prudent in patients with questionable renal function or dialysis dependence to determine electrolyte status, in patients with poorly controlled diabetes, patients who are taking medication that could alter electrolytes, or if a new arrhythmia has been noted.

○ Urinalysis: Not routinely recommended. May be necessary for surgical procedures involving prosthetic implants or procedures involving the urinary tract.

○ Pregnancy testing: Not mandatory as data is not strong regarding effects of anesthesia on early pregnancy. May be offered to the patient or be required by certain hospitals preoperatively.

1.1.4 Risk Calculators

• Risk calculators have been developed to more accurately define a specific patient's risk when undergoing a surgical intervention. The calculators take into account the patient's underlying illnesses and general health, as well as the type of surgery being performed.

• Two of the more well-known risk calculators will be discussed: The American College of Surgery's National Surgery Quality Improvement Program (ACS NSQIP) Risk Calculator and the Revised Cardiac Risk Index.

• NSQIP risk calculator (http://riskcalculator.facs.org/RiskCalculator/):

○ Developed using data entered from surgeons at 393 hospitals, encompassing 1.4 million patients and 1,557 surgical procedures (identified by Current Procedural Terminology (CPT) code).[13]

○ Twenty-one data fields, including demographics, pertinent health history, and planned procedure.

○ Twelve outcomes are predicted based on the above information, including the following: Any complication, serious complication, pneumonia, cardiac complication, surgical site infection, urinary tract infection, venous thromboembolism, renal failure, readmission, return to the operating room, discharge to rehab or nursing facility, and death. Predicted length of hospital stay has been a recent addition.

○ In one small study ($n = 75$), the accuracy of the NSQIP calculator in emergent versus nonemergent colorectal surgery was studied. Predicted outcomes were compared to actual outcomes. Based on this study, in nonemergent surgeries, NSQIP appears to be accurate. In emergent surgeries, NSQIP appears to underestimate the perioperative risk.[14]

• Revised Cardiac Risk Index (RCRI):

○ Developed using a prospective cohort study of 4,300 patients.

○ Established six independent risk factors for major cardiac complication only, which include: High-risk surgery, history of previously diagnosed ischemic heart disease, CHF, cerebrovascular accident (CVA), preoperative insulin use, and preoperative serum creatinine > 2.0 mg/dL.[15]

○ The overall rate of adverse cardiac outcome in this study was 2%.

○ In those with 0 risk factors, risk of perioperative major adverse cardiac event was 0.4%, 1 risk factor 1.3%, 2 risk factors 4%, and 3 risk factors 9%.[16]

○ The RCRI has been utilized since its publication in 1999, and has been validated since that time.[16]

1.2 Perioperative Medical Optimization

Michael Karsy

• Introduction:

○ Critical to document preoperative medications and establish timing on medication stoppage prior to surgery.

○ Preoperative and postoperative pain management plans can be more effective in pain control and improving recovery.

- ○ Review of discharge medications performed to avoid polypharmacy.
- ○ Significant perioperative holding of medications in surgical patients[17,18]:
  - – Up to 50% of surgical patients may take medications prior to surgery with an average of 2.1 drugs per patient; cardiac medications account for the highest proportion of medications.
  - – 50% of medications are held on the day of surgery; 33% of medications are held on postoperative day 1.
  - – Reasons medications are held: Fasting (49%), failure to prescribe (29%), drug withhold on purpose (10%), drug unavailable in the pharmacy (1%), gastrointestinal tract operation (3%), unknown (8%).
- ○ Utilization of inpatient or outpatient anesthesia clearance prior to surgical procedures can help with intraoperative risk reduction.
- • Specific management[19]:
  - ○ Cardiovascular:
    - – Beta-blockers should be continued in the perioperative period to reduce risk of ischemia and mortality; highest risk of myocardial infarction from postoperative to day 5; ischemia can present atypically in 50% of cases; thus, patients at risk should undergo continued telemetry monitoring.
    - – Nitroglycerin, clonidine, and calcium channel blockers can be continued the day before surgery.
    - – Patients with severe congestive heart failure, valvular disease, or arrhythmias often require expert consultation for medical management.
    - – Aspirin is typically discontinued 1 week before surgery but can be continued through some surgeries after discussion with the surgical team and a patient's cardiologist.
    - – Antiplatelet (e.g., clopidogrel, prasurgrel) treatments should be discontinued 1 week before surgery.
    - – Dual antiplatelet medications are continued for 6–12 months after placement of a DES but with controversy on the optimal duration in patients with acute coronary syndrome.
    - – Elective noncardiac surgery should be delayed for 30 days after a bare metal stent implantation and 6 months after a DES implantation; emergent cases with discontinuation of a platelet inhibitor should have aspirin continued if possible.
    - – Transitioning of warfarin to heparin drip performed for valvular prostheses, heparin stopped 6 hours before surgery and usually restarted 12–24 hours after surgery, enoxaparin can also be used for bridging with last dose 12 hours before surgery, bridging highly dependent on recommendations from cardiology and assessment of patient risk.
    - – Patients with pacemakers or internal cardiac defibrillators require device interrogation and reprogramming prior to surgery reprogramming prior to surgery; see Chapter 6.6 Implantable Cardiovert Defibrillators and Pacemakers.
  - ○ Hypertension:
    - – All antihypertensive medications except ACE inhibitors and ARBs can be continued the day before and the day of surgery in patients with significant hypertension.
    - – Diuretics are generally stopped the day before surgery but volume resuscitation can be easily performed in most patients on the day of surgery if needed.
    - – Patients with mild postoperative hypertension can wait to restart medications until taking oral intake.
  - ○ Arrhythmia:
    - – Digitalis is usually continued the night before surgery but can be discontinued 12 hours before surgery due to risk of toxicity and perioperative arrhythmia.
    - – Disopyramide and amiodarone are stopped the night before surgery.
    - – Quinidine, procainamide, and tocainide are administered the night before surgery.
    - – Verapamil is administered the morning of surgery.
    - – Intravenous procainamide or lidocaine can be used in perioperative period; other antihypertensive medications can be used for rate control.
  - ○ Respiratory:
    - – Beta-agonists and bronchodilators are continued for asthma.
    - – Beta-agonists and atropine are continued for chronic obstructive pulmonary disease; increased steroid doses for 1–2 weeks preoperatively can be used.
    - – Discontinuation of smoking for 2 months can reduce postoperative pulmonary complication rates.

- ○ Hypolipidemic agents:
  - – Niacin, gemfibrozil, and fenofibrate increase the risk of myopathy and rhabdomyolysis perioperatively; these are discontinued on the day before surgery.
  - – Cholestyramine and colestipol can interfere with medication absorption perioperatively; these are discontinued on the day before surgery.
  - – Statins are continued for surgery.
- ○ Diabetes:
  - – Target blood glucose of 100–200 mg/dL is recommended on the day of surgery; levels > 300 mg/dL warrant cancelation of surgery.
  - – Increased risk of wound complications, perioperative deaths, myocardial infarction, and other poor outcomes are seen across various subspecialties in diabetic patients.
  - – Patients with type 1 diabetes require insulin perioperatively.
  - – Patients with type 2 diabetes on insulin are treated with 50% of usual morning isophane on the day of surgery or intravenous infusion of 1 U/h along with dextrose.
  - – Serum glucose is monitored q1–2 hours during surgery and q2–4 hours before surgery.
  - – Metformin is discontinued on the day of surgery due to risk of renal dysfunction and lactic acidosis; sulfonylureas are discontinued on the day of surgery.
  - – Inhaled general anesthetics suppress insulin secretion.
- ○ Hypothyroidism:
  - – Thyroid replacement can be discontinued for up to 7 days due to long half-life; monitoring for hypothermia, hypoventilation, hyponatremia and hypoglycemia is performed.
  - – Severe hypothyroidism is treated with intravenous L-thyroxine and possible corticosteroids.
  - – Thyrotoxicosis is treated with iodine 10 days prior to surgery and perioperative propranolol.
- ○ Hormonal therapy:
  - – Contraceptives are discontinued for 4–6 weeks prior to surgery and perioperatively due to increased risk of venous thromboembolism; these can be controversial.
  - – Estrogen is recommended for postmenopausal hormonal therapy at lower dose than oral contraceptives but can increase the risk of venous thromboembolism; it is discontinued 4–6 weeks preoperatively.
  - – Selective estrogen receptor modulators (e.g., tamoxifen, raloxifene) increase the risk of venous thromboembolism; can be continued for low-moderate risk surgery; discontinued for high-risk surgery without increasing the risk of breast cancer recurrence.
- ○ Perioperative steroids:
  - – Suppression of the hypothalamic-pituitary-adrenal axis occurs in supraphysiologic doses (i.e., prednisone: 5 mg/d long term, 7.5–10 mg/d for 1 month, > 20 mg/d for 1 week, high-dose inhaled corticosteroids).
  - – Steroid potency can be converted from one type to another (▶ Table 1.3).
  - – Minor surgery, > 10 mg/d of prednisone treated with 25–100 mg of hydrocortisone at induction followed by resumption of home corticosteroid the following day.
  - – Major surgery, 100 mg every 8 hours for 24 hours followed by 50% reduction per day to usual steroid dose.

Table 1.3 Steroid potency conversion

Medication	Equivalent dose (mg)	Glucocorticoid potency	Mineralocorticoid potency	Biologic half-life (h)
Cortisone	25	0.8	0.8	8–12
Hydrocortisone	20	1	1	8–12
Prednisone	5	4	0.8	18–36
Prednisolone	5	4	0.8	18–36
Methylprednisolone	5	5	0.5	18–36
Dexamethasone	0.75	25	0	36–54

- ○ Osteoporosis:
  - – Bisphosphonates can be discontinued on the day of surgery, but no change is needed for dental surgery.
- ○ Epilepsy:
  - – Lower threshold for epilepsy is seen during general anesthesia.
  - – Controlled epilepsy does not require modification of medications; many medications can be administered intravenously.
  - – Phenytoin and phenobarbital are effective for all types of seizures except absence seizures.
- ○ Parkinson disease:
  - – Levodopa/carbidopa should be continued perioperatively, no intravenous formulation exists, significant risk of freezing can occur with missed doses, placement of nasogastric feeding tube can be needed in cases to ensure doses are received.
- ○ Antiretroviral medications:
  - – Antiretroviral medications are continued perioperatively; stopping for few days does not worsen effectiveness.
- ○ Psychiatric medications:
  - – Serotonin reuptake inhibitors, selective norepinephrine reuptake inhibitors, and bupropion can be continued.
  - – Tricyclic antidepressants held before surgery and resumed with resumption of oral intake, tapering over 1–2 weeks may be required.
  - – Monoamine oxidase inhibitors (MAOIs) held before surgery when able, controversial if interaction with narcotics, meperidine contraindicated with MAOIs.
  - – Antipsychotic medications are continued perioperatively due to risk of exacerbating psychoses by withholding medications.
  - – Methylphenidate can be continued perioperatively.
  - – Lithium is discontinued 2–3 days before major surgery but can be continued before minor surgery.
  - – Benzodiazepines are discontinued before surgery and can be resumed postoperatively, which have the potential for hypotension and myocardial depression.
- ○ Deep vein thrombosis:
  - – See Chapter 5.2 Venous Insufficiency and Occlusion.
  - – Prophylactic anticoagulation with heparin or enoxaparin is generally withheld before surgery; some patients with planned abdominal surgeries or orthopedic surgeries undergo anticoagulation the day before surgery (e.g., enoxaparin 30 mg q12h subcutaneously starting the night before surgery).
  - – Lab monitoring of enoxaparin is performed in high-risk patients.
- ○ Pain medications:
  - – Nonsteroidal anti-inflammatory drugs (NSAIDs) inhibit cyclooxygenase-1, blocking the formation of thromboxane A2 which can impair platelet aggregation; thromboxane A2 inhibition varies with the type of agent.
  - – NSAIDs are withheld 3–7 days before surgery depending on the type of surgery and drug half-life.
  - – Patients with chronic narcotic use often require preoperative pain plans along with continuation of baseline medications and use of multimodality perioperative pain treatment; use of corticosteroids, neuroleptic medications (e.g., gabapentin), and non-narcotic medications is recommended in addition to adequate narcotic treatment.
  - – Naltrexone should be discontinued preoperatively when pain regiment is implemented.
- ○ Rheumatologic treatments:
  - – Controversial whether methotrexate impacts wound complications; it is metabolized within 2 days; however, it is generally held for 2 weeks preoperatively; can be held for up to 1 month in the setting of orthopaedic fusion.
  - – Cyclophosphamide is held few days before surgery.
  - – Hydroxychloroquine, colchicine, sulfasalazine, and azathioprine are held few days before surgery but there is limited evidence.
  - – Colchicine is held the morning of surgery due to potential for weakness or polyneuropathy, and acute flare can be treated with corticosteroids.

○ Gastrointestinal treatments:
  – Treatments for gastroesophageal reflux disorder are continued perioperatively; anticholinergics, H2 receptor antagonists, antacids, and drugs promoting gastric motility have all been investigated to reduce the risk of aspiration pneumonitis; H2 receptor antagonists and proton pump inhibitors remain the most commonly used.
  – See Chapters 1.3 Fundamentals of Anesthesiology and 10.1 Pediatric Physiology and Surgical Preparation, regarding preoperative fasting times.
○ Benign prostatic hypertrophy:
  – Terazosin, doxazosin, tamsulosin, alfuzosin can be continued preoperatively; potential for intraoperative floppy iris syndrome with use in cataract surgery but medications not typically stopped.
○ Herbal medications:
  – Review of medications should be performed to provide recommendations; due to the heterogeneity of supplements, herbal medications should be stopped 1 week before surgery.
  – Ephedra and Kava should be stopped 24 hours before surgery; Ginkgo should be stopped 36 hours before surgery; garlic, ginseng, St. John's wort, and Valerian should be stopped 7 days before surgery.
○ Anticoagulation:
  – See Chapters 2.8 Hematology and Coagulation and 16 Medications and Rapid Access Information.
  – Limited high-level data are available in the decision making of specific anticoagulants in surgical subspecialties; most recommendations are from retrospective studies and expert opinion.
  – Generally, thromboembolic risk (▶ Table 1.4) is balanced against bleeding risk (▶ Table 1.5)[20] in order to decide duration of anticoagulation disruption and/or restart.
  – Some specialized scores for thrombosis risk exist in certain diseases (e.g., CHADS2-VASc score for atrial fibrillation; see Chapter 2.5 Cardiac Arrhythmia in Surgical Patients).
  – Surgical procedures are delayed, if possible, in patients with transiently increased thromboembolic risk (e.g., stroke, pulmonary embolism).
  – Timing of anticoagulation interruption varies depending on specific agent and patient metabolism.

Table 1.4 Estimation of procedural bleeding risk

High risk (2–4%)[a]	Low risk (0–2%)[a]
Major operation > 45 min	Abdominal hernia repair
Abdominal aortic aneurysm repair	Abdominal hysterectomy
Coronary artery bypass or heart valve replacement	Arthroscopic surgery < 45 min
Endoscopic needle aspiration	Bronchoscopy
Orthopaedic joint surgery or replacement	Carpal tunnel surgery
Spine surgery including lumbar puncture	Cataract surgery
Neurosurgical/urological/otolaryngological surgery	Central venous catheter removal
Polyp	Cholecystectomy
Transurethral prostate resection	Cutaneous lymph node biopsies
Vascular surgical procedure	Dilatation and curettage
Transjugular intrahepatic portosystemic shunts	Gastrointestinal endoscopy, enteroscopy, biliary/pancreatic stenting, endosonography without fine-needle aspiration
Lung interventions	Hemorrhoidal surgery
Solid organ biopsies or drainage	Hydrocele repair
	Noncoronary angiography
	Cardiac defibrillator insertion
	Tooth extraction
	Endovascular procedures (e.g., angioplasty, catheter ablation, atherectomy)

[a] Estimation of 2-d major bleeding in the absence of anticoagulation.

- Anticoagulation reversal depends on agent, clinical factors, and often institutional policy/preference.
- Bridging anticoagulation is considered for patients with very high thromboembolic risk due to increased bleeding risk with bridging medications; bridging weight against risk of thromboembolism in patients with high or moderate risk (▶ Table 1.6); bridging depends on agent being used; warfarin bridge is initiated 5 days before a procedure.
- Risk of hemorrhage from bridging is higher than risk of thromboembolic complication.
- Temporary vena cava filters can be considered for patients with recent acute venous thromboembolism in past 3–4 weeks with anticipated delay in anticoagulation for > 12 hours.

Table 1.5 Estimation of major bleeding risk with anticoagulation for atrial fibrillation via HAS-BLED score[4]

Category	Point
Hypertension (systolic blood pressure > 160 mm Hg)	+ 1
Abnormal liver function (chronic liver disease, impaired liver function)	+ 1
Abnormal renal function (chronic dialysis, renal transplantation, creatinine ≥ 2.26 mg/dL)	+ 1
Previous history of stroke	+ 1
Bleeding tendency or predisposition requiring hospitalization or transfusion	+ 1
Labile INRs in patients taking warfarin	+ 1
Age > 65	+ 1
Concomitant antiplatelet agents (e.g., aspirin, antiplatelet agents, nonsteroidal anti-inflammatory agents)	+ 1
Excessive alcohol use	+ 1
HAS-BLED score interpretation	
0 points	1.13 bleeds/100 patient-years
1 point	1.02 bleeds/100 patient-years
2 points	1.88 bleeds/100 patient-years
3 points	3.74 bleeds/100 patient-years
4 points	8.70 bleeds/100 patient-years
5–9 points	Insufficient data

Table 1.6 Conditions with potential need for bridging therapy

Very high thrombotic risk	High thrombotic risk	Moderate thrombotic risk
• Any mitral valve prosthesis • Any caged-ball or tilting disc aortic valve prosthesis • Stroke or TIA within 6 mo • CHADS2-VASc score 5–6 • Rheumatic valvular heart disease • VTE within 3 mo • Severe thrombophilia[a]	• Bileaflet aortic valve prosthesis with additional risk factor (atrial fibrillation, prior stroke/TIA, hypertension, diabetes, congestive heart failure, age > 75 y) • CHADS2-VASc of 4–5 • VTE within 3–12 mo • Nonsevere thrombophilia[b] • Recurrent VTE • Active cancer within last 6 mo	• Bileaflet aortic valve prosthesis without atrial fibrillation or other risk factors • CHADS2-VASc of 2–3 • VTE > 12 mo without other risk factors

Abbreviations: CHADS2-VASc, congestive heart failure, hypertension, age > 75 y, diabetes mellitus, stroke, valvular disease, age 65–74, female; TIA, transient ischemic attack; VTE, venous thromboembolism.

[a] Deficiency of protein C, protein S, antithrombin; antiphospholipid antibodies; multiple coagulation abnormalities.

[b] Heterozygous factor V Leiden, prothrombin mutation.

1.3 Fundamentals of Anesthesiology

Jeffrey B. Horn, Mark Harris, and Stephen Sams

1.3.1 Standards for Basic Anesthesia Monitoring[21]

- Standards for basic anesthesia monitoring (▶ Table 1.7):
  - American Society for Anesthesia (ASA) adopted the Standards for Basic Anesthesia Monitoring in 1986.
  - The standards are updated over time due to evolution of medical equipment and practice.
  - These are the framework of minimal acceptable criteria for patient monitoring.
  - Each patient monitoring modality is subject to discretion of the provider.
- Nothing per os (NPO) (▶ Table 1.8)[22,23,24]:
  - ASA guidelines recommend lengths of preoperative fasting prior to monitored anesthesia care (MAC), neuraxial anesthesia, or general anesthesia.
  - Recommendations (NOT standards or absolute requirements) are based on expert consensus when contemplating the adverse physiologic effects associated with pulmonary aspiration after the use of sedative pharmacologic agents.
  - Although the incidence of pulmonary aspiration is rare, significant morbidity and mortality has been associated with the composition of the aspirate (content high in particulate matter, volume, and acidity).

Table 1.7 Standards for basic anesthesia monitoring

Standard 1		Qualified anesthesia personnel should present in the operating room throughout ALL surgical cases involving general anesthesia, regional anesthesia, and monitored anesthesia care
Standard 2		Any anesthesia technique decided on by the provider shall assess a patient's oxygenation, ventilation, circulation, and temperature
	Oxygenation	Oxygen concentration of inspired gas (general anesthesia)
		Observation of patient's skin and mucous membrane color
		Use of pulse oximetry with low threshold alarm
		Observation of patient and reservoir bag (general anesthesia)
		Mechanical ventilation circuit disconnection alarms (general anesthesia)
	Ventilation	Auscultation of breath sounds
		Continuous end-tidal carbon dioxide measurement ($ETCO_2$)
		Quantification of the volume of expired gas
		Continuous electrocardiogram display
	Circulation	Heart rate and blood pressure (measured ≥ 5 min)
		Evaluation of the circulation (auscultation of heart sounds, palpation of pulse, plethysmography, pulse oximetry)
	Temperature	Continual temperature monitoring (when significant changes are anticipated or suspected)

Table 1.8 Nothing per os status

Food/Fluid intake	Minimum fasting period
Clear liquids	2 h
Breast milk	4 h
Infant formula	6 h
Nonhuman milk	
Light meal	6 h
Heavy meals (fatty or fried, alcohol)	8 h

- ○ Guidelines focus on reducing or eliminating particulate matter, decreasing the volume (gastric stimulants), and reducing the acidity (alkaline solution) of any content remaining in the stomach and/or gastrointestinal tract.
- Oxygenation (▶ Table 1.9)[25,26]:
  - ○ Intermittent assessment of arterial oxyhemoglobin (SaO_2): Most sensitive and specific method of quantifying a patient's blood oxygenation. However, this analysis is invasive and has limited utility in a regular setting.
  - ○ Continuous pulse oximetry:
    - – Convenient, noninvasive method, used as a surrogate based on the Beer–Lambert law (correlation of solute concentration to intensity of light displayed through solution).
    - – A probe containing two light-emitting diodes (LEDs) is attached to a translucent part of the body (commonly a fingertip or an ear lobe). The LED emits a red (660 nm) and infrared wavelength (940 nm) of light that is preferentially absorbed by either oxygenated (infrared light) or deoxygenated (red light) hemoglobin. The proportion of light absorbed by each hemoglobin type is analyzed as a ratio and displayed on a monitor as a percentage of oxygenated hemoglobin.
    - – The percentage of hemoglobin accepted representing adequate tissue oxygenation is > 92%.
- Hypoxemia (▶ Table 1.10):

Table 1.9 Oxygenation

Pulse oximetry	2 Wavelengths of light emitted (red 660 nm and infrared 940 nm)
	Displayed as percentage of total hemoglobin existing as oxyhemoglobin (SpO_2)
	$SPO_2 = (O_2HGB \ / \ (O_2HGB + DEOXYHGB)) \times 100$
Limitations	Decreased blood flow
	Movement artifact
	Electrocautery
	Inaccurate estimation of arterial oxygenation: dyes, nail polish, extreme hypothermia, hemoglobinopathies

Table 1.10 Hypoxemia differential diagnosis

Decreased delivery of inspired oxygen	Decreased transportation of oxygen	Artifacts
Kinked circuit tubing		
Kinked endotracheal tube		
Decreased oxygen flow		Blue dyes (methylene blue)
Inadequate ventilation	Decreased cardiac output	Electrocautery
(obesity, decreased respiratory rate, right mainstem intubation, bronchospasm, pneumothorax)	Hypotension	Cold hands
		Raynaud's phenomenon
Ventilation/perfusion mismatch		Decreased perfusion
(atelectasis, pneumonia, aspiration, pulmonary embolus, pulmonary edema, cardiac shunt)		
Management		
100% oxygen		
Check $ETCO_2$ and peak airway pressure		
Ventilate by hand with large volumes		
Look at the patient for adequate chest rise, and auscultate for breath sounds		
Check endotracheal tube and circuit		
Suction airway		
Check pulse oximeters and color of patient (artifact?)		
Reintubate?		

- Hypoxemia: Decreased levels of oxygen in the blood, oxygen saturation of less than 90%, or a decrease of more than 5% (as opposed to hypoxia, which is the reduction of oxygen supply at the tissue level).
  - Hypoxia: Insufficient oxygen supply for the metabolic demands of the body as a whole, or a particular tissue or organ.
  - Can adversely affect every tissue in the body.
  - Organs particularly susceptible to hypoxia are the brain (< 3 minutes), the kidneys, and liver (15–20 minutes).
  - Until proven otherwise, low oxygen saturation indicates hypoxemia (i.e., don't assume it's an artifact).
- Temperature (core vs. peripheral) (▶ Table 1.11)[27]:
  - Euthermia is vital to normal homeostatic physiologic function (coagulation, wound healing, organ function).
  - Surgical environment (ambient/cold room temperature; disrobed patients) of the operating room impedes the body's ability to maintain or conserve heat (lack of shivering under general anesthesia).
  - Vast majority of anesthetic agents are known to alter thermoregulation (vasodilation) by transferring body heat from the core to periphery.
  - Although heat is not literally lost from the core, redistribution of body heat to the periphery is the main method of temperature reduction via radiation, conduction, convection, and evaporation (decreases approximately 1.5 °C during the first hour of surgery).
- Hypothermia (▶ Table 1.12):
  - Definition: Core body temperature < 35 °C.
  - Best avoided in the operating room by increasing room temperature, using warm blankets, preheated intravenous fluids, and heated anesthetic circuit humidifier, and decreasing flow of gases to the patient.
  - Metabolic oxygen requirements of the patient are decreased approximately 9% per 1 °C drop in core body temperature (if shivering is absent); other physiological changes are also seen.
- Noninvasive blood pressure[25,26]:
  - Automated sphygmomanometers are the standard of care in the operating room to assess a patient's blood pressure.
  - Appropriate sizing of blood pressure cuffs is crucial to ensure accurate measurements.
  - According to the American Heart Association,[28] the proper bladder length of a blood pressure cuff recommended is 80% of the circumference of the patient's arm while the ideal width is 40.
  - A cuff that is too small will erroneously overestimate blood pressure while oversized cuffs will underestimate blood pressure.
- Electrocardiogram (EKG)[25,26]:
  - EKG interpretation is crucial for perioperative assessment of patient circulation.
  - According to the ACC/AHA 2007 guidelines, patients with at least one cardiovascular risk factor undergoing intermediate risk surgery (vascular, known coronary artery disease or cerebrovascular accident) require a perioperative EKG.
  - Intraoperative EKG interpretation can provide integral patient information such as but not limited to anesthetic depth related to surgical stimulation, dysrhythmias, and electrolyte abnormalities.

Table 1.11 Temperature regulation

Core temperature monitoring sites	Peripheral heat loss mechanisms
Blood (pulmonary artery)	Radiation (most common): transfer of heat from one substance to another without physical contact
Distal esophagus	
Tympanic membrane	Conduction: direct transfer of heat from one object to another
Oropharynx	Convection: heat transfer to a small layer of air moving around the body
Nasopharynx	Evaporation: transfer of heat from water to gas (sweating)
Bladder (variable)	
Rectum (variable)	

Table 1.12 Physiologic changes associated with hypothermia

Oxygen delivery	Hemoglobin-oxygen curve shifted to the left (decreased release of oxygen to the tissues)
	Decreased systemic vascular resistance → peripheral hypoperfusion
Acid-base status	Metabolic acidosis
Hematology	Decreased blood viscosity
	Increased prothrombin time
	Decreased fibrinogen activity
	Decreased platelet aggregation
Cardiovascular	Increased systemic vascular resistance (vasoconstriction)
	Decreased heart rate leads to decreased myocardial contractility leads to decreased cardiac output
	Ventricular fibrillation at 23–28 °C
	Asystole at 20 °C
Pulmonary	Increased pulmonary vascular resistance
	Decreased hypoxic pulmonary vasoconstriction leads to increased ventilation-perfusion mismatch leads to decreased ventilatory drive
Hepatic	Decreased renal blood flow leads to decreased drug metabolism
	Glucose/citrate not metabolized leads to hyperglycemia
Renal	Cold diuresis (decreased renal blood flow due to increased renin–angiotensin–antidiuretic hormone secretion)
	Anuria leads to < 20 °C
Central nervous system	Decreased cerebral blood flow
	Decreased evoked potential latency
	Decreased anesthetic requirement
Endocrine	Increased epinephrine
	Increased adrenocortical hormones
	Increased adrenocorticotropic hormone

1.3.2 Anesthesia Basics

- Sedation continuum (▶ Table 1.13)[29]:
  - Four levels of sedation are demarcated by the ASA.
  - Sedation levels include minimal sedation/anxiolysis, moderate sedation/analgesia, deep sedation/analgesia, and general anesthesia described by four distinctive criteria (responsiveness, airway, spontaneous ventilation, and cardiovascular function).
  - Detailed understanding of the criteria exclusive to each level of sedation is integral with regard to patient safety.
  - A given dose of sedative medication will not reliably yield a repeatable and distinctive level of consciousness for each patient.
  - Commonplace for patients to progress to deeper than intended levels of sedation, even when a comparatively lower amount of medication is used. Therefore, any provider that administers sedation should be adept in airway management, and basic and advanced cardiac life support.
- ASA's physical classifications status (▶ Table 1.14):
  - Its purpose is to stratify the overall health of patients to determine the anesthetic and/or surgical strategy.
  - It is a universally accepted system that allows members of different medical specialties to communicate in a collective syntax as well as create a persistent system of record-keeping and classification for statistical analysis.[30]
  - Not intended to predict perioperative risk, but there is evidence to suggest that an increased ASA score correlates with an increased risk of perioperative mortality.[31,32]
  - Inter-rater variability scores of the ASA's physical classification status are significant across medical specialties and between anesthesia providers.[33]

Table 1.13 Sedation continuum

Clinical findings	Minimal sedation/ anxiolysis	Moderate sedation/ analgesia	Deep sedation/ analgesia	General anesthesia
Responsiveness	Normal response to verbal stimulation	Purposeful response to verbal or tactile stimulation	Purposeful response following repeated or painful stimuli[a]	Unarousable to painful stimuli
Airway		No intervention required	Intervention may be required	Intervention often required
Spontaneous ventilation	Unaffected	Adequate	May be inadequate	Frequently inadequate
Cardiovascular function		Usually maintained	Usually maintained	May be impaired

[a] Reflex withdrawal from a painful stimulus is not considered a purposeful response.

Table 1.14 American Society for Anesthesia (ASA) physical classification status

APA class	Features	
I	Normal healthy patient	
II	Patient with mild systemic disease	Controlled hypertension
		Diabetes mellitus without systemic disease
		Smoking without chronic obstructive pulmonary disease
		Social alcohol use
III	Severe systemic disease that is *not* incapacitating	Stable angina
		Controlled heart failure
IV	Incapacitating disease that is a *constant* threat to life	Symptomatic heart failure
		Symptomatic chronic obstructive pulmonary disease
		Cerebrovascular accident/transient ischemic attack
V	Moribund patient that is *not* expected to live 24 h without the surgery	Multiorgan failure
		Massive trauma
VI	Declared brain dead patient whose organs are being harvested for transplant	
E	Denotes emergent surgical action	

1.3.3 Neuraxial Anesthesia

- Types and purpose of neuraxial anesthesia (▶ Table 1.15)[25,26]:
  - Several neuraxial analgesia and anesthesia techniques are commonly used for various medical indications.
  - The decision to choose one technique over the other is dependent on a host of factors such as the individual pharmacodynamic and pharmacokinetic properties of each pharmacologic agent, the natural and comorbid attributes of each patient, technical aspects distinctive to the various neuraxial methods, and the risks and benefits of the procedure to the patient.
  - Knowledge of spinal anatomy, dermatomal and sensory distribution, and the type and duration of the surgical procedure are vital to the anesthesia provider when determining the spinal segment(s) that should be anesthetized.
  - Advantages include the ability to target specific and localized anatomic areas over longer duration of time, and disadvantages include symptomatic hypotension after sympathectomy and postdural puncture headache.
- Physiologic alterations after neuraxial anesthesia (▶ Table 1.16)[25,26]:
  - Safe and effective patient treatment with neuraxial anesthesia requires knowledge of potential physiologic.

Table 1.15 Neuraxis anesthesia and analgesia

Type of anesthesia/analgesia	Definition	Structures traversed
Spinal anesthesia	Direct injection of medication directly into the thecal sac	Skin
		Subcutaneous fat
		Supraspinous ligament
		Intraspinous ligament
		Ligamentum flavum
		Dura mater
Epidural anesthesia	Placement of catheter and delivery of continuous medication to the epidural space	Skin
		Subcutaneous fat
		Supraspinous ligament
		Intraspinous ligament
		Ligamentum flavum
Combined spinal and epidural anesthesia	Single injection of medication directly into the thecal sac; with placement of catheter and delivery of continuous medication into the epidural space	Skin
		Subcutaneous fat
		Supraspinous ligament
		Intraspinous ligament
		Ligamentum flavum
		Dura mater

Surgical procedures	Dermatomal level of anesthesia/analgesia
Upper abdominal surgery	T_4
Caesarian section	T_4
Transurethral resection of the prostate	T_{10}
Hip surgery	T_{10}
Foot and/or ankle surgery	L_2

Table 1.16 Physiologic changes after neuraxial anesthesia and analgesia

System	Physiological ramifications
Cardiovascular	Hypotension (decreased systemic vascular resistance, venous > arterial)
	Heart block (first, second, or third)
	Decreased stroke volume
	Bradycardia
	Decreased preload
	Increased afterload
Pulmonary	Minimally decreased (not clinically significant):
	• Forced expiratory volume in one-second
	• Maximum inspiratory volume
	• Expiratory reserve volume
	• Vital capacity
Central nervous system	Decreased regional cerebral blood flow
	(Increased elderly and preexisting hypertension)
Renal	+/− Neurogenic bladder (questionable)
	Decreased renal blood flow
Gastrointestinal	Decreased hepatic blood flow (decreased mean arterial pressure)
	Increased incidence of nausea and vomiting
	Hyperperistalsis (T_6–L_1)
Other; progression of block effect	Temperature then vasomotor tone then sensory then motor

- ○ Local anesthetic inhibits both the sympathetic and somatic divisions of the central nervous system in a dose- and concentration-dependent manner by sequentially blocking small unmyelinated sympathetic fibers prior to larger myelinated fibers.
- ○ Sympathetic blockade can effectively anesthetize two successive dermatomes when compared to sensory and motor inhibition.
- ○ Virtually every organ system in the human body is affected by neuraxial anesthesia (e.g., sympathetic blockade of the cardiac accelerator (T_1–T_4) fibers can lead to unopposed parasympathetic activity with subsequent decreased stroke volume and bradycardia).
- Spinal anesthesia (▶ Table 1.17)[25,26]:
  - ○ Spinal anesthesia (aka spinal block or a spinal) is a primary neuraxial anesthetic technique and is typically chosen for lower extremity (lower abdomen, limbs, genital, perineum) procedures lasting less than 3–4 hours in duration.
  - ○ Spinal needle is inserted between vertebral levels L_3 and L_4, through the dura mater, and the medication (local anesthetic) is injected directly into the thecal sac; local anesthetic exerts its

Table 1.17 Spinal anesthesia

Features	Notes
Benefits	Decreased morbidity and mortality in high-risk patients
	Decreased incidence of thromboembolic complications
	Decreased stress response to surgical stimulation
	Increased intraoperative blood loss
Relative contraindications	Preexisting neurologic conditions
	Moderate stenotic valvulopathy
	Severe spinal deformity
	Uncooperative patient
	Sepsis
Additives that prolong analgesic effect	Epinephrine
	Phenylephrine
	Clonidine
Absolute contraindications	Anaphylaxis to local anesthetics
	Severe aortic or mitral stenosis
	Infection at injection site
	Elevated intracranial pressure
	Severe hypovolemia
	Patient refusal
	Coagulopathy
Controversial contraindications	Prolonged surgical procedures
	Major blood loss anticipation
	Compromised ventilation
	Language barrier
Factors affecting height of analgesia	Patient posture related to the natural curvature of the spine
	Dose, concentration, and volume of local anesthetic
	Baricity of local anesthetic
	Age (increased age results in increased block height)
	Gender (males have decreased block height)
	Site of injection
	Patient height
	Pregnancy

pharmacologic effects on the ventral and dorsal spinal nerve roots, and the diffusive spread of local anesthetic depends on several variables such as the baricity and lipophilicity of the local anesthetic and the size and/or myelination of the neural fibers.

○ Onset of block is within minutes of injection, time to peak varies with agent and from 10–20 minutes, and duration depends on dose, concentration, and/or addition of adjuvant medication (phenylephrine, clonidine).

○ Compared with general anesthesia, spinal anesthesia results in decreased intraoperative blood loss, decreased incidence of deep vein thrombosis, and decreased pulmonary aspiration, especially in patients with potential airway problems and comorbid pulmonary pathology.

○ Spinal anesthetic creates denser block than epidural anesthetic.

○ Spinal anesthetic must be administered below conus medullaris (L1).

○ Disadvantages are high-spinal postdural puncture headache, transient neurologic syndrome, cauda equina syndrome, spinal hematoma, backache, infection, and cardiac death.

• Epidural anesthesia (▶ Table 1.18)[25,26]:

○ Epidural anesthesia is a primary neuraxial anesthesia or analgesia technique with a catheter placed in close proximity to the spinal dura mater in an area called the epidural space.

○ Epidural space is a potential anatomic space filled with spinal nerve roots, epidural fat, blood vessels, and lymphatic tissue.

○ Anesthesia is administered intermittently or continuously.

○ Boundaries: Anterior—posterior longitudinal ligament; lateral—pedicles and intervertebral foramina; posterior—ligamentum flavum (yellow ligament).

○ Anesthesia acts on ventral and dorsal nerve roots.

○ It can be administered anywhere along the length of vertebral column, allows targeting of specific vertebral segments.

• Neuraxial anesthesia complications (▶ Table 1.19):

○ Postdural puncture headache (PDPH)[25,26]:

– It occurs after inadvertent or intentional perforation of the dural membrane.

– Hypothesized etiology: Net loss of cerebrospinal fluid (CSF) leading to resultant cerebral vasodilation and stretching of the meninges, can cause cranial nerves palsies with most commonly cranial nerve VI (abducens nerve) palsy or visual disturbance (lateral rectus muscle palsy).[34]

– Incidence 0.1–50% from dural violation depending on needle size and tip style (pencil-point vs. beveled).

Table 1.18 Epidural anesthesia

Features	Notes
Absolute contraindications	Anaphylaxis to local anesthetics
	Infection at the injection site
	Elevated intracranial pressure
	Severe coagulopathy
	Patient refusal
	Severe hypovolemia
Relative contraindications	Mild-to-moderate coagulopathy
	Sepsis
	Spinal deformity
	Uncooperative patient
Diffusion of medication	Epidural space to systemic circulation
	Across meninges to spinal cord → Paravertebral space → Epidural fat → Systemic circulation
Epidural test dose	Rules out intravascular catheter placement
	Typical dose: 3 mL of 1.5% lidocaine with 1:200,000 epinephrine

Table 1.19 Neuraxial anesthesia complications

Features	Notes
Postdural puncture headache (PDPH)	
Risk factors	History of previous PDPH
	Cutting needle (Quincke)
	Increased diameter of needle
	Female gender
	Pregnancy
	Decreased age
Signs and symptoms	Bilateral frontal or occipital scalp pain
	Positional headache (increased severity sitting or standing)
	Diplopia (stretching of cranial nerve VI)
	12–48 h after dural perforation
	Stiffness of the neck
	Photophobia
	Tinnitus
	Nausea
Medical management	Intravenous hydration
	Epidural blood patch
	Acetaminophen
	Caffeine
	Bed rest
	Nonsteroidal anti-inflammatory drug (NSAID)
Transient neurological symptoms	
Pathophysiology	Unclear etiology
	Ephemeral pain and/or sensory irregularities of the lower back emanating to the lower extremities and/or buttocks after subarachnoid injection
Signs and symptoms	Burning radicular pain
	Within 24 h after spinal anesthetic
	Not associated with sensory loss, motor weakness, or bowel and bladder dysfunction
Risk factors	Subarachnoid local anesthetic injection (lidocaine)
	Ambulatory surgical procedures
	Lithotomy position
Medical management	Self-limited
	Complete resolution ~3–10 d after spinal anesthetic
	NSAIDs
	Trigger point injections
Spinal anesthesia complications	
Pathophysiology	Chemical injury (local anesthetic) to the lumbosacral nerve roots
Signs and symptoms	Lower back and buttock pain
	Lower extremity motor weakness
	Saddle anesthesia
	Bowel and bladder dysfunction
Risk factors	Continuous infusion (microcatheter)
	Lithotomy position
	Increased concentration of lidocaine
	Repeated use of lidocaine

(Continued)

Table 1.19 (*Continued*) Neuraxial anesthesia complications

Features	Notes
Medical management	Mild improvement with time but likely a permanent disability
Hematoma	
Facts	Increased incidence with epidural *or* combined spinal–epidural neuraxial anesthesia
	Progressive motor and sensory block
Signs and symptoms	Bowel and/or bladder dysfunction
	Back pain
	Increased age
	Female gender
	Coagulopathy
Risk factors	Difficult neuraxial procedure
	Multiple attempts at catheter placement
	Spinal abnormalities
	Vascular malformations
	Neoplasm
Medical management	Immediate surgical decompression

- Risk factors in increasing likelihood are female gender, gravidity, thin body habitus, and history of prior headache or PDPH.
- Obesity is considered a protective attribute, as increased intra-abdominal pressure decreases the diameter or altogether closes the dural perforation to retain CSF and obviate meningeal stretching.
- It is important to differentiate PDPH from other types of headaches (cluster, migraine).
- Characteristic symptoms include symmetric and bilateral (frontal, occipital) dull or aching pain/pressure, positional (worse when standing or sitting; relieved when recumbent), and associated nausea, photophobia, neck stiffness, and/or tinnitus.
- Symptoms are usually self-limited, present within 12–48 hours after dural puncture, and resolve 1–7 days after onset of the initial symptoms.[35]
- Conservative treatment includes bed rest in recumbent position, intravenous fluids, acetaminophen, NSAIDs, and/or oral caffeine (anecdotal, lack of empiric evidence).
- Invasive treatments include epidural blood patch (EBP); injection of autologous blood into the epidural space at the level of dural perforation; proposed mechanisms of pain relief are the autologous blood clotting and plugging the dural hole; complications include inadvertent dural reuncture or increase in epidural space pressure restarting CSF leak by dislodging clot.
- Continued symptoms suggest need for neurologic consultation or imaging.
○ Transient neurologic symptom (TNS)[25,26]:
- Potential neuraxial complication attributed to the placement of local anesthetic in the CSF, especially after the use of lidocaine (RR = 7.31)[36] or mepivacaine, arises within 24 hours, resolves spontaneously without impediment approximately 5 days after the procedure.
- The etiology has not been clearly illuminated; an accepted but controversial hypothesis was that TNS was attributed to the toxic effects of local anesthetics on neuronal tissue.[37]
- Neurologic examination, magnetic resonance imaging, and electropathological testing reveal normal physiology.[38]
- TNS presents with sensory deficits and/or intermittent pain in the lower back radiating to the pelvic girdle and/or lower extremities, absence of motor symptoms, and bowel/bladder dysfunction.
- Risk factors are high lithotomy position and ambulatory surgical procedures.
- TNS is self-limiting, and is treated with NSAIDs and trigger point injection.
○ Cauda equina syndrome (CES)[25,26,39]:

- Spinal nerve roots below the level of the conus medullaris (L1) known as the cauda equina (aka horse's tail); provides sensory and motor functions of the lower extremities, bowel, and bladder.
- CES is a rare medical and/or surgical emergency that occurs when spinal nerves below the conus medullaris, either individually or collectively, are injured due to external compression, entrapment, and direct chemotoxic insult resulting from trauma, tumors, stenosis, hemorrhage/hematoma, arteriovenous malformations, and local anesthetics.[40]
- Early recognition of the signs/symptoms (excruciating lower back pain, saddle anesthesia and sphincter, sexual, bowel, and bladder dysfunction) with definitive diagnosis (MRI, myelography) is paramount to minimizing long-term neurologic sequelae such as permanent paralysis.
- Incidence of CES after spinal anesthesia was greatest after continuous infusion of high-dose lidocaine (5%) through a microcatheter.[41]
- CES has been reported after intrathecal injection through larger catheters (epidural) and local anesthetics other than lidocaine.
- Etiology of CES after spinal anesthesia was theorized to be direct neurotoxic chemical insult to the spinal nerves associated with the maldistribution or "pooling" of local anesthetics in the lumbosacral region. Unlike surgical decompression after a compressive or entrapment origin of CES, the neurotoxic insult to the cauda equina associated with local anesthetics lacks definitive treatment. Therefore, recommended guidelines have been established in attempt to minimize the likelihood of CES: lidocaine dosing should not exceed 60 mg and 2% concentration and bupivacaine or mepivacaine should be used to prolong the block.[42]
- ○ Spinal hematoma[25,26]:
  - It is a rare but potentially devastating complication associated with neuraxial anesthesia.
  - Highest incidence is after epidural or combined spinal–epidural neuraxial anesthesia, and is more likely to occur when the catheter is removed compared to insertion.
  - Hematoma symptoms are more likely to be unilateral and associated with back pain, and sensory and motor dysfunction.
  - Risk factors: Older females (> 70 years of age), history of coagulopathy or spinal deformity, multiple attempts, failure to discontinue anticoagulation agent, and other factors.
  - Treatment involves urgent recognition and decompression.
- ○ Local anesthetic systemic toxicity (LAST) (▶ Table 1.20 and ▶ Table 1.21):

Table 1.20 Local anesthetic toxicity

Features	Notes
Pathophysiology	Injection of local anesthetic directly into systemic circulation *or* peripheral systemic uptake
Risk factors that increase toxicity	Decreased protein binding
	Systemic acidosis
	Hypercarbia
Progression of symptoms	Tinnitus, circumoral numbness → Facial tingling → Seizure → Hypotension → Cardiovascular collapse
Medical management	Early endotracheal intubation
	100% oxygen
	Hyperventilation
	(decreased cerebral blood flow, conversion to nonionized lidocaine)
	Benzodiazepine (0.5–1 mg/kg)
	Intralipid
	(bolus: 1.5 mL/kg; infusion: 0.25 mL/kg; upper limit of dosing: 10 mL/kg)
Signs and symptoms	Central nervous system
	Circumoral numbness, tonic–clonic seizure, slurred speech, restlessness, tinnitus, vertigo
Rate of local anesthetic systemic absorption	Intravenous (fastest) > tracheal > intercostal > caudal > paracervical > epidural > brachial plexus > sciatic/femoral > subcutaneous tissue (slowest)

Table 1.21 Local anesthetic properties

Type	Maximum allowable dose (mg/kg)	Potency	Onset of action (min)	Duration of action (min)	Metabolism	Excretion
Chloroprocaine	12	1	1–3	30–60	Plasma hydrolysis	Urine
Procaine	12	1	5–10	45–90	Plasma esterase	Urine
Cocaine	3	2				
Tetracaine	3	8	10	420–480	Plasma esterase	Unclear
Lidocaine	4–5 (7 with epinephrine)	2	1–3	30–120	Hepatic (90%)	Urine
Mepivacaine	4–5 (7 with epinephrine)	2	2–5	120–150	Hepatic	Urine
Prilocaine	8	2	1–2	20–120	Hepatic/Renal	Urine
Bupivacaine	3	8	5–10	120–480	Hepatic	Urine
Ropivacaine	3	8	3–15	120–480	Hepatic	Urine

Source: Local anesthetic pharmacologic data[45]

- Local anesthetics uses: Regionally (subcutaneous) or systemically (intravenous) analgesia, decreased pain perception, alleviation of ventricular dysrhythmia or reduction of intracranial pressure associated with direct laryngoscopy and endotracheal intubation.
- LAST results in neurologic dysfunction (restlessness, tinnitus, circumoral numbness, seizure) and cardiovascular collapse (hypotension, cardiac arrest).
- Each local anesthetic has a characteristic weight-based amount that can be safely administered to a patient determined by the potency, lipid solubility, degree of protein binding, and clearance from systemic circulation.
- Factors impacting toxicity: Systemic aberrations (e.g., metabolic or respiratory acidosis; affect lipid solubility and protein binding, can result in anesthetic toxicity even at appropriate doses), site of local anesthetic injection, vascularity of the region (increases the risk of LAST; intercostal > caudal > epidural).
- Treatment: 100% oxygenation, early intubation prior to central nervous and cardiovascular collapse, hyperventilation to decrease the effects of acidosis associated with increased carbon dioxide, benzodiazepines to decrease the risk of seizure (caution: oversedation can lead to hypoxia and acidosis), intralipid (propofol is NOT an acceptable substitute) to decrease circulating levels of local anesthetic.
- In the event of cardiac arrest, code-dose epinephrine (1 mg) should be substituted for low-dose epinephrine (< 1 µg/kg) and vasopressin should be avoided due to evidence associated with worse outcomes.[43,44]
- Cases of LAST refractory to epinephrine should incorporate the use of cardiopulmonary bypass.
- The American society of regional anesthesia and pain management (ASRA) has made several recommendations regarding the prevention of LAST, including but not limited to, using the lowest possible dose of local anesthetic, addition of an intravascular marker (epinephrine), and the use of ultrasound when applicable.[44]

1.3.4 Other Anesthesia Complications

- Surgical airway fire (▶ Table 1.22)[25]:
  - Awareness and preparation are important to prevention, and quick identification and a coordinated management plan are vital to minimize harm; discussed in American Society of Anesthesiologist updated Practice Advisory on the Prevention and Management of Operating Room Fires in 2013.[45]
  - Exact incidence of airway fires in the United States is not precisely known; ~500–600 annual cases with 10% being associated with serious injury or death.[46]
  - Fire triad: Oxidizer-enriched atmosphere, ignition source, fuel.

Table 1.22 Surgical airway fire

Features	Notes	
Airway fire triad	Ignition source	Electrocautery, drills, lasers, fiberoptic cables
	Oxidizing agent	Oxygen, nitrous oxide
	Fuel	Sponges, drapes, gauze, alcohol prepping solutions, tracheal tubes, nasal cannula, dressings, patient's hair
High-risk procedure properties	Potential for ignition source to be in proximity to an oxidizer-enriched atmosphere	
	Increase in oxidizer concentration at the surgical site	
Treatment of airway fire	Stop procedure	
	Call for help	
	Announce airway fire	
	Simultaneously remove the endotracheal tube and stop gases/disconnect circuit	
	Pour saline into airway	
	Remove burning materials	
	Mask ventilate patient	
	Assess injury	
	Consider bronchoscopy	
	Reintubate (airway swelling)	
Treatment of fire on patient	Turn off gases	
	Remove drapes and burning materials	
	Extinguish flames with water, saline, or fire extinguisher	
	Assess patient's status	
	Assess for smoke inhalation	

- High-risk procedures:
  - Include any procedure in which there is a potential for an ignition source to be in proximity to an oxidizer-enriched atmosphere or a procedure when there is an increase in the oxidizer concentration at the surgical site.
  - Procedures that involve lasers, when ignition sources and surgery are inside the airway, cases that involve moderate or deep sedation, and when an ignition source and surgery occur around the face, head, or neck.
- Prevention[47]: Minimizing and avoiding an oxidizer-enriched atmosphere near the surgical site if possible, surgical drapes should be configured in a way that minimizes the accumulation of oxidizers, allow time for flammable skin preparations to dry before draping, moisten gauze and sponges that are near an ignition source, scavenging with suction around the airway should be used, constant communication between the anesthesiologist and surgeon during cases to determine when high-risk portions of the procedure are occurring so that steps can be taken to reduce the risk of airway fires.
- Multistep management strategy is used by surgeon and anesthesiologist (▶ Table 1.20).[47]
- Postoperative vision loss (POVL) (▶ Table 1.23)[48,49]:
  - Rare, devastating, unexpected complication.
  - Higher risk in spine and cardiac surgery compared to other nonocular operative procedures.
  - Incidence: in spine surgery (prone position) from 0.017 to 0.1%, and in cardiac surgery from 0.06 to 0.113%.[48]
  - Mechanisms: Retinal ischemia from branch or central retinal artery occlusion; ischemic optic neuropathy (sudden visional loss from either anterior or posterior optic neuropathy), brain injury rostral to the optic nerve resulting in cortical blindness.
  - Preoperative evaluation should be aimed at identifying patients with increased risk factors including preoperative anemia, vascular risk factors (hypertension, diabetes, peripheral vascular disease, coronary artery disease, carotid artery stenosis, tobacco use, and obesity).[48]

Table 1.23 Postoperative vision loss

Type	Mechanism	Characteristics	Causes	Risk factors	Prevention
Retinal ischemia branch and central retinal artery occlusion	Localized injury to portion of the retina or decreased blood supply to the retina	Unilateral, painless visual loss, abnormal pupil reactivity, branch: (cholesterol emboli), central: (cherry red macula)	External compression of eye, decreased arterial supply to the retina, impaired venous drainage of retina, arterial thrombosis	Direct pressure, improper positioning, horseshoe headrest, prone position	Foam headrest with eyes in opening, intermittent examination of eyes, use of pin head holder, avoid direct pressure to orbit
Ischemic optic neuropathy (anterior and posterior)	Temporary hypoperfusion or nonperfusion of the vessels supplying the anterior and/or posterior portion of the optic nerve	Painless visual loss, afferent pupil defect, nonreactive pupils. AION: Optic disc edema and hemorrhage. PION: Optic disc appears normal although patient has vision loss	Increased ocular venous pressure, hemodilution, hypotension, release of endogenous vasoconstrictors	AION: CABG, thoracovascular procedures. PION: Spinal surgery. Both: Increased length of surgery, increased blood loss	Decreased surgical time, decreased blood loss, treat hypotension, avoid massive fluid replacement, decreased pressure to eye, avoid increased venous ocular pressure, maintain neutral head position
Cortical blindness	Damage beyond the visual cortex in the occipital lobe	Bilateral visual loss with absence of optokinetic nystagmus and decreased eyelid reflex response. Normal optic nerve and retina	Global ischemia, cardiac arrest, hypoxemia, intracranial hypertension, thrombosis, vasospasm, and emboli	CABG, aortic atherosclerosis, preexisting cerebrovascular disease, cerebral edema, decreased perfusion, and systemic blood pressure	Prevent progression of stroke, decreased intraoperative manipulation of aorta, removal of air during cardiovascular bypass

Abbreviations: AION, anterior ischemic optic neuropathy; CABG, coronary artery bypass graft; PION, posterior ischemic optic neuropathy.

- ○ Intraoperative management involves the following factors: (1) appropriate blood pressure management, (2) management of blood loss and appropriate administration of fluids, (3) use of vasopressors when necessary to correct for hypotension, (4) head positioning to ensure the head is level when possible, (5) avoiding direct pressure to eye, and (6) periodically checking patient positioning during surgery.
- Pseudocholinesterase deficiency/butyrylcholinesterase (BChE) deficiency[25,26] (► Table 1.24):
  - ○ Rare hazard of depolarizing neuromuscular blocker succinylcholine use in patients with pseudocholinesterase deficiency, which results in prolonged paralysis not reversible by conventional methods.
  - ○ If unrecognized, it can result in patient paralysis without anesthesia, inquired by asking patient or family member response to anesthesia.
  - ○ Succinylcholine is a depolarizing neuromuscular blocker that works at the neuromuscular junction to cause paralysis. It is broken down in the plasma by butyrylcholinesterase (BChE) also known as plasma cholinesterase or pseudocholinesterase. BChE is synthesized in the liver and influences the duration of action of succinylcholine. Mutations in the gene coding for BChE give rise to a variety of biochemical phenotypes which can cause prolonged paralysis and apnea.
  - ○ Incidence of approximately 1 in 2,500 patients overall.
  - ○ Few preoperative qualitative tests are available to assess BChE enzyme levels: dibucaine number is most commonly used; variation in BChE abnormalities and the duration of depolarizing agent effects (► Table 1.24).
- Malignant hyperthermia (MH) (► Table 1.25):
  - ○ Incidence of MH is 1:15,000; mostly in older children and adults under 30 years old.
  - ○ Results in patients with mutations encoding for abnormal Ryanodine receptor 1 (RYP1) or dihydropyridine receptor (DHP) receptors; triggered by inhalational anesthetics (e.g., succinylcholine and phenothiazines); MH results in unregulated passage of calcium from the sarcoplasmic reticulum into the intracellular space leading to sustained muscle contraction; complete mechanism of anesthetic agents triggering is unclear.

Table 1.24 Pseudocholinesterase/butyrylcholinesterase (BChE) deficiency

Common BChE phenotypes

BChE type	Prevalence	Succinylcholine sensitivity	Dibucaine number	Response to succinylcholine
Homozygous typical usual (U/U)	96% of population	None	70–80	5–8 min
Heterozygous atypical (U/A)	1/480 patients	Some	50–60	Increases 50–100%
Homozygous atypical (A/A)	1/3,200 patients	Very high	20–30	Increases for 4–8 h

Change in BChE activity

Physiologic	Decreased in third trimester of pregnancy, decreased activity in newborn
Acquired decrease	Liver disease, cancer, malnutrition, hypothyroidism, ECMO, burns, plasmapheresis
Acquired increase	Obesity, alcoholism, hyperthyroidism, electroconvulsive therapy
Drug related	Neostigmine, pyridostigmine, monoamine oxidase inhibitors, pancuronium, oral contraceptives, esmolol

Management of BChE deficiency

Presentation	Prolonged paralysis after succinylcholine; history or family history of reintubation after surgery or failure to emerge from anesthesia; prolonged apnea after surgery
Treatment	Supportive → mechanical ventilatory support; extended PACU or ICU stay until return of neuromuscular function
Laboratory testing	Dibucaine number, genetic testing (for the medical record → future anesthetics)

Abbreviations: ECMO, extracorporeal membrane oxygenation; ICU, intensive care unit; PACU, postanesthetic care unit.

Table 1.25 Malignant hyperthermia

Direct association	Signs	Labs	Treatment	Late complications
Central core disease King-Denborough	Hypercarbia (earliest and most sensitive) Skeletal muscle rigidity (most specific) Tachycardia (most consistent sign) Hyperthermia (late sign) Dysrhythmias Unstable blood pressure Tachypnea Cyanosis/mottling	Decreased mixed venous oxygen saturation Mixed metabolic and respiratory acidosis Increased calcium Hyperkalemia Increased creatinine kinase Myoglobinuria	Discontinue succinylcholine or volatile anesthetic 100% oxygen Cool patient Arterial line Dextrose-insulin infusion Sodium bicarbonate Diuresis with furosemide/mannitol IV Dantrolene 2–5 mg/kg q5 min until decrease in symptoms (directly interferes with muscle contraction by inhibiting calcium release from the sarcoplasmic reticulum)	Renal failure Consumptive coagulopathies Pulmonary edema Cerebral edema Hyperkalemia hypothermia

- ○ MH results in increased aerobic metabolism that produces carbon dioxide and cellular acidosis, depleting oxygen and adenosine triphosphate (ATP).
- ○ Signs of MH are hypercarbia and a mixed respiratory/metabolic acidosis; continued crisis results in worsening acidosis, hyperkalemia, and myoglobinuria; some develop clinically evident hyperkalemia.
- ○ Muscle contraction generates more heat than the body is able to eliminate, core temperature may rise 1 °C every few minutes, hyperthermia can occur in minutes to hours after symptom onset, severe hyperthermia (up to 45 °C) can result in vital organ dysfunction and disseminated intravascular coagulation.
- ○ Treated with dantrolene which binds to the RYR1 receptor inhibiting the release of calcium from the sarcoplasmic reticulum.
- ○ Mortality: 70% if untreated, 5% if treated with dantrolene.

1.3.5 Postanesthetic Care Unit (PACU)

- It provides a safe place for patients to recover from after anesthesia and surgery where they can be continually monitored and assessed; monitoring of the hemodynamic effects of surgery and alterations to physiology from anesthetic medications is performed; it serves as a waypoint between surgery and hospital discharge.[25,26]
- ASA House of Delegates standards for postanesthesia care:
  - ○ All patients who have received anesthesia shall receive appropriate postanesthesia management.
  - ○ A patient transported to the PACU shall be accompanied by a member of the anesthesia care team and continually evaluated, monitored, and treated.
  - ○ Upon arrival, the patient shall be re-evaluated and verbal report given to the PACU nurse by a member of the anesthesia care team.
  - ○ The patient's condition shall be evaluated continually in the PACU.
  - ○ A physician is responsible for the discharge of the patient from the PACU.
- Postoperative nausea and vomiting (PONV):
  - ○ This is one of the most common and challenging side effects of anesthesia encountered in the PACU.
  - ○ Avoiding PONV is advantageous in attempts to improve patient satisfaction as well as decreases institutional financial burden from prolonged or unanticipated hospital stay.
  - ○ Risk factors: Ophthalmic, ENT, and gynecological surgeries; prior history of PONV; motion sickness; menstruating females; obesity; nonsmokers; use of volatile anesthetics (compared to total intravenous anesthetic techniques [TIVA]).

Table 1.26 Modified Aldrete scoring system

Findings	2 Points	1 Point	0 Points
Respiration	Deep breath and cough	Dyspnea/shallow breathing	Apnea
O_2 saturation	$SpO_2 > 92\%$ on room air	Needs supplemental to maintain saturation $> 90\%$	Oxygen saturation $< 90\%$ with supplemental oxygen
Consciousness	Awake	Arousable	No response
Circulation	Blood pressure ±20 mm Hg preoperatively	Blood pressure ±20–50 mm Hg preoperatively	Blood pressure ±50 mm Hg preoperatively
Activity	Able to move four extremities voluntarily	Able to move two extremities	Unable to more extremities

Score ≥ 9 for discharge.

- Treatment: 5-HT3 receptor antagonists (e.g., ondansetron), dexamethasone, perioperative hydration, and other antiemetic medications.
- Postoperative pain management[50,51]:
  - Top priority for patients, severity of pain varies among surgical procedure and anesthetic techniques, numeric pain scales have been developed to help evaluate patients' pain after surgery. Mainstay for treatment of surgical pain is intravenous opioids given at the start of the anesthetic.
  - Intravenous nonopioid medication is an important part of multimodal anesthesia and should be used whenever possible.
  - Regional techniques as well as peripheral nerve blocks and catheters should also be deployed when appropriate.
- Safe discharge/transfer from PACU:
  - Each patient should be oriented, able to communicate needs, and have appropriate hemodynamics, airway protection, and pain control.
  - Scoring systems such as the Modified Aldrete Score (▶ Table 1.26) or Post-anesthesia Discharge Scoring System are commonly used in an attempt to simplify and standardize patient discharge criteria.[51]
  - Each patient should be evaluated and discharged based on their coexisting medical condition, severity of their surgery, their recovery in the PACU, and the anesthetic technique.

1.3.6 Anesthesia Postoperative Management

- Hypotension (▶ Table 1.27):
  - Defined as a decrease in mean arterial pressure of more than 20% below baseline.
  - Oxygen supply is affected by oxygen content of the blood, and blood flow to the tissue.
  - Blood flow is affected by blood pressure, vascular resistance, and blood viscosity.
  - Blood pressure is the proxy measure we use for blood flow.
  - Hypotension implies compromised blood flow, and, therefore, oxygen supply.
  - Normotensive reading may not connote normal blood flow (e.g., the vascular resistance has been increased by the use of alpha-agonists).
  - Various factors impact preload (filling pressure of heart at end of diastole), afterload (pressure against which heart must work to eject blood in systole), and cardiac contractility (▶ Table 1.26).
  - Treatment is geared toward maintaining tissue oxygenation (e.g., supplemental oxygenation) while improving blood pressures (e.g., crystalloid fluids, decreasing anesthesia, utilizing vasopressors).
- Hypertension (▶ Table 1.28):
  - Defined as an increase in blood pressure more than 20% above baseline.
  - Symptom of easily remediable problem (e.g., light anesthesia), or a sign of an underlying pathology (e.g., increased intracranial pressure).
  - Perioperative hypertension requires immediate BP reduction to prevent or limit end organ damage (e.g., hypertensive encephalopathy, intracerebral hemorrhage, acute renal dysfunction, unstable angina, myocardial infarction, heart failure, and aortic dissection).
  - Broken down into various etiologies; numerous medications can be used for treatment (▶ Table 1.27).

- Hyponatremia (▶ Table 1.29):
  - Defined as serum sodium < 135 mmol/L.
  - Higher frequency in females, the elderly, and in hospitalized patients.
  - Usually asymptomatic until sodium level falls below 130 mmol/L.
  - Symptoms are nonspecific and include muscle weakness, cramps, lethargy, dizziness, nausea, and headache, but can also present as confusion, ataxia, seizure, and death.
  - Various forms of treatment are available but are rarely indicated to completely correct in perioperative period.
- Hypernatremia (▶ Table 1.30):
  - Defined as sodium > 145 mmol/L.
  - Caused by a decrease in total body water relative to electrolyte content.
  - In addition to thirst, other clinical manifestations are primarily neurologic due to an osmotic shift of water out of brain cells, e.g., confusion, neuromuscular excitability, seizures, and coma.
  - Correction of hypernatremia requires the administration of dilute fluids to correct the water deficit and replace ongoing water losses and, if necessary, the limitation of further water loss. In general, a net positive balance of 3 mL of electrolyte-free water per kilogram of lean body weight will lower the serum sodium by approximately 1 mEq/L.
- Hypokalemia (▶ Table 1.31):
  - Symptoms include muscle weakness and cardiac dysrhythmias. Symptoms generally do not manifest until the serum potassium is below 3.0 mEq/L or if the serum potassium falls quickly or the patient has a predisposition to dysrhythmias (e.g., taking digoxin).
  - Symptoms usually resolve with the correction of hypokalemia.
- Hyperkalemia (▶ Table 1.32):
  - Potentially life-threatening condition in which serum potassium exceeds 5.5 mmol/L.

Table 1.27 Postoperative hypotension

Etiology of hypotension			
Preload		**Afterload**	**Contractility**
True hypovolemia	**Relative hypovolemia**	Neuraxial anesthesia	Myocardial infarction
Ongoing hemorrhage	Positive pressure ventilation	Spinal shock	Myocardial ischemia
Inadequate resuscitation	Tension pneumothorax Cardiac tamponade	Release of aortic cross-clamp	Dysrhythmias
Fluid sequestration		Anaphylaxis	Congestive heart failure
Vomiting/diarrhea	Caval compression (pregnancy, tumor, surgical packing)	Transfusion reaction	Hypothermia (<32°C)
Osmotic/diuretic polyuria		Systemic inflammation	Hypothyroidism
Chronic hypertension	Pulmonary hypertension	Sepsis	Malignant hyperthermia/sepsis
	Pulmonary embolism	Liver failure	Hypocalcemia
	Valvular disease	Hypothyroid	Severe acidosis/alkalosis
	Head up position	Drugs:	Local anesthetic toxicity
		• Antihypertensives	Drugs:
		• Antidysrhythmias	• Anesthetics
		• Anticonvulsants	• Antidysrhythmias
		• Inhalational agents	• Calcium/adrenergic blockers
Management			
Assess blood pressure reading (is someone leaning on blood pressure cuff?)			
Assess other vital signs (heart rate, CO_2, oxygenation)			
Assess blood loss or persistent surgical venous compression			
Increase intravenous (crystalloids) fluids			
Decrease or stop anesthetic			
Increase inspired FiO_2			
Inotropes/vasopressors (ephedrine/phenylephrine/epinephrine/vasopressin)			

Table 1.28 Postoperative hypertension

Etiology of hypertension			
Preexisting disease	**Surgical**	**Anesthesia**	**Drugs**
Hypertension	Aortic cross-clamping	Pain/light anesthesia	Vasopressors
Heart failure	Prolonged tourniquet time	Increased temperature	Systemic absorption of vasoconstrictors
Acute myocardial infarction	Postmyocardial revascularization	(malignant hyperthermia)	Monoamine oxidase inhibitors/tricyclic antidepressants
Aortic dissection	Postcarotid endarterectomy (denervation of carotid baroreceptors)	Hypoxemia	
Autonomic hyperreflexia		Hypercarbia	
Increased intracranial pressure		Metabolic acidosis	Cocaine/ketamine
Autonomic instability	Hypervolemia (TURP syndrome)	Hypervolemia	Naloxone (reverses opiates)
Alcohol withdrawal		Vasoconstriction	Intravenous indigo carmine dye
Hyperthyroid		Small blood pressure cuff small	Rebound hypertension (i.e., clonidine/β-blocker cessation)
Hypoglycemia		Emergence delirium	
Pheochromocytoma			
Carcinoid syndrome			
Pre-eclampsia			

Management
Assess blood pressure (is someone leaning on blood pressure cuff?)
Assess other vital signs (heart rate, CO_2, oxygenation)
Assess sources of anesthetic (vaporizer)
Increase anesthetic (vaporizer/epidural/local)
Labetalol: 5 mg increments
Nitroglycerine: 0.1–2 µg/kg/min
Nitroprusside: 0.1–3 µg/kg/min
Nifedipine: 10 mg sublingual

Abbreviation: TURP, transurethral resection of the prostate.

Table 1.29 Postoperative hyponatremia

Isotonic	Hypertonic			Hypotonic
Lab error	Check volume status of patient			Presence of glycine, sorbitol, or mannitol
(hyperlipidemia or hyperproteinemia)	(history, physical exam, urine sodium, urine osmolality)			
	Isovolemic	**Hypovolemic**	**Hypervolemic**	
	Decreased solute intake			
	Primary polydipsia			
	Symptom of inappropriate diuretic hormone (SIADH) secretion	Renal and extrarenal loss of Na	Cirrhosis	
			Heart failure	
	Hypothyroidism		Nephrosis	
	Adrenal insufficiency			

Hyponatremia treatment goals
Prevent further decreases in the serum sodium concentration
Decreased intracranial pressure in patients at risk for developing brain herniation
Relieve symptoms of hyponatremia
Avoid excessive correction of hyponatremia in patients at risk for osmotic demyelination syndrome (formerly central pontine myelinolysis)

- ○ Symptoms are nonspecific and predominantly related to muscular or cardiac dysfunction.
- ○ Rare in normal individuals.
- Prolonged emergence/extubation (▶ Table 1.33, ▶ Fig. 1.2):
  - ○ Can be defined as delayed return to normal level of responsiveness and arousal, usually delayed if persists for 15–90 minutes in normal individuals, depends on specific patient.
  - ○ Prolonged emergence divided into causes from drugs, metabolic abnormalities, or neurological injury.
  - ○ Prolonged neuromuscular blockade divided into causes from drugs, and acid-base, metabolic, or neurologic causes.
- Anesthetic medication reference (▶ Table 1.34 and ▶ Table 1.35).

Table 1.30 Postoperative hypernatremia

Free water losses	Free water intake deficit	Sodium overload
Renal concentration effect (osmotic diuresis, diabetes insipidus)	Inability to drink/access water	Hypertonic fluid administration
Gastrointestinal	Impaired thirst mechanism	Ingestion of increased amounts of salt
Insensible losses		Mineralocorticoid excess
Sweating		

Table 1.31 Postoperative hypokalemia

Shift into cells	Total depletion			
Alkalosis	Decreased intake	Increased loss		
Hypothermia		Renal		External
β-Stimulation		Mineralocorticoid	Tubular	Vomiting
Insulin	Malnutrition	Hyperaldosteronism	Diuretics	Diarrhea
Xanthines (e.g., theophylline/caffeine)	Malabsorption	Cushing disease	Hypomagnesemia	Nasogastric suction
		Licorice	Penicillin	Laxatives
		Renal artery stenosis	Renal tubular acidosis	Burns
		Hypertensive	Hypo/normotensive	

Table 1.32 Postoperative hyperkalemia

Increased intake	Distribution between cells and extracellular fluid	Reduced excretion
IV bolus of K-containing injectate	Pseudohyperkalemia (lab artifact)	Decreased aldosterone secretion/responsiveness
Accidental ingestion of K-containing salt substitute	Metabolic acidosis	Acute or chronic kidney disease
Red cell transfusion	Insulin deficiency	Significant arterial volume depletion
Moderate increased intake with hypoaldosteronism or renal insufficiency	Hyperglycemia	(reduced delivery of Na/water to kidneys)
	Increased tissue catabolism (tumor lysis syndrome, severe hypothermia)	Gordon syndrome
	β-Blockers	Ureterojejunostomy
	Exercise	
	Hyperkalemic periodic paralysis	
	Digitalis overdose	
	Succinylcholine	
	Arginine hydrochloride	
	Adenosine triphosphate–dependent potassium channels activation	
	(calcineurin inhibitors, diazoxide, minoxidil, and some volatile anesthetics)	

Table 1.33 Emergence and criteria for extubation

Prolonged emergence	
Causes	**Etiology**
Prolonged drug action	Overdose
	Hypothermia (< 33 °C)
	Increased sensitivity
	Increased protein binding
	Redistribution
	Drug interaction
	Hypoxia/hypercapnia
	Organ dysfunction (hepatic, renal, endocrine)
Metabolic causes	Hypo/hyperglycemia
	Hyperglycemic hyperosmolar nonketotic coma/diabetic ketoacidosis
	Electrolyte imbalance (hyponatremia, hypocalcemia, hypomagnesemia)
	Hypothermia (< 33 °C)
	Sepsis
	Alcohol
Neurologic injury	Intracranial (hemorrhage, contusion)
	Cerebral embolus/ischemia
	Seizure (subclinical, postictal)
	Increased intracranial pressure
	Pneumocephalus
Prolonged neuromuscular blockade	
Causes	**Etiology**
Drugs	Excess neuromuscular blockade
	Echothiophate eye drops
	Aminoglycoside antibiotics (decrease in acetylcholine formation)
	Magnesium/lithium (decrease in acetylcholine release)
	Furosemide (decreased acetylcholine release)
	Local anesthetics (decreased propagation of action potentials)
	Antidysrhythmic medication
	Calcium channel blockers
	Common culprits: steroids; dantrolene; beta-blockers; monoamine oxidase inhibitors; inhalational agents; alkylating chemotherapy agents
Acid-base	Metabolic alkalosis (from respiratory acidosis)
	Pseudocholinesterase deficiency
	Liver disease/uremia
	Pregnancy (third trimester)
	Malignancy
	Malnutrition
Metabolic	Collagen vascular disease
	Hypothyroidism
	Neostigmine/pyridostigmine
	Phenelzine
	Cyclophosphamide
	Liver disease (decreased metabolism)

(Continued)

Table 1.33 (*Continued*) Emergence and criteria for extubation

Prolonged neuromuscular blockade	
Causes	**Etiology**
	Renal failure (decreased excretion)
	Hypothermia (decreased metabolism/excretion)
	Plasmapheresis
	Amyotrophic lateral sclerosis
	Malignant hyperthermia
	Muscular dystrophy
Neurologic	Familial periodic paralysis
	Hereditary hepatic porphyria
	Myasthenia gravis
	Lambert-Eaton
	Hypokalemia
	Hypocalcemia
Electrolyte	Hypermagnesemia
	Hypernatremia

1.4 Wound Closure and Infection

Michael Karsy

1.4.1 Preoperative Antibiotics

- Surgical site infections (SSIs) involve superficial or deep infection occurring within 30–90 days postoperatively depending on surgery.
- Various guidelines on SSIs: Surgical Care Improvement Project (SCIP) (https://manual.jointcommission.org); American College of Surgeons[52]; World Health Organization (http://www.who.int); Infectious Disease Society of America and Surgical Infection Society[53]; and Centers for Disease Control[54] (▶ Table 1.36).
- Surgical Care Improvement Project (SCIP):
  - National partnership of multiple organizations aimed at reducing surgical complications.
  - Antibiotic administration within 1 hour prior to surgical incision.
  - Use of first- or second-generation cephalosporins for most operations and addition of anaerobic coverage for colorectal surgery. Vancomycin is not recommended for routine use because of development of antibiotic resistance. Fluoroquinolones, clindamycin, and vancomycin are acceptable in patients with beta-lactam allergies.
  - Discontinuation of antibiotics within 24 hours of surgery and 48 hours of cardiac surgery.
- SSIs account for 38% of iatrogenic infections and occur in 1:24 patients undergoing surgery in the United States (http://hcupnet.ahrq.gov/). Annual cost of SSI is $3.5–10 billion because of complications, increased length of stay, and antibiotic treatment.
- Wounds are divided into clean (nonviscous surgery such as respiratory, alimentary, genital, or urinary tract surgery), clean-contaminated (viscous surgery), contaminated (fresh trauma, gross spillage from viscous), and dirty (old trauma, foreign bodies, fecal contamination, existing infection).
- Rate of SSIs: Clean (1.3–2.9%), clean-contaminated (2.4–7.7%), contaminated (6.4–15.2%), and dirty (7.1–40.0%).
- Causative bacteria for SSI include skin flora (*Staphylococcus aureus*, coagulase-negative staphylococci); gram-negative rods and enterococci are potentials in viscous surgery.

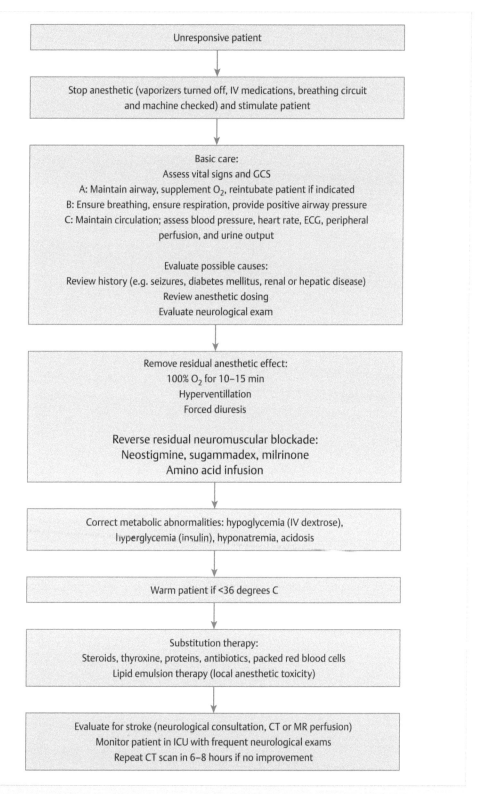

Fig. 1.2 Stepwise approach to the evaluation and management of prolonged emergence/extubation. CT, computerized tomography; ECG, electrocardiogram; GCS, Glasgow coma scale; ICU, intensive care unit; MRI, magnetic resonance imaging.

Table 1.34 Anesthetic considerations

Inhaled anesthetic agents

	CMRO2	Cardiac output	CBF	ICP	SVR	BP	Bronchodilation	Respiratory rate
Halothane	↓	↓	↑	↑	↓	↓	+	↑
Isoflurane	↓	Maintain	↑	↑	↓	↓	+	↑
Sevoflurane	↓	↓	↑	↑	↓	↓	+	↑
Desflurane	↓	↓	↑	↑	↓	↓	+	↑
Nitrous oxide	↑	− / ↑	↑	−	− / ↑	−/− ↑	+	↑

Depolarizing neuromuscular blocking agent

Succinylcholine	Onset of action: 30–60 s
	Duration: 10 min
	Metabolism: Plasma pseudocholinesterase
	Results in histamine release, potassium release, increased intracranial and intraocular pressure, myalgia
	Potential for malignant hyperthermia

Nondepolarizing neuromuscular blocking agents

Type	Mechanism of action	Dosing (mg/kg)	Duration of action	Metabolism	Histamine release
Pancuronium	Acetylcholine antagonist at the postsynaptic nicotinic receptor	0.1	40–60 min	Hepatic	No
Vecuronium		0.1	20–30 min	Hepatic	No
Rocuronium		0.6	30–40 min	Hepatic	No
Atracurium		0.5	20–30 min	Renal: 10% / Hoffman elimination: 30% / Ester hydrolysis: 60%	Yes
Cis-atracurium		0.1	30–40 min	Hoffman elimination: 30% / Ester hydrolysis: 60%	No

Abbreviations: BP, blood pressure; CBF, cerebral blood flow; CMRO$_2$, cerebral metabolic rate of oxygen; ICP, intracranial pressure; SVR, systemic vascular resistance.

Table 1.35 Commonly used intravenous anesthetic agents

Features	Propofol	Thiopental	Midazolam	Etomidate	Ketamine	Dexmedetomidine
Mechanism of action	GABA$_A$ receptor agonist	GABA$_A$ receptor agonist	GABA$_A$ receptor agonist	GABA$_A$ receptor agonist	NMDA receptor antagonist / μ- and κ-opioid receptors (high doses) / Acetylcholine muscarinic antagonist / GABA potentiation	Central α$_2$-agonist
Myocardial depressant	Yes	Yes	Yes	No	Yes (with catecholamine depletion)	Yes

(Continued)

Table 1.35 (*Continued*) Commonly used intravenous anesthetic agents

Features	Propofol	Thiopental	Midazolam	Etomidate	Ketamine	Dexmedetomidine
Heart rate response	~↑	↑	↓	Maintained	↑	↓
Systemic vascular resistance (SVR)	↓	↓	+/−	Maintained	↑	↓
Cardiac output	↓	↓	↓	Maintained	↑	↓
Cerebral perfusion pressure	↓	↓	↓	Maintained	↑	↓
Cerebral metabolic rate of oxygen (CMRO$_2$)	↓	↓	↓	↓	↑	↓
Intracranial pressure	↓	↓	↓	↓	↑	↓
SSEP amplitude	↓	↓	↓	↑	↑	No change
SSEP latency	↑	↑	—	↑	—	No change
Burst suppression	Yes	Yes	No	Yes	No	Yes
Respiratory depression	Yes	Yes	No	No	No	No
Bronchorelaxation	Yes	No	No	No	Yes	Yes
Nausea and vomiting	No	Yes	No	Yes	No	No
Continuous infusion	Yes	No	Yes	No	Yes	Yes
Analgesia	No	No	No	No	Yes	Yes
Thrombophlebitis	Yes	No	Yes	Yes	No	No
Adrenocortical suppression	No	No	No	Yes	No	Yes
Myoclonus	Yes (children)	No	No	Yes	No	Yes
Pain on injection	Yes	No	No	Yes	No	No
Histamine release	No	No	No	No	No	No
Hypnosis	Yes	Yes	Yes	Yes	No	Yes
Duration of action (min)	3–8	5–10	15–20	3–8	5–10	5–15
Protein binding	↑ (99%)	↑ (83%)	↑ (94%)	↑ (77%)	↓ (12%)	↑ (94%)
Anterograde amnesia	No	No	Yes	No	No	No
Active metabolite	No	No	Yes	No	Yes	No
Reversal agent	No	No	Yes	No	No	No

Abbreviations: GABA, gamma aminobutyric acid; NMDA, N-methyl-D-aspartate; SSEP, somatosensory evoked potential.

- Rates of methicillin-resistant *S. aureus* (MRSA), other antibiotic-resistant organisms, and fungi have increased over time because of antibiotic use, greater severity of illness, and immunocompromise in patients undergoing surgery.
- Nonmodifiable risk factors include age, radiation treatment, and infection; modifiable risk factors include diabetes, obesity, alcoholism, smoking, albumin < 3.5 mg/dL, total bilirubin > 1.0 mg/dL, immunosuppression, surgical technique, and facility protocols.

Table 1.36 Selection of perioperative antibiotics

Procedure	Primary drug	Alternative drug[a]
Spine, orthopaedic, thoracic, vascular, plastic, and neurosurgery	Cefazolin	Clindamycin
Joint replacements	Cefazolin (MRSA negative) or cefazolin and vancomycin (MRSA positive)	Clindamycin ± vancomycin
Cardiac	Cefazolin or cefuroxime, vancomycin added for patients from facilities	Clindamycin
Ventricular assist devices	Aztreonam, vancomycin, and fluconazole	
Colorectal	Cefazolin and metronidazole	Levofloxacin and metronidazole or cefoxitin
Gynecology, obstetrics	Cefazolin	Clindamycin and gentamicin (gyn/ob) or ciprofloxacin/levofloxacin and metronidazole (gyn)
Gynecologic oncology	Cefazolin and metronidazole	Levofloxacin and metronidazole
Open gastric and biliary Low vs. high (biliary stent, implant)	Cefazolin (low risk) or cefoxitin (high risk)	Ciprofloxacin and gentamicin or clindamycin and ciprofloxacin/levofloxacin
Genitourinary Low vs. high (nonsterile urine, implant, entry into urinary tract) risk	Cefazolin (low risk) or ciprofloxacin (high risk) or cefazolin and gentamicin (implants) or metronidazole and gentamicin (multiple UTI)	Clindamycin (low risk) or gentamicin and clindamycin (high risk, implants) or cefazolin and metronidazole (high risk) or ampicillin and gentamicin (high risk) or cefazolin and aztreonam (prosthesis) or ertapenem (multiple UTI)
Head and neck Low vs. high (oral mucosa incision) risk	Cefazolin (low risk) or cefazolin and metronidazole (high risk)	Clindamycin or ampicillin/sulbactam (high risk)
Kidney transplant	Cefazolin	Clindamycin and Levaquin
Pancreas/kidney-pancreas	Meropenem and caspofungin	Levofloxacin and metronidazole ad caspofungin
Heart/lung/heart-lung transplant	Cefuroxime	Vancomycin
Liver transplant	Piperacillin-tazobactam	Ceftriaxone and vancomycin
Prostate biopsy	Ciprofloxacin	
Other: laparoscopic cholecystectomy, laparoscopic gastric and biliary, breast biopsy, inguinal hernia without mesh, anorectal surgery, percutaneous endoscopic gastrostomy placement	Cefazolin	Clindamycin

Abbreviations: MRSA, methicillin-resistant Staphylococcus aureus; UTI, urinary tract infection.

[a] Penicillin allergy—defined as a documented history of anaphylaxis or other serious reactions (angioedema, hives, bronchospasm, Stevens-Johnson syndrome, or toxic epidermal necrolysis)—is a contraindication to cephalosporins.

1.4.2 Surgical Wound Closure

- Primary intention healing:
  - *Phase 1.* First few days: Inflammatory response, coagulation cascade activated, accumulation of fibroblasts, increased blood supply to wound, leukocyte-mediated debridement.
  - *Phase 2.* Day 3 onwards: Laying down of collagen, occurs up to 12 months.
  - *Phase 3.* Day 3–4 onwards: Wound retraction and remodeling.

- Delayed primary closure for dirty wounds, trauma, or wounds with high risk of infection involves leaving wounds open and packing twice daily with gauze packing changes before closure within 3–5 days after debridement if wound shows no infection and good granulation.
- Secondary intention healing:
  - Open wound that heals from formation of granulation tissue mediated by myofibroblasts.
  - Wound irrigation and debridement can reduce bacterial load and remove excessive granulation.
- Wound closure:
  - Selection of suture material depends on tissue type, surgeon preference, and institutional practice (▶ Table 1.37). No evidence to support one material over another.[55]
  - Multilayer closure (skin, subcutaneous tissue, fascial layers) improves healing by reducing wound tension and closing dead space.
  - Superficial wounds < 5 cm in size that can be easily approximated may be amenable to Steri-Strips or adhesive.
  - Suture techniques available via online videos: Simple square knots, subcuticular, vertical mattress, horizontal mattress, figure of 8, purse string, running continuous, laparoscopic methods, instrument ties, deep knots with knot driver.
  - Tetanus immunization indicated for patients with traumatic wounds without prior immunization within 10 years.
  - Topical bacitracin can reduce wound infection; relative risk 0.61 equating to 20 fewer SSI per 1,000 patients, with a number needed to treat of 50.[56]
  - Dressings for 24 hours can allow for coagulation; suture removal depends on site and type of suture material. Absorbable sutures used for pediatric patients can eliminate need for later removal (▶ Table 1.38).
  - Wound washing within 12–24 hours has not been shown to worsen SSI but most surgeons will wait longer.[57,58]

1.4.3 Postoperative Fevers: Categories of Causes

- Immediate: Within few hours of surgery; medications, blood products, trauma, infections before surgery, malignant hyperthermia.
- Acute: Within 7 days of surgery; upper respiratory infection, SSI, pneumonia, urinary tract infection (UTI), intravascular catheters, atelectasis, aspiration.
- Subacute: > 7 days of surgery; catheters, iatrogenic infections (e.g., *Clostridium difficile*), thrombophlebitis, deep vein thrombosis, nosocomial infection.
- Delayed: Weeks after surgery; deep infection, viral infection, parasites, SSI from indolent microorganisms, delayed cellulitis.
- Specialty-specific considerations for infection exist along with workup strategies and thresholds for antibiotic treatment.
- Helpful mnemonic for causes: Wind (pulmonary, aspiration, atelectasis), water (UTI), wound (SSI), walking (thromboembolism), wonder drug (drug fever), what did we do? (iatrogenic, nosocomial).

1.4.4 Wound Infection, Dehiscence, and Management

- Evaluation of wound vascularity (redness) vs. necrosis, purulent material (pus, foul odor), size (length × width × depth), tunneling (depth with sterile swab), granulation tissue.
- Initial management to clean and irrigate wound if clean and reapproximate; wound cultures can be contaminated by skin flora; delayed primary closure can be performed by twice-daily wound packing or wet-to-dry dressing changes.
- Risk factors for poor wound healing: Infection, smoking, age, malnutrition, immobilization, diabetes, vascular disease, immunosuppressive therapy.
- Antibiotic for wounds:
  - Selected in consultation with infectious disease specialists and clinical pharmacists while treatment effect is carefully monitored.

Table 1.37 Suture material types

Suture	Type	Material	Tensile strength	Absorption rate	Usage
Absorbable					
Surgical gut (i.e., catgut, fast gut)	Plain, chromic	Collagen from beef and sheep	Variable	Variable, proteolysis	Face (fast-absorbing), mouth, tongue (chromic)
Monocryl	Monofilament	Copolymer of glycolide and epsilon-caprolactone	50–60% at 1 wk, 20–30% at 2 wk, 0% at 3 wk	91–119 d, hydrolysis	Face, deep contaminated wounds
Vicryl	Braided, monofilament	Copolymer of lactide and glycoside, plus with polyglactin 910, rapid type pretreated for earlier absorption	75% at 2 wk, 50% at 3 wk, 25% at 4 wk	56–70 d, hydrolysis	Face, scalp, cast/splint, deep closure, mouth
Polyglycolic acid (Dexon)	Monofilament	Polyglycolic acid polymer	50% at 10 d	30 d	Deep closure
Polydioxanone (PDS)	Monofilament	Polyester polymer	70% at 2 wk, 50% at 4 wk, 25% at 6 wk	180 d, hydrolysis	Deep closure
Polyglyconate (Maxon)	Monofilament	Polyglyconate polymer	50% at 3 wk	45–60 d	Deep closure
Nonabsorbable					
Silk	Braided	Fibrin	Some with fiber degradation	None	Skin, securing lines
Surgical steel	Monofilament or multifilament	316 L stainless steel	None	None	Back, chest, extremity, sternum
Nylon	Monofilament or braided	Aliphatic polymers of nylon	Some fiber degradation with hydrolysis	None	Superficial and deep closure
Polyester	Monofilament or braided	Polyethylene terephthalate	None	None	Superficial and deep closure
Polypropylene	Monofilament	Polypropylene	None	None	Superficial and deep closure

Table 1.38 Time until suture removal depending on surgical site

Site	Days
Eyelids	3
Neck	3–4
Face	5
Scalp	7–14
Trunk and upper extremities	7
Lower extremities	8–10

- Nonpurulent cellulitis without systemic inflammatory response syndrome (SIRS) criteria: Penicillin, amoxicillin, cephalexin, clindamycin, trimethoprim–sulfamethoxazole.
  - Nonpurulent cellulitis with SIRS criteria: Cefazolin, ceftriaxone, clindamycin.
  - Nonpurulent cellulitis with clinical progression: Vancomycin or daptomycin (MRSA); cefazolin, nafcillin, oxacillin, or clindamycin (methicillin-susceptible *S. aureus* [MSSA]).
  - Purulent with concern for MSSA or MRSA: Trimethoprim–sulfamethoxazole, doxycycline and amoxicillin, minocycline and amoxicillin, clindamycin; escalated to vancomycin or daptomycin for MRSA coverage or clinical progression.
- Negative-pressure wound therapy:
  - Benefits are reduced need for wound changes, micro- and macro-deformation of wound tissue, fluid and wound exudate removal, beneficial alteration of wound cellular microenvironment.
  - Wound filled with porous foam for vacuum-assisted closure (VAC); used from −50 to 150 mm Hg; pore sizes on foam vary for tissue (smaller pore foam used to protect structures).
  - Limited level I and meta-analysis evidence for improved wound healing in a variety of wounds.[59,60,61]
- Wound dressings and adjuvants can be used for acute or chronic wounds (▶ Table 1.39).
- Wound staging: Useful for decubitus ulcers or other types of wounds to assess severity of injury, healing, and urgency for pursuing surgical debridement.
  - Stage 1: Intact skin, red skin, nonblanchable, painful or firm skin.
  - Stage 2: Open wound through epidermis and part of the dermis; tissue blistering can be seen.
  - Stage 3: Deep, crater wound with some loss of skin fat; cellular debris can be seen.
  - Stage 4: Exposure of bone, muscle, or tendon; necrotic/eschar can be seen; wound can extend beneath surface to healthier tissue.

1.5 Surgical Instruments

Michelle D. Ford

1.5.1 Instrument Categories[62,63]

- Instruments are typically categorized by their basic function and purpose.
- Most instruments are the same in every surgical specialty.
- Cutting and dissecting: Knives, scissors, biopsy tools, elevators, etc., that are designed to cut, dissect, elevate, or remove tissue (▶ Fig. 1.3).
  - Scissors:
    - Designed for re-sharpening but some brands are sharper than others such as black-handled scissors (e.g., Microgrind, Super Cut).
      Made of stainless steel (SS) or tungsten carbide.
    - Can be straight, curved, sharp, blunt, short, long, or various angles.
    - Types: Mayo, Metzenbaum, tenotomy.
  - Elevators:
    - Can be straight, curved, various angles and sizes, single or double ended, and are service specific.
    - Types: Chandler, Cobb, Freer, Key, McGlamry, Penfield.
- Grasping and holding: Forceps that are used to grasp and hold tissue (▶ Fig. 1.4).
  - Variety of lengths, rigid or flexible, with or without teeth, straight or bayonetted.
  - Types: Adson, DeBakey, Bonney, Ferris-Smith.
- Clamping and occluding: Clamps and hemostats that are used to hold or occlude (▶ Fig. 1.5 and ▶ Fig. 1.6).
  - Variety of lengths, straight or curved, delicate or heavy, with or without teeth.
  - Types of hemostats: Mosquito, Crile, Kelly, Kocher, Right Angle.
  - Types of occlusion clamps: DeBakey, Henly, Javid, Profunda.
- Exposing and retracting: Retractors that allow for increased view of the surgical field (▶ Fig. 1.7 and ▶ Fig. 1.8).

Table 1.39 Wound care adjuvants

Type	Examples	Purpose
Hydrocolloid	DuoDERM, Tegasorb	Dressings with ability to absorb moisture from wounds
Silicone	Mepiform silicone dressing	Padded dressing for absorbing exudate and maintaining moisture
Transparent	Tegaderm	Waterproof, permeable to moisture and oxygen, impermeable to bacteria, allow wound observation, facilitates autolytic debridement, not useful for infected or necrotic wounds
Alginate	Aquacel Ag	Seaweed derived, allow moisture absorption
Antimicrobial	Silver, iodine, antimicrobial dressings, honey, hydrofera, miconazole	Antimicrobial treatment of wounds
Collagen	Promogran prisma	Encourages formation of collagen in wounds, used in partial- or full-thickness wounds
Hydrogel	DuoDERM hydroactive gel	Water-retaining gels used for maintaining moisture in dry wounds, facilitate autolytic debridement, improve pain

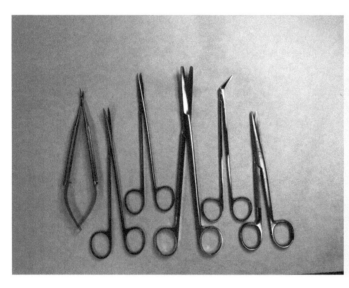

Fig. 1.3 Cutting instruments. Left to right: Castroviejo, Metzenbaum, Tenotomy, long curved Mayo, 45 degrees Potts, straight Mayo.

- ○ Allow for increased view of surgical field and either held or self-retaining.
- ○ Hand-held retractors: Senn, Army/Navy (USA), Richardson, Deaver (▶ Fig. 1.7).
- ○ Self-retaining retractors: Weitlaner Retractor, Gelpi Retractor, Balfour Retractor, Bookwalter Retractor (▶ Fig. 1.8).
- • Most common procedures based on specialty specific instruments:
  - ○ General surgery:
    - – Bowel resection: Pean, Allis, Babcock, and tonsil clamps; Metzenbaum scissors; DeBakey forceps; Army-Navy, Richardson, and Bookwalter retractors; various disposable endomechanical stapling devices.
    - – Herniorrhaphy: Curved Criles and Pean clamps; curved Metzenbaum scissors; Adson and DeBakey forceps; Army-Navy, Goelet, and Weitlaner retractors; ½" Penrose drain; vendor-specific mesh.
    - – Laparoscopic cholecystectomy: Curved Pean, straight Kocher, and tonsil clamps; penetrating towel clamps; curved Metzenbaum scissors; Adson forceps and forceps with teeth; Army-Navy and S-shaped retractors for cut-down; 5-mm Maryland dissector; 5-mm atraumatic graspers; 10-mm spoon forceps; 10-mm claw graspers; laparoscopic scissors; laparoscopic endoscopes; HD camera and light cord; vendor-specific irrigating/suction instruments; laparoscopic clip appliers; insufflation tubing.

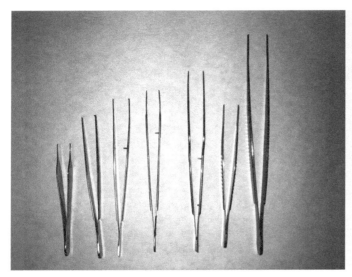

Fig. 1.4 Grasping and holding instruments. Left to right: Adson, rat tooth, Cushing with teeth, Gerald without teeth, bayonet, heavy DeBakey, 11" DeBakey.

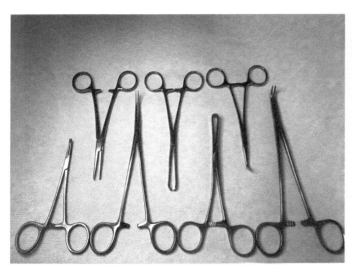

Fig. 1.5 Clamping and occluding instruments. Left to right: mosquito, Crile, tonsil, Allis, Lahey, short and long right angles.

○ Orthopaedic surgery:
 – Total knee replacement: Kocher clamps; curved Mayo scissors; Freer elevator; Bonney forceps; Mayo-Hegar needle holders; Leksell rongeurs; Meyerding and Hohmann retractors; Lewin bone clamp; Moreland knee spreader; sagittal saw; vendor-specific implants and sets.
 – Shoulder arthroscopy: 5.5-mm arthroscopy cannulas and obturators; pressure-sensing scope sheath; probes; rotator cuff and suture retriever graspers; Fiberwire knot cutters; curved suture hooks; arthroscopic shavers; arthroscopic scopes; HD camera and light cord.
 – Wrist fracture: Crile clamps; curved Metzenbaum scissors; Adson forceps and forceps with teeth; curettes; Freer, Key, and Chandler elevators; Hohmann and Weitlaner retractors; vendor-specific mini- or small-fragment implant sets.
○ Obstetrics/Gynecology:
 – Vaginal hysterectomy: Allis Adair, Allis Willauer, and Heaney clamps; Schroeder tenaculum; Heaney needle holder; Russian and 10" tissue forceps; Heaney retractors; Auvard vaginal speculum.
 – Cesarean section: Curved Kelly, curved Pean, Kocher, Allis, and sponge clamps; curved Metzenbaum, curved Mayo, and bandage scissors; Mayo-Hegar and Heaney needle holders; Adson, Russian, and tissue forceps with teeth; Kelly and DeLee retractors; Simpson fenestrated forceps.

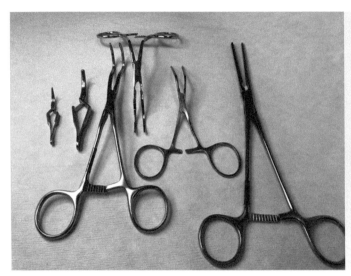

Fig. 1.6 Vascular instruments. Left to right: small and large bulldogs, Satinsky, profunda, angled, and straight DeBakey clamps.

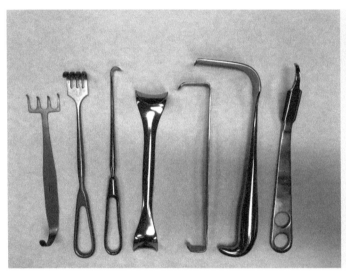

Fig. 1.7 Hand-held retractors. Left to right: Paws Rake, Vein, Goelet, Army-Navy, Meyerding, Hohmann.

- Dilation and curettage: Single- or double-toothed tenaculum; uterine sound; sponge clamps, Russian, or tissue forceps with teeth; Hegar uterine dilators; Kevorkian endocervical curette and sharp Sims uterine curettes; Auvard vaginal speculum.
  ○ Vascular surgery:
  - Carotid endarterectomy: Hemostats and right-angle clamps; 60° DeBakey, Profunda, and Javid clamps (for shunt); DeBakey forceps; Castroviejo needle holders; Metzenbaum and Potts scissors; Army-Navy and Weitlaner retractors.
  - Abdominal aortic aneurysm repair: Various-length hemostat; right-angle and tonsil clamps; Metzenbaum and Potts scissors; various-length DeBakey and Gerald forceps; Profunda, DeBakey, Glover, Wylie, Satinsky, and other aortic aneurysm clamps based on anatomical needs; Freer elevator; nerve hooks, No. 4 Penfield dissector; Crile Wood, Ryder, and Castroviejo needle holders; Richardson and Bookwalter retractors; vascular Doppler probe; vendor-specific graft and suture material.
  - Arteriovenous fistula: Mosquito and Crile Clamps; Adson and DeBakey forceps; DeBakey and angled bulldog clamps; Metzenbaum and Potts scissors; Heiss and Weitlaner retractors; vascular Doppler probe; vendor-specific grafting material as needed.

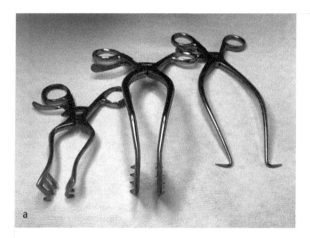
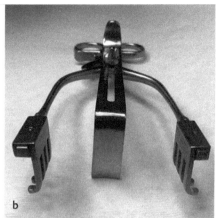
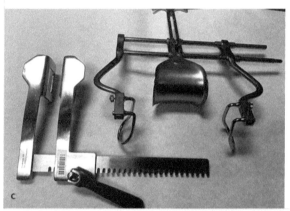

Fig. 1.8 Self-retaining retractors. (a) Left to right: blunt Weitlaner, Adson cerebellar, Gelpi retractors. **(b)** Henly vascular retractor. **(c)** Left to right: Finochietto and Balfour retractors.

○ Neurosurgery:
 – Craniotomy for tumor: Raney clip applier; hemostats; Metzenbaum and bayonet microvascular scissors; No. 1, 3, and 4 Penfield dissectors and Langenbeck elevators; bipolar coagulators; Cushing and Gerald forceps with teeth; Kerrison rongeurs; Decker and tumor forceps; Frazier and Fukushima suctions; Fukushima retractor; Castroviejo needle holder; perforator drill and footed drill attachments.
 – Endoscopic transsphenoidal hypophysectomy: Freer and Cottle elevators; No. 4 Penfield dissector; bayonet forceps; bayonet osteotome and mallet; angled spinal curettes; ebony Cottle and Rhoton speculums; up-biting and down-biting Kerrison rongeurs of various sizes; Noyes and Decker forceps; Cushing rongeur; long suctions; Hardy bayonet curettes; enucleators; and bayonet knife handles; Jannetta dissectors.
 – Ventriculoperitoneal shunt: Raney clip applier; hemostat; tonsil, right-angle, and Bozeman clamps; Metzenbaum scissors; Adson, Cushing, and Gerald forceps with teeth; bayonet forceps; No. 1, 3, and 4 Penfield dissectors; Woodson dural separator; Weitlaner and cerebellar retractors; Kerrison rongeurs; shunt passer; vendor-specific shunt implants and supplies.
○ Otolaryngology:
 – Functional endoscopic sinus surgery: Ballenger knife; Cottle and Freer elevators; Noyes, Blakesley, Takahashi, and Jansen Middleton forceps; Cottle speculums; sinus cannulas; Sofferman needle holder; Ostium probes.

43

– Thyroidectomy: Curved mosquito and Crile clamps; right-angle and tonsil clamps; curved Mayo, Metzenbaum, and tenotomy scissors; Adson, DeBakey, and bipolar forceps; Army-Navy, Green, Lahey thyroid, Weitlaner, and Beckman retractors; small and medium Ligaclip appliers; nerve stimulator.

– Translabyrinthine approach for acoustic neuroma: Weitlaner, cerebellar, and Perkins retractors; electric or pneumatic drill with various-sized diamond and cutting round burrs; bayonet forceps and coagulators; Freer and Lempert elevators, No. 4 Penfield dissector; Fukushima retractor; Rosen needle; House sickle knife; Sheehy knife/curettes; Antoli Candela elevator; 90-degree House hook; alligator forceps and scissors; curved bayonet microscissors; nerve stimulator; CUSA or Sonopet; possible soft tissue graft set-up (Allis clamps, curved Metzenbaum or Mayo scissors; Weitlaner retractor).

1.5.2 Qualities of Surgical-Grade Stainless Steel

- Grades of SS determine the strength, durability, sharpness, and flexibility. Martensitic and austenitic are most common chemical compositions for surgical steel.[64,65]
  - Martensitic SS alloy contains chromium:
    - Least expensive material.
    - Most widely used, strong but brittle, magnetic, good corrosion resistance.
    - 400 Series SS used for surgical instruments.
  - Austenitic SS alloy contains nickel and may contain chromium:
    - Most expensive material.
    - Most malleable, tough, nonmagnetic, corrosion resistant.
    - 300 Series SS used in probes, dilators, and retractors.
- Manufacturers differentiate instruments SS grade and product lines such as OR, Mid-Grade, Physician's Grade, Floor Grade, and Disposable.
- Customized instruments must be made from high-quality SS by a manufacturer and provide Instructions for Use on sterilization requirements per regulatory standards. Alterations to products may render the warranty void, decrease life expectancy, and may present potential liability.

1.5.3 Instrument Maintenance

- Quality instruments are essential during surgical procedures[62,63]:
  - Higher life expectancy, durability, and improved performance.
  - Instruments fail due to extreme or repeated stress:
    - Box lock: Fails from stress and torque; prevents effective occlusion, clamping or grasping of tissue.
    - Instrument tips: Fail from dullness, broken, or overlapping; may tear delicate tissue or not adequately grip or occlude.
    - Toothed instruments: Fail when teeth stick, click, or overlap; may cause local tissue damage or tears.
    - Ratcheted handles: Fail because of stress and torque or overlapping; may not allow for complete locking of instrument.
    - Spring joints: Fail on forceps because of unstable closing and opening tension; may cause tips of forceps to overlap or tear tissue.

1.5.4 Sterilization Methods

- Sterilization is the process that renders instruments free of biological contaminants and safe for use within the surgical environment.[66,67]
  - Manual and mechanical decontamination is essential to sterilization.
    - Uses chemical detergents.
    - Manual only renders instrument free of gross debris.
    - Mechanical decontamination uses washer sterilizer units.
- Steam sterilization is oldest and safest form and uses pressurized saturated steam.
  - Biological indicator is Geobacillus stearothermophilus.
  - Prevacuum sterilization cycle:

- – Vacuum empties air from the chamber rapidly.
- – Temperatures rise quickly reducing exposure and drying time.
- – 134 °C has 3-minute exposure and 6- to 99-minute drying times.
  - ○ Gravity sterilization cycles:
    - – Gravity is used to empty the chamber of air slowly.
    - – It is ideal for nonporous items with direct steam contact, laboratory media, and glassware.
    - – 134 °C has 10-minute exposure and 20- to 60-minute drying times.
  - ○ Immediate use steam sterilization (IUSS):
    - – Pre-vac or gravity.
    - – Primarily used in the operating room.
    - – Decontamination of instruments prior per hospital guidelines.
    - – Sterilization at 134 °C requires 3-minute exposure and 4- to 10-minute drying times.
- • Hydrogen peroxide gas plasma:
  - ○ Gas plasma via electrical fields created by radio frequencies.
  - ○ Biological indicator is *G. stearothermophilus.*
  - ○ Water vapor and oxygen are the byproducts.
  - ○ Low-temperature sterilization at 37–44 °C with a 75-minute cycle time.
- • Ethylene oxide (ETO):
  - ○ Biological indicator is *Bacillus atrophaeus.*
  - ○ Requires safety considerations because of carcinogenic risks.
  - ○ Low-temperature sterilization with 1- to 6-hour cycle time and 8- to 12-hour aeration.
- • Peracetic acid:
  - ○ Biological indicator is *G. stearothermophilus* spore strips.
  - ○ Commonly used for flexible endoscopic equipment.
  - ○ Sterilization at 50 °C with a 12-minute exposure time.
- • Various factors can negatively influence the sterilization process:
  - ○ Time: Inadequate processing times or interrupted cycles.
  - ○ Temperature: Inadequate maintenance of temperature during the exposure time.
  - ○ Accessibility: An improperly cleaned lumen or gross debris remaining on item.
  - ○ Moisture: Certain sterilization methods will fail if moisture remains on items.
- • Microorganisms:
  - ○ Sterilization kills all organisms, including fungi and spores if properly decontaminated and sterilization parameters are met.
  - ○ No sterilization cycles kill prions, and all items, including instruments, must be properly disposed of when there is concern for prion contamination (e.g., brain biopsies).

1.5.5 Electrosurgery

- • Electrosurgery: Electric current used at high frequency (100 kHz–5 MHz) alternating current at various voltages (200–10,000 V) passed through tissue to generate heat; electrosurgical unit consists of generator, handpiece, and one or more electrodes.
  - ○ Bipolar electrosurgery (▶ Fig. 1.9): Active and return electrode at site of surgery, can work in high fluid environment, tissue grasped and coagulated.
  - ○ Monopolar electrosurgery: Active electrode at surgical site, return electrode at dispersive pad on body.
    - – Cutting mode: High power density used to vaporize water.
    - – Coagulation mode: Lower power density causing coagulation and desiccated.
  - ○ Return electrode should not be used over metallic implants or bony prominences to reduce injury; return should be placed on large tissue areas (e.g., buttocks, thigh); pacemakers and internal cardiac defibrillators interrogated before use; patient jewelry removed to avoid current leakage.
- • Electrocautery: Electrical current used to heat a metal wire then applied to target tissue to coagulate a specific area; utilized in superficial situations (e.g., dermatology, ophthalmology, plastic surgery, urology).

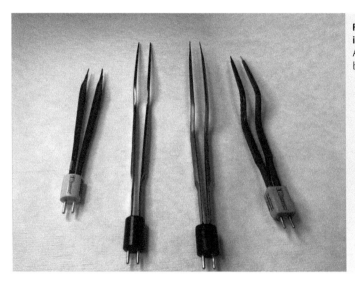

Fig. 1.9 Bipolar electrosurgery instruments. Left to right: insulated Adson bipolar, Cushing and Gerald bipolar, insulated irrigating bipolar.

References

[1] Sabaté S, Mases A, Guilera N, et al. ANESCARDIOCAT Group. Incidence and predictors of major perioperative adverse cardiac and cerebrovascular events in non-cardiac surgery. Br J Anaesth. 2011; 107(6):879–890

[2] Fleisher LA, Fleischmann KE, Auerbach AD, et al. American College of Cardiology, American Heart Association. 2014 ACC/AHA guideline on perioperative cardiovascular evaluation and management of patients undergoing noncardiac surgery: a report of the American College of Cardiology/American Heart Association Task Force on practice guidelines. J Am Coll Cardiol. 2014; 64(22):e77–e137

[3] Banerjee S, Angiolillo DJ, Boden WE, et al. Use of antiplatelet therapy/DAPT for post-PCI patients undergoing noncardiac surgery. J Am Coll Cardiol. 2017; 69(14):1861–1870

[4] Kazmers A, Cerqueira MD, Zierler RE. Perioperative and late outcome in patients with left ventricular ejection fraction of 35% or less who require major vascular surgery. J Vasc Surg. 1988; 8(3):307–315

[5] Xu-Cai YO, Brotman DJ, Phillips CO, et al. Outcomes of patients with stable heart failure undergoing elective noncardiac surgery. Mayo Clin Proc. 2008; 83(3):280–288

[6] Matyal R, Hess PE, Subramaniam B, et al. Perioperative diastolic dysfunction during vascular surgery and its association with postoperative outcome. J Vasc Surg. 2009; 50(1):70–76

[7] Neelankavil JP, Thompson A, Mahajan A. Managing cardiac implantable electronic devices (CIEDs) during perioperative care. Anesth Patient Saf Found 2013;28(2). Available at: https://www.apsf.org/article/managing-cardiovascular-implantable-electronic-devices-cieds-during-perioperative-care. Accessed January 10, 2020

[8] American Society of Anesthesiologists. Practice advisory for the perioperative management of patients with cardiac implantable electronic devices: pacemakers and implantable cardioverter-defibrillators: an updated report by the American Society of Anesthesiologists Task Force on perioperative management of patients with cardiac implantable electronic devices. Anesthesiology. 2011; 114 (2):247–261

[9] Chia PL, Foo D. A practical approach to perioperative management of cardiac implantable electronic devices. Singapore Med J. 2015; 56(10):538–541

[10] Kash BA, Zhang Y, Cline KM, Menser T, Miller TR. The perioperative surgical home (PSH): a comprehensive review of US and non-US studies shows predominantly positive quality and cost outcomes. Milbank Q. 2014; 92(4):796–821

[11] American Society of Anesthesiologists. Practice advisory for preanesthesia evaluation: an updated report by the ASA Task Force on preoperative evaluation. Anesthesiology. 2012; 116:1. https://anesthesiology.pubs.asahq.org/article.aspx?articleid=2443414

[12] Feely MA, Collins CS, Daniels PR, Kebede EB, Jatoi A, Mauck KF. Preoperative testing before noncardiac surgery: guidelines and recommendations. Am Fam Physician. 2013; 87(6):414–418

[13] Bilimoria KY, Liu Y, Paruch JL, et al. Development and evaluation of the universal ACS NSQIP surgical risk calculator: a decision aid and informed consent tool for patients and surgeons. J Am Coll Surg. 2013; 217(5):833–42.e1, 3

[14] Lubitz AL, Chan E, Zarif D, et al. American College of Surgeons NSQIP risk calculator: accuracy for emergent and elective colorectal operations. J Am Coll Surg. 2017; 225(5):601–611

[15] Lee TH, Marcantonio ER, Mangione CM, et al. Derivation and prospective validation of a simple index for prediction of cardiac risk of major noncardiac surgery. Circulation. 1999; 100(10):1043–1049

[16] Cohn SL, Fernandez Ros N. Comparison of 4 cardiac risk calculators in predicting postoperative cardiac complications after noncardiac operations. Am J Cardiol. 2018; 121(1):125–130

[17] Kluger MT, Gale S, Plummer JL, Owen H. Peri-operative drug prescribing pattern and manufacturers' guidelines: an audit. Anaesthesia. 1991; 46(6):456–459

[18] Zafirova Z, Vázquez-Narváez KG, Borunda D. Preoperative management of medications. Anesthesiol Clin. 2018; 36(4):663–675

[19] Kerridge RK. Perioperative patient management. Best Pract Res Clin Obstet Gynaecol. 2006; 20(1):23–40

[20] Lip GY. Implications of the CHA(2)DS(2)-VASc and HAS-BLED scores for thromboprophylaxis in atrial fibrillation. Am J Med. 2011; 124 (2):111–114

[21] Committee of Origin: Standards and Practice Parameters. Standards of Basic Anesthetic Monitoring. American Society of Anesthesiologists. 1986; revised October 28, 2015. Available at: https://www.asahq.org/~/media/Sites/ASAHQ/Files/Public/Resources/standards-guidelines/standards-for-basic-anesthetic-monitoring.pdf. Accessed January 10, 2020

[22] Warner MA, Warner ME, Weber JG. Clinical significance of pulmonary aspiration during the perioperative period. Anesthesiology. 1993; 78(1):56–62

[23] Practice guidelines for preoperative fasting and the use of pharmacologic agents to reduce the risk of pulmonary aspiration: application to healthy patients undergoing elective procedures: an updated report by the American Society of Anesthesiologists Task Force on preoperative fasting and the use of pharmacologic agents to reduce the risk of pulmonary aspiration. Anesthesiology. 2017; 126 (3):376–393

[24] James CF, Modell JH, Gibbs CP, Kuck EJ, Ruiz BC. Pulmonary aspiration: effects of volume and pH in the rat. Anesth Analg. 1984; 63(7): 665–668

[25] Barash PG. Clinical Anesthesia, 7th ed. Philadelphia, PA: Lippincott Williams & Wilkins; 2013

[26] Miller RD. Miller's Anesthesia, 7th ed. Philadelphia, PA: Elsevier; 2010

[27] Sessler DI. Perioperative heat balance. Anesthesiology. 2000; 92(2):578–596

[28] Smith L. New AHA recommendations for blood pressure management. Am Fam Physician. 2005. Oct1; 72(7):1391–1398

[29] Committee on Quality Management and Departmental Administration. Continuum of depth of sedation: definition of general anesthesia and levels of sedation/analgesia. American Society of Anesthesiologists Standard and Guidelines. Last amended October 15, 2014. Available at: https://www.asahq.org/standards-and-guidelines/continuum-of-depth-of-sedation-definition-of-general-anesthesia-and-levels-of-sedationanalgesia. Accessed January 10, 2020

[30] Anesthesia Physical Classification System. Cleveland Clinic. Available at: https://my.clevelandclinic.org/health/articles/12976-anesthesia-physical-classification-system. Accessed January 10, 2020

[31] Lemmens LC, Kerkkamp HE, van Klei WA, et al. Implementation of outpatient preoperative evaluation clinics: facilitating and limiting factors. Br J Anaesth. 2008; 100(5):645–651

[32] Hopkins TJ, Raghunathan K, Barbeito A, et al. Associations between ASA physical status and postoperative mortality at 48 h: a contemporary dataset analysis compared to a historical cohort. Perioper Med (Lond). 2016; 5:29

[33] Sankar A, Johnson SR, Beattie WS, Tait G, Wijeysundera DN. Reliability of the American Society of Anesthesiologists physical status scale in clinical practice. Br J Anaesth. 2014; 113(3):424–432

[34] Smith L. New AHA recommendations for blood pressure management. Am Fam Physician. 2005; 72(7):1391–1398

[35] Harrington BE, Reina MA. NYSORA Post-dural puncture headache. Available at: https://www.nysora.com/foundations-of-regional-anesthesia/complications/postdural-puncture-headache/. Accessed January 10, 2020

[36] Zaric D, Pace NL. Transient neurologic symptoms (TNS) following spinal anaesthesia with lidocaine versus other local anaesthetics. Cochrane Database Syst Rev. 2009(2):CD003006

[37] Ilias WK, Klimscha W, Skrbensky G, Weinstabl R, Widhalm A. Continuous microspinal anaesthesia: another perspective on mechanisms inducing cauda equina syndrome. Anaesthesia. 1998; 53(7):618–623

[38] Douglas MJ. Neurotoxicity of lidocaine: does it exist? Can J Anaesth. 1995; 42(3):181–185

[39] Pollock JE, Burkhead D, Neal JM, et al. Spinal nerve function in five volunteers experiencing transient neurologic symptoms after lidocaine subarachnoid anesthesia. Anesth Analg. 2000; 90(3):658–665

[40] American Association of Neurological Surgeons. Cauda equina syndrome. Available at: https://www.aans.org/en/Patients/Neurosurgical-Conditions-and-Treatments/Cauda-Equina-Syndrome. Accessed January 10, 2020

[41] Drasner K. Lidocaine spinal anesthesia: a vanishing therapeutic index? Anesthesiology. 1997; 87(3):469–472

[42] Spinal Anesthesia. Available at: https://www.nysora.com/techniques/neuraxial-and-perineuraxial-techniques/spinal-anesthesia/. Accessed January 10, 2020

[43] El-Boghdadly K, Pawa A, Chin KJ. Local anesthetic systemic toxicity: current perspectives. Local Reg Anesth 2018; 11:35–44

[44] Neal JM, Bernards CM, Butterworth JF, IV, et al. ASRA practice advisory on local anesthetic systemic toxicity. Reg Anesth Pain Med. 2010; 35(2):152–161

[45] Open Anesthesia. Local Anesthetics: Systemic Toxicity. Available at: https://www.openanesthesia.org/local_anesthetics_systemic_toxicity/. Accessed March 3, 2019

[46] ECRI Institute. New clinical guide to surgical fire prevention. Patients can catch fire: here's how to keep them safer. Health Devices. 2009; 38(10):314–332

[47] Apfelbaum JL, Caplan RA, Barker SJ, et al. American Society of Anesthesiologists Task Force on Operating Room Fires. Practice advisory for the prevention and management of operating room fires: an updated report by the American Society of Anesthesiologists Task Force on Operating Room Fires. Anesthesiology. 2013; 118(2):271–290

[48] Practice Advisory for Perioperative Visual Loss Associated with Spine Surgery. Practice Advisory for Perioperative Visual Loss Associated with Spine Surgery 2019: an updated report by the American Society of Anesthesiologists Task Force on Perioperative Visual Loss, the North American Neuro-Ophthalmology Society, and the Society for Neuroscience in Anesthesiology and Critical Care. Anesthesiology. 2019; 130(1):12–30

[49] Committee on Standards and Practice Parameters (CSPP). Standards for Postanesthesia Care. Approved by the ASA House of Delegates on October 27, 2004, and last amended on October 15, 2014. Available at: https://www.asahq.org/standards-and-guidelines/standards-for-postanesthesia-care. Accessed January 10, 2020

[50] Hsu DC. Subcutaneous infiltration of local anesthetics. Last updated April 3, 2018

[51] Lexi Comp Drug Information Handbook. 27th ed. New York: Wolters Kluwer; 2018

[52] Ban KA, Minei JP, Laronga C, et al. American College of Surgeons and Surgical Infection Society: Surgical Site Infection Guidelines, 2016 update. J Am Coll Surg. 2017; 224(1):59–74

[53] Bratzler DW, Dellinger EP, Olsen KM, et al. American Society of Health-System Pharmacists (ASHP), Infectious Diseases Society of America (IDSA), Surgical Infection Society (SIS), Society for Healthcare Epidemiology of America (SHEA). Clinical practice guidelines for antimicrobial prophylaxis in surgery. Surg Infect (Larchmt). 2013; 14(1):73–156

[54] Berríos-Torres SI, Umscheid CA, Bratzler DW, et al. Healthcare Infection Control Practices Advisory Committee. Centers for Disease Control and Prevention Guideline for the Prevention of Surgical Site Infection, 2017. JAMA Surg. 2017; 152(8):784–791

[55] Xu B, Xu B, Wang L, et al. Absorbable versus nonabsorbable sutures for skin closure: a meta-analysis of randomized controlled trials. Ann Plast Surg. 2016; 76(5):598–606

[56] Heal CF, Banks JL, Lepper PD, Kontopantelis E, van Driel ML. Topical antibiotics for preventing surgical site infection in wounds healing by primary intention. Cochrane Database Syst Rev. 2016; 11:CD011426

[57] Heal C, Buettner P, Raasch B, et al. Can sutures get wet? Prospective randomised controlled trial of wound management in general practice. BMJ. 2006; 332(7549):1053–1056

[58] Toon CD, Sinha S, Davidson BR, Gurusamy KS. Early versus delayed post-operative bathing or showering to prevent wound complications. Cochrane Database Syst Rev. 2015(7):CD010075

[59] Webster J, Scuffham P, Stankiewicz M, Chaboyer WP. Negative pressure wound therapy for skin grafts and surgical wounds healing by primary intention. Cochrane Database Syst Rev. 2014(10):CD009261

[60] Dumville JC, Owens GL, Crosbie EJ, Peinemann F, Liu Z. Negative pressure wound therapy for treating surgical wounds healing by secondary intention. Cochrane Database Syst Rev. 2015(6):CD011278

[61] AN, Khan WS, JP. The evidence-based principles of negative pressure wound therapy in trauma & orthopedics. Open Orthop J. 2014; 8:168–177

[62] Shultz R. Inspecting surgical instruments: an illustrated guide. 2nd ed. RMPS Publishing LLC; 2005

[63] Lind N. Instrumentation resource course: identification, handling and processing of surgical instruments. International Association of Healthcare Central Service Material Management. 2005

[64] Types of Stainless Steel used in Medical Instruments. Available at: https://medical-tools.com/shop/blog/post/types-of-stainless-steel-used-in-medical-instruments/. 2019. Accessed January 28, 2019

[65] Brendle TA. Reducing the risk of cross-contamination from transmissible spongiform encephalopathies. AORN J. 2005; 82(3):442–446

[66] Rutala WA, Weber DJ. Guideline for disinfection and sterilization in healthcare facilities. Centers for Disease Control; 2008. Available at: https://www.cdc.gov/infectioncontrol/guidelines/disinfection/index.html. Accessed January 28, 2019

[67] AAMI ST79: Comprehensive Guide to Steam Sterilization and Sterility Assurance in Health Care Facilities. Association for the Advancement of Medical Instrumentation; 2017. Available at: http://www.aami.org/standards/downloadables/aamirevf.pdg. Accessed August 12, 2018

2 Critical Care for Surgeons

Edited by Milos Buhavac

2.1 Organ System–Based Assessment in the SICU

Dorothea Rosenberger

2.1.1 Summary

- Patients admitted to the surgical intensive care unit (SICU) for high-acuity care require a physiologic system–based assessment approach to minimize the risk of data omission.
- All essential information representing all organ systems needs to be exchanged with a multidisciplinary critical care team on daily morning and/or evening rounds.
- Critical care medicine is goal-oriented based on the physiologic systems involved, requiring "intensive," invasive, and medically complex multidisciplinary attention. Once all organ system–specific goals are met, patients are considered for transfer to care areas with less acuity.
- Scoring systems are useful for describing unbiased severity of critical illness at different time points during the patient's stay in the SICU, predicting mortality and length of stay in the SICU depending on the score used.

2.1.2 Common Indications for Admissions to the SICU

- Perioperative complications caused by comorbidities, surgical procedure, or intraoperative events:
  - Shock: Septic, hemorrhagic, distributive, and combination of different shock forms in the perioperative and trauma setting.
  - Respiratory insufficiency and respiratory failure.
  - Hemodynamic instability and cardiac arrest.
  - Neurologic compromise and brain attack.
  - Gastrointestinal complications with hemorrhage or ileus.
  - Acute renal failure, metabolic and electrolyte dysregulation.
  - Immunocompromised state with organ transplant or hematologic disease.

2.1.3 Pathways of Admission to the SICU

- Patients admitted to the SICU require high-intensity, close hemodynamic, neurological, and organ system–based monitoring by specialty trained medical and nursing staff that cannot be provided on general surgical floors.
- Depending on the pathway of admission, the patient may require specific assessment, additional laboratory work-up, and invasive procedures.
- Patients can come from various areas within the same hospital and from outside the hospital.
  - Emergency department: Transfer for management of an acute severe illness. Causes of that illness may or may not be known upon admission to the SICU (e.g., acute trauma or burn patients may arrive with a series of diagnostic tests, imaging, and history in the ICU and require further assessment for patient management plans).
  - Postoperative admission from operating room (OR) or postanesthesia care unit (PACU): Surgical patients with need for higher level of care such as invasive hemodynamic monitoring, ventilator management, fluid and blood resuscitation, correction of coagulopathy with complex surgery, intraoperative complications, or substantial comorbidities affecting outcomes in the perioperative period may be transferred directly to the SICU postoperatively.
  - General surgical or medical hospital floor: Surgical and medical patients with acute changes such as respiratory failure, hemodynamic instability, cardiopulmonary arrest, any form of shock, acute renal failure with severe electrolyte disturbances, or any other critical pathophysiologic diagnosis perioperatively or during the hospital stay may require higher acuity of care in an SICU setting.

○ Referral and transfer from outside facilities for higher acuity care: Other hospitals or outside care facilities that cannot provide the level of critical care medicine required for their patient. For example, level 1 trauma, burn, transplant, stroke, and cardiac care centers with specialized critical care units are accepting referrals from other hospitals directly.

2.1.4 Physiologic System–Based Assessment

- General approach for assessment includes a first exam focused on the acute critical problem or problems the patient is presenting with in the SICU. Evaluation of the key issue is followed by a system-based assessment from "head to toe," covering all physiological systems, medications, and procedures applied, including results of invasive and noninvasive monitoring and laboratory values. All communication in the ICU setting is system-based and presented in standardized physiologic order to assure all ICU team members have a full all-inclusive report.[1,2]
- "FAST HUG" became a mnemonic for seven key care components in critically ill patients. The concept is tied into organ system assessment and systematic evaluation on an at least daily basis for multidisciplinary critical care rounds.[3]
  ○ FAST: Feeding—analgesia—sedation—thromboembolic prevention
  ○ HUG: Head of bed elevated—stress ulcer prophylaxis—glucose control
- Admission to specific surgical ICU will determine which standardized assessment and evaluation focus is most appropriate: Neurocritical care and head trauma will have a greater focus on monitoring of intracranial pressure (ICP) and cerebral perfusion pressure (CPP) compared with other disciplines like plastic surgery and burn. Visceral-abdominal, surgical oncology, cardiothoracic, cardiovascular, and disciplines like transplant (with either abdominal or cardiothoracic focus) all differ in the emphasis of key issues and detailed organ system–based assessment, procedures, medications required, and patient management plan.
- Point of care ultrasound (POCUS) is also increasingly used in critically ill patients as a fast bedside imaging technique to assess patients in a system-based approach to guide therapy plans (e.g., volume status, need for inotropic support, identifying pneumothorax). Ultrasound techniques complement physical exam, data and invasive device driven monitoring tools and are indicated for arterial and venous line placement.
- Pediatric surgical ICU assessment will be discussed under Chapter 10 Pediatrics.

2.1.5 Neurologic System

- Clinical presentation: Functional neurologic exam with cranial nerves, complete motor and sensory system, strengths and deficits, pain score (visual analog scale 0–10), sedation level using appropriate standardized sedation scores like Richmond Agitation-Sedation Score (RASS) and/or Glasgow Coma Score (GCS).
- General intervention: Frequency of neurological testing, changes in neurological exam, analgesic control, and required sedation type/route/amount, "sedation vacation" trials or wake-up trials.
- Specific intervention: ICP monitoring, extraventricular drainage, epidural pain catheters, wound drainage, electroencephalogram (EEG), transcranial Doppler (TCD). Subarachnoid hemorrhage (SAH) with Hunt Hess classification for severity of initial level of neurological presentation and Fisher grading as a computer tomography (CT)–based assessment of subarachnoid blood found in the head CT, traumatic brain injury (TBI) with severity of intracranial hemorrhage (ICH) score, spinal trauma assessment using American Spinal Injury Association (ASIA) criteria.

2.1.6 Cardiovascular System

- Clinical presentation: Heart rate, rhythm, type, systolic, diastolic, mean arterial blood pressure (ABP), maximum, minimum, and average over 12/24-hour period, auscultation, electrocardiogram (EKG) findings and echocardiographic results, laboratory work-up results, including complete blood count (CBC), basic or comprehensive metabolic panel (BMP/CMP), coagulation results.
- General intervention: Vasoactive medication (pharmacologic vasopressors, vasodilators, inotropic, antiarrhythmic, chronotropic support) including type/route/dosing and laboratory work-up, drug levels,

anticoagulation and antithrombotic medication, volume demands and resuscitation requirements (blood products and crystalloid versus colloid replacement), drainages in place and output.
- Specific intervention: Data obtained by specific invasive hemodynamic monitoring:
  - Central venous pressure (CVP) by central venous line, systolic and diastolic pulmonary artery pressures calculated and measured by pulmonary artery catheter (PAC), stroke volume determination by invasive hemodynamic cardiac output monitoring.
  - Pacemaker/defibrillator with mode and need for intervention.
  - Assist device management:
    - Temporary or permanent left ventricular, right ventricular assist devices, extracorporeal membrane oxygenation (ECMO), intra-aortic balloon pumps.
    - Includes report of device settings and parameters and specific laboratory work-up required for monitoring (anticoagulation and antithrombotic therapy).

2.1.7 Pulmonary/Respiratory System

- Clinical presentation: Respiratory status, breathing pattern, and supplemental oxygen or ventilatory support requirements, auscultation, signs of secretion retention, pulmonary infiltration, atelectasis.
- General intervention: Oxygen demands in liters/min and oxygen saturation, specific intervention with ventilator support including mode with settings, calculated and measured parameters, specific pharmacologic bronchodilator and mucolytic intervention, chest X-ray results, arterial blood gas data, end-tidal CO_2 monitoring, chest tubes, suction level and output.
- Specific intervention:
  - Ventilation mode and adjustments (escalation to full support, de-escalation to spontaneous breathing), spontaneous breathing trials and parameters obtained, endotracheal tube placement with size and depth of tube, endotracheal tube removal, tracheostoma size, and date of procedure.
  - P/F ratio, PaO_2, and fraction of oxygen for grading of acute lung injury.
  - Bronchoscopy, bronchoalveolar lavage and results, chest tube placement with reasons for indication, venovenous ECMO with device settings, and results.

2.1.8 Renal and Genitourinary System with Fluid Status and Electrolytes

- Clinical presentation: Body weight, results for creatinine (Cr)/blood urea nitrogen (BUN), urine output, and fluid input (with breakdown in crystalloid, colloid, and blood products), drainage output.
- General intervention: Removal or placement of urinary drainage catheters, forced diuresis with diuretics (route/dose), electrolytes.
- Specific intervention:
  - Renal failure staging, renal replacement therapy (continuous or intermittent) with fluid removal goals and specific dialysis mode, intravenous access versus permanent shunt/peritoneal dialysis.
  - Electrolyte replacement therapy.

2.1.9 Gastrointestinal and Nutrition Status

- Clinical presentation: Nutritional status, abdominal examination (auscultation/palpation), bowel movements, vomitus/nausea.
- General intervention: Nasogastric/orogastric tube, bowel protocol with prokinetics and laxatives, frequency and quality of bowel movements, fecal management systems, swallow evaluation, abdominal drains, stress ulcer prophylaxis.
- Specific intervention: Enteral feeding access (temporary, route/rate of nutrition, gastric/postpyloric), parenteral nutrition, amount of calories per hour or in 24 hours, type of nutrition and duration, enteral stoma, stoma care, gastroscopy/endoscopy.

2.1.10 Metabolic, Endocrine System

- Clinical presentation: Body mass index and body habitus, weight loss and weight gain history, jaundice.

- General intervention:
  - Electrolytes, hormone levels, comprehensive/basic metabolic panel, and liver function testing.
  - Blood sugar control, hyperglycemia, hypoglycemia, antihyperglycemic agents, and insulin requirements (continuous vs. scheduled).
  - Hormone/steroid replacement therapy (e.g., stress dose steroids, testosterone, thyroxine).
- Specific intervention: Insulin pump, diabetes insipidus and intervention, Cushing syndrome, endocrine tumor suppression, liver replacement therapy.

2.1.11 Infection, Hematologic System, Skin, and Wound Healing

- Clinical presentation:
  - Fever, hypothermia, systemic inflammatory response syndrome (SIRS), sepsis/septic shock criteria (specific and/or multiple organ system failure).
  - Hemorrhagic shock, coagulopathy, active hemorrhage with or without cardiovascular instability.
  - Surgical wound inspection and wound-healing assessment, drainage, skin condition, perfusion status.
- General intervention:
  - White blood cell (WBC) count, differential blood cell count, pan culture assessment, and results of bacterial/viral/fungal/parasitic infectious processes with gram stain, antibiogram, polymerase chain reaction (PCR), quantification, virus load, temperature control.
  - Hemorrhage, anemia, and coagulopathy, test results in CBC and coagulation laboratory assessment.
  - Antithrombotic/anticoagulation medication:
    – Prophylactic versus therapeutic.
    – Continuous infusion (dose and monitoring effectiveness with laboratory tests).
    – Scheduled subcutaneous injections.
    – International normalized ratio (INR)/partial thromboplastin time (PTT)/prothrombin time (PT).
  - Drainage output, drainage sampling and culture results, skin condition, ulcer, erythema, eczema, delayed wound healing, wound defects requiring special wound care, burned surface.
- Specific intervention:
  - Active cooling therapy, contact isolation, empiric broad-spectrum antibiotics/anti-infectious medication, sepsis markers.
  - Disseminated intravascular coagulopathy, coagulopathy due to medication requiring reversal therapy with coagulation factors, noncoagulopathy hemorrhage requiring transfusion, intervention other than surgery, e.g., interventional radiology for coiling or clipping of blood vessels.
  - Advanced coagulation laboratory testing using rotational thromboelastometry, thromboelastography (TEG), coagulation factor blood results, platelet aggregation testing.
  - Burned body surface area and degree and depth of burn, calculation of fluid demands and infection prevention measures.

2.1.12 Severity of Illness: Scoring Systems in the SICU

Scoring systems are tied into organ system–based assessment in adult critically ill surgical patients for documentation of severity of disease as well as for predicting patients' mortality risk and outcome, less so in guiding management of the critical ill patient. The most commonly used scoring systems in surgical critically ill patients are presented in their latest updated versions.

- APACHE IV (Acute Physiology and Chronic Health Evaluation):
  - Predicts SICU length of stay and hospital mortality.
  - Complex score collecting data on first SICU day.
  - Data include acute physiologic data upon SICU admission following an organ-based assessment:
    – Neurological data with GCS.
    – Cardiac data with mean ABP, heart rate per minute.
    – Respiratory data with respiratory rate per minute, mechanical ventilation yes/no, and fraction of inspired oxygen in percent, arterial blood gas data for oxygen and carbon dioxide, as well as arterial pH.
    – Renal and fluid status data with urine output, sodium level, Cr, and urea.

- Nutritional and metabolic data using albumin and bilirubin.
- Infectious data with WBC count.
- Also included are age of patient, and chronic health variables (renal failure, cirrhosis, hepatic failure, lymphoma, leukemia, immunosuppression, metastatic carcinoma, AIDS). Further information required for this score are location of hospital and length of stay before admission, emergency surgery, readmission, nonoperative and operative admission diagnosis, and thrombolytic therapy.[4]
- SAPS 3 (Simplified Acute Physiology Score):
  - Predicts SICU length of stay and hospital mortality.
  - The score is an arithmetic sum of three subscores covering the following data:
    - Subscore 1: Patient characteristics before SICU admission (age, health status, comorbidities, location before SICU admission, length of stay before SICU admission, e.g., vasopressor demands).
    - Subscore 2: Circumstances about the SICU admission (if applicable anatomic site of surgery, planned or unplanned admission to SICU, reasons for admission to SICU following organ-based assessment, surgical status and infection at SICU admission).
    - Subscore 3: Presence and degree of physiologic derangement at SICU admission, within 1 hour before or after admission. Data are organ-based, including, e.g., GCS, total bilirubin, body temperature, Cr, heart rate.
  - Scoring follows a point system, based on rating and grading of the affected organ and site of surgery, leading to a prediction of severity of illness and mortality risk.[5,6]
- MPM0-III (Mortality Prediction Model)
  - Predicts hospital mortality, customized for seven different geographic regions.
  - Data collection at SICU admission (±1 hour).
  - Data include physiologic data (heart rate, systolic blood pressure, GCS), acute diagnosis, anatomical site of surgeries, chronic diagnoses (e.g., renal insufficiency acute vs. chronic, cirrhosis, metastatic cancer, cardiac arrhythmia, cerebrovascular accident, gastrointestinal bleeding, intracranial mass effect, mechanical ventilation within first hour of admission), age, hospital location and length of stay before SICU admission, type of admission, and resuscitation status of the patient and whether cardiopulmonary resuscitation prior to admission was required.[7]

2.2 Neurological Monitoring

Michael Karsy and Gregory W.J. Hawryluk

2.2.1 Neurological Status in Critically Ill Patients

- Consciousness: Awareness of state and environment, requires state of arousal.
- Coma: Disruption of arousal by impairment of reticular activating system, diencephalic structures, or diffuse bilateral hemisphere damage; can be caused by unilateral cerebral injury with brainstem compression; varying spectrum of arousal (e.g., inattentiveness, stupor, obtundation).
- Medical causes of coma: Cerebrovascular disease (50%), hypoxia–ischemia (20%), metabolic and encephalopathic conditions (30%).
- Descending level of injury accounts for motor exam findings, injury above diencephalon yields withdrawal or localization, and brainstem injury above red nucleus results in decorticate posturing and decerebrate posturing.
- Work-up: Clinical examination to localize lesion if able; serial monitoring of Glasgow Coma Scale (GCS); metabolic evaluation; computed tomography (CT) imaging used to evaluate for acute neurological changes (GCS change ≥ 2 points) but only in hemodynamically stable patients, electroencephalography and MRI of brain used for further evaluation, and monitoring should be considered with mass-occupying lesions and GCS ≤ 8.
- Treatment: Supportive therapy, treatment of primary condition, and expert consultation for prognostication and further management.

2.2.2 Monitoring Indications

- Fourth edition of *Guidelines for the Management of Severe Traumatic Brain Injury* help guide indications for intracranial monitoring.[8]
- Level IIB evidence for ICP monitoring in patients with severe TBI to reduce in-hospital and 2-week postinjury mortality rates.[9,10,11,12]
- ICP monitoring indications:
  - ○ Patients with severe TBI (GCS 3–8) and an abnormal CT scan of the head (e.g., scan with hematoma, contusions, herniation, or compressed basal cisterns).
  - ○ Severe TBI with normal CT scan of the head and two or more of the following: age ≥ 40 years, unilateral or bilateral motor posturing, systolic blood pressure < 90 mm Hg.
- Monro-Kellie hypothesis suggests cranial vault is a closed compartment made of brain + cerebrospinal fluid (CSF) + blood; a mass-occupying lesion decreases volume for the brain.
- Level III evidence that external ventricular drain (EVD) zeroed at the midbrain with continuous drainage lowers ICP as opposed to intermittent drainage.
- Optimization of intracranial monitoring parameters (▶ Table 2.1) varies by provider and institution.
- Medical and surgical management strategies are used to lower ICP (▶ Fig. 2.1).
- Newer approaches have advocated multimodality neurological monitoring (▶ Table 2.1) as improving understanding of different components of neurological injury to optimize treatment; limited evidence supports a uniform treatment strategy using multiple monitors.[13]

Table 2.1 Neurological parameters for monitoring

Parameters	Measurement	Treatment threshold	Significance
Intracranial pressure (ICP)	External ventricular drain, intracranial pressure bolt	22–25 mm Hg	Marker of cerebral edema, impending herniation, and impacts neurological function
Cerebral perfusion pressure (CPP)	MAP–ICP	< 60 mm Hg	Indirect marker of cerebral blood flow
Cerebral blood flow (CBP)	Transcranial Doppler	> 200 cm/s or LR > 6	Detects vasospasm and ischemia
	Thermal dilution probe (e.g., Bowman perfusion monitor)	< 20 mL/100 g/min	Differentiates hyperemia from vasospasm
			Evaluates regional ischemia
Cerebral oxygenation	Jugular vein oximetry	< 50% or > 80%	Evaluates global ischemia or hyperemia
	Licox	< 20 mm Hg	
Cerebral metabolic rate of oxygen (CMRO$_2$)	Microdialysis	Glucose < 0.4 µmol/L, lactate > 3.0 µmol/L, lactate to pyruvate ratio > 40, glutamate > 10 µmol/L, glycerol > 90 µmol/L	Evaluates metabolic brain function
Electroencephalography (EEG)	Continuous EEG	Epileptic spikes, focal or global synchronization, periodic lateralizing epileptic discharges, abnormal waveform slowing	Evaluates subclinical nonconvulsive seizures, monitors status epilepticus

Abbreviations: LR, Lindegaard ratio (ratio of mean velocity in middle cerebral artery vs. internal cerebral artery); MAP, mean arterial pressure.

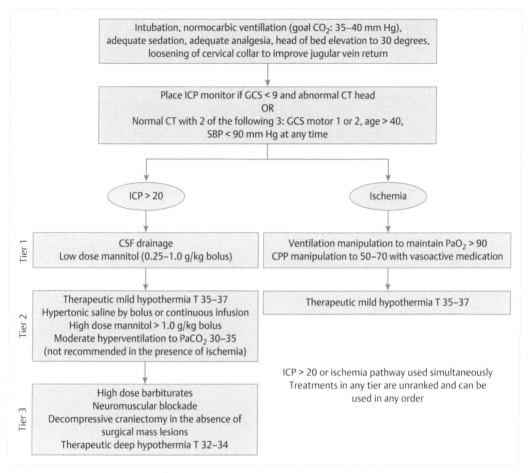

Fig. 2.1 Intracranial pressure management algorithm.[8]

2.2.3 Intracranial Pressure Management

- EVD:
  - Catheter placed into the lateral ventricle using surface anatomy for monitoring of ICP and drainage of CSF (▶ Fig. 2.2a).
  - CSF production ranges from 500 to 600 mL/d, and drainage of 10–20 mL/h is appropriate for most patients.
  - Various locations for placement by provider in patients without medical contraindications (e.g., anticoagulation): Entry site at Kocher's point (10–11 cm posterior to the nasion and 3 cm lateral; in line with the midpupillary line, 1–2 cm anterior to the coronal suture), trajectory to a plane intersecting the external auditory meatus and nasion.
  - Complications of hemorrhage (2–10%), infection (5–20%), failure, inadvertent placement,[14] hemorrhages rarely of clinical significance (0.5–1%), risk of upward herniation in patients with mass-occupying lesions of the posterior fossa.
  - EVD leveled with the patient tragus and height in cm H_2O used to establish a relief pressure setting; continuous or intermittent draining strategies can be used; evaluation of pressure, drainage amounts and patency performed hourly.

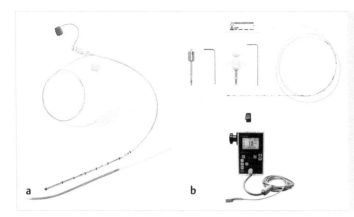

Fig. 2.2 Example of bolt and external ventricular drain (EVD) monitoring. (a) Dual EVD and bolt system. (b) Bolt system with skull mount and pressure monitor. Reproduced with permission from Integra Life Science (Plainsboro, New Jersey).

- Pressure monitoring can be used for guiding clinical treatment.
- Antibiotic-impregnated catheters, reduced access of the system, and adherence to placement protocols can reduce risk of infection although not shown in all studies.[15,16]
- Intracranial bolt:
  - Intraparenchymal or subdural pressure transducer anchored into the bone or secured to the skin (▶ Fig. 2.2b).[17]
  - Provides continuous ICP monitoring without ability for CSF drainage.
  - Evaluation of pressure values and waveform performed hourly; intermittent provocative maneuvers (e.g., pressing on abdomen, suctioning) performed to ensure monitor responsiveness.
  - Lower complication risk than EVDs, risk of hemorrhage (1–2%).

2.2.4 Elevated Intracranial Pressure Management

- Cerebral autoregulation maintains constant blood flow over a large range of blood pressures, loss of blood flow at low blood pressures, as well as pathologic hyperemia at high blood pressures.
- ICP waveform (▶ Fig. 2.3): Comprised of P1, P2, and P3 components, with P1 resulting from arterial pulsations, P2 from brain tissue compliance, and P3 from closure of the aortic valve (dicrotic notch).
- Worsening ICP waveform shows increase in P2 wave.
- Lundberg waves: Waveform changes over longer time period.
  - Lundberg A: Plateau waves, periodic sustained ICP > 50 mm Hg for > 15 minutes, predicts poor prognosis.
  - Lundberg B: ICP 20–50 mm Hg for 1–2 minutes.
  - Lundberg C: ICP 20 mm Hg every 4–8 minutes, unknown significance.

2.2.5 Other Neurological Monitors

- Lumbar drain:
  - Tunneled lumbar catheter used for draining CSF from the thecal sac.
  - Inserted at L3/4 or L4/5 level in patients with appropriate anatomy and without medical contraindications (e.g., infection, anticoagulation), tunneled up to 20 cm at the skin and secured to the skin.
  - Used for treatment of CSF leaks, reduction of subarachnoid blood, and less often ICP monitoring or evaluation (e.g., normal pressure hydrocephalus).
  - Drainage strategies aimed at the rate of 5–10 mL/h, patient laid flat and drain not lowered below level of the mattress to avoid over drainage regardless of hourly output goals.
  - Patient monitored hourly for tonsillar herniation resulting in increased nausea/vomiting and altered mental status.

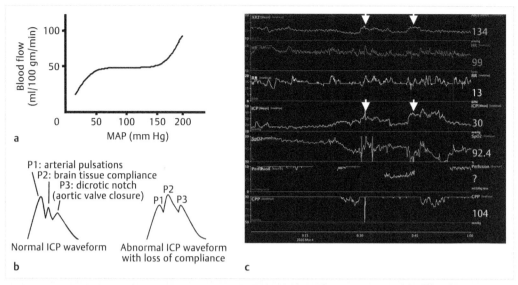

Fig. 2.3 Example of intracranial pressure waveform, multimodal monitoring, and poor cerebral autoregulation.
(a) Cerebral autoregulation results in maintenance of constant cerebral blood flow over a range of mean arterial pressures. **(b)** Intracranial pressure (ICP) waveforms show loss with abnormal brain compliance. **(c)** Patient with severe traumatic brain injury showing elevation of ICP with increases of mean arterial pressures, suggesting poor autoregulation (*arrows*).

- Electroencephalography:
  - Evaluation of regional electrical brain activity using surface contacts.
  - Used for evaluation of epileptic activity, nonconvulsive status epilepticus, and brain activity during induction of coma for treatment of ICP.
  - International 10–20 system uses 19 contacts, 1 ground, and 1 reference, differences between two adjacent electrodes represent a channel waveform, and series of channels are termed a montage.
  - EEG activity evaluates rhythmic activity and transient, episodic events.
  - EEG rhythmic activity is divided into frequencies:
    - Delta: < 4 Hz, seen in frontally during slow-wave sleep, deep/subcortical lesions, deep midline disorders, diffuse lesions, metabolic encephalopathy, hydrocephalus.
    - Theta: 4–7 Hz, seen during drowsiness, focal subcortical lesions, metabolic encephalopathy, deep midline disorders, hydrocephalus.
    - Alpha: 8–15 Hz, seen posteriorly during eye closure and coma.
    - Beta: 16–31 Hz, seen during wakeful state.

2.3 Ventilator Management

Michael Karsy

- Positive pressure ventilation used to support breathing, oxygenation, and tissue perfusion.[18]
- Ventilation controlled by trigger (flow vs. pressure), limit (factor determining breath size), and cycle (factor ending breathing).
- Indications for ventilation can be suggestive but are not definitive (▶ Table 2.2).
- Ventilation divided into volume-, pressure-, or dual-controlled modes.
- Basic ventilation modes:
  - Volume-controlled ventilation modes:
    - Inflation volume is preselected and ventilator adjusts pressure to deliver volume.
    - Peak airway pressure is pressure needed to overcome resistive airway and elastic lung forces to fill to volume.

Table 2.2 Indications for mechanical ventilation

$PaO_2 < 50$ mm Hg with $FiO_2 > 0.6$

$PaO_2 > 50$ mm Hg with pH < 7.25

Vital capacity $< 2 \times$ tidal volume

Negative inspiratory force < 25 cm H_2O

Respiratory rate > 35/min

Glasgow coma scale < 8

Physical signs of respiratory distress (hyperventilation, confusion, agitation, diaphoresis, decline in mental status, use of accessory muscles, increased work of breathing, thoracic retractions)

Upper airway burns or trauma

Cervical spine injury

Pulmonary contusion

Diagnostic procedures in combative/uncooperative patients

- Inflation hold occurs for 1 second after peak pressure is achieved at the plateau pressure before deflation.
- Assist-control ventilation (ACV)/continuous mandatory ventilation (CMV): Breath triggered ventilation which is mechanically assisted or patient controlled, undesirable for hyperventilating patients.
- Synchronized intermittent-mandatory ventilation (SIMV): Set number of breaths, patient controls rate of breathing, reduced risk of hyperinflation or alkalosis but increased work of breathing and reduced cardiac output in left-ventricular dysfunction.
  ○ Pressure-controlled ventilation modes:
  - Inflation pressure and duration are selected.
  - No air flow occurs at the end of inspiration, end-inspiratory pressure equals alveolar pressure.
  - Pressure-controlled ventilation (PCV): Pressure utilized to deliver breaths, reduced risk of barotrauma by modulating desired pressure compared to ACV or SIMV, ventilation waveform reduces peak pressures and improves gas exchange, preferred for neuromuscular disease but normal lungs.
  - Pressure support ventilation (PSV): Patient determines inflation volume and respiratory rate, augments spontaneous breathing, utilized during ventilation weaning.
  - Pressure-controlled inverse ratio ventilation (PCIRV): Elevated inspiratory time (reversed I:E ratio) with increased airway pressure and slightly improved oxygenation, risk of hemodynamic compromise.
  - Airway pressure release ventilation (APRV): Variation of continuous positive airway pressure (CPAP) with pressure release on exhalation, higher airway pressures, allows ventilation at both low and high pressures, risk of hemodynamic compromise.
  ○ Other modes:
  - Pressure-regulated volume control: Volume target backup added to pressure assist-control mode.
  - Proportional assist ventilation: % work of breathing set by clinician, ventilator utilizes feedback loop requiring knowledge of thoracic resistance and elastance.
  - CPAP: Positive pressure utilized to maintain airway; aids in obstructive sleep apnea, to delay intubation or to treat acute exacerbation.
  - Bilevel positive airway pressure (BIPAP): Positive airway pressure at both inspiration and exhalation set, useful to improve tidal volumes or decrease CO_2.
  - Prone or rotatory ventilation: May be useful in treatment of acute respiratory distress syndrome (ARDS) by redistributing pulmonary blood flow to improve oxygenation, decreases brain oxygenation in neurosurgical patients with elevated ICP.
  - High-frequency oscillatory ventilation: Multiple short breaths at high frequency, utilized more often in neonates.
- Positive end-expiratory pressure (PEEP):
  ○ Minimum pressure in alveoli during ventilator cycle.
  ○ Applied PEEP at the end of an expiratory limb aims to prevent airway collapse and overcome mechanical resistance.

- Occult PEEP can occur during continued airflow at the end of expiration not allowing lung emptying due to an obstructive event (e.g., asthma, chronic obstructive pulmonary disease) or ventilator settings (e.g., high inflation volumes, decreased time for exhalation compared to inhalation).
- Other factors:
  - Mean airway pressure: Average pressure in airway during ventilator cycle; depends on peak airway pressure, contour of waveform, PEEP level, respiratory rate, and inflation time; higher airway pressures can increase mechanical force needed for ventilation which can compromise hemodynamic function.
  - Thoracic compliance: Change in volume versus pressure of lung and chest.
  - Airway resistance: Inspiratory or expiratory resistance.
- Ventilation settings:
  - Ventilator initiation: Set tidal volume (10–15 mL/kg predicted body weight), set FiO_2 to minimum required to maintain PaO_2 80–100 mm Hg, set ventilator mode, adjust sensitivity to trigger with minimum effort (2 mm Hg negative inspiratory force), inspiratory flow rate 60–80 mL/min used, I:E ratio ≥ 1:2 used, respiratory rate < 35 breaths/min used, record arterial blood gas to make adjustments, tidal volume reduced by 6 mL/kg over next 2 hours as possible, flow rate at end of expiration evaluated to detect occult PEEP.
  - Lung protective ventilation initiation: Set tidal volume (8 mL/kg predicted body weight), maintain plateau pressure ≤ 30 cm H_2O, PEEP minimum 5 cm H_2O, permissive hyperapnea allowed as long as arterial pH > 7.3.
- Ventilation complications:
  - Ventilation failure:
    - Ventilation machine failure, increased airway pressures, poor oxygenation in the setting of otherwise reasonable ventilator setting.
    - Troubleshooting: Recheck ventilator settings, clear condensation from ventilator, re-evaluate patient clinical condition, suction airway, auscultate lungs to ensure ventilation, manually bag patient.
  - Ventilator-associated pneumonia (VAP):
    - Pulmonary infection due to ventilation, occurs 48–72 hours after intubation, accounts for 50% of all hospital-acquired pneumonias (HAPs), occurs in 9–27% of mechanically ventilated patients.
    - Diagnosed by clinical signs (e.g., fever, increased work of breathing) and laboratory studies (e.g., elevated white blood count, respiratory cultures showing infection, chest X-ray) (▸ Table 2.2 and ▸ Table 2.3).[19]
    - Quantitative culture is most predictive with colony-forming unit (CFU) cutoffs depending on the method (e.g., 103 CFU/mL for protected specimen brushing vs. 104 for bronchoalveolar lavage [BAL]).
    - Highest risk within first 5 days if ventilation (3% risk/day) and then declines to 1%/day risk.
    - Variable mortality due to other underlying conditions.
    - Top three causes: *Pseudomonas* (24.4%), *S. aureus* (20.4%), Enterobacteriaceae (14.1%).
    - Treatment: Divided into early-onset (< 4 days from intubation) to late-onset, treated with broad-spectrum antibiotics.
    - Prevention methods: Hand washing, early discontinuation of invasive devices, reduced intubation and early extubation, head of bed elevation to 30–45 degrees, early tracheostomy, small bowel feeding compared to gastric feeding, probiotics, maintaining cuff > 20 cm H_2O.
    - No full proof method of eliminating VAP; thus, extubation as early as possible is encouraged.
  - Ventilator-induced lung injury:
    - Volutrauma: General term describing injury tidal volumes > 5–7 mL/kg, results in barotrauma, air leak, pulmonary infiltration, and edema.
    - Atelectrauma: Repetitive opening and closing of small airways resulting in alveolar sheer injury, can be reduced via PEP.
    - Biotrauma: Proinflammatory cytokine release due to mechanical ventilation.
    - Barotrauma: Air leaks from ruptured alveoli can result in pneumomediastinum, subcutaneous emphysema, and pneumoperitoneum.
    - Oxygen toxicity: Inflammatory infiltration and fibrosis due to prolonged exposure to high FiO_2, FiO_2 > 0.6 avoided.
    - Lung protective ventilation strategies using ARDSNet protocols for treatment of ARDS.

Table 2.3 Clinical pulmonary infection score

Parameter	Result	Score
Temperature (°C)	36.5–38.4	0
	38.5–38.9	1
	≤ 36 or ≥ 39	2
Leukocytes in blood (cells/mm³)	4,000–11,000	0
	< 4,000 or > 11,000	1
	≥ 500 band cells	2
Tracheal secretions	None	0
	Mild/nonpurulent	1
	Purulent	2
Radiographic findings (excluding CHF or ARDS)	No infiltrate	0
	Diffuse/patchy infiltrate	1
	Localized infiltrate	2
Culture results (endotracheal aspirate)	No/mild growth	0
	Moderate/florid growth	1
	Moderate/florid growth and pathogen consistent with Gram stain	2
Oxygenation status (PaO_2:FiO_2)	> 240 or ARDS	0
	≤ 240 and absence of ARDS	2

Abbreviations: ARDS, acute respiratory distress syndrome; CHF, congestive heart failure.

Note: Sensitivity, 65%; specificity, 64%; score ≥ 6 shows good correlation with ventilator-associated pneumonia.[19]

Table 2.4 Extubation criteria

Breathing frequency < 30 breaths/min

Maximum inspiratory pressure < –20 cm H_2O

Vital capacity > 15 mL/kg

Tidal volume > 6 mL/kg

Absence of copious secretions

Able to maintain airway postextubation

Resolution of pathology necessitating initial intubation

Glasgow coma scale > 8 or able to follow commands

Hemodynamic stability without significant vasopressor support

Adequate gas exchange (O_2 saturation ≥ 93%)

Adequate neuromuscular block reversal

Rapid shallow breathing index (RSBI) = frequency/tidal volume; RSBI < 105 predicts better extubation

Adequate leak on cuff deflation

Note: No single criteria adequate predicts extubation success.

- Extubation strategies[20]:
  - Multiple strategies can be used to evaluate patient readiness for extubation (▶ Table 2.4).
  - Weaning to pressure support ventilation can be a transition to extubation.
  - Sedation, especially narcotics, should be reduced to decrease risk of airway compromise.
  - Planning for reintubation important as high-risk airways should involve notification of anesthesia and obtaining necessary equipment.
  - Airway edema can be treated with short courses of corticosteroids.
- ECMO[21]:
  - Temporary, artificial oxygenation by an external system in patients with severe cardiopulmonary failure refractory to medical management or ventilation.

Table 2.5 Indications for extracorporeal membrane oxygenation

Indications	Criteria
Acute respiratory distress syndrome	$PaO_2/FiO_2 < 150$ with $FiO_2 > 90\%$ and positive end-expiratory pressure 15–20 cm H_2O
	Inability to maintain airway plateau pressure ≤ 30 cm H_2O
Bridge to lung transplant, heart transplant, or ventricular-assist device implantation	
Primary graft failure of lung or heart transplant	
Exacerbation of chronic obstructive pulmonary disease or status asthmaticus	$PaCO_2 > 80$ mm Hg
	pH < 7.15
	Inability to maintain airway plateau pressure ≤ 30 cm H_2O
Cardiogenic shock from myocardial infraction, postcardiotomy, or post–heart transplant	
Myocarditis	
Sepsis-associated myocardial dysfunction	

- Can be utilized for oxygenation, reduction of carbon dioxide, and support of perfusion.
- Initially utilized in children and now increasingly used in adults with respiratory or cardiac failure.
- Two configurations: Venoarterial ECMO vs. venovenous ECMO.
- Venoarterial ECMO:
  - Complete or partial cardiopulmonary support.
  - Deoxygenated blood from venous system returned as oxygenated blood to arterial circulation.
  - Central configuration: Right atrium → proximal ascending aorta.
  - Peripheral configuration: Right atrium → ipsilateral or contralateral femoral artery *or* axillary artery.
- Venovenous ECMO:
  - Complete or partial pulmonary support, used for isolated respiratory failure with preserved cardiac function.
  - Double lumen catheter placed in internal jugular vein allows continuous recirculation of blood.
  - Variation of technique using pumpless system can be used for carbon dioxide removal.
- Indications generally involve cases where mortality is > 50% without ECMO (▶ Table 2.5), several scoring systems (e.g., RESP, PIPER) have been developed.
- Absolute contraindications include uncontrolled active hemorrhage, terminal illness, or end-stage heart or lung failure for patients not candidates for transplantation.
- Relative contraindications include > 7 days of mechanical ventilation with high FiO_2 or pressure, nonpulmonary organ dysfunction (e.g., renal failure), irreversible central nervous system (CNS) injury, malignancy, immunosuppression, inability to use anticoagulation, older age, obesity.
- Controllable parameters:
  - Blood flow: Depends on revolutions per minute of pump, circuit preload, and circuit afterload.
  - Fraction of oxygen in sweep gas: Blender of oxygen and air used to control partial pressure of oxygen in the blood.
  - Sweep gas flow rate: Utilized to remove carbon dioxide by diffusion and control partial pressure of carbon dioxide in the blood.
- Monitoring of arterial blood gases in patient, before ECMO circuit and after ECMO circuit, lactate (marker of tissue perfusion), plasma free hemoglobin (marker of hemolysis).
- Weaning of mechanical ventilation, judicious fluid use, monitoring of organ dysfunction, anticoagulation levels, and early ambulation are encouraged.
- Weaning:
  - Venovenous: Improvement of lung function, ECMO circuit flow rate < 3 L/min.
  - Venoarterial: Improvement of cardiac function based on pulse pressure and echocardiography, flow reduced 0.5–2 L/min over 24–36 hours.
- Complications: Hemorrhage (43%), infection, renal failure, thromboembolism, lower limb ischemia.

2.4 Hemodynamics

Landon Blumel and David Dorsey

2.4.1 Importance

- Maintenance of physiologic blood pressure is critically important for patient outcomes.
- Morbidity and mortality increase with inadequate hemodynamic management in many clinical situations.
- All organs are dependent on adequate blood pressure to ensure proper perfusion. In addition, patients exhibit a wide range of baseline blood pressures as outpatients that correlate with very different hemodynamic needs during the perioperative period. Certain surgical procedures demand strict blood pressure goals outside of the patient's physiologic needs.

2.4.2 Prevalence

- Prevalence of hypotension and shock varies substantially based on patient population and presenting diagnosis.
- Will be a common subject of many pages during residency and practice.

2.4.3 Noninvasive Blood Pressure Monitoring Techniques

- Intermittent:
  - Automated oscillometry (automatic blood pressure cuff).
  - Manual sphygmomanometer with auscultation.
- Continuous:
  - Arterial applanation tonometry: A small transducer at the wrist detects radial artery pulsation to provide systolic and diastolic pressures among other information. Has very limited use due to expense, need for constant monitoring and assessment by provider, patient movement, and invalidation by peripheral vascular disease.
  - Volume clamp: A small blood pressure cuff is placed on the finger to detect arterial pulsation. Often advertised as noninvasive cardiac output monitoring. Similar limitations as above.

2.4.4 Invasive Monitoring Techniques

- ABP:
  - A small catheter is placed in an artery and pressure is transduced directly.
  - Advantages are low cost, easily understood, minimal impact from patient movement, long history of safety, can be used to assess more than blood pressure alone.
- CVP:
  - After placement of a central venous catheter (CVC) or central line, a single lumen is connected to a pressure transducer for measurement.
  - Advantages are many: Since many critically ill patients already have central venous access it is easy and doesn't increase cost, requires no proprietary equipment, and has minimal risk.
  - However, many studies show CVP alone is not an accurate surrogate for volume status and may be more useful taken as a trend and in conjunction with other clinical markers.
- PAC (or Swan-Ganz):
  - Advantages include ability to evaluate cardiac output and index, ability to assess systemic vascular resistance, and measurement of mixed venous oxygen content.
  - Disadvantages include risk of pulmonary artery rupture, studies showing use doesn't improve outcomes in critically ill patients and may worsen them.[22] Use is more common in the cardiac surgery population.

- Transesophageal echocardiography (TEE):
  - Visual assessment of cardiac contractility, valve function, calculation of cardiac output, and assessment of volume status allow provider to rule out other causes of hypotension such as cardiac tamponade, right ventricular strain in the setting of pulmonary embolism.
  - Disadvantages include cost, need for highly trained operator, risk for esophageal injury, need for sedation to ensure patient comfort.

2.4.5 Indications for Invasive Hemodynamic Monitoring

- Need for instantaneous blood pressure or cardiac output monitoring in hemodynamically unstable patients (i.e., aortic dissection, unstable aneurysm, shock states, large and ongoing fluid shifts).
- Frequent blood draws which will affect treatment (i.e., invasive mechanical ventilation, use, and titration of vasoactive medications).
- Inability to measure blood pressure via noninvasive techniques due to body habitus (i.e., morbid obesity).

2.4.6 Treatment of Hemodynamic Derangements

- Assessment and treatment of hemodynamic derangements can be broken down to assessment of preload (volume status), afterload (vascular tone), and contractility (cardiac output).
- This then lends itself to treatment through the following tools:
  - Optimization of fluid status.
  - Vasopressor support.
  - Mechanical support devices.

2.4.7 Assessment of Volume Status and Volume Responsiveness

- Ensuring appropriate volume status is critical to quality hemodynamic management.
- Requires a complex combination of physical examination, monitor values, clinical history, and response to initial therapies to guide decision making.
- High-degree of variability between providers.
- Optimization of fluids status helps to maximize cardiac contractility which further leads to normalization of cardiac output and blood pressure regardless of underlying physiological status (▶ Fig. 2.4).

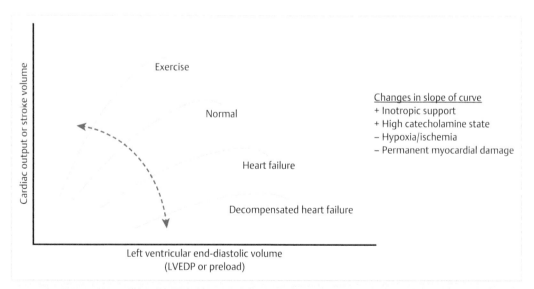

Fig. 2.4 Frank–Starling curve of cardiac output.

- Invasive:
  - Pulse pressure variation (PPV):
    - Assesses the change in peak ABP during inspiration and expiration during mechanical ventilation.
    - Used as a measure of volume responsiveness,[23] and considered positive if > 12% change.
    - Important to note that volume responsiveness indicates that blood pressure will improve with volume administration but not necessarily that more volume is needed.
    - Disadvantages include need for arterial line and mechanical ventilation to use.
  - CVP:
    - Has been found in many studies to be a poor predictor of fluid responsiveness and volume status.[24]
    - Use with caution and in conjunction with other factors. May be more useful at extreme values.
  - Pulmonary capillary wedge pressure (PCWP):
    - Estimate of left atrial pressure and left ventricular filling pressures. Limitations are described in Chapter 2.4.4.
- Noninvasive:
  - A number of proprietary devices are currently available, but use is limited.

2.4.8 Autoregulation and Individualized Approach to Hemodynamic Management

- As each patient is unique, so also are their hemodynamic needs.
- Autoregulation is the range of blood pressures under which the organs are able to regulate blood pressure to meet the metabolic demands needed in each organ (▶ Fig. 2.5).
- Autoregulation is altered in patients based on baseline hemodynamics:
  - For example, a patient with longstanding, poorly controlled hypertension may have significant rightward shift in autoregulation, necessitating different mean arterial pressure (MAP) goals than a patient with normal baseline blood pressures.
- In a study of septic patients, high target blood pressures were associated with arrhythmias, and low target blood pressures were associated with increased need for renal replacement,[25] further supporting idea that a one-size-fits-all approach is inadequate and need for individualized blood pressure treatment based on individual patient factors and current clinical picture.

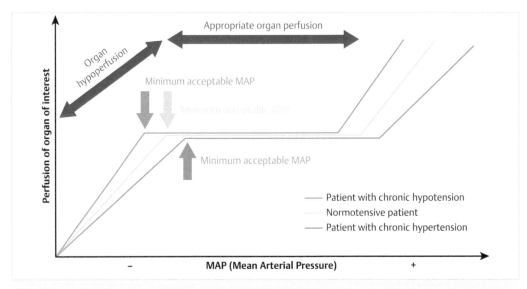

Fig. 2.5 Autoregulation of tissue perfusion.

2.4.9 Conditions Necessitating Elevated Maps

- There are many conditions in which an otherwise acceptable MAP of 65 mm Hg is not adequate to assure proper perfusion; some brief examples are as follows:
  - Aortic stenosis: In long-standing aortic stenosis, hypertrophy of the left ventricle (LV) with elevated LV filling pressures requires higher arterial pressures at the aortic root to ensure adequate coronary perfusion. Avoid tachycardia to ensure adequate time for LV filling.
  - Coronary artery disease: Coronary perfusion pressure is diastolic blood pressure (DBP) minus left ventricular end-diastolic pressure (LVEDP). To ensure adequate coronary flow, a higher systemic pressure is needed.
  - Elevated ICP: In the case of trauma or mass effect causing elevation of ICP, the CPP is determined by the equation CPP = MAP − CVP or ICP (whichever is highest), with a desired CPP of at least 60 mm Hg and may require norepinephrine to maintain a supranormal MAP in the setting of elevated ICP.
  - Spinal cord injury: In the case of spinal cord injury, especially anterior cord injury where blood flow is more limited, an elevated MAP is important to assure adequate cord perfusion. This can be achieved with fluid administration or with vasopressors, often phenylephrine infusion. A goal MAP of ≥ 85 mm Hg is common.
  - Pulmonary hypertension: Low systemic MAP is not sufficient to assure perfusion of the right ventricle (RV), which is perfused during systole and diastole. Poor perfusion of the RV leads to RV failure, low cardiac output, and marked hypotension with equalization of pulmonary pressures and systemic pressures potentially leading to hemodynamic collapse.
  - Arterial disease with threatened flow: A greater than average pressure gradient is needed to overcome stenosis and optimize flow to threatened area in any number of organ systems (e.g., brain, bowel, kidney, peripheral vascular disease).

2.4.10 Conditions Necessitating Lower than Expected MAP

- Heart failure:
  - In heart failure with reduced ejection fraction, patients are treated with vasodilators to reduce afterload and allow the weak ventricular to empty more fully (increasing stroke volume and cardiac output).
  - Diuretics are used to combat hypervolemia and overfilling of the ventricle. In the perioperative period, a temptation to hold home medications and aggressively raise blood pressure can cause increased cardiac workload and lead to decompensation of heart failure.
  - MAP goals should mirror the patient's outpatient MAPs as much as possible, but can lead to challenging clinical dilemmas when these patients develop an indication for higher MAPs (e.g., spinal cord injury).
- Threatened rupture/contained rupture of aneurysm: In patients admitted with ruptured or threatened abdominal, thoracic, or intracranial aneurysms, strict avoidance of hypertension is critical (arterial line placement with intravenous vasodilators).

2.4.11 When Is Treatment/Resuscitation Adequate?

- Endpoints to resuscitation include:
  - Hemodynamic stability.
  - Improvement in mental status.
  - Normalization of urine output.
  - Downtrending of lactate:
    - Early clearance of lactate indicates a resolution of inadequate oxygen delivery and cessation of anaerobic metabolism.
    - Associated with increased survival.[26]

2.4.12 Shock

- Shock (▶ Table 2.6) is a state of inadequate delivery of oxygen to end organs which is often marked by low blood pressure, and other signs of end organ hypoperfusion such as elevated lactate, low urine output, altered mental status, etc. While shock state is spoken of generally it is important to properly diagnose the cause as the treatment for different causes of shock are quite unique.
- Early physical exam includes assessment of volume status as well as "warm" versus "cold" extremities which provides critical information about the patient's systemic vascular resistance and subsequent treatment pathway. For example, patients in cardiogenic shock will manifest with cold, poorly perfused extremities due to low cardiac output and compensatory peripheral vasoconstriction. Unlike in sepsis patients, these patients will do poorly with large volume resuscitation.
- Hypovolemic shock (▶ Table 2.7):
  - Most commonly caused by hemorrhage but can also result from severe dehydration induced by extreme diarrhea, vomiting, or exposure to heat without adequate fluid intake.
  - Cause will guide treatment with hemorrhagic shock necessitating source control, and crystalloid, possible colloid, or blood product administration.
  - Other causes are treated with crystalloid with a focus on electrolyte and metabolic correction.
- Distributive shock:
  - Distributive shock is a shock type with many different root causes that leads to an inappropriate distribution of blood flow to peripheral and small blood vessels at the expense of vital organs.
  - Septic shock results from an infectious pathogen which causes widespread inflammation and loss of vascular tone ultimately causing fluid loss from the vascular space and low blood pressures.
    - Septic shock has a high mortality rate in some studies ranging up to 50%.
    - Treatment has evolved over time and was revolutionized by movement to early goal-directed therapy (EGDT) as pioneered by Dr. Manny Rivers greatly improved outcomes and with a marked decrease in mortality.[27]
    - Includes: Crystalloid administration (30 mL/kg); blood cultures; initiation of broad-spectrum antibiotics within 60 minutes of presentation; initiation of vasopressors if hypotension persists.
    - Nevertheless, this continues to be an area of active research and change including high-dose vitamin C, vitamin B12, thiamine, and corticosteroid administration being recent discoveries that are not yet mainstream treatment at this time.[28]

Table 2.6 Types of shock

Shock type	CO	Warm vs. cold	SVR	MVO$_2$	LVEDP/ PCWP	Treatment principles
Pump failure						
• Impaired forward flow → vascular tone increases to support blood pressure → slow moving blood leads to overextraction of oxygen						
• Goal to optimize heart function						
Hypovolemic	↓↓	Cold	↑↑↑	↓	↓	Resuscitate
Obstructive	↓↓	Cold	↑↑	↓	↑	Clear obstruction
Cardiogenic	↓↓↓	Cold	↑↑↑	↓	↑↑	Inotropes, later diuresis
Vasodilatory						
• Primary vasodilation problem → vascular tone unable to support adequate blood pressure → CO increases to compensate if it can						
• Goal to increase afterload						
Septic	↑↔↓[a]	Warm	↓↓↓	↑ (sometimes ↓)	↓↔	Volume/pressors
Anaphylactic	↑	Warm	↓↓	↔	↔	Volume/pressors
Neurogenic	↑ or ↓[b]	Warm	↓↓	↓	↔	Volume/pressors

Abbreviations: CO, cardiac output; LVEDP, left ventricular end diastolic pressure; MVO$_2$, myocardial oxygen consumption; PCWP, pulmonary capillary wedge pressure; SVR, systemic vascular resistance.

[a] Often high CO with appreciable cardiac dysfunction on echo.

[b] If associated with bradycardia, cervical sympathetic injury likely.

Table 2.7 Hemorrhagic shock classification

Findings	Class I	Class II	Class III	Class IV
Blood loss (mL)	<750 mL	750–1,500 mL	1,500–2,000 mL	>2,000 mL
(% Blood volume lost)	15%	15–30%	30–40%	>40%
HR (bpm)	Normal	>100	>120	>140
RR	Normal	20–30	30–40	>35
Systolic BP	Normal	Normal	Decreased	Markedly decreased
Urine output	Normal	20–30	5–15	Negligible
CNS function	Normal	Mild anxiety	Anxious	Lethargy, confusion
Capillary refill	Normal	Delayed	Delayed	Delayed
Treatment strategies	Aggressive crystalloid resuscitation and hemorrhage control sufficient for management		Blood product administration required	Impending death without immediate intervention

Abbreviations: BP, blood pressure; BPM, beats per minute; CNS, central nervous system; HR, heart rate; RR, respiratory rate.

- – Also, there is concern for the complications associated with over-resuscitation after a "one-size-fits-all" approach to fluid administration.[29]
    - – Early initiation of pressors after reasonable fluid administration guided by physical exam and comprehensive volume assessment is now advocated.[30]
- Neurogenic shock:
    - ○ Results from cervical spine injuries which disrupt the cervical sympathetic trunk causing an abrupt decrease in sympathetic tone.
    - ○ This results in dramatically decreased systemic vascular resistance, pooling of blood in the lower extremities, and lower than expected HR given the degree of hypotension.
    - ○ Low heart rate is due to cord injury above cardiac accelerator fibers (T1–T4).
    - ○ Neurogenic shock is treated with crystalloid administration along with vasopressors if crystalloid alone is insufficient.
- Anaphylactic shock:
    - ○ Results from either immunologic (IgE mediated) or nonimmunologic mast cell degranulation which leads to inflammatory cascade of cytokines and other mediators which leads to marked vasodilation, hypotension, tachycardia, bronchospasm, cutaneous manifestations, angioedema, etc.
    - ○ Treated with epinephrine, fluid administration, potential airway management, as well as adjuncts such as antihistamines and corticosteroids.
- Cardiogenic shock:
    - ○ Cardiac dysfunction that results in inadequate delivery of oxygen to end organs.
    - ○ Causes including acute myocardial infarction, decompensated cardiomyopathy, arrhythmia induced cardiogenic shock.
    - ○ Important note: Cardiogenic shock is inadequate cardiac function despite adequate volume status (also known as normal LV filling pressures).
    - ○ Physical exam findings: Cold extremities, jugular venous distension, pulmonary or lower extremity edema based on left versus right ventricular dysfunction.
    - ○ Treatment will vary based on the cause of cardiogenic shock; the complete scope is beyond the detail included in this text. However,
        - – In acute myocardial infarction the mainstay is expeditious angiography with percutaneous revascularization and possible mechanical support device utilization.
        - – In decompensated heart failure, diuresis allows patients to get back onto the ascending portion of the starling curve and inotropes allow for improved cardiac contractility.
        - – Arrhythmia-induced cardiogenic shock is treated with defibrillation or cardioversion depending on the arrhythmia, pharmacologic management, or transvenous pacing in complete heart block refractory to conservative management.

- Obstructive shock:
  - As the name implies it is a consequence of obstruction to the flow of blood which subsequently causes a dramatic decrease in cardiac output.
  - Classic causes are cardiac tamponade, tension pneumothorax, massive (often saddle) pulmonary embolism, and left ventricular outflow tract (LVOT) obstruction from hypertrophic cardiomyopathy.
  - Respective treatments being pericardiocentesis, needle thoracostomy vs. thoracostomy tube, thrombolytics vs. pulmonary thrombectomy, and volume loading, increased intravascular volume, and increasing systemic vascular resistance.

2.4.13 Vasoactive Agents

- Appropriate understanding and use of vasoactive medications, often called vasopressors, is an important part of hemodynamic management of critically ill patients. As detailed above, first accurate assessment of volume status and management of volume status should be completed prior to initiation of vasopressors (▶ Table 2.8).
- The importance of correct medication selection and dose cannot be overstated. Much has been learned about vasopressor selection, such as the increased rate of arrhythmias when dopamine was used for septic shock compared to norepinephrine.[31]
- However, it is also important to note that use of vasoactive medications differs greatly regionally and based on a variety of practice patterns. Contained below is a table with basic information for quick reference on vasopressor selection, it is not intended to be comprehensive but is a great starting point for vasoactive medication selection.

2.5 Cardiac Arrhythmia in Surgical Patients

Michael Karsy

2.5.1 Introduction

- New-onset, postoperative dysrhythmia affects 10–40% of patients after cardiothoracic surgery and 4–20% after noncardiothoracic surgery; incidence varies depending on type and study (▶ Table 2.9, ▶ Fig. 2.6)[32,33]; incidence of 40–90% in critically ill patients depending on underlying condition.
- Nonvascular abdominal surgery is an independent risk factor for postoperative supraventricular arrhythmia.
- New-onset arrhythmias increase length of stay and may increase mortality.
- Arrhythmia after cardiothoracic surgery due to mechanical irritation of pericardium or myocardium.
- Arrhythmia after noncardiothoracic surgery due to systemic inflammatory response, subclinical infection, sepsis, acid/base or electrolyte disturbances, volume shifts, stress, or complications of surgery (e.g., stroke, wound infection, pulmonary embolism, gastrointestinal bleeding).
- 80% arrhythmias revert to normal sinus rhythm prior to discharge, 20–30% of cases require no treatment.
- Preoperative risk factors: Age, male, congestive heart failure, valvular heart disease, asthma, history of supraventricular arrhythmia, premature atrial rhythms on preoperative EKG, left anterior hemiblock, American Society of Anesthesiologists (ASA) Classification class III or IV, hypertension, low preoperative potassium.

2.5.2 Treatment

- Tachyarrhythmias are classified by anatomical origin:
  - Supraventricular arrhythmias: Sinus tachycardia, atrial flutter, atrial fibrillation, ectopic atrial tachycardia, multifocal atrial tachycardia, junctional tachycardia, atrioventricular nodal re-entrant tachycardia, accessory pathway reciprocating tachycardia.
  - Ventricular arrhythmia: Premature ventricular complexes, ventricular tachycardia, ventricular fibrillation.
- Rhythm evaluation:
  - Evaluate rate and cardiac axis.

Table 2.8 Selection of vasopressors

Clinical findings				Pharmacologic effects						Physiologic effects		
Drug	Trade name	Common use	Dose range[a]	α	β1	β2	D	V	PDE (inhibition)	CO	HR	SVR
Phenylephrine	Neo-synephrine	Spinal cord injury/neurogenic shock, Septic shock 4th line	0.1–0.5 µg/kg/min	+++	–	–	–	–	–	↓/↔	↓↑	↑↑
Norepinephrine	Levophed	Septic shock, 1st line	0.2–1.5 µg/kg/min	+++	++	–	–	–	–	↕	↑/↕	↑↑
Dopamine	Intropin	Cardiogenic shock, neurogenic shock, 1st line pediatric pressor	2–5 µg/kg/min	+	++	–	+++	–	–	↕	↕	↑
Epinephrine	Adrenalin	Septic shock 3rd line, anaphylactic shock, cardiogenic shock	0.2–1.0 µg/kg/min	+++	+++	+++	–	–	–	↑↑	↑	↑
Dobutamine	Dobutrex	Cardiogenic shock, rarely septic shock	2–10 µg/kg/min	–	++	++	–	–	–	↑	↑	↓
Isoproterenol	Isuprel	Cardiac transplant, bradyarrhythmias, heart block	1–10 µg/kg/min	–	+++	++	–	–	–	↑	↑↑	↓↑
Vasopressin	Vasostrict	Septic shock 2nd line	0.01–0.04 units/min	–	–	–	–	++++	–	↕	↓/↕	↑↑
Milrinone	Primacore	Cardiogenic shock, RV failure	0.4–0.8 µg/kg/min	–	–	–	–	–	+++	↑	↕	↓

Abbreviations: CO, cardiac output; HR, heart rate; PDE, phosphodiesterase; SVR, systemic vascular resistance.

[a] Dosing of vasoactive medications is most appropriately done in a dose per units of weight and time, though in some locations it is performed dose per time only.

Table 2.9 Summary of common tachyarrhythmias in surgical patients and management

Arrhythmia	Finding	Incidence in surgical patients	Treatment	Potential complications
Atrial fibrillation	Chaotic atrial rhythm, normal QRS, irregularly irregular RR interval	4.4%	Rate control in acute settings using β-blockers, calcium channel blockers, amiodarone or digoxin (▶ Table 2.10); rhythm control or anticoagulation in chronic settings; echo to evaluate thrombus; cardiac ablation	Increase risk of stroke, dementia
Atrial flutter	Saw tooth waves in leads II, III, aVF; normal QRS, regular RR interval; 2:1 atrial to ventricular rate	0.4%		
Paroxysmal or macroreentrant atrial tachycardia	Various locations and durations of atrial tachycardia, form of supraventricular tachycardia, rate > 100 bpm, P–R interval normal or prolonged	0.3%	Can be difficult to distinguish from paroxysmal supraventricular tachycardias and adenosine can be helpful; β-blockers, calcium channel blockers, amiodarone, dofetilide or class IC antiarrhythmias can be used	Untreated can result in cardiomyopathy, heart failure, or recurrence
Focal vs. multifocal atrial tachycardia		0.4%		
Paroxysmal supraventricular tachycardia	Re-entrant cardiac rhythms, short QRS widths	3%	ACLS pathway (Chapter 16.2); adenosine or cardioversion, β-blockers, calcium channel blockers can be used, cardiac ablation	Digoxin, diltiazem, or verapamil can lead to atrial fibrillation
A–V nodal reentry	P-wave in or after QRS			
Ectopic atrial tachycardia	Abnormal P-wave, normal PR interval			
Ventricular ectopy	Common, benign, electrographic changes; higher risk in patients with heart disease, right ventricle outflow tract tachycardia, or worsened exercise-induced arrhythmia	0.3%	Reassurance in patients without heart disease, β-blockers, or implantable cardiac defibrillators for higher risk patients	Risk of sudden cardiac death from malignant ectopic beats or trigger of malignant ventricular arrhythmia
Ventricular tachycardia	Monomorphic or polymorphic ventricular pattern	0.13%	ACLS pathway (Chapter 16.2); defibrillation or cardiac thump in sustained ventricular tachycardia or pulseless arrests; stable patients treated with procainamide, sotalol, lidocaine, β-blockers, and amiodarone; magnesium used for Torsades de pointes; implantable cardiac defibrillator considered	Untreated ventricular tachycardia can result in pulseless arrest or ventricular fibrillation
Ventricular fibrillation		0.02%		
Any dysrhythmia		7.84%		

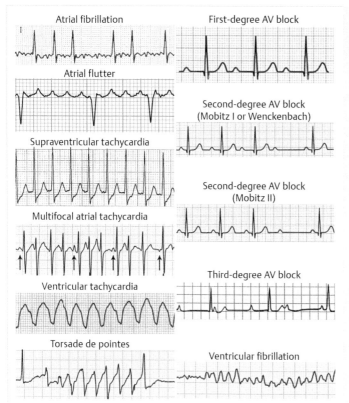

Fig. 2.6 Summary of tachyarrhythmias. (Adapted from Wikipedia.org under a Creative Commons license 2.0.)

- ○ Identify P-waves, P-wave rate, and P-wave morphology.
- ○ Number of P-waves > QRS (atrioventricular block), P-wave < QRS (junctional or ventricular rhythm), P-wave=QRS (measure PR interval).
- ○ Evaluate QRS morphology, < 0.12 ms indicates supraventricular arrhythmia, wide QRS represents ventricular tachycardia, supraventricular tachycardia with another cardiac condition, or anterograde condition via an accessory pathway.
- • Treatment algorithm:
  - ○ Evaluation of EKG to identify arrhythmia and causation of patient's problem.
  - ○ Evaluate urgency of arrhythmia, initiate ACLS protocol if necessary (see Chapter 16.2)
    - – ACLS protocol for bradycardia (heart rate < 40 bpm), and tachycardia (heart rate > 150 bpm).
    - – ACLS arrest protocol for patients without a pulse with division between shockable (VT/VF) and nonshockable rhythms (asystole/PEA).
    - – Cardioversion is performed for symptomatic patients (e.g., chest pain, hypotension, ischemia on EKG, altered consciousness) with supraventricular arrhythmia.
  - ○ If nonemergent, evaluate location of tachycardia and goal for electroconversion, chemical conversion, rate control, or rhythm control.
  - ○ Consider evaluation of secondary sequela (e.g., thromboembolism, stroke).
  - ○ Work-up: Chest radiograph used to evaluate pulmonary disease or cardiac enlargement, transthoracic or transesophageal echocardiogram used to evaluate cardiac function and thrombus formation, electrophysiology studies used selectively to further evaluate certain rhythms, B-type natriuretic peptide, sleep apnea testing, stress testing, cutaneous or implantable halter monitoring.
- • Arrhythmia types:
  - ○ Bradycardia:
    - – Sinus node dysfunction resulting in slowed heart rate.

- Can be exacerbated by increased vagal tone (e.g., epidural anesthesia, laryngoscopy, surgical intervention).
  - Treatment: ACLS bradycardia pathway.
- Atrial fibrillation[34]:
  - 4% major noncardiothoracic surgery, more common in elderly.
  - Irregular and rapid atrial beating can become symptomatic if driving rapid ventricular rhythm, no P-waves seen on ECG and irregular ventricular rate.
  - Presents: Fatigue, heart palpitations, dyspnea, hypotension, syncope, heart failure.
  - Types: Paroxysmal (terminates spontaneously or within 7 days); persistent (sustained > 7 days); long-standing persistent (continuous for > 12 months); permanent (defines when patients no longer seeking rhythm control); nonvalvular (occurs in the absence of mitral stenosis, heart valve, or valvuloplasty).
  - Treatment: Acute events lasting > 15 min treated with ventricular rate control (▶ Table 2.10), use of β-blockers followed by diltiazem and amiodarone can be used, digoxin can be used but is ineffective in acute control; events ongoing for > 48 hours require anticoagulation for 3 weeks before cardioversion and 4 weeks after; chronic management involves anticoagulation for prevention of stroke, consideration of endovascular and open ablative, or surgical procedures to reduce thromboembolism risk (e.g., Watchman device).
  - Calculation of CHA2DS2-VASc (▶ Table 2.11) can be useful in evaluating stroke risk during stopping, bridging, and restarting of anticoagulation; anticoagulation is recommended with score ≥ 2 with target INR 2–3, target INR 2–3 or 2.5–3.5 depending on valve type.
  - Bridging anticoagulation with heparin or Lovenox is recommended in patients with mechanical valves or CHA2DS2-VASc scores ≥ 2 depending on bleed risk, limited evidence supporting decision-making.

Table 2.10 Medication strategy for rate control of atrial fibrillation

Tier	Agent	IV dosage	Oral maintenance
1st	Metoprolol	2.5–5 mg IV bolus every 2 min up to three doses	25–100 mg BID
	Esmolol	500 μg/kg IV bolus over 1 min, 50–300 μg/kg/min IV	None
	Propranolol	1 mg IV over 1 min every 2 min up to three doses	10–40 mg TID or QID
2nd	Verapamil	0.075–0.15 mg/kg IV bolus over 2 min, additional 10 mg after 30 min if no response then 0.005 mg/kg/min infusion	180–480 QD extended release
	Diltiazem	0.25 mg/kg IV bolus over 2 min then 5–15 mg/h	120–360 mg QD extended release
3rd	Amiodarone	300 mg IV over 1 h, 10–50 mg/h over 24 h	100–200 mg QD
	Digoxin	0.25 mg IV with repeated dosing, max 1.5 mg over 24 h	0.125–0.25 mg QD

Table 2.11 CHADS$_2$-VASc score and stroke risk

	Risk	Points	Score = annual stroke risk (%)
C	Congestive heart failure, ejection fraction ≤ 40%	1	1 = 1.3
H	Hypertension	1	2 = 2.2[a]
A	Age ≥ 75	2	3 = 3.2
D	Diabetes	1	4 = 4
S$_2$	Stroke/transient ischemic attack/thromboembolism	2	5 = 6.7
V	Vascular disease	1	6 = 9.8
A	Age 65–74	1	7 = 9.6
S	Sex (female)	1	8 = 6.7
			9 = 15.2

[a] Anticoagulation recommended with score ≥ 2.

- HAS-BLED score can quantify bleed risk (▶ Table 2.12); scores ≥ 3 indicate higher risk for bleeding warranting closer monitoring of INRs, differential oral anticoagulant dose, or aspirin.
- Multiple anticoagulants potentially useable (see Chapter 16), no role for stroke primary prevention with aspirin.
○ Sinus tachycardia:
  - Common postoperatively and can be an appropriate response (e.g., pain, anxiety, fever, hypovolemia, anemia, hypoxemia, medications, alcohol withdrawal).
  - Treatment: ACLS tachycardia pathway, rates > 130 bpm may be poorly tolerated by elderly patients and should involve evaluation and treatment of underlying causes; β-blockers and calcium channel blockers can be used.
○ Atrial tachycardia:
  - Automatic focus or re-entrant pathway, 8% of paroxysmal supraventricular tachycardia (SVT).
  - Various types, considered a supraventricular tachycardia.
  - Show different P-wave morphology from sinus rhythm.
  - Multifocal atrial tachycardia (≥ 3 P-wave morphologies, irregularly irregular rhythm) more common in acutely ill patients.
  - Treatment: Evaluation and management of underlying causes; β-blockers and calcium channel blockers can be used; amiodarone, dofetilide, or class IC antiarrhythmics can be useful to refractory cases.
○ Heart blocks:
  - First-degree heart block: Prolonged PR interval > 120 ms.
  - Mobitz I: Progressive PR interval before nonconducted P-wave.
  - Mobitz II: Unchanged PR interval with nonconducted P-wave, higher likelihood of progression to third-degree heart block.
  - Third-degree heart block: Independent atrial (P-wave) and ventricular (QRS) contraction.
  - Treatment: Atropine, transcutaneous pacing, placement of permanent pacemaker.
○ Atrioventricular nodal re-entry:
  - Dual A–V nodal pathways with differing conduction velocities and refractory periods, P-waves cannot be seen due to simultaneous retrograde and anterograde ventricular activity, 60% paroxysmal SVT.
  - Orthodromic atrioventricular reciprocating tachycardia: Conduction retrograde along bypass tract and anterograde down A–V node, narrow QRS complex.
  - Antidromic tachycardia: Pre-excitation tachycardia with anterograde accessory pathway conduction and normal retrograde conduction via His-Purkinje system and A–V node.
  - Wolf-Parkinson-White: Conduction anterograde along accessory pathway, delta wave present, QRS wide.
  - Treatment: ACLS tachycardia pathway, carotid sinus massage or vagal maneuvers, infusion of 6–12 mg of IV adenosine, cardioversion if decompensating, β-blockers can be used, calcium channel

Table 2.12 HAS-BLED score and hemorrhage risk

	Risk	Points	Score= bleeds per 100 patient-years
H	Hypertension	1	0 = 1.13
A	Abnormal renal function[a]	1	1 = 1.02
	Abnormal liver function[a]	1	2 = 1.88
S	Stroke	1	3 = 3.74[b]
B	Bleeding source	1	4 = 8.7
L	Labile international normalized ratio (INRs)	1	5 = 12.5
E	Elderly > 65 years	1	
D	Drugs[a]	1	
	Alcohol[a]	1	

[a] 1 point each.

[b] Scores ≥ 3 indicate higher risk for bleeding.

blockers can be used cautiously as conduction down accessory pathway can lead to atrial fibrillation; digoxin, diltiazem, and verapamil block A–V node, resulting in rapid conduction down bypass track and potential development of atrial flutter/fibrillation; cardiac ablation can be used to target re-entrant pathway.

- ○ Ventricular tachycardia:
  - – Monomorphic type most common 48 hours after myocardial infarction or in cardiomyopathy due to scar.
  - – Polymorphic type most commonly due to muscle repolarization dysfunction.
  - – Long QT syndrome: Congenital prolongation of QTc interval (> 440 ms) with risk of progression to ventricular tachycardia.
  - – Acquired QTc prolongation can be due to a number of medications.
  - – Torsades de pointes: Specific type of polymorphic ventricular tachycardia associated with QT prolongation, treated with magnesium empirically otherwise may require pharmacological treatment or temporary pacing.
  - – Nonsustained (< 30 seconds) vs. sustained (> 30 seconds).
  - – Treatment: ACLS tachycardia pathway, pulseless ventricular tachycardia can be treated with synchronized defibrillation or a cardiac thump in an attempt to prevent degeneration to ventricular defibrillation, pharmacological treatments in stable patients include procainamide, sotalol, lidocaine, β-blockers, and amiodarone; implantable cardiac defibrillator may prevent death due to ventricular tachycardia or fibrillation.
- ○ Ventricular fibrillation:
  - – Disorganized electrical activity of the heart, associated with diseased hearts, myocardial infarction, major trauma, or metabolic derangements.
  - – Treatment: ACLS tachycardia pathway, tachycardia can be treated with asynchronous defibrillation or a cardiac thump; cardiac defibrillator may prevent death due to ventricular tachycardia or fibrillation.

2.5.3 Perioperative Cardiac Risk Assessment

- • Guidelines aim for identification and management of major adverse cardiac events (MACE).[35]
  - ○ Patients with emergent cases are optimized as best as possible and proceed with surgery.
  - ○ Patients with prior history of acute coronary syndrome (symptomatic heart failure, arrhythmia, coronary artery disease, or myocardial infarction) are referred to cardiology.
  - ○ Perioperative risk of MACE calculated using various scales (e.g., American College of Surgeons NSQIP risk calculator; riskcalculator.facs.org), perioperative metabolic equivalents (MET) calculated with Duke Activity Status Index with MET ≤ 4 correlated to higher cardiac risk.
    - – Examples of MET > 4 activity: Climbing a flight of stairs, walking up a hill, walking at 4 mph on level ground, performing heavy work around the house.
  - ○ Patients with low surgical risk (< 1%), elevated risk, and MET (> 4) do not require additional testing and can proceed to surgery; routine EKG or echo testing has poor evidence that it improves management or outcomes but can be optional especially in asymptomatic patients.
  - ○ Patients with MET ≤ 4 can undergo additional testing if potential to modify perioperative care, can include pharmacological testing with coronary revascularization.
  - ○ Noncardiac surgery should be delayed 14 days after balloon angioplasty, 30 days after bare metal stent, and 1 year after drug eluting stent at a minimum (level I evidence).
  - ○ Antiplatelet agents should be continued for 4–6 weeks after bare metal stent or drug-eluting stent unless risk of bleeding outweighs risk of in-stent thrombosis; patients discontinued from $P2Y_{12}$ platelet receptor-inhibiting therapy should be started on aspirin and restarted as soon as possible (level I evidence).
  - ○ Continuation of perioperative aspirin may show some benefit for patients with stent but requires evaluation of bleeding risk.
  - ○ β-Blockers and statins should be continued in patients continued in patients with long-term use (level I evidence).
  - ○ Patients with implantable cardiac defibrillators should undergo continuous cardiac monitoring with available external defibrillation equipment (level I evidence).

2.5.4 Myocardial Infarction

- 5% of patients ≥ 45 years undergoing noncardiac surgery undergo in-hospital cardiac death, nonfatal myocardial infarction, heart failure, or ventricular tachycardia; rate of 15% in patients > 65 years with symptomatic events increasing 30-day mortality by 9% and 1-year mortality by 22%.
- Myocardial injury: Elevation of cardiac troponin above 99th percentile.
- Myocardial injury after noncardiac surgery:
  - Troponin elevation within first 30 days from noncardiac surgery.
  - Due to supply-demand mismatch, plaque rupture, or acute thrombus.
  - Independently associated with increased mortality.
  - Symptomatic or asymptomatic.
- Goldman cardiac risk index is most predictive of perioperative cardiac complications; six factors: high-risk surgery, history of ischemic heart disease, heart disease, cerebrovascular disease, insulin-dependent diabetes mellitus, or perioperative Cr > 2.0 mg/dL.
- Presents: Rapid onset chest pain worse with activity, dyspnea, dizziness, diaphoresis.
- Work-up: EKG, troponin with evaluation of trend can be used with symptoms or high-risk patient screening.
  - ST-elevation MI criteria: New ST-elevation at J-point in two continuous leads of 1–2.5 mm depending on lead, gender, and age.
  - Non-ST-elevation MI or unstable angina criteria: New horizontal or downsloping ST-depression ≥ 0.5 mm, T inversion > 1 mm with prominent R-wave in two continuous leads or R/S ratio > 1.
- Treatment: Antiplatelet agents and statins, early involvement of expert consultation, consideration of oral anticoagulation and percutaneous coronary intervention.

2.6 Nutrition of the Critical Care and Postsurgical Patient

Michael Karsy

2.6.1 Nutrition Overview

- Acute critical illness results in metabolic catabolism rather than anabolism, whereby carbohydrates are the main energy source, fat mobilization is impaired, and adequate and not excessive protein supplementation is designed to prevent muscle breakdown.[36,37,38,39,40]
- Adequate but not excess enteral nutrition within 48–72 hours is the general goal; parenteral nutrition is used after 1–2 weeks for patients unable to receive enteral nutrition.
- Adequate nutrition results in reduced risk of surgical complications, infection, and mortality, but benefit is unclear in some studies.[41,42,43,44]
- Parenteral nutrition may increase risk of infection, rates of mechanical ventilation, and mortality, increased risk of adverse events with early (< 48 hours) parenteral nutrition compared with late parenteral nutrition (> 8 days).
- Enteral nutrition may reduce infection without impacting mortality compared to parenteral nutrition.
- Monitoring malnourished patients for electrolyte deficiencies and refeeding syndrome (e.g., hypophosphatemia, rhabdomyolysis, cardiovascular collapse, respiratory failure, seizures, delirium) required.
- Obese patients treated with same indications as other critical care patients.
- Malnourishment definition is variable and can include BMI < 18.5 kg/m^2, unintentional loss of 5% body weight over 1 month or 10% over 6 months, insufficient energy intake, loss of muscle mass, loss of subcutaneous fat, local or general fluid accumulation, diminished functional status (e.g., handgrip strength).
- Poor nutrition in surgical patients increases risk of susceptibility to infection, poor wound healing, pressure wounds, overgrowth of bacteria in the gastrointestinal tract, worsened nutrient loss through the stool.

- Nutritional surrogates:
  - Albumin: Half-life 18–20 days, < 2.2 g/dL marker of negative catabolic state; levels affected by surgical stress, hepatic disease, and renal disease.
  - Transferrin: Half-life 8–9 days, marker of nutrition only with normal serum iron.
  - Prealbumin/transthyretin: Half-life 2–3 days, responds rapidly to protein intake, can be altered in acute or chronic inflammation.
  - Other: BUN/Cr, glucose, electrolytes, vitamin levels.
- Nutrition is based on resting energy expenditure (REE) or dosing weight, indirect calorimetry can predict REE; goal 18–25 kcal/kg/d.
- Indirect calorimetry:
  - Noninvasive method of determining REE.
  - Indirectly correlates with heat production by monitoring O_2 consumption and CO_2 production over a period of time; volume of gases converted using Weir formula: metabolic rate (kcal/d) = 1.44 (3.94 VO_2 + 1.11 VCO_2).
  - Respiratory quotient (RQ) = VCO_2/VO_2; RQ for carbohydrates = 1, RQ for protein = 0.8–0.9, underfeeding induces lipogenesis and lowers RQ < 0.85, overfeeding increases RQ > 1.0.

2.6.2 Enteral Nutrition

- Nutrition via oral or feeding tubes (▶ Table 2.13).
- Oral diets:
  - Regular, diabetic (reduced glycemic index), cardiac (low sodium), renal (low in sodium, phosphorous, and protein).
  - National Dysphagia Diets (NDD): standardized terminology published in 2002 by the American Dietetic Association:
    - NDD Level 1: Dysphagia-pureed (homogenous, very cohesive, pudding-like, requiring very little chewing ability).
    - NDD Level 2: Dysphagia-mechanical altered (cohesive, moist, semisolid foods, requiring some chewing).
    - NDD Level 3: Dysphagia-advanced (soft foods that require more chewing ability).

Table 2.13 Overview of enteral supplements and formulas

Feeding type	kcal/mL	Indication
Boost, Ensure, Juven, Resource		Oral supplements
Promote (with or without fiber)	1.0, 1.2, or 1.5	General feeding, lower calorie needs but higher protein needs
Osmolite	1.0, 1.2, 1.5	
Isocal	1.0	
Jevity	1.0, 1.2 or 1.5	
TwoCal HN, NovaSource, Deliver, Nutren	2.0	High-calorie feed with reduced volume
Glucerna, Choice DM, DiabetiSource AC, Glytrol, Resource Diabetic	1.0 or 1.5	Designed for diabetic patients with lower amount of total carbohydrate and a higher amount of fat
Nepro, Magnacel Renal, NovaSource Renal, Suplena, Nutri-Renal	2.0	Design for renal disease with lower protein, potassium, magnesium, and phosphorous content; more calorie dense
NutriHep, Hepatic-Aid II	1.5	Designed for hepatic disease with increased amounts of branched chain amino acids: valine, leucine, and isoleucine; and reduced amounts of aromatic amino acids to reduce cerebral amino acid uptake and hepatic encephalopathy
Pulmocare, Nutrivent, NovaSource Pulmonary, Respalor	1.5	Designed for chronic obstructive pulmonary disease with reduced carbohydrate composition to reduce CO_2 production
Oxepa	1.5	Designed for acute respiratory distress syndrome with modified lipid component to reduce production of proinflammatory eicosanoids (e.g., thromboxane A2, leukotrienes, prostaglandin E2)

- No evidence to support that dysphagia diets reduce aspiration risk, but can improve quality of life in patients.[45]
- Tube feeding types:
  - Gastric: Nasogastric, percutaneous endoscopic gastrostomy (PEG), percutaneous radiologic gastrostomy, surgical gastrostomy, gastrostomy with jejunal adapter.
  - Duodenal: Postpyloric nasoduodenal.
  - Jejunal: Nasojejunal, percutaneous endoscopic jejunal.
- Postpyloric placement of tubes can improve feeding tolerance, reduce reflux and risk of aspiration with higher feeding rates, and potential for uninterrupted feeding for patients receiving procedures or surgeries.
- Types:
  - Standard: Isotonic, 1 kcal/mL, lactose-free, protein 40 g/1,000 mL, nonprotein calorie:nitrogen ratio 130, mixture of simple and complex carbohydrates, long-chain fatty acids, vitamins and minerals to 100% of recommended daily dose with a minimum of 1,000 calories/d, carb/fat ratio 50%/30%, 1.2–2 g/kg protein per day.
  - Concentrated: 1.2–2.0 kcal/mL.
  - Predigested/elemental: 1–1.5 kcal/mL, protein hydrolyzed to short-chain peptides, more simple carbohydrates, lower amount of fat; useful for thoracic duct leak, digestive defects, and intolerance to standard enteral nutrition.
  - Studied enteral supplements: Omega-3 fatty acids, glutamine, ornithine ketoglutarate, arginine, prebiotics/probiotics, fiber, additional vitamin/mineral supplementation.
- Tube feeding selection in consultation with registered dietician and indirect calorimetry when able.
- No clinical difference between continuous or enteral feeding, although one or the other may be more tolerated by patients.
- Goal rate 10–30 mL/h incrementally increased to goal, feeding stopped for gastrointestinal intolerance based on physical examination (e.g., nausea, vomiting, gastric distension) or residuals > 500 mL, feeds provide 70–80% of daily water.
- Complications: Aspiration, diarrhea (15–18%), hyperglycemia, nutrient deficiencies, refeeding syndrome, placement of feeding tube, gastrointestinal reflux.
- Aspiration risk reduced but not eliminated by siting patients upright, postpyloric feeding, and placement of PEG tube.
- Bowel motility agents (e.g., metoclopramide, erythromycin) not shown to reduce mortality or risk of pneumonia.

2.6.3 Parenteral Nutrition

- Types (▶ Fig. 2.7):
  - Total parenteral (TPN)/central: Administered via CVC, high osmotic load.
  - Peripheral parenteral (PPN): Lower osmotic load (< 900 mOsm), larger volume.
- Composed of: Dextrose stock solution (40–70%), amino acids and electrolytes, lipid emulsion infused separately or added to mixture, vitamins and trace elements, mineral supplementation, glutamine.
- Weaned when patient able to receive > 60% of needs enterally.
- Complications: Blood stream infections, hyperglycemia, electrolyte disturbance, refeeding disturbance, hepatic dysfunction, Wernicke encephalopathy.

2.7 Fluids, Electrolytes, and Acid-Base Abnormalities

Michael Karsy

2.7.1 Fluids

- Fluid imbalance can increase mortality, reduce organ function, and increase intensive care unit (ICU) length of stay.[46,47,48]

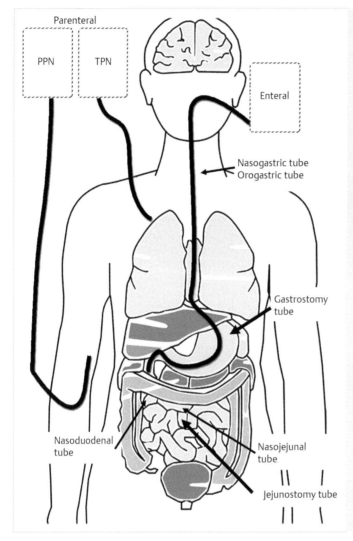

Fig. 2.7 Overview of enteral and parenteral nutrition.

- Body fluid approximated distributions:
  - Total body water (TBW) = intracellular fluid (2/3 TBW) + extracellular fluid (1/3 TBW).
  - Extracellular fluid = plasma (1/5 extracellular fluid) + interstitial fluid (4/5 extracellular fluid) + transcellular fluid/third spacing (~2.5%).
  - Third spaced fluid can be found inside gastrointestinal, cerebrospinal, peritoneal, ocular, and pleural spaces among others.
  - TBW can be approximated as 0.6 × ideal body weight.
- Fluid status remains difficult to assess, each method has strengths and weaknesses.
  - Noninvasive measurements: Clinical exam, chest radiograph, echocardiogram, bioimpedance, vena cava diameter, passive leg raising.
    - Clinical exam: MAP, heart rate, orthostatic changes, mentation, capillary refill, skin turgor, skin perfusion, temperature, urinary output, fractional excretion of sodium or urea, serum lactate, mixed venous oxygen saturation.
  - Invasive measurements: CVP, PCWP, esophageal Doppler, arterial waveform analysis.

- Maintenance fluids account for insensible fluid loss but vary depending on patient status.
- Maintenance fluids calculations typically use 4–2–1 rule: add 4 mL/kg/h (for first 0–10 kg) + 2 mL/kg/h (10–20 kg) + 1 mL/kg/h (> 20 kg).
- Postoperative hormone responses affecting TBW include: vasopressin/antidiuretic hormone (results in water retention), aldosterone (increases sodium and water retention), cortisol (promotes hyperglycemia), catecholamines (increased cardiac output, hypertension, and hyperglycemia), inflammatory cytokines/IL-1/IL-6.
- Fluids types:
  - 0.9% saline: 154 mEq/L Na, approximates serum osmolarity, reverses contraction alkalosis, used with blood products and head injury, large volumes can cause hyperchloremic acidosis and renal vasoconstriction.
  - Lactated Ringers: 130 mEq/L, avoided in hyperkalemia and poor renal function.
  - Plasma-Lyte: 140 mEq/L, avoided in hyperkalemia and poor renal function.
  - Bicarbonate added when lost (e.g., pancreatic fluid, pancreatic transplant).
  - 3%/hypertonic saline: Used resuscitation of trauma patients with temporary abdomen closure devices to reduce volume overload, used in head trauma for reducing ICP.
  - 0.5% dextrose/0.45% saline: Isotonic solution used to stimulate basal insulin secretion and prevent muscle breakdown in patients without shock, effects last for 5 days.
  - Colloids (e.g., albumin): Maintains oncotic pressure by remaining in plasma longer but effects last a few hours, no evidence to improve outcome over crystalloids.
  - Blood products: 1:1:1 ratio for plasma:platelets:red blood cells recommended for resuscitation.

2.7.2 Electrolytes

- Varied diagnosis (▶ Fig. 2.8, ▶ Fig. 2.9, ▶ Fig. 2.10, and ▶ Fig. 2.11) and correction (▶ Table 2.14).[49,50]

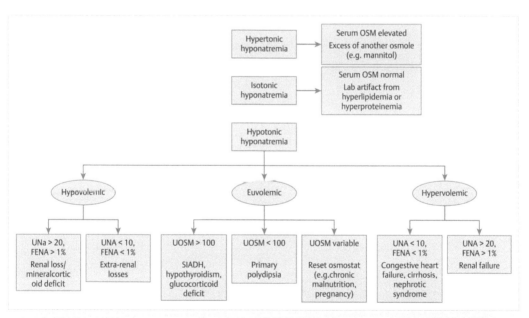

Fig. 2.8 Algorithm for hyponatremia management. UNA, urinary sodium excretion; FENA, fractional excretion of sodium = (serum creatinine × urinary sodium)/(serum sodium × urinary creatinine) × 100; UOSM, urinary osmole excretion.

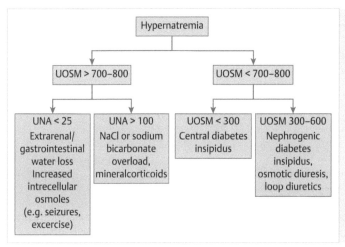

Fig. 2.9 Algorithm for hypernatremia management. UNA, urinary sodium excretion; UOSM, urinary osmole excretion.

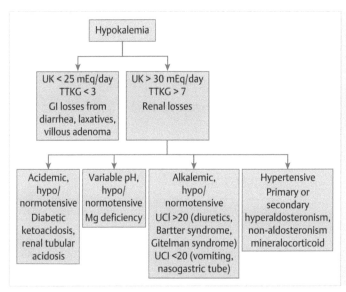

Fig. 2.10 Algorithm for hypokalemia management. TTKG, transtubular potassium gradient = (urinary potassium/plasma potassium)/(urinary osmoles/plasma osmoles); UCl, urinary calcium excretion; UK, urinary potassium excretion.

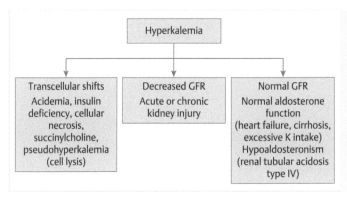

Fig. 2.11 Algorithm for hyperkalemia management.

Table 2.14 Summary of electrolyte changes and treatments

Electrolyte	Treatment	Notes
Hyponatremia (Na < 135 mEq/L)	• Salt tablets (1–3 g TID) • Free water restriction (1–2 L/d) • Fludrocortisone 0.2 mg q12 • 3% saline (0.5–1 mL/kg bolus or 30–50 mL/h) • Conivaptan (20 mg load IV then 20 mg IV/24 h)	• Free water excess = $[140 - Na_{serum}]/140 \times TBW$ • Free water deficit = $[Na_{serum} - 140]/140 \times TBW$ • Sodium correction 0.5 mEq/L/h and < 10 mEq total in 24-h period
Hypernatremia (Na > 145 mEq/L)	• Free water (e.g., orally or with NGT feeds) • Hypotonic IV fluids (e.g., LR, 0.5% NS)	
Hypokalemia (K < 3.5 mEq/L)	• KCl (20–80 mEq IV at 10 mEq/h with Mg replacement)	• Peaked T-waves and widened QRS in hyperkalemia; increased ectopy, increased P-wave amplitude and width, T-wave flattening, U-wave, long QT interval in hypokalemia • Priority to stabilize cardiac conduction in hyperkalemia • Preferred treatment with calcium gluconate and insulin
Hyperkalemia (K > 5.5 mEq/L)	• Calcium gluconate (1–2 g IV) • Calcium chloride (1–2 g IV) • Insulin (10–20 U in 500 mL 10% dextrose) • Bicarbonate (150 mEq in 1 L 5% dextrose) • Beta-2 agonists/albuterol (10–20 mg nebulized) • Kayexalate • Diuretics (Lasix 40 mg q12h) • Hemodialysis	
Hypomagnesemia Hypermagnesemia	• Magnesium sulfate (1–2 g IV q2h)	• Can be cause of refractory hypokalemia or hypocalcemia • Treatment for torsades de pointes
Hypophosphatemia Hyperphosphatemia	• NeutraPhos (1 packet q4–8h) • Potassium phosphate (15–30 mmol IV)	• Levels regulated by parathyroid hormone and vitamin D • Hypophosphatemia seen with decreased absorption, increased excretion, or movement into cells • Levels important in hypophosphatemia to avoid refeeding syndrome in acutely ill patients
Hypocalcemia Hypercalcemia	• Calcium gluconate (1–2 g IV) • Calcium chloride (1–2 g IV)	• Levels regulated by parathyroid hormone and vitamin D • Concurrent hypomagnesemia seen in hypercalcemia can be seen and requires correction • Shortened QT, Osborn or J wave with hypercalcemia; Chvostek/Trousseau sign with prolonged QT in hypocalcemia

Abbreviations: LR, lactated ringers; NS, normal saline; TBW, total body water.

2.7.3 Acid/Base Evaluation

• Identify primary disorder (▶ Table 2.15) then determine if degree of compensation is appropriate (▶ Table 2.16, ▶ Fig. 2.12, ▶ Fig. 2.13, and ▶ Fig. 2.14).
• Metabolic acidosis:
  ○ Identify anion gap: AG = Na − (Cl − HCO₃); identifies unmeasured anions (increased AG) or cations (decreased AG).

Table 2.15 Diagnosis acid/base abnormalities

Disorder	pH	HCO₃	PaCO₂
Normal	7.4	24 mEq/L	40 mm Hg
Metabolic acidosis	↓	↓	↓
Metabolic alkalosis	↑	↑	↑
Respiratory acidosis	↓	↑	↓
Respiratory alkalosis	↑	↓	↑

Table 2.16 Compensation for acid/base abnormalities

	Acidosis	Alkalosis
Metabolic	$1.25 \times \Delta HCO_3$	$0.75 \times \Delta HCO_3$
Respiratory	$0.4 \times \Delta PaCO_2$ (chronic)	$0.4 \times \Delta PaCO_2$ (chronic)
	$0.1 \times \Delta PaCO_2$ (acute)	$0.2 \times \Delta PaCO_2$ (acute)

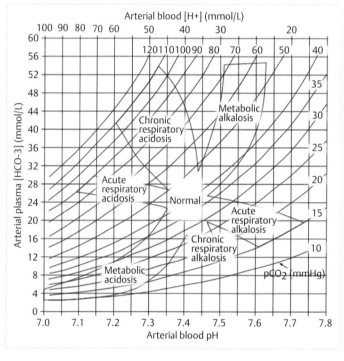

Fig. 2.12 Evaluation of acid/base disorders. Source: Huckfinne (Public domain).

- Delta-delta gap: $\Delta\Delta = \Delta AG/\Delta HCO_3 =$ (calculated AG – expected AG)/(24-HCO₃), $\Delta\Delta$ 1–2 suggests pure AG metabolic acidosis, $\Delta\Delta < 1$ suggests AG metabolic acidosis and non-AG acidosis, $\Delta\Delta > 2$ suggests AG metabolic acidosis and metabolic alkalosis.
- Correction of diabetic ketoacidosis (DKA) with insulin, intravenous fluids, dextrose, and electrolyte repletion.
- Correction of lactic acid with improving tissue perfusion.
- Correction of renal failure with hemodialysis.
- Correction of ingestions with antidotes if available or hemodialysis.

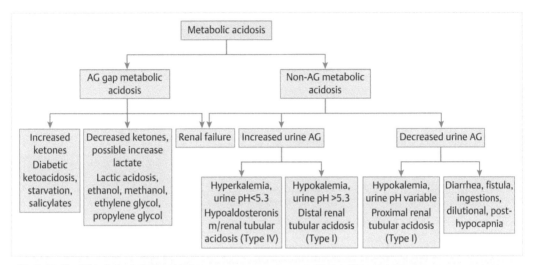

Fig. 2.13 Algorithm for metabolic acidosis.

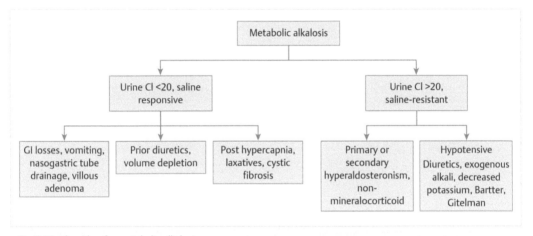

Fig. 2.14 Algorithm for metabolic alkalosis.

- Metabolic alkalosis:
  - Saline-responsive types treated with volume-deficit correction using isotonic saline.
  - Patients with cardiopulmonary disease treated with KCl, acetazolamide, or HCl.
  - Removal of proton-pump inhibitors can improve treatment when nasogastric tubes cannot be removed.
- Respiratory acidosis:
  - CNS depression, neuromuscular disorders, upper or lower airway abnormalities all treated with improving ventilation and possible intubation.
  - Bicarbonate can be used in select patients with limited ability to increase minute ventilation.
- Respiratory alkalosis:
  - Hypoxia induced (e.g., pulmonary embolism, pneumonia) or other primary (e.g., CNS disorders, pain, salicylates, sepsis, pregnancy) hyperventilation treated with improving underlying disease.

2.8 Hematology and Coagulation

Michael Karsy

2.8.1 Hematology

- Anemia[51]:
  - Decrease in red blood cells. Diagnosis includes history, CBC, reticulocyte index, peripheral smears, and bone marrow aspirates (▶ Fig. 2.15).
  - Microcytic anemia:
    - Iron deficiency anemia: ↓iron, ↑total iron-binding capacity (TIBC), ↓ferritin.
    - Thalassemia: Decreased synthesis of alpha or beta hemoglobin chains.
    - Anemia of chronic inflammation: ↓iron, ↓TIBC, ↑ferritin.
    - Sideroblastic anemia: ↑iron, normal TIBC, ↑ferritin.
    - Aplastic anemia: Pancytopenia from hematopoietic stem cell disruption (e.g., toxicity, viruses, immunological, congenital).
    - Hemolytic anemia: Hereditary (e.g., Glucose-6-phosphate dehydrogenase (G6PD) deficiency, sickle cell anemia, thalassemia, hereditary spherocytosis, paroxysmal nocturnal hemoglobinuria) or acquired (autoimmune, drug induced, microangiopathic hemolytic anemia, prosthetic valves, malaria, hypersplenism).
- Leukocytes:
  - Neutrophilia: Seen in bacterial infections, inflammatory states, drugs, stress conditions, marrow stimulation, asplenia, paraneoplastic syndromes, and leukemoid reaction.
  - Lymphocytosis: Seen in viral infections, drug hypersensitivity, stress conditions, autoimmune reactions, and neoplasms (e.g., acute lymphocytic leukemia [ALL], chronic lymphocytic leukemia [CLL], lymphoma).
  - Monocytosis: Seen in tuberculosis, bacterial, or parasite infections, inflammatory conditions, and neoplasms (e.g., Hodgkin disease, leukemia).
  - Eosinophilia: Seen in parasitic infections, allergies, collagen vascular diseases, endocrine issues, neoplasms, cholesterol emboli syndrome, and hypereosinophilic syndrome.
  - Basophilia: Seen in neoplasms, alterations in bone marrow, or inflammatory conditions.

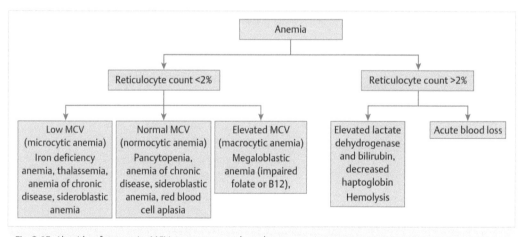

Fig. 2.15 Algorithm for anemia. MCV, mean corpuscular volume.

2.8.2 Platelets and Clotting Factors

Coagulation

- Coagulation regulated by platelets and coagulation factors (▶ Fig. 2.16).[52]
- Pharmacological anticoagulation and coagulation discussed in Chapter 16.
- Platelet cascade:
  - Damage to endothelium exposes underlying collagen to platelet glycoprotein Ia/IIa surface receptors.
  - von Willebrand factor (vWF) released from endothelium and platelets forms links between glycoproteins and collagen fibrils.
  - Glycoprotein VI activates platelet integrins and induces release of stored granules containing ADP, serotonin, platelet-activating factor, vWF, platelet factor 4, and thromboxane A2, which activate further platelets in a G-protein mediated manner.
  - Platelets change shape and promote fibrinogen cross-linking with glycoprotein IIb/IIIa.
- Thrombocytopenia:
  - Bleeding risk with platelet count ($\times 10^3/\mu L$):
    - \> 100,000: No risk of hemorrhage.
    - 50–100,000: Risk with major trauma, general surgery acceptable.
    - 20–50,000: Risk with minor trauma or surgery.
    - < 20,000: Risk of spontaneous bleeding.
    - < 10,000: Risk of life-threatening bleeding.
  - Aplastic anemia: Pancytopenia due to decreased bone marrow production.
  - Idiopathic thrombocytopenia: Immune mediated, platelet count < 50,000/μL, treated with steroids, intravenous immunoglobulin (IVIG), splenectomy and immune-suppressant medications.
  - Infection-mediated thrombocytopenia: Various sources (e.g., human immunodeficiency virus (HIV), herpes, viruses, viral hepatitis).
  - Autoimmune-mediated thrombocytopenia: Seen in collagen vascular diseases, antiphospholipid syndrome, lymphoproliferative disorders.
  - Drug-related thrombocytopenia: Heparin or other types.
  - Heparin-induced thrombocytopenia (HIT): Antibody-mediated thrombocytopenia, increased risk of thrombosis, screened with PF4-heparin enzyme-linked immunosorbent assay (ELISA) and confirmed with serotonin-release assay; treated with discontinuation of heparin and use of nonheparin anticoagulation (e.g., fondaparinux, argatroban); risk of HIT can be predicted with the 4Ts score evaluating the level and timing of thrombocytopenia.
  - Hemolytic uremic syndrome (HUS): Triad of thrombocytopenia, anemia, and renal failure; mediated by autoimmune causes (e.g., Shiga toxin).

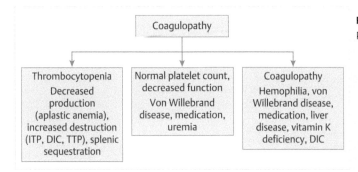

Fig. 2.16 Algorithm for thrombocytopenia and coagulopathy.

- ○ Thrombotic thrombocytopenic purpura (TTP): Pentad of HUS, mental status changes, and fever; mediated by decreased ADAMTS13 protease activity from drug, and autoimmune or idiopathic causes.
  - ○ Uremic platelets: Decreased aggregation, treated with desmopressin, cryoprecipitate, and correction of anemia.
- Coagulation cascade:
  - ○ Contact activation/intrinsic pathway and tissue factor/extrinsic pathways that merge at the final common pathway (▶ Fig. 2.17); primary pathway in blood is the extrinsic pathway but separation between the two pathways is artificial and based on lab testing; factors are activated in sequence.
  - ○ Damage to endothelium causes factor VII to leave circulation and contact tissue factor expressed on fibroblasts and leukocytes.
  - ○ Factor activation proceeds until factor Va forms prothrombinase complex, activating prothrombin to thrombin.
  - ○ Thrombin activates factors V, VIII, and XIII; thrombin releases VIII from vWF; thrombin converts fibrinogen to fibrin.
  - ○ Fibrin is cross-linked by factor XIIIa.
- Coagulopathy:
  - ○ Hemophilia: Deficiency of factor VIII (hemophilia A) or factor IX (hemophilia B) most common; diagnosed with elevated PTT that normalizes with mixing studies; treated with repletion of coagulation factor using recombinant factors, cryoprecipitate (hemophilia A only), desmopressin (mild disease), and/or aminocaproic acid.
  - ○ Coagulation factor–inhibiting drugs (e.g., vitamin K antagonists) and liver failure can cause acquired coagulopathy.
  - ○ Von Willebrand disease: Disruption of plasma carrier for factor VIII; results in ↑ PT, ↓ PTT, and ↓ fibrinogen; three types with varying levels of severity, treated with fresh frozen plasma, cryoprecipitate, platelets, desmopressin.

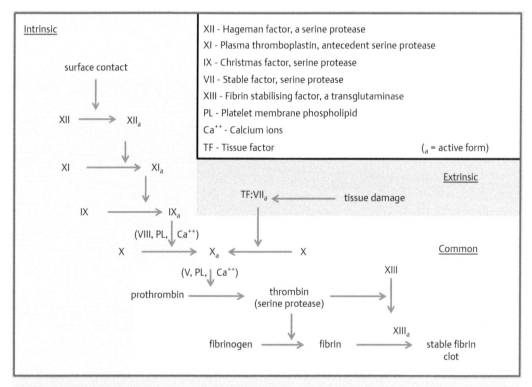

Fig. 2.17 Coagulation cascade. Source: Dr Graham Beards (CC BY-SA 3.0 [https://creativecommons.org/licenses/by-sa/3.0]).

- ○ Vitamin K deficiency: Decreased coagulation production from malnutrition, decreased vitamin K absorption, or liver disease.
- Hypercoagulopathy:
  - ○ Spontaneous/primary and acquired/secondary types (▶ Table 2.17); requires expertise for testing and interpretation.[53]
  - ○ Nongenetic acquired types can be due to malignancy, venous stasis, hormonal causes (e.g., oral contraceptives), or nephrotic syndrome.
- Prophylactic anticoagulation:
  - ○ "Antithrombotic Therapy and Prevention of Thrombosis, 9th ed: American College of Chest Physicians Evidence-Based Clinical Practice Guidelines" has summarized the available literature well.[54,55]
  - ○ Grade 1B recommendations for no pharmacological prophylaxis in patients with < 0.5% of venous thromboembolism.
  - ○ Grade 2B recommendation for unfractionated heparin or low-molecular-weight heparin for preventative treatment of deep vein thrombosis in surgical patients.
  - ○ Anticoagulation used in combination with pneumatic compression stockings, early ambulation, and inferior vena cava filters when indicated.
  - ○ Unclear guidelines on timing of anticoagulation due to variation in surgical patients and practice patterns.
  - ○ Various modalities of screening for deep vein thrombosis via venous duplex ultrasound of the leg and D-dimer have been described.

Table 2.17 Acquired hypercoagulability diseases

Type	Prevalence	Testing[a]	Relative risk of venous thrombosis[b]
Antiphospholipid syndrome	3–5%, spontaneous or acquired	Antiphospholipid antibodies (e.g., cardiolipin, beta-2 glycoprotein 1) or lupus anticoagulant	9
Activated protein C resistance/Factor V Leiden	3–7%, spontaneous or acquired	Activated protein C resistance testing or genotyping	4–8 (heterozygote) 24–80 (homozygote)
Prothrombin G202010A mutation	2–4%	PCR testing	3
Protein C deficiency	0.14–0.5%	Autosomal-dominant, clot-based, chromogenic-based, and antigenic protein C assay	3.1–3.4
Protein S deficiency	0.01–1%	Clot-based and immunological-based assays	2
Antithrombin III deficiency	0.05–0.1%, highest VTE risk	Autosomal-dominant, chromogenic and immunoassays, confirmed by quantitative methods	5
Hyperhomocysteinemia	5–10%	Methylenetetrahydrofolate reductase genetic testing, evaluation of nutritional status (vitamin B6, B12, folate) or other medical conditions and drugs	1.5–2.5
Elevated factor VIII	20–25% in patients with VTE	Activated PTT-based clotting or chromogenic assay, quantified by ELISA	2.6–4.8
Fibrinogen defects/dysfibrinogenemia	0.8% of patients with VTE	Clauss method functional assay	

Abbreviations: VTE, venous thromboembolism; PTT, partial thromboplastin time; ELISA, enzyme-linked immunosorbent assay.

[a] Testing can be impacted by other concurrent medical conditions and drugs.

[b] Relative risks of venous thrombosis for comparison to genetic predisposition: hospitalization (9–11), pregnancy (4.2), postpartum (14), surgery (6), oral contraceptives/hormone replacement (2–4), malignancy (7).

- Therapeutic anticoagulation:
  - "Antithrombotic Therapy for VTE Disease: CHEST Guideline and Expert Panel Report" has summarized the available literature.[56]
  - Therapeutic anticoagulation used for patients with deep vein thrombosis above the knee (e.g., large veins) or pulmonary embolism as these can be life-threatening.
  - Grade IB recommendation for 3-month anticoagulation therapy.
  - Grade 2B recommendation for dabigatran, rivaroxaban, apixaban, or edoxaban over vitamin K antagonists.
  - Grade 2C recommendations for vitamin K antagonists over low-molecular-weight heparin.
  - Grade 2C recommendations for low-molecular-weight heparin over vitamin K antagonists, dabigatran, rivaroxaban, apixaban, or edoxaban for VTE and cancer.

2.8.3 Transfusion

- Guidelines and cutoffs for transfusion have evolved rapidly based on newer studies.[57,58]
- Transfusion of blood products used judiciously and for specific end goals, typically hemoglobin/hematocrit transfused if lower than 7.0/22.0 while platelet and coagulation factor transfusion titrated to specific patient goals of care (▶ Table 2.18).
- Thromboelastogram (TEG):
  - Viscoelastic test that involves monitoring clotting of blood via mechanical testing by using a sensitive needle to monitor for physical clot formation; indirectly can be used to interpret the status of platelets, coagulation factors, and drugs influencing coagulation.
  - Two commercial types: TEG and rotational thromboelastogram (ROTEM).
  - Can be a useful method to identify coagulation disorders and target resuscitation efforts (▶ Fig. 2.18).
  - Used in trauma surgery, cardiothoracic surgery, organ transplantation, and spine surgery.
- Transfusion reactions:
  - Acute hemolytic: Fever, hypotension, flank pain, and renal failure; occurs within 24 hours of transfusion; due to ABO incompatibility; treated with support.
  - Delayed hemolytic: Occurs in 5–7 days due to antibodies against minor antigens; no treatment required.
  - Febrile nonhemolytic: Fevers within 0–6 hours; common in 1:100 patients; due to antibodies against donor WBCs and cytokine release; treated with acetaminophen; rule out blood-borne infection which is extremely rare; rule out hemoglobinemia or hemoglobinuria.
  - Allergic: Urticarial or anaphylaxis, rare, can be seen in IgA-deficiency patients, treated with support.

Table 2.18 Blood products for transfusion

Product	Notes
PRBCs	Transfusion if Hb < 7 g/dL or Hb < 9 g/dL in coronary ischemia, 1 U PRBC increases Hb by 1 g/dL, large volume transfusion will require 1:1:1 RBC:platelets:FFP
Platelets	Transfused per specific patient goal, typically > 50,000 acceptable if patient is not bleeding, 1 U increases platelet count by 30–60,000, contraindicated in TTP/HUS, HELLP, HIT
FFP	Enriched in all coagulation factors, used in reversing vitamin K antagonists but requires multiple units in conjunction with vitamin K
Cryoprecipitate	Enriched in fibrinogen, vWF, factor VIII, and factor XIII
Irradiated products	Prevents donor T-cell proliferation, used if risk of transfusion associated graft vs. host disease
Leukoreduced products	Reduced WBC concentration in patients with history of febrile nonhemolytic transfusion reaction

Abbreviations: FFP, fresh frozen plasma; Hb, hemoglobin; HELLP, hemolysis, elevated liver enzymes, low platelet count syndrome; HIT, heparin-induced thrombocytopenia; HUS, hemolytic uremic syndrome; PRBC, packed red blood cell; RBC, red blood cell; TTP, thrombotic thrombocytopenic purpura; vWF, von Willebrand factor; WBC, white blood cells.

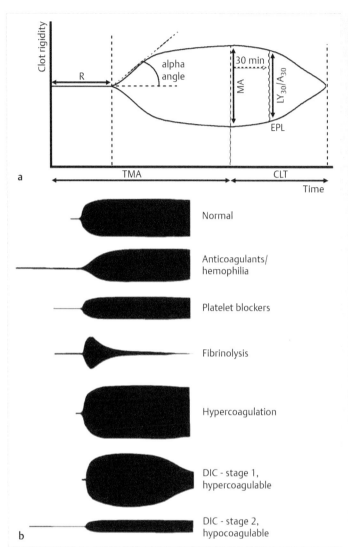

Fig. 2.18 Thromboelastography and diagnosis of coagulation disorders.
(a) Representative image of a thromboelastography tracing is shown. A_{30} or LY_{30}: amplitude at 30 minutes, measure of fibrinolysis; alpha angle: slope between reaction R and time indicating the speed of fibrin formation; CLT: clot lysis time; EPL: estimated percentage lysis, rate of clot fibrinolysis; MA: maximum amplitude, overall strength of fibrin clot; R-value: reaction time, time from test start to fibrin formation (e.g., amplitude of 2 mm); TMA: time to maximum amplitude. **(b)** Various examples of abnormal coagulation tracings. Increased R time (e.g., wine glass) suggests clotting factor dysfunction and should be treated with fresh frozen plasma. Decreased alpha angle (e.g., champagne flute) suggests fibrinogen deficiency and should be treated with cryoprecipitate. Decreased MA (e.g., test tube) suggests clot weakness as a function of fibrin and platelets, which should be treated with platelets. Elevated EPL (e.g., upside down martini glass) suggests increased fibrinolysis and should be treated with tranexamic acid, aprotinin, or aminocaproic acid.

- Transfusion-related acute lung injury (TRALI): noncardiogenic pulmonary edema (e.g., ARDS); due to donor antibodies against recipient WBCs; treated with support.
- Graft-versus-host disease: donor leukocyte attacking recipient tissue; treated with support and leukocyte-depleted blood products.

2.9 Acute Kidney Injury

Michael Karsy

- Introduction[59]:
  - AKI can be defined by 2012 Kidney Disease: Improving Global Outcomes (KDIGO) Clinical Practice Guideline for Acute Kidney Injury; one or more criteria:
    - Rise in serum Cr of 0.3 mg/dL over 48-hour period.

- – ≥ 1.5 × baseline value of Cr within previous 7 days.
- – ≤ 0.5 mL/kg urine output for 6 hours.
- • Epidemiology:
  - ○ AKI seen in 9% of hospitalized patients and 50% of ICU patients.
- • Etiology:
  - ○ Can be a common problem in postoperative patients.
  - ○ Most common inpatient causes: Acute tubular necrosis (ATN; 45%), prerenal disease (21%), acute on chronic renal failure (13%), urinary tract obstruction (10%), glomerulonephritis/vasculitis (4%), acute interstitial nephritis (2%), atheroemboli (1%).
  - ○ Prerenal:
    - – Renal ischemia from decreased tissue perfusion.
    - – Occurs form systemic hypoperfusion, focal renal ischemia, or drugs decreasing glomerular function (e.g., nonsteroidal anti-inflammatory drugs, angiotensin-converting enzyme inhibitors, angiotensin II receptor blockers).
    - – Commonly form volume depletion or poor intravascular volume (e.g., heart failure, cirrhosis, nephrotic syndrome).
  - ○ ATN:
    - – Necrosis of kidneys with epithelial destruction and tubular occlusion by casts and cell debris.
    - – Can occur by prerenal disease, renal ischemia, sepsis, or nephrotoxins (e.g., vancomycin, aminoglycosides, heme, cisplatin, radiocontrast, certain antiviral medications, IV immunoglobulins, mannitol, hetastarch, synthetic cannabinoids) damage.
- • Diagnosis:
  - ○ History and physical can help identify potential source; evaluate for poor intravascular volume, heart failure, cirrhosis, abdominal compartment syndrome; evaluation of antecedent causes (e.g., hypotension, drug exposure).
  - ○ Urinalysis used to evaluate for casts and superimposed infection, normal urinalysis does not rule out ATN.
  - ○ Fractional excretion of sodium (FENa = [UNa × SCr]/[SNa × UCr]) can be high in ATN due to tubular dysfunction and low in patients with prerenal disease; low FENa can be seen in ATN with renal ischemia, glomerulonephritis, vasculitis, and contrast-induced nephropathy.
  - ○ Response to fluid in depleted patients can narrow diagnosis to prerenal disease.
  - ○ Other ancillary tests include BUN/serum Cr ratio (10–15:1 in ATN, > 20:1 in prerenal disease), rate of serum Cr rise (rises > 0.3–0.5 mg/dL per day in ATN), urine electrolytes and osmolality (UOsm < 450 mOsm/kg in ATN).
  - ○ Urinary obstruction evaluated by bladder ultrasound.
  - ○ Renal ultrasound used for evaluating unknown causes of AKI.
  - ○ Renal biopsy used after normal renal imaging, minimal proteinuria, benign urinalysis evaluation, and unknown cause of AKI.
- • Management:
  - ○ Staging by RIFLE (risk, injury, failure, loss, ESDR), Acute Kidney Injury Network (AKIN), or KDIGO criteria performed (► Table 2.19); previously multiple classification systems for AKI were utilized.

Table 2.19 Staging of acute kidney injury

RIFLE staging criteria	Equivalence to AKIN/KDIGO	Definition
Risk	Stage 1	Increase serum creatinine 50–99% *or* urine output < 0.5 mL/kg/h for 6–12 h
Injury	Stage 2	Increase serum creatinine 100–199% *or* urine output < 0.5 mL/kg/h for 12–24 h
Failure	Stage 3	Increase serum creatinine ≥ 200% increase serum creatinine by 0.5–4 mg/dL *or* urine output < 0.3 mL/kg/h for 24 h *or* no urine output for > 12 h *or* initiation of renal replacement therapy
Loss		Need for renal replacement for > 4 wk
End stage		Need for renal replacement for > 3 mo

○ Treatment involves elimination of nephrotoxic medications, review of medication dosing for glomerular filtration rate, correction of hypovolemia with 1–3 L of crystalloid when indicated.

○ Loop diuretics can be used to treat some patients with hypervolemia and AKI who produce urine; diuretics should be used with caution in patients with prerenal causes of AKI or poor perfusion.

○ Urgent nephrology referral recommended after initial treatments fail to improve kidney injury, glomerulonephritis suspected (e.g., AKI, hematuria, proteinuria), or future nephrology follow-up may be needed.

○ Emergency evaluation:
  – Patients with stage 1 AKI with unclear etiology, duration, or worsening trajectory.
  – Patients with stage 2 or 3 AKI recommended for emergency evaluation.
  – Patients requiring evaluation of obstruction or other intervention.

○ Renal replacement therapy indications: Pulmonary edema, hyperkalemia with or without signs/symptoms (e.g., cardiac conduction abnormalities, rhabdomyolysis), uremia, metabolic acidosis (pH < 7.1) with hypervolemia, or poisoning.

2.10 Infections in the Surgical ICU

Adrienne Carey and Emily Spivak

Antibiotic recommendations made in this chapter are based on local epidemiology and antimicrobial susceptibility patterns at the University of Utah Health. Please consult your institution's local antibiogram and antimicrobial formulary before making any decisions based on recommendations presented here.

2.10.1 Nosocomial Fever and Leukocytosis

• Fever[60]:
  ○ Detected in approximately 50% of patients admitted to adult intensive care units (ICUs).
  ○ Based on a recent literature review, the algorithm in ▸ Fig. 2.19 details the causes of fever in immunocompetent patients in the ICU.[61]
  ○ Relative lack of data regarding the approach to the febrile ICU patient.
  ○ Poor association between fever and the likelihood of a positive culture.
  ○ Presence of shaking chills and rigors is predictive of bacteremia, whereas the absence of SIRS is the strongest predictor of negative blood cultures.
  ○ Thoughtful review of the most likely causes, paired with history and physical examination should be performed before ordering cultures, imaging, and broad-spectrum antibiotics.

• Tips for evaluating a hospitalized patient with fever:
  ○ Obtain a history if the patient is able to communicate to direct the workup for fever.
  ○ Perform a comprehensive physical exam including skin examination, specifically paying attention to all peripheral intravenous line (PIV) and CVC insertion sites.
  ○ When obtaining blood cultures, obtain two sets of cultures drawn peripherally:
    – The role of two blood culture sets is to increase the sensitivity of detecting bacteremia as well as paired cultures to rule out contamination with growth of a common contaminant in one set.
    – 1 set = 1 needle stick = 1 aerobic bottle and 1 anaerobic bottle.
  ○ Restrict urine cultures to patients with symptoms of urinary tract infection (UTI), and those with indwelling urinary catheters with no other obvious source of fever. Utility of urinalysis/microscopy for UTI diagnosis is to rule out UTI based on absence of pyuria (< 10 WBC/high-power field [hpf] or negative leukocyte esterase). Presence of bacteriuria and pyuria is common in hospitalized patients and not diagnostic of a UTI.

• Leukocytosis:
  ○ Recent retrospective review of hospitalized patients with WBC count ≥ 30 × 10^9/μL showed that infection was the most common cause (47.9%) followed by ischemia/stress (27.7%), inflammation (6.9%), and obstetric diagnoses (6.9%)—about half were due to causes other than infection.[62]
  ○ Higher WBC counts are associated with positive blood cultures or *Clostridioides* (formerly *Clostridium*) *difficile* infection (CDI).

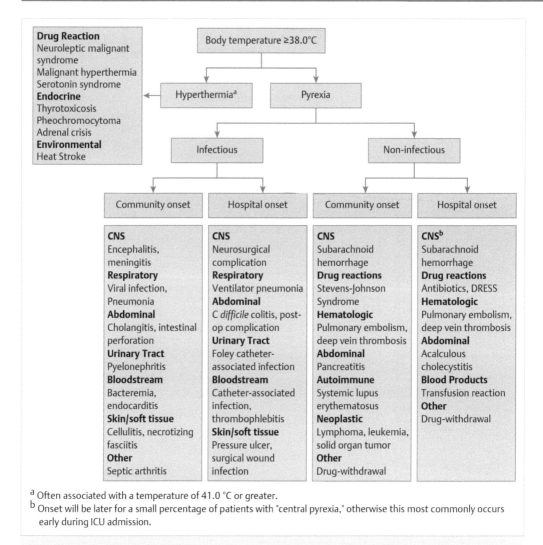

Drug Reaction
Neuroleptic malignant syndrome
Malignant hyperthermia
Serotonin syndrome
Endocrine
Thyrotoxicosis
Pheochromocytoma
Adrenal crisis
Environmental
Heat Stroke

Body temperature ≥38.0°C

Hyperthermia[a] ← Pyrexia

Infectious | Non-infectious

Community onset | Hospital onset | Community onset | Hospital onset

CNS
Encephalitis, meningitis
Respiratory
Viral infection, Pneumonia
Abdominal
Cholangitis, intestinal perforation
Urinary Tract
Pyelonephritis
Bloodstream
Bacteremia, endocarditis
Skin/soft tissue
Cellulitis, necrotizing fasciitis
Other
Septic arthritis

CNS
Neurosurgical complication
Respiratory
Ventilator pneumonia
Abdominal
C difficile colitis, post-op complication
Urinary Tract
Foley catheter-associated infection
Bloodstream
Catheter-associated infection, thrombophlebitis
Skin/soft tissue
Pressure ulcer, surgical wound infection

CNS
Subarachnoid hemorrhage
Drug reactions
Stevens-Johnson Syndrome
Hematologic
Pulmonary embolism, deep vein thrombosis
Abdominal
Pancreatitis
Autoimmune
Systemic lupus erythematosus
Neoplastic
Lymphoma, leukemia, solid organ tumor
Other
Drug-withdrawal

CNS[b]
Subarachnoid hemorrhage
Drug reactions
Antibiotics, DRESS
Hematologic
Pulmonary embolism, deep vein thrombosis
Abdominal
Acalculous cholecystitis
Blood Products
Transfusion reaction
Other
Drug-withdrawal

[a] Often associated with a temperature of 41.0 °C or greater.
[b] Onset will be later for a small percentage of patients with "central pyrexia," otherwise this most commonly occurs early during ICU admission.

Fig. 2.19 Flowchart for causes of fever.

○ Medications associated with leukocytosis: Glucocorticoids (up to 2 weeks after administration), granulocyte-macrophage colony-stimulating factor (GM-CSF) such as Neupogen, catecholamines (epinephrine), lithium, and carbamazepine.
• Tips for work-up of leukocytosis in a hospitalized patient:
   ○ See "Tips for evaluating a hospitalized patient with fever" above.
   ○ Review medications.
   ○ Evaluate for diarrhea, if present, with no other alternative explanation (e.g., laxative use, tube feeds) and other signs/symptoms of infection, consider work-up for CDI.

2.10.2 Catheter-Related Blood Stream Infection (CRBSI)

• Epidemiology[63]:
   ○ About 80,000 CVC-related blood stream infections in ICUs per year.
   ○ Most common organisms for percutaneously inserted CVCs: Coagulase-negative staphylococci, *Staphylococcus aureus*, *Candida* species, and enteric gram-negative bacilli.

- Most common organisms for surgically implanted or peripherally inserted CVCs (PICCs): Coagulase-negative staphylococci, enteric gram-negative bacilli, *Staphylococcus aureus*, and *Pseudomonas aeruginosa*.
- Risk factors:
  - Type of catheter and intended use.
  - Insertion site.
  - Experience/education of the individual who places the catheter.
  - Frequency with which the catheter is accessed.
  - Duration of catheter placement.
- Diagnosis:
  - CVC should be examined daily and if there is more than minimal erythema or any purulence at the exit site, the catheter is likely infected and should be removed.
  - Obtain two sets of peripheral blood cultures at minimum, and potentially one additional set of blood cultures from the CVC. Institutional policies vary regarding drawing blood cultures from CVCs.
  - Blood cultures from CVCs are more likely to yield contaminants.
  - If two sets of peripheral blood cultures cannot be collected, at least one peripheral blood culture set should be attempted in addition to a blood culture set from the CVC.
  - Cultures of the catheter tip (upon removal) should only be sent when there are positive blood cultures with no alternative source of bacteremia.
  - Routinely culturing CVC tips is not recommended; must be accompanied by two sets of blood cultures as detailed above.
- Management:
  - Varies depending on if CVC is short-term (in situ < 14 days) versus long term (in situ ≥ 14 days).

2.10.3 Indwelling Catheters

- Short-term catheters (in situ < 14 days; ▶ Fig. 2.20a).
- Long-term catheters (in situ ≥ 14 days; ▶ Fig. 2.20b).
- Preferred empiric therapy depending on pathogen, as identified by rapid blood culture diagnostics (this is dependent on your institution, please consult your institution's antibiogram and/or consult with Infectious Diseases and Antimicrobial Stewardship in addition to using this guide):
  - *Staphylococcus aureus*, −*mecA* gene (methicillin-sensitive *Staphylococcus aureus*, MSSA)—Cefazolin.
  - *Staphylococcus aureus*, +*mecA* gene (methicillin-resistant *Staphylococcus aureus*, MRSA)—Vancomycin.
  - *Enterococcus* species, −*vanA/B* gene (*Enterococcus faecalis*, *Enterococcus faecium*, not VRE)—Ampicillin.
  - *Enterococcus* species, + van A/B (VRE)—Linezolid.
  - Coagulase-negative Staphylococcus (CoNS, *Staphylococcus* species)—no treatment if a suspected contaminant; if suspected to be real, Vancomycin.
  - Group B *Streptococcus* (GBS, *Streptococcus agalactiae*)—Penicillin.
  - Group A *Streptococcus* (GAS, *Streptococcus pyogenes*)—Penicillin.
  - *Streptococcus pneumoniae*—Penicillin
  - *Escherichia coli*—Ceftriaxone; if history of extended-spectrum beta-lactamase (ESBL), Meropenem.
  - *Enterobacter cloacae* complex—Meropenem.
  - *Pseudomonas aeruginosa*—Cefepime.
  - *Klebsiella oxytoca/pneumoniae*—Ceftriaxone; if history of ESBL, Meropenem.
  - *Proteus* species—Ceftriaxone.
  - *Serratia marcescens*—Cefepime.
  - *Acinetobacter baumannii*—Meropenem.

2.10.4 Catheter-Associated Urinary Tract Infection (CA-UTI)

- Background[64]:
  - Definition—Infection occurring in a person whose urinary tract is currently catheterized or has been catheterized within the previous 48 hours.
  - Most effective way to reduce the incidence of CA-UTI is to reduce the use of urinary catheterization by only using in patients who have clear indications and remove the catheter as soon as it is no longer necessary.

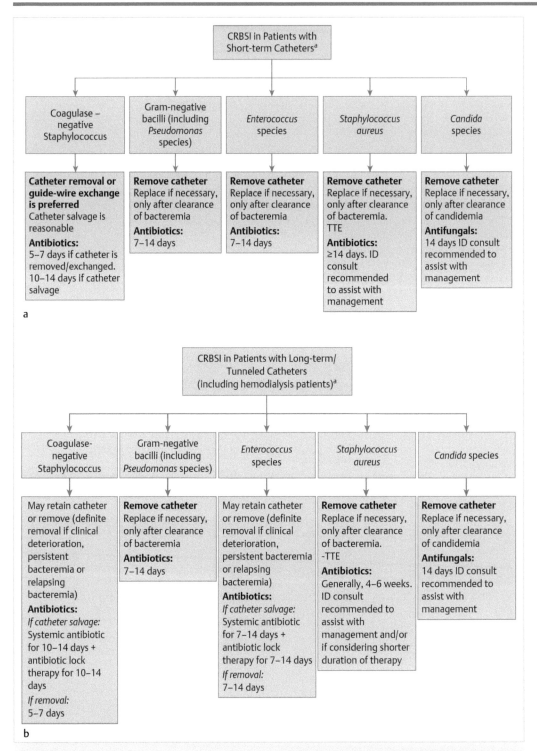

Fig. 2.20 Treatment algorithm for catheter-related blood stream infection (CRBSI) in patients with **(a)** short-term and **(b)** long-term catheters.
[a] Treatment recommendations apply in situations where the infection is uncomplicated—blood steam infection and fever resolve within 72 hours in a patient who has no intravascular hardware and no evidence of endocarditis or suppurative thrombophlebitis.

- Epidemiology:
  - 15–25% of patients have a urinary catheter inserted during their hospitalization.
  - Incidence of bacteriuria with indwelling catheterization is 3–8% per day.
  - *E. coli* is the most frequently isolated organism followed by *Klebsiella, Serratia, Citrobacter, Enterobacter, Pseudomonas aeruginosa,* CoNS, and *Enterococcus* species.
- Diagnosis:
  - Patients with catheters do not manifest symptoms classic for urinary tract infections (dysuria, urinary frequency/urgency), although these symptoms may occur after the catheter has been removed.
  - Symptoms appropriate for obtaining a culture in a patient with an indwelling catheter include the following: Costovertebral angle (CVA) tenderness, flank pain; fever ≥ 38.3 °C, rigors without a clear source; symptoms not localized to the urinary tract and leukocytosis have less predictive value for the diagnosis of CA-UTI.
  - When CA-UTI is suspected, culture specimens should not be obtained from the catheter drainage bag—it is preferable to remove the current catheter, obtain a fresh urine specimen, and then replace the catheter if it has been in place ≥ 2 weeks and cannot be permanently removed.
  - Signs and symptoms help distinguish between cystitis versus pyelonephritis.
  - Cystitis: Dysuria, frequency, urgency, suprapubic pain/tenderness; generally do NOT have fever or leukocytosis.
  - Pyelonephritis: CVA tenderness, flank pain; fever ≥ 38.3 °C, rigors; nausea, vomiting without another explanation; may or may not have cystitis symptoms; leukocytosis, WBC casts on urinalysis.
- Consult local antibiogram and antimicrobial formulary.
- Antibiotics choice depends on if signs and symptoms are consistent with cystitis or pyelonephritis.
- Empiric choice for cystitis (in order of preference):
  - Nitrofurantoin 100 mg PO q12h (do not use if CrCl ≤ 30 mL/min).
  - Trimethoprim-sulfamethoxazole (TMP-SMX) 160/800 mg (DS) 1 tab PO q12h (if no exposure in last 3 months).
  - Cephalexin 500 mg PO q6h *or* cefuroxime 500 mg PO q12h *or* amoxicillin/clavulanate 875/125 mg PO q12h.
  - If intravenous (IV) therapy is necessary, cefazolin 2 g IV q8h.
  - When final culture information returns, select an agent from list above based on susceptibility.
  - Fluoroquinolones should be reserved for when alternatives cannot be used (Levofloxacin 500 mg PO q24h; Ciprofloxacin 500 mg PO q12h).
- Empiric choice for pyelonephritis (in order of preference):
  - Ceftriaxone 1 g IV q24h.
  - Aztreonam 1 g IV q8h (use if life-threatening allergy to penicillins/cephalosporins).
  - Piperacillin-tazobactam 4.5 g IV q6h; history of *Pseudomonas aeruginosa* in the last year *or* ICU admission for UTI + indwelling urinary catheter *or* immunosuppression *or* urologic procedure in the last month.
  - Ertapenem (or inpatient carbapenem formulary equivalent) 1 g IV q24h if ESBL within 1 year.
  - When final culture information returns, select an agent from list below based on susceptibility (in order of preference):
    – TMP-SMX 160/800 mg (DS) 1 tab PO q12h.
    – Amoxicillin 1,000 mg PO q8h *or* amoxicillin/clavulanate 875/125 mg PO q12h.
    – Cefpodoxime 400 mg PO q12h *or* cefuroxime 500 mg PO q12h.
    – Levofloxacin 750 mg PO q24h *or* ciprofloxacin 750 mg PO q12h.
- Notes with regard to antibiotic choice:
  - Aztreonam, amoxicillin/clavulanate, cefazolin, cefpodoxime, cefuroxime, cephalexin, ciprofloxacin, levofloxacin, TMP-SMX all require dose adjustment based on renal function.
- Duration:
  - 7 days: Prompt response (fever and symptom duration 48–72 hours).
  - 10 days: Delayed response (fever and symptom duration > 72 hours).
  - Females: 3–5 days if catheter is removed and no signs of pyelonephritis (flank pain/CVA tenderness).
  - Based on a recent randomized controlled trial, if gram-negative bacteremia is also present as a result of the UTI, treatment is only needed for 7 days.[65]

2.10.5 Hospital-Acquired Pneumonia/Ventilator-Associated Pneumonia

- Definition[66]:
  - Hospital-acquired pneumonia (HAP)—pneumonia occurring ≥ 48 hours after admission to the hospital; pneumonia not associated with mechanical ventilation.
  - Ventilator-associated pneumonia (VAP)—pneumonia occurring ≥ 48 hours after endotracheal intubation.
- Epidemiology:
  - 22% of all hospital-acquired infections are due to HAP/VAP.
  - About 10% of mechanically ventilated patients are diagnosed with VAP.
  - Estimated mortality directly due to VAP is 13%.
- HAP:
  - Diagnosis: Sputum should be sent for respiratory culture to guide antibiotic therapy; growth of *Candida* species from respiratory secretions usually indicates colonization and rarely requires treatment with antifungal therapy.
  - Empiric regimen for HAP should include coverage for *Staphylococcus aureus*, *Pseudomonas aeruginosa*, and other gram-negative bacilli.
  - Antibiotic choice depends on if the patient is at high risk of mortality (requiring ventilatory support for pneumonia, septic shock) and if they have risk factors that increase the likelihood of MRSA (IV antibiotic treatment during the previous 90 days, and treatment in a unit where the prevalence of MRSA among *Staphylococcus aureus* isolates is not known or is > 20%).
  - Not at high risk of mortality and no factors increasing the likelihood of MRSA:
    - Piperacillin-tazobactam 4.5 g IV q6h *or*
    - Cefepime 2 g IV q8h *or*
    - Levofloxacin 750 mg PO/IV q24h.
  - Not at high risk of mortality but with risk factors for MRSA:
    - Piperacillin-tazobactam 4.5 g IV q6h *or*
    - Cefepime 2 g IV q8h *or*
    - Levofloxacin 750 mg PO/IV q24h; Ciprofloxacin 400 mg IV q8h *or*
    - Imipenem 500 mg IV q6h; Meropenem 1 g IV q8h *or*
    - Aztreonam 2 g IV q8h (severe cephalosporin/penicillin allergy) PLUS Vancomycin 15 mg/kg IV q8–12h, consider a loading dose 20 mg/kg IV × 1 dose for severe illness *or* Linezolid 600 mg PO/IV q12h.
  - High risk of mortality or receipt of intravenous antibiotics during the prior 90 days:
    - Piperacillin-tazobactam 4.5 g IV q6h *or*
    - Cefepime 2 g IV q8h *or*
    - Imipenem 500 mg IV q6h; Meropenem 1 g IV q8h *or*
    - Aztreonam 2 g IV q8h (severe cephalosporin/penicillin allergy) *or*
    - Amikacin 15–20 mg/kg IV q24h, Gentamicin 5–7 mg/kg IV q24h, Tobramycin 5–7 mg/kg IV q24h *or* Levofloxacin 750 mg PO/IV q24h; Ciprofloxacin 400 mg IV q8h *or* Choice of an aminoglycoside or a fluoroquinolone should be based on local antibiotic susceptibility pattern PLUS Vancomycin 15 mg/kg IV q8–12h, consider a loading dose 20 mg/kg IV × 1 dose for severe illness *or* Linezolid 600 mg PO/IV q12h.
  - Treatment duration for HAP: 7 days.
  - Lack of growth of *Staphylococcus aureus* and *Pseudomonas aeruginosa* on respiratory cultures rules out these organisms and should be used to guide antibiotic de-escalation.
  - Nasal MRSA PCR (MRSA nares swab) has an excellent negative predictive value (> 95%) for ruling out MRSA pneumonia and should be used to facilitate vancomycin de-escalation.[67]
- VAP:
  - Risk factors for a multidrug-resistant (MDR) pathogen: Prior IV antibiotic use within 90 days; septic shock at the time of VAP; ARDS preceding VAP; five or more days of hospitalization prior to occurrence of VAP; acute renal replacement therapy prior to VAP onset
  - Diagnosis: Clinical findings suggestive of VAP[68] (fever ≥ 38.5 °C; WBC count ≥ 15,000/mm^3; chest imaging with worsening infiltrates; worsening gas exchange), AND noninvasive sampling (endotracheal aspiration) to send respiratory cultures is the preferred method for microbiologic diagnosis (vs. BAL or mini-BAL).

- Growth of *Candida* from respiratory secretions usually indicates colonization and rarely requires treatment with antifungal therapy.
- Empiric antibiotic regimen for VAP should include coverage for *Staphylococcus aureus*, *Pseudomonas aeruginosa*, and other gram-negative bacilli.
- If MRSA is a concern (see above risk factors), vancomycin or linezolid should be used:
  - Vancomycin 15 mg/kg IV q8–12h, consider a loading dose 20 mg/kg IV × 1 dose for severe illness.
  - Linezolid 600 mg PO/IV q12h.
- If MRSA is not a concern, the following are appropriate choices given the clinical scenario:
  - Piperacillin-tazobactam 4.5 g IV q6h *or*
  - Cefepime 2 g IV q8h *or*
  - Imipenem 500 mg IV q6h *or* Meropenem 1 g IV q8h *or*
  - Levofloxacin 750 mg PO/IV q24h.
- In situations where two antipseudomonal antibiotics should be used (see above for risk factors for MDR pathogen, patients in units where > 10% of gram-negative isolates are resistant to an agent being considered for monotherapy), addition of one of the following should be considered:
  - Aminoglycosides: Amikacin 15–20 mg/kg IV q24h; Gentamicin 5–7 mg/kg IV q24h; Tobramycin 5–7 mg/kg IV q24h *or*
  - Polymixins: Colistin 5 mg/kg IV 1 (loading dose) followed by 2.5 mg × (1.5 × CrCl + 30) IV q12h (maintenance dose), Polymyxin B 2.5–3.0 mg/kg/d divided in 2 daily IV doses (should be reserved for settings where there is a high prevalence of multidrug resistance and local expertise in using this medication).
- Both aminoglycosides and polymyxins require drug levels and adjustment of doses and/or intervals; suggest consulting with infectious diseases.
- Treatment duration for VAP is 7 days; however, there exist situations where shorter or longer courses may be indicated depending on the rate of clinical improvement.

2.10.6 Clostridioides (formerly Clostridium) Difficile Colitis

- Epidemiology[69]:
  - Most commonly recognized cause of infectious diarrhea in health care settings.
  - Estimates suggest there are close to 500,000 infections annually in the United States.
  - 15,000–30,000 US deaths and inpatient costs $4.8 billion per year.
- Risk factors:
  - Recent broad-spectrum antibiotic use (high-risk antibiotics such as clindamycin, fluoroquinolones, and cephalosporins).
  - Health care exposure.
  - Gastrointestinal procedure.
  - Proton pump inhibitor (PPI) use.
  - Chemotherapy.
  - Age ≥ 65 years.
- Diagnosis:
  - Depending on your institution, *C. difficile* testing may be PCR based or glutamate dehydrogenase (GDH) antigen/EIA toxin based.
  - Testing for *C. difficile* should be considered if the following criteria are met:
    - One or more risk factors for CDI are present (see above).
    - Presence of acute diarrhea (≥ 3 unformed Bristol category 7 stools within 24 hours).
    - Absence of another cause of diarrhea (i.e., laxative use within 48 hours, current or recent tube feeds).
    - No *C. difficile* testing in the previous 7 days or positive *C. difficile* test in the previous 14 days.
- Management:
  - Patients with suspected CDI must be placed on pre-emptive contact precautions pending the test results; those with positive results remain in contact precautions.

○ Metronidazole is no longer considered first-line therapy for nonsevere CDI. Studies have shown that oral vancomycin is superior to metronidazole with regard to resolution of diarrhea at end of treatment and with regard to recurrence rates 21–30 days after treatment.

○ Initial (▶ Table 2.20) and recurrent (▶ Table 2.21) treatment for *C. difficile*.

Table 2.20 Initial treatment of *Clostridioides difficile*

Clinical definition	Supportive clinical data	Recommended treatment
Initial episode, nonsevere	WBC < 15,000 cells/mL and serum creatinine (SCr) < 1.5 mg/dL	Vancomycin 125 mg PO QID × 10 d *or* Fidaxomicin[a] 200 mg PO BID × 10 d If above are unavailable, metronidazole 500 mg PO TID × 10 d
Initial episode, severe	WBC ≥ 15,000 cells/mL or SCr ≥ 1.5 mg/dL	Vancomycin 125 mg PO QID × 10 d *or* Fidaxomicin[a] 200 mg PO BID × 10 d
Initial episode, fulminant	Hypotension/shock, ileus[b], megacolon	Vancomycin 500 mg PO (not IV) QID *and* Metronidazole 500 mg IV q8h *and* ID consult recommended

[a] At some institutions, Fidaxomicin is a restricted antibiotic and must be approved by Antimicrobial Stewardship or through ID consult.

[b] If ileus, consider adding rectal administration of vancomycin (500 mg PR QID).

Table 2.21 Treatment of *Clostridioides difficile* recurrence

Clinical definition	Recommended treatment
First recurrence	*If metronidazole was used for the initial episode:* Vancomycin 125 mg PO QID × 10 d *If vancomycin was used for the initial episode:* Vancomycin taper Example: 125 mg PO QID × 10 d, BID × 7 d, once daily for 7 d, every other day for 2–8 wk[b] *or* Fidaxomicin 200 mg PO BID × 10 d[a]
Second or subsequent recurrence	Vancomycin taper Example: 125 mg PO QID × 10 d, BID × 7 d, once daily for 7 d, every other day for 2–8 wk[b] *or* Fidaxomicin 200 mg PO BID × 10 d[a] *or* Vancomycin 125 mg PO QID × 10 d followed by rifaximin 400 mg PO TID for 20 d *or* Fecal microbiota transplantation (FMT)[c]

[a] At some institutions, Fidaxomicin is a restricted antibiotic and must be approved by Antimicrobial Stewardship or through ID consult.

[b] Duration of vancomycin pulse dosing is unclear based on the literature and should be based on individual patient circumstances. Suggest ID consult.

[c] At least two recurrences (i.e., three CDI episodes) should be tried prior to offering FMT.

2.10.7 Candidemia

- Epidemiology[70]:
  - Third to fourth most common cause of health care–associated blood stream infections.
  - Associated with up to 47% attributable mortality.
  - Most common species of *Candida* yeast in ICU patients: *Candida albicans, Candida glabrata, Candida parapsilosis, Candida krusei, Candida tropicalis.*
- Risk factors:
  - CVCs; present in at least 70% of patients diagnosed with candidemia.
  - Exposure to broad-spectrum antibiotics.
  - Recent major surgery, specifically abdominal surgery.
  - Necrotizing pancreatitis.
  - Dialysis.
  - Total parenteral nutrition (TPN).
  - Corticosteroids.
  - Severity of illness.
- Rule for prediction of candidemia[71]:
  - Any systemic antibiotic for 1–3 days (1 point) *or* presence of a CVC for 1–3 days (1 point) AND at least TWO of the following (1 point for each):
    - TPN for 1–3 days
    - Any dialysis for 1–3 days
    - Any major surgery within the last 7 days
    - Pancreatitis within the last 7 days
    - Any use of steroids within the last 7 days
    - Use of other immunosuppressive agents within the last 7 days
  - If 3 points are not achieved, 97% negative predictive value for candidemia.
- Diagnosis:
  - Blood cultures are the gold standard for diagnosis; you do not need to order fungal blood cultures as *Candida* will grow well in traditional blood cultures.
  - (1,3)-beta-D-glucan is a nonspecific fungal cell wall marker that can be elevated in cases of invasive candidiasis. However, it has largely been studied in hematologic patients whom are neutropenic. It can also be falsely positive for a variety of reasons including continuous renal replacement therapy (CRRT), intermittent hemodialysis, transfusions of blood products, albumin, and IVIG, among others.
- Management:
  - Recommend consulting infectious diseases service for help in management.
  - Remove all CVCs as early as possible in the course of infection.
  - Repeat blood cultures every 24–48 hours until clear.
  - Echocardiography should be considered if the patient has persistent candidemia.
  - Consult ophthalmology for a dilated eye exam to assess for endophthalmitis/retinitis.
  - First-line empiric therapy: Echinocandins (caspofungin, micafungin).
  - Most patients can be transitioned to fluconazole depending on *Candida* species and antifungal susceptibilities.
  - Recommended duration of therapy is 14 days following documented clearance of blood cultures. Patients with persistent fungemia or metastatic complications need a longer duration of therapy.

2.10.8 Complicated Intra-abdominal Infections, Peritonitis

- Definition[72]:
  - Complicated intra-abdominal infection (IAI) extends beyond the hollow viscus of origin into the peritoneal space and is associated with either abscess formation or peritonitis.
- Epidemiology:
  - IAI is the second most common cause of infectious mortality in the ICU.
  - The most common organisms isolated in complicated IAIs are *E. coli* (71%), anaerobes including *Bacteroides fragilis*, other *Bacteroides* species, *Clostridium* species (30–70%), and *Streptococcus* species (38%).

- Diagnosis:
  - CT scan is the imaging modality of choice for evaluation.
  - Obtain blood cultures if the patient is hemodynamically unstable, appears toxic, or is immunocompromised.
  - Send aerobic, anaerobic, and fungal cultures from intra-abdominal fluid/abscess drainage—if there is concern for infected tissue, tissue cultures rather than swabs of tissue is the preferred method for diagnosis.
- Management:
  - Source control is the most important component for management of complicated IAIs—closure of the perforated viscus or drainage of an infected fluid collection.
  - Therapy based on severity of infection and community versus health care associated.
  - Community-acquired, mild-to-moderate severity:
    - Cefazolin 2 g IV q8h + Metronidazole 500 mg PO/IV q8h; Ceftriaxone 2 g IV q24h + Metronidazole 500 mg PO/IV q8h.
    - If cephalosporin allergy, Ciprofloxacin 400 mg IV q12h + Metronidazole 500 mg PO/IV q8h.
    - Do not use a fluoroquinolone as first line unless the antibiogram at your institution indicate > 90% susceptibility of *E. coli* to quinolone.
    - Do not use ampicillin-sulbactam because of wide spread resistance of *E. coli.*
    - Adjust empiric antibiotic regimen based on culture information and susceptibilities.
  - Community-acquired, severe, *or* health care associated:
    - Severe infections include those with Acute Physiology and Chronic Health Evaluation (APACHE II) score ≥ 15, advanced age, presence of malignancy/immunocompromised state, high degree of organ dysfunction.
    - Piperacillin-tazobactam 4.5 g IV q6h.
    - If life-threatening penicillin allergy, cefepime 1 g IV 8 hours + metronidazole 500 mg PO/IV q8h; this regimen will not provide coverage for *Enterococcus* species so if this is a concern, consider the addition of vancomycin.
    - Adjust empiric antibiotic regimen based on culture information and susceptibilities.
  - MRSA coverage: Should only be provided to patients with postoperative peritonitis who are known to be colonized with MRSA; it should be discontinued if MRSA does not grow in culture after 48 hours.
  - Antifungal coverage (targeting *Candida*): Should be considered for patients with clinical evidence of IAI and significant risk factors for candidiasis, including recent abdominal surgery, anastomotic leaks, or necrotizing pancreatitis; Fluconazole 400 mg PO/IV q24h should be used first line; echinocandin if the patient is critically ill.
  - Duration of treatment[73]: 4 days, unless adequate source control is not achieved defined as ongoing contamination and/or undrained collection of infection; 7 days if the patient is also bacteremic from IAI.
  - Durations longer than 7 days have not been associated with improved outcome.
  - Treatment of *Enterococcus* and *Candida* in polymicrobial intra-abdominal infections remains controversial but should be considered in critically ill or immunocompromised patients, or when they are the dominant organism in peritoneal culture.

2.10.9 Necrotizing Fasciitis

- Epidemiology[74]:
  - High mortality rate, 30–70%.
  - Approximately two-third of the cases will present in the lower extremities.
- Diagnosis:
  - Can develop from a break in the skin related to trauma or surgery; however, nearly 50% of patients with necrotizing fasciitis caused by *Streptococcus pyogenes* have no portal of entry but develop deep infection at the site of nonpenetrating trauma such as bruise or muscle strain.
  - Monomicrobial (streptococci, MRSA, *Aeromonas hydrophila*, *Vibrio vulnificus*) versus polymicrobial (aerobic and anaerobic bacteria, e.g., Fournier's gangrene).
  - Wooden, hard induration of the subcutaneous tissues; underlying tissues are firm and the fascial planes, muscle groups cannot be distinguished by palpation.

○ Other features:
  – Hypotension, toxic appearance with cellulitis.
  – Severe pain disproportional to the clinical findings.
  – Edema or tenderness extending beyond the erythema.
  – Crepitus (gas in the tissues).
  – Anesthesia over the affected area.
  – Skin necrosis or bullae.
○ Clinical judgment is the most important component for diagnosis; imaging (CT or MRI) can help but may cause delay in treatment. Surgical exploration is the preferred diagnostic test.
• Immediate surgical debridement upon recognition.
• Empiric antibiotic regimen:
○ Vancomycin 15 mg/kg IV q12h (maintenance dose), 20 mg/kg IV (1 loading dose) AND Piperacillin-tazobactam 4.5 g IV q6h OR Cefepime 2 g IV q8h (if penicillin allergy) ALL WITH clindamycin 900 mg IV q8hr
○ Aztreonam 2 g IV q8h (if severe/life-threatening allergy to penicillins/cephalosporins) AND clindamycin 900 mg IV q8h.
○ Continue treatment until no further need for debridement and afebrile for 2–3 days.
○ The efficacy of IVIG as an antitoxin has not been definitively established.

2.10.10 Penicillin Allergy

• Penicillin allergies are reported in 10–20% of patients.[75]
• Only 1–8% of patients with a reported penicillin allergy test positive when a penicillin skin test is performed.
• Important to conduct a history about the allergy if one is reported:
○ When was the reaction?
○ How long after beginning the penicillin/beta-lactam did the reaction occur?
○ What was the reaction?
○ Were there any signs of swelling of the tongue, throat, or lips? Did you develop hives?
○ If a rash occurred, what was the nature of the rash? Where was it, and what did it look like?
○ Has the patient received another penicillin or cephalosporin since the reaction?
○ Ask about "ceph" drugs or trade names (Augmentin, Keflex, Ceftin, Omnicef).
○ Check the patient's chart to see if they have ever received cefazolin (Ancef) for perioperative antibiotics.
• Reaction types associated with penicillin/beta-lactam allergy:
○ Immediate (type 1)—anaphylaxis, hypotension, laryngeal edema, angioedema, wheezing, urticaria (hives); onset almost always within an hour.
○ Accelerated (type 1)—laryngeal edema, angioedema, wheezing, urticaria, NOT hypotension; onset is usually within 1–72 hours of administration.
○ Late (rash)—maculopapular/morbilliform rash or contact dermatitis-like appearance; onset almost always >72 hours after administration.
○ Late (other)—thrombocytopenia, anemia, eosinophilia, neutropenia, interstitial nephritis, hepatitis, serum sickness; onset almost always >72 hours after administration; Stevens-Johnson Syndrome (SJS)—exfoliative dermatitis (skin layer detachment, peeling) with mucous membrane involvement; onset almost always >72 hours after administration.
○ If the patient has a clear history of type 1 reactions (as above), especially anaphylaxis, the patient should not receive a beta-lactam without undergoing testing for the allergy. Penicillin skin testing predicts type 1, IgE-mediated reactions.
○ Patients who report a rash consistent with a late reaction (as above), and the rash is not consistent with SJS, are not at risk for severe adverse reaction. They can receive penicillins or beta-lactams but should be monitored for rash.
○ Patients who report gastrointestinal symptoms (diarrhea, nausea) do not have a penicillin allergy.
○ Cross-reactivity rates for type 1 reactions:
  – Cephalosporins (with true penicillin allergy): 2%.
  – Carbapenems (with true penicillin allergy): 0.3%.

– Cephalosporins are often a reasonable choice for patients with documented penicillin reactions of unclear clinical significance. Please consult with Infectious Diseases or your Antimicrobial Stewardship Program.
• See recent Toolkits published by Journal American Medical Association (JAMA) for handouts on conducting a penicillin allergy history and instructions for performing amoxicillin challenge for low- and moderate-risk patients.[76]

References

[1] Medical Student's Guide to Intensive Care Medicine. DesPlaines, IL: Society of Critical Care Medicine; 2005
[2] Artis KA, Bordley J, Mohan V, Gold JA. Data omission by physician trainees on ICU rounds. Crit Care Med. 2019; 47(3):403–409
[3] Vincent JL. Give your patient a fast hug (at least) once a day. Crit Care Med. 2005; 33(6):1225–1229
[4] Zimmerman JE, Kramer AA, McNair DS, Malila FM. Acute Physiology and Chronic Health Evaluation (APACHE) IV: hospital mortality assessment for today's critically ill patients. Crit Care Med. 2006; 34(5):1297–1310
[5] Moreno RP, Metnitz PG, Almeida E, et al. SAPS 3 Investigators. SAPS 3: From evaluation of the patient to evaluation of the intensive care unit. Part 2: Development of a prognostic model for hospital mortality at ICU admission. Intensive Care Med. 2005; 31(10):1345–1355
[6] Metnitz PG, Moreno RP, Almeida E, et al. SAPS 3 Investigators. SAPS 3: From evaluation of the patient to evaluation of the intensive care unit. Part 1: Objectives, methods and cohort description. Intensive Care Med. 2005; 31(10):1336–1344
[7] Higgins TL, Teres D, Copes WS, Nathanson BH, Stark M, Kramer AA. Assessing contemporary intensive care unit outcome: an updated Mortality Probability Admission Model (MPM0-III). Crit Care Med. 2007; 35(3):827–835
[8] Carney N, Totten AM, O'Reilly C, et al. Guidelines for the management of severe traumatic brain injury, fourth edition. Neurosurgery. 2017; 80(1):6–15
[9] Gerber LM, Chiu YL, Carney N, Härtl R, Ghajar J. Marked reduction in mortality in patients with severe traumatic brain injury. J Neurosurg. 2013; 119(6):1583–1590
[10] Farahvar A, Gerber LM, Chiu YL, Carney N, Härtl R, Ghajar J. Increased mortality in patients with severe traumatic brain injury treated without intracranial pressure monitoring. J Neurosurg. 2012; 117(4):729–734
[11] Chesnut RM, Temkin N, Carney N, et al. Traumatic brain injury in Latin America: lifespan analysis randomized control trial protocol. Neurosurgery. 2012; 71(6):1055–1063
[12] Alali AS, Fowler RA, Mainprize TG, et al. Intracranial pressure monitoring in severe traumatic brain injury: results from the American College of Surgeons Trauma Quality Improvement Program. J Neurotrauma. 2013; 30(20):1737–1746
[13] Tasneem N, Samaniego EA, Pieper C, et al. Brain multimodality monitoring: a new tool in neurocritical care of comatose patients. Crit Care Res Pract. 2017; 2017:6097265
[14] Fried HI, Nathan BR, Rowe AS, et al. The insertion and management of external ventricular drains: an evidence-based consensus statement: a statement for healthcare professionals from the Neurocritical Care Society. Neurocrit Care. 2016; 24(1):61–81
[15] Kestle JR, Holubkov R, Douglas Cochrane D, et al. Hydrocephalus Clinical Research Network. A new Hydrocephalus Clinical Research Network protocol to reduce cerebrospinal fluid shunt infection. J Neurosurg Pediatr. 2016; 17(4):391–396
[16] Jamjoom AAB, Joannides AJ, Poon MT, et al. British Neurosurgical Trainee Research Collaborative. Prospective, multicentre study of external ventricular drainage-related infections in the UK and Ireland. J Neurol Neurosurg Psychiatry. 2018; 89(2):120–126
[17] Marcus HJ, Wilson MH. Videos in clinical medicine: insertion of an intracranial-pressure monitor. N Engl J Med. 2015; 373(22):e25
[18] Kalanuria AA, Ziai W, Mirski M. Ventilator-associated pneumonia in the ICU. Crit Care. 2014; 18(2):208
[19] Shan J, Chen HL, Zhu JH. Diagnostic accuracy of clinical pulmonary infection score for ventilator-associated pneumonia: a meta-analysis. Respir Care. 2011; 56(8):1087–1094
[20] Thille AW, Richard JC, Brochard L. The decision to extubate in the intensive care unit. Am J Respir Crit Care Med. 2013; 187(12):1294–1302
[21] Kulkarni T, Sharma NS, Diaz-Guzman E. Extracorporeal membrane oxygenation in adults: a practical guide for internists. Cleve Clin J Med. 2016; 83(5):373–384
[22] Sandham JD, Hull RD, Brant RF, et al. Canadian Critical Care Clinical Trials Group. A randomized, controlled trial of the use of pulmonary-artery catheters in high-risk surgical patients. N Engl J Med. 2003; 348(1):5–14
[23] Hofer CK, Müller SM, Furrer L, Klaghofer R, Genoni M, Zollinger A. Stroke volume and pulse pressure variation for prediction of fluid responsiveness in patients undergoing off-pump coronary artery bypass grafting. Chest. 2005; 128(2):848–854
[24] Marik PE, Baram M, Vahid B. Does central venous pressure predict fluid responsiveness? A systematic review of the literature and the tale of seven mares. Chest. 2008; 134(1):172–178
[25] Marik PE. Early management of severe sepsis: concepts and controversies. Chest. 2014; 145(6):1407–1418
[26] Nguyen HB, Rivers EP, Knoblich BP, et al. Early lactate clearance is associated with improved outcome in severe sepsis and septic shock. Crit Care Med. 2004; 32(8):1637–1642
[27] Rivers E, Nguyen B, Havstad S, et al. Early Goal-Directed Therapy Collaborative Group. Early goal-directed therapy in the treatment of severe sepsis and septic shock. N Engl J Med. 2001; 345(19):1368–1377
[28] Marik PE, Khangoora V, Rivera R, Hooper MH, Catravas J. Hydrocortisone, vitamin C, and thiamine for the treatment of severe sepsis and septic shock: a retrospective before-after study. Chest. 2017; 151(6):1229–1238
[29] Kelm DJ, Perrin JT, Cartin-Ceba R, Gajic O, Schenck L, Kennedy CC. Fluid overload in patients with severe sepsis and septic shock treated with early goal-directed therapy is associated with increased acute need for fluid-related medical interventions and hospital death. Shock. 2015; 43(1):68–73

[30] Asfar P, Meziani F, Hamel JF, et al. SEPSISPAM Investigators. High versus low blood-pressure target in patients with septic shock. N Engl J Med. 2014; 370(17):1583–1593

[31] De Backer D, Biston P, Devriendt J, et al. SOAP II Investigators. Comparison of dopamine and norepinephrine in the treatment of shock. N Engl J Med. 2010; 362(9):779–789

[32] Hollenberg SM, Dellinger RP. Noncardiac surgery: postoperative arrhythmias. Crit Care Med. 2000; 28(10) Suppl:N145–N150

[33] Walsh SR, Tang T, Wijewardena C, Yarham SI, Boyle JR, Gaunt ME. Postoperative arrhythmias in general surgical patients. Ann R Coll Surg Engl. 2007; 89(2):91–95

[34] January CT, Wann LS, Alpert JS, et al. American College of Cardiology/American Heart Association Task Force on Practice Guidelines. 2014 AHA/ACC/HRS guideline for the management of patients with atrial fibrillation: a report of the American College of Cardiology/American Heart Association Task Force on Practice Guidelines and the Heart Rhythm Society. J Am Coll Cardiol. 2014; 64(21):e1–e76

[35] Fleisher LA, Fleischmann KE, Auerbach AD, et al. 2014 ACC/AHA guideline on perioperative cardiovascular evaluation and management of patients undergoing noncardiac surgery: executive summary: a report of the American College of Cardiology/American Heart Association Task Force on practice guidelines. Developed in collaboration with the American College of Surgeons, American Society of Anesthesiologists, American Society of Echocardiography, American Society of Nuclear Cardiology, Heart Rhythm Society, Society for Cardiovascular Angiography and Interventions, Society of Cardiovascular Anesthesiologists, and Society of Vascular Medicine Endorsed by the Society of Hospital Medicine. J Nucl Cardiol. 2015; 22(1):162–215

[36] Mehta NM, Skillman HE, Irving SY, et al. Guidelines for the provision and assessment of nutrition support therapy in the pediatric critically ill patient: Society of Critical Care Medicine and American Society for Parenteral and Enteral Nutrition. Pediatr Crit Care Med. 2017; 18(7):675–715

[37] McClave SA, Taylor BE, Martindale RG, et al. Society of Critical Care Medicine, American Society for Parenteral and Enteral Nutrition. Guidelines for the provision and assessment of nutrition support therapy in the adult critically ill patient: Society of Critical Care Medicine (SCCM) and American Society for Parenteral and Enteral Nutrition (A.S.P.E.N.). JPEN J Parenter Enteral Nutr. 2016; 40(2):159–211

[38] Heyland DK, Dhaliwal R, Drover JW, Gramlich L, Dodek P, Canadian Critical Care Clinical Practice Guidelines Committee. Canadian clinical practice guidelines for nutrition support in mechanically ventilated, critically ill adult patients. JPEN J Parenter Enteral Nutr. 2003; 27(5):355–373

[39] Reintam Blaser A, Starkopf J, Alhazzani W, et al. ESICM Working Group on Gastrointestinal Function. Early enteral nutrition in critically ill patients: ESICM clinical practice guidelines. Intensive Care Med. 2017; 43(3):380–398

[40] Rice TW, Wheeler AP, Thompson BT, et al. National Heart, Lung, and Blood Institute Acute Respiratory Distress Syndrome (ARDS) Clinical Trials Network. Initial trophic vs full enteral feeding in patients with acute lung injury: the EDEN randomized trial. JAMA. 2012; 307(8):795–803

[41] Heidegger CP, Berger MM, Graf S, et al. Optimisation of energy provision with supplemental parenteral nutrition in critically ill patients: a randomised controlled clinical trial. Lancet. 2013; 381(9864):385–393

[42] Harvey SE, Parrott F, Harrison DA, et al. CALORIES Trial Investigators. Trial of the route of early nutritional support in critically ill adults. N Engl J Med. 2014; 371(18):1673–1684

[43] Doig GS, Simpson F, Sweetman EA, et al. Early PN Investigators of the ANZICS Clinical Trials Group. Early parenteral nutrition in critically ill patients with short-term relative contraindications to early enteral nutrition: a randomized controlled trial. JAMA. 2013; 309(20):2130–2138

[44] Casaer MP, Mesotten D, Hermans G, et al. Early versus late parenteral nutrition in critically ill adults. N Engl J Med. 2011; 365(6):506–517

[45] O'Keeffe ST. Use of modified diets to prevent aspiration in oropharyngeal dysphagia: is current practice justified? BMC Geriatr. 2018; 18(1):167

[46] Vincent JL, Sakr Y, Sprung CL, et al. Sepsis Occurrence in Acutely Ill Patients Investigators. Sepsis in European intensive care units: results of the SOAP study. Crit Care Med. 2006; 34(2):344–353

[47] Wiedemann HP, Wheeler AP, Bernard GR, et al. National Heart, Lung, and Blood Institute Acute Respiratory Distress Syndrome (ARDS) Clinical Trials Network. Comparison of two fluid-management strategies in acute lung injury. N Engl J Med. 2006; 354 (24):2564–2575

[48] Kalantari K, Chang JN, Ronco C, Rosner MH. Assessment of intravascular volume status and volume responsiveness in critically ill patients. Kidney Int. 2013; 83(6):1017–1028

[49] Lee JW. Fluid and electrolyte disturbances in critically ill patients. Electrolyte Blood Press. 2010; 8(2):72–81

[50] Kraft MD, Btaiche IF, Sacks GS, Kudsk KA. Treatment of electrolyte disorders in adult patients in the intensive care unit. Am J Health Syst Pharm. 2005; 62(16):1663–1682

[51] Drews RE. Critical issues in hematology: anemia, thrombocytopenia, coagulopathy, and blood product transfusions in critically ill patients. Clin Chest Med. 2003; 24(4):607–622

[52] Palta S, Saroa R, Palta A. Overview of the coagulation system. Indian J Anaesth. 2014; 58(5):515–523

[53] Nakashima MO, Rogers HJ. Hypercoagulable states: an algorithmic approach to laboratory testing and update on monitoring of direct oral anticoagulants. Blood Res. 2014; 49(2):85–94

[54] Gould MK, Garcia DA, Wren SM, et al. Prevention of VTE in nonorthopedic surgical patients: antithrombotic therapy and prevention of thrombosis, 9th ed. American College of Chest Physicians Evidence-Based Clinical Practice Guidelines. Chest. 2012; 141(2) Suppl: e227S–e277S

[55] Falck-Ytter Y, Francis CW, Johanson NA, et al. Prevention of VTE in orthopedic surgery patients: antithrombotic therapy and prevention of thrombosis, 9th ed. American College of Chest Physicians Evidence-Based Clinical Practice Guidelines. Chest. 2012; 141(2) Suppl:e278S–e325S

[56] Kearon C, Akl EA, Ornelas J, et al. Antithrombotic therapy for VTE disease: CHEST guideline and expert panel report. Chest. 2016; 149 (2):315–352

[57] Valentine SL, Bembea MM, Muszynski JA, et al. Pediatric Critical Care Transfusion and Anemia Expertise Initiative (TAXI), Pediatric Critical Care Blood Research Network (BloodNet), and the Pediatric Acute Lung Injury and Sepsis Investigators (PALISI) Network. Consensus recommendations for RBC transfusion practice in critically ill children from the pediatric critical care transfusion and anemia expertise initiative. Pediatr Crit Care Med. 2018; 19(9):884–898

[58] Napolitano LM, Kurek S, Luchette FA, et al. EAST Practice Management Workgroup, American College of Critical Care Medicine (ACCM) Taskforce of the Society of Critical Care Medicine (SCCM). Clinical practice guideline: red blood cell transfusion in adult trauma and critical care. J Trauma. 2009; 67(6):1439–1442

[59] Khwaja A. KDIGO clinical practice guidelines for acute kidney injury. Nephron Clin Pract. 2012; 120(4):c179–c184

[60] Rehman T, deBoisblanc BP. Persistent fever in the ICU. Chest. 2014; 145(1):158–165

[61] Niven DJ, Laupland KB. Pyrexia: aetiology in the ICU. Crit Care. 2016; 20:247

[62] Potasman I, Grupper M. Leukemoid reaction: spectrum and prognosis of 173 adult patients. Clin Infect Dis. 2013; 57(11):e177–e181

[63] Mermel LA, Allon M, Bouza E, et al. Clinical practice guidelines for the diagnosis and management of intravascular catheter-related infection: 2009 update by the Infectious Diseases Society of America. Clin Infect Dis. 2009; 49(1):1–45

[64] Hooton TM, Bradley SF, Cardenas DD, et al. Infectious Diseases Society of America. Diagnosis, prevention, and treatment of catheter-associated urinary tract infection in adults: 2009 International Clinical Practice Guidelines from the Infectious Diseases Society of America. Clin Infect Dis. 2010; 50(5):625–663

[65] Yahav D, Franceschini E, Koppel F, et al. Seven versus fourteen days of antibiotic therapy for uncomplicated gram-negative bacteremia: a non-inferiority randomized controlled trial. Clin Infect Dis. 2019 Sep 13; 69(7):1091–1098

[66] Kalil AC, Metersky ML, Klompas M, et al. Executive summary: management of adults with hospital-acquired and ventilator-associated pneumonia: 2016 clinical practice guidelines by the Infectious Diseases Society of America and the American Thoracic Society. Clin Infect Dis. 2016; 63(5):575–582

[67] Parente DM, Cunha CB, Mylonakis E, Timbrook TT. The clinical utility of methicillin-resistant Staphylococcus aureus (MRSA) nasal screening to rule out MRSA pneumonia: a diagnostic meta-analysis with antimicrobial stewardship implications. Clin Infect Dis. 2018; 67(1):1–7

[68] Kirtland SH, Corley DE, Winterbauer RH, et al. The diagnosis of ventilator-associated pneumonia: a comparison of histologic, microbiologic, and clinical criteria. Chest. 1997; 112(2):445–457

[69] McDonald LC, Gerding DN, Johnson S, et al. Clinical practice guidelines for Clostridium difficile infection in adults and children: 2017 update by the Infectious Diseases Society of America (IDSA) and Society for Healthcare Epidemiology of America (SHEA). Clin Infect Dis. 2018; 66(7):987–994

[70] Pappas PG, Kauffman CA, Andes D, et al. Infectious Diseases Society of America. Clinical practice guidelines for the management of candidiasis: 2009 update by the Infectious Diseases Society of America. Clin Infect Dis. 2009; 48(5):503–535

[71] Ostrosky-Zeichner L, Sable C, Sobel J, et al. Multicenter retrospective development and validation of a clinical prediction rule for nosocomial invasive candidiasis in the intensive care setting. Eur J Clin Microbiol Infect Dis. 2007; 26(4):271–276

[72] Solomkin JS, Mazuski JE, Bradley JS, et al. Diagnosis and management of complicated intra-abdominal infection in adults and children: guidelines by the Surgical Infection Society and the Infectious Diseases Society of America. Clin Infect Dis. 2010; 50(2):133–164

[73] Sawyer RG, Claridge JA, Nathens AB, et al. STOP-IT Trial Investigators. Trial of short-course antimicrobial therapy for intraabdominal infection. N Engl J Med. 2015; 372(21):1996–2005

[74] Stevens DL, Bisno AL, Chambers HF, et al. Infectious Diseases Society of America. Practice guidelines for the diagnosis and management of skin and soft tissue infections: 2014 update by the Infectious Diseases Society of America. Clin Infect Dis. 2014; 59(2):e10–e52

[75] Joint Task Force on Practice Parameters; American Academy of Allergy, Asthma and Immunology; American College of Allergy, Asthma and Immunology; Joint Council of Allergy, Asthma and Immunology. Drug allergy: an updated practice parameter. Ann Allerg Asthma Immunol. 2010; 105(4):259–273

[76] Shenoy ES, Macy E, Rowe T, Blumenthal KG. Evaluation and management of penicillin allergy: a review. JAMA. 2019; 321(2):188–199

3 Trauma

Edited by Rebecca Kim and Milos Buhavac

3.1 Advance Trauma Life Support (ATLS) and General Approach to Trauma

Michael Karsy, Austin Cannon, Andrea Weitz, and Milos Buhavac

3.1.1 Epidemiology

- Trauma is the leading cause of death in young adults (age 1–46 years); accounts for 10% of all annual deaths, 50 million annual medical visits, 50 million patients with moderate-to-severe disability annually, and 30% of intensive care unit (ICU) admissions.
- Most commonly unintentional (2/3) followed by suicide/homicide (1/3).
- Annual cost to health care and lost productivity of over $700 billion.
- Variation in cause based on region of the USA.[1]
- Recent overall reduction in rate of injury globally from different causes.[2]

3.1.2 Triage and Assessment

- Golden hour: Need for early intervention in trauma patients to reduce mortality after major trauma; unclear correlation timing of emergency medical services (EMS) and intervention with mortality.[3]
- Trimodal mortality curve (▶ Fig. 3.1): At scene within minutes (prevention/education is only way to influence these), early deaths within hours (chance for successful intervention by both EMS teams and early stabilization/decision making/ATLS/golden hour), late deaths weeks after event from sepsis/complications/ICU care/multiple organ failure.
- ATLS training aims to update and standardize clinical treatment of trauma patients[4] and also ensure that trauma patients are able to be effectively cared for in both high- and low-resource environments in the United States and globally, with obvious limitations in low-income countries.
- Educating the general public with courses such as "Stop the Bleed" has also been shown to decrease out-of-hospital morbidity and mortality.
- Phases of care:
  - Prearrival/prehospital: EMS involved in assessing patient, stabilizing patient, providing information to the receiving hospital; relevant information can be remembered by MIST mnemonic (M: mechanism and time of injury, I: injuries found and suspected, S: symptoms and signs, T: treatment initiated).

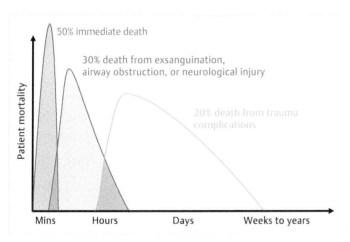

Fig. 3.1 Diagram of trauma timing and risk of mortality/morbidity.

- Injuries requiring trauma level I or II admission: Penetrating injuries to head, neck, torso, extremities proximal to elbow and knee, two or more long-bone fractures, severely injured extremities, depressed level of consciousness, pelvic fractures, open or depressed skull fractures, paralysis, falls > 20 feet for adults or > 10 feet for children, high-risk autocrash (intrusion, ejection, death within the passenger compartment, high-speed impact > 20 mph), motorcycle crash > 20 mph, high-risk patients (older adults, children, anticoagulation use, burns, pregnancy > 20 weeks), or EMS provider judgment.
  - Care should not be delayed to transport a patient to a higher-level trauma center. Injuries that can be dealt with by the closest hospital should be stabilized first before transferring the patient to a higher level of care.
  - Treatment before transfer can involve stabilization of airway/breathing/circulation (ABCs), administration of medications for reducing intracranial pressure, administration of blood products,[5] diagnostic studies if time permits without delaying transfer, dressing of wounds, and extremity splinting/traction.
  - Trauma team/hospital: Evaluation of patient at appropriate trauma-level designated hospital involves teams of individuals with clearly assigned roles and an assigned leader; patients can always be escalated to a higher level of care once stabilized.
  - Specialty teams: Evaluation and triaging of patient for specific medical and surgical treatment.
  - Critical care: Management of patients for continued resuscitation and hemodynamic/respiratory monitoring, polytraumas too unstable for the operating room, pre- and postsurgical care when necessary and appropriate, and other initial and follow-up issues; increasing evidence supports long-term cognitive decline of critically ill patients with delirium in the ICU even if patients start off with normal cognitive function.
  - Rehabilitation care: Follow-up of patients for improving of function, anticipation and management of long-term sequelae from trauma. Of particular importance when applicable are nutrition/toleration of diet, intensive work with physical, occupational, and speech therapists, which may include prostheses or assistive devices, family support/involvement, and long-term disposition.
- Primary survey:
  - Role of the primary survey is to quickly diagnose and treat traumatic injuries that constitute an immediate threat to life. Each section should be broken down into evaluation and intervention; ABCDE.
  - Airway and cervical spine control:
    - Evaluation: Airway patency, airway protection, and cervical spine protection; patients with facial fractures, neck injury, airway obstruction or Glasgow Coma Scale (GCS) score ≤ 8, nonpurposeful motor movement require a definitive airway (cuffed tube placed below the vocal cords).
    - If the mechanism of injury is such that an oral airway cannot be placed (penetrating injuries to the face and neck and massive swelling), rapid recognition and placement of a surgical airway should ensue.
    - Cervical spine injury should be assumed in patients with blunt multisystem trauma, altered level of consciousness, or blunt injury above the clavicle.
    - LEMON mnemonic can be used to assess airway accessibility (L: look for face/neck injuries and foreign bodies; E: evaluate size of mouth [3 finger breadths], mandible [3], and neck [2]; M: Mallampati score; O: obstruction/obesity; N: neck mobility).
    - If massive hemorrhage is seen during this part of the evaluation, it should be controlled with direct pressure, packing, or a tourniquet and not in the circulation section of the ABCDEs.
    - Intervention: Should proceed in logical stepwise fashion. Airway maneuvers such as jaw-thrust should be performed first. We do not advocate the use of the head tilt/chin lift because of concerns for cervical spine injury. Next oral-pharyngeal and in some cases nasopharyngeal (not in traumas where basilar skull fractures are suspected) airway devices can be used to improve oxygenation and ventilation.
    - Nondefinitive airways such as laryngeal mask airways and supraglottic tubes can be used especially if no other airway is available and the patient is hypoxic. Definitive airways in the form of endotracheal tubes are ideal. As a final resort, trauma providers should be familiar with and able to perform a surgical cricothyroidotomy and tracheostomy.
    - Failure to recognize and place airway can quickly lead to patient hypoxia, decompensation, irreversible end organ damage, and death.

- Breathing:
  - Evaluation: Assess patient's ability to oxygenate and ventilate; inspect chest excursion by visualization, palpation, and auscultation; assess pulse oximetry and if available end-tidal CO_2. Monitor arterial blood gases.
  - Intervention: Administration of supplemental oxygen and ventilation by hand with bag valve mask or ventilator.
  - If identified, tension pneumothorax should be treated initially by needle decompression and then tube thoracotomy placement. Hemothorax, simple pneumothorax, and open pneumothorax should be treated with tube thoracostomy and, if necessary, with intubation in an unstable patient.
  - In patients who are intubated and ventilated, but are struggling to oxygenate and ventilate despite chest tube placement, a tracheobronchial injury should be suspected and immediate bronchoscopy should be performed and the endotracheal tube advanced beyond the injury.
- Circulation:
  - Evaluation: All trauma patients are assumed to be bleeding until proven otherwise. Assess hemodynamic status, intravascular access, and degree of hemorrhage control; altered level of consciousness, pale skin, hypotension, and rapid pulse suggest shock, sources of which may be varied but hemorrhagic shock must be assumed on presentation.
  - Intervention: As discussed previously, direct compression, packing, and tourniquets of bleeding sources can temporize hemorrhage; if no external sources of bleeding are found, a high suspicion for internal hemorrhage may be necessary.
  - Classic signs of hypovolemia may not be present in elderly or pediatric patients.
  - 1–2 L bolus of warmed intravenous (IV) solution can be an initial step followed by product transfusion in a balanced fashion with and definitive hemorrhage control, including surgically when necessary, as an ultimate step.
- Disability:
  - Evaluation: Neurological status by GCS evaluation. Multiple reasons for decreased GCS may be present (e.g., hypoxia, hemorrhagic shock, hypoglycemia, elicit substances, mass-occupying lesions, blunt/penetrating head trauma).
  - Intervention: The goal is to prevent hypoxia and hypotension and worsen any existing neurologic injuries. Management may be complex in the setting of polytrauma but for isolated head injuries maintaining adequate perfusion pressures and oxygenation is the first step.
- Exposure/Environment:
  - Evaluation: Undressing of patient for complete visual assessment and physical examination, in addition to the assessment of hypothermia.
  - Intervention: Warm patient to prevent coagulation dysregulation and ensure no other injuries are missed.
- Asking patient to state name and what happened can evaluate the status of ABC.
- Monitors and lines: Pulse oximetry, noninvasive and invasive blood pressure, rapid infusion IVs or other adequate IV/intraosseous access, gastric tubes except for patients with facial or skull base fracture, transurethral catheterization except in patients with blood at the urethral meatus, perineal ecchymosis or high-riding or nonpalpable prostates.
- Esophageal intubations occur in 0.5–6% of prehospital intubations and all intubated patients should be evaluated by an end-tidal carbon dioxide detector, or alternatively direct visualization or esophageal pressure monitor can be employed.
- Constant re-evaluation of patients is required to detect injuries that are initially unapparent on physical or imaging studies; the primary survey should always be revisited when a patient becomes unstable.
- Resources and team sizes vary by institution. Many higher-level trauma centers have large teams and many of the steps of ATLS happen concurrently. If a small team or single provider is all that is available, remember to not proceed to the next step in the primary survey until the current step has been thoroughly evaluated and appropriate treatment initiated.
- Secondary survey:
  - Head-to-toe evaluation of injuries involving the head, face, ears, eyes, nose, throat, chest, abdomen, pelvis, genitourinary, extremities, and pulses.

- AMPLE: Allergies, medications currently used, past illness/pregnancy, last meal, events/environment related to the injury.
  - AMPLE answers obtained from patient, EMS, and family when able.
  - Reversal of medications and anticoagulation performed when these are known about and a patient is experiencing ongoing hemorrhage or an intracranial lesion.
  - Emergency laboratory studies include complete blood count, basic or complete metabolic panel, coagulation profile (e.g., prothrombin time, partial thromboplastin time, international normalized ratio, thromboelastography), blood typing and crossmatching, arterial blood gas, and toxicology screen; additional labs are used depending on patient indications.
- Pitfalls of trauma evaluation include delay in diagnosis and initiating life-saving interventions such as intubation, tube thoracostomy, product transfusion, and early transfer to a higher level of care when necessary and patient has been stabilized. Focusing on obvious extremity injuries and deformities and foregoing the primary survey is also a common misstep.
- Shock:
  - Inadequate delivery of oxygen to meet the metabolic demands of the body; cardiac output = heart rate × stroke volume; vascular tone maintained by blood volume, blood vessel compliance, and neurologic control.
  - Initial shock can be compensated but if not reversed results in cellular death.
  - Identified by clinical exam (cool skin, tachycardia, hypotension, narrow pulse pressure [systolic − diastolic pressure < 0.25 × systolic]), blood pressure limited for diagnosis since can compensate with < 30% blood loss.
  - Different types of shock require recognition and treatment (▶ Table 3.1).

Table 3.1 Types of shock

Types	Example	CO	SVR	Other findings	Treatment
Hypovolemic/ hemorrhagic	Hemorrhage, burns, pancreatitis	↓	↑	*Hypotension*, ↓ preload, tachycardia, weak thread pulse, cool and pale skin, ↓ UOP	Repletion of vascular volume, fluid boluses and PRCB administration, control of hemorrhage
Cardiogenic	Myocardial infarction, arrhythmia, myocarditis	↓	↑	↑ Preload and afterload, cool and pale skin, ↓ UOP, weak thread pulse, tachypnea	Vasopressors, cardiac revascularization, aortic balloon pump, ventricular assistance device
Obstructive	Tension pneumothorax, cardiac tamponade, pulmonary embolism	↓	↑	↑ Afterload, ↓ cardiac contractility (cardiac index/stroke volume)	Correction of obstruction
Distributive					
Neurogenic	Spinal cord injury	↓	↓	Bradycardia, *hypotension*, warm dry skin, not seen in isolated intracranial injury	Vasopressors, limited fluid boluses
Anaphylactic	Drug or environmental allergy	↓	↓	*Hypotension*, tachycardia, cough, dyspnea, pruritus, urticaria, angioedema	Steroids, airway protection, antihistamines, fluid boluses
Septic	Septic shock, bacteremia, urosepsis, penetrating abdominal injury	↓	↓	*Hypotension*, tachycardia, bounding pulses, tachypnea, pink flushed skin, ↓ UOP, fever	Vasopressors, sepsis protocol, broad spectrum antibiotics, fluid boluses

Abbreviations: CO, cardiac output; SVR, systemic vascular resistance; UOP, urine output; PRBC, packed red blood cells.

Note: Italicized physiological parameter indicates initial change for type of shock.

Table 3.2 Types of hemorrhagic shock

Class	Blood loss (mL)	Pulse rate	Systolic blood pressure	Pulse pressure	Respiratory rate	Urine output (mL/h)	Mental status	Treatment
I	<750	<100	Normal	Normal or ↑	14–20	>30	Anxious	Crystalloid
II	750–1500	100–120	Normal	↓	20–30	20–30	Anxious	Crystalloid
III	1500–2000	120–140	↓	↓	30–40	5–15	Confused	Crystalloid and blood
IV	>2000	>140	↓	↓	>35	Minimal	Lethargic	Crystalloid and blood

Note: Parameters for 70-kg male; blood volume for female is roughly 10% lower than a male.

- ○ Different classes of hemorrhage can estimate blood volume depletion but differ based on patient's age, injury severity, time lapse of injury, medications, and treatment (▶ Table 3.2); treatment preemptively performed.
- ○ Estimated adult male blood volume is 7% of body weight (70 mL/kg) and female is 6% of body weight (60 mL/kg), children have blood volumes of 8–9% of body weight, infants have blood volumes of 9–10% of body weight.
- ○ Two large 16-gauge antecubital IVs can be used more effectively than a central venous line, rate of flow is proportional to the fourth power of the radius of the cannula and inversely related to its length (Poiseuille law); warmed fluid should be used during massive infusion; intraosseous lines can be beneficial in situations that IV access is delayed and can be used in ALL age groups.
- ○ Initial fluid bolus is 1–2 L for adults and 20 mL/kg for pediatric patients with close monitoring of response.
- ○ Hemorrhagic shock may require a high index of suspicion in patients who do not respond to initial fluid boluses.
- ○ Only body cavities that can hold enough blood to cause hemorrhagic shock are the chest, abdomen, pelvis/retroperitoneum, and thigh; external bleeding can result in large and rapid blood volume losses.
- ○ Adequate resuscitation: >0.5 mL/kg urine output (UOP) in adults, >1 mL/kg for pediatric patients, >2 mL/kg for children under 1 year of age.
- ○ Transfusion ratio of blood:platelets:fresh frozen plasma is 1:1:1 with monitoring for coagulopathy in large volume transfusion (PROPER Trial[6]: Evaluated 680 patients randomized to 1:1:1 vs. 1:1:2 transfusion after polytrauma, showed no difference in 24-hour and 30-day outcomes but 1:1:1 transfusion showed lower rate of exsanguination and improved rate of hemostasis).
- ○ Tranexamic acid (1 g prehospital, 1 g in emergency department) may reduce mortality (CRASH-2 Trial[7]: Evaluated 20,211 patients to receive 1 g tranexamic acid within 10 minutes and 1 g over 8 hours vs. placebo, reduced all-cause mortality at 28 days was observed with tranexamic acid (14.5 vs. 16.0%, $p = 0.0035$), treatment beyond 3 hours may be ineffective, criticism over small effect size, small mortality benefit in hemorrhagic shock subgroup, randomization process, and generalizability; CRASH-3 trial ongoing).
- ○ Crucial to avoid lethal triad of coagulopathy, acidosis, and hypothermia to prevent ongoing bleeding during massive transfusions.

3.1.3 Imaging

- Initial imaging:
  - ○ Chest X-ray (▶ Fig. 3.2): Assessment of ABCDE (in this case, airway, breathing, cardiac, diaphragm, and edges). (A) Airway and endotracheal tube position; (B) pneumo- or hemothorax, rib fractures; (C) cardiac silhouette, pulmonary and vascular markings; (D) diaphragm shape and position; (E) edges of pleura and costophrenic recesses.

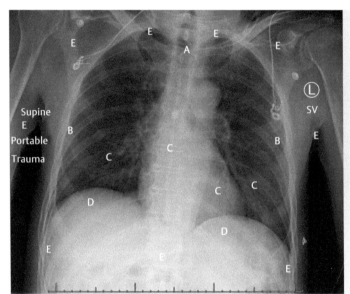

Fig. 3.2 Rapid evaluation of chest X-rays. A, Airway and endotracheal tube position; B, pneumo- or hemothorax, rib fractures; C, cardiac silhouette, pulmonary and vascular markings; D, diaphragm shape and position; E, edges of pleura and costophrenic recesses.

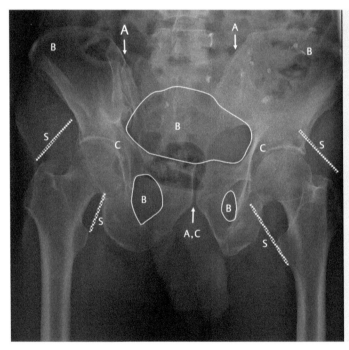

Fig. 3.3 Rapid evaluation of pelvic X-rays. A, Pubic symphysis symmetrical and sacroiliac joints intact; B, three pelvic rings and pelvic ala intact; C, distance of pubic symphysis and femoral cartilage, symmetric soft tissues; S, obturator internus, perivesical fat plane, gluteus medius, and psoas fat planes.

- Pelvic X-rays (▶ Fig. 3.3): Assessment of ABCS (alignment, bones, cartilage, soft tissue). (A) Pubic symphysis symmetrical and sacroiliac joints intact; (B) three pelvic rings and pelvic ala intact; (C) distance of pubic symphysis and femoral cartilage, symmetric soft tissues; (S) obturator internus, perivesical fat plane, gluteus medius, and psoas fat planes.
- Radiographs of the chest and pelvis are used to evaluate trauma; X-rays of the cervical spine show 70–80% sensitivity for injury and thus computed tomography (CT) imaging is more definitive for suspected injuries.

- Focused Assessment with Sonography for Trauma (FAST):
  - Used to detect pericardial and intraperitoneal free fluid, which is concerning for hemorrhage when positive.
  - Standardized order of evaluation can ensure not missing an area, one protocol is: (1) pericardial, (2) right flank/hepatorenal view/Morison's pouch, (3) left flank/perisplenic view, (4) pelvic/retrovesical view, and (5) thoracic view.
  - 63–75% sensitivity for intraperitoneal hemorrhage; however, suspected injuries may require additional CT imaging or diagnostic peritoneal lavage (DPL).
  - FAST cannot identify diaphragm tears, pancreatic injuries, bowel perforations, mesenteric trauma, chronic pericardial effusions, and injuries with free fluid < 200 mL or distinguish blood from urine or ascites; limited ability to detect kidney and retroperitoneal injuries; limited ability in pregnant women and the morbidly obese.
  - DPL: Used when ultrasound or CT unavailable; 98% sensitive for detection of intraperitoneal bleeding; contraindicated in patients with prior abdominal operations, morbid obesity, advanced cirrhosis, and coagulopathy; infraumbilical entry in most patients, supraumbilical entry in patients with pelvic hematoma or pregnancy; immediate gross aspiration of blood (> 10 mL) or gastrointestinal contents is a positive test; lavage with 1,000-mL warmed crystalloid (10 mL/kg) is positive if > 100,000 red blood cells (RBC)/mm^3, 500 white blood cells (WBC)/mm^3, or bacteria on Gram stain, or positive for elevated bilirubin or amylase.
- Secondary imaging (CT imaging):
  - Widely available resource used for initial assessment of trauma.[8,9,10,11,12,13]
  - Performed in focused manner depending on area of injury, but only after patient stabilization and in a timely manner.
  - CT imaging should be obtained at facilities where treatment can be initiated and should not delay transfer to a higher level of care.

3.2 Specific Injury Patterns in Trauma

Michael Karsy, Austin Cannon, Andrea Weitz, and Milos Buhavac

- Vascular trauma[4]:
  - Common vessel injury patterns: Aorta (deceleration at ligamentum arteriosum), carotid/vertebral (flexion/extension), brachial (proximal humeral fracture), popliteal (posterior knee dislocation).
  - Permissive hypotension (systolic ≤ 90 mm Hg) can reduce risk of dislodging hemostatic plug.
  - Arteriography used for difficult areas: Axillary/subclavian, zone 3 carotid injuries, thoracic inlet neck injuries.
  - Treatment options: Direct pressure, direct clamping, balloon occlusion, vessel ligation, end-to-end repair (1–2 cm), interposition graft, and endovascular repair.
  - Tolerated ligation: Venous ligation in extremities, subclavian artery, radial or ulnar if palmar arch present, internal iliac, single tibial artery, superficial femoral.
- Thoracic injuries:
  - Tension pneumothorax: Development of air entrainment into the pleural cavity through a one-way valve from the lung or chest wall; results in mediastinal compression, decreased venous return and obstructive shock; most common in positive-pressure ventilation with visceral pleural injury but can be seen with penetrating or blunt chest injury; diagnosed with respiratory failure, air hunger, tracheal deviation, neck vein distension, and unilateral absence of breath sounds progressing to hypotension and cardiac arrest; treated with needle decompression (4/5th intercostal space between anterior and mid axillary lines) or chest tube; can be exacerbated if patient is intubated without chest tube first; chest tube maintained for 24–48 hours at 10–20 cm H_2O suction until air leak (e.g., bubbles) resolve, water sealed for 4 hours to evaluate recurrent pneumothorax, output < 100 mL/24 hours before discontinuing; repeat chest X-ray unnecessary. Should not be diagnosed radiographically.

- Open pneumothorax/sucking chest wound: Air entrapment from penetrating chest wall injury; treated with occlusive dressing secured on three sides and intubation when necessary in trauma bay; ultimately requires operative repair.
- Closed pneumothorax: Lung tissue disruption causing air leak into pleural space; causes ventilation/perfusion mismatch.
- Flail chest: Segment of chest wall not in continuity with the thoracic cage, three or more contiguous ribs broken in two places; creates a flail segment that results in paradoxical motion of the chest wall and is typically associated with an underlying pulmonary contusion; if causing significant ventilatory compromise will need emergent intubation; fixation results in less time on ventilator but no changes in morbidity or mortality.
- Hemothorax: Blood in chest cavity can accumulate > 1,500 mL or 1/3 of the patient's blood volume and compromises cardiopulmonary function; most commonly from penetrating injury of the systemic or hilar vessels; chest tube size does not impact drainage; drainage of 1,500 mL immediately or > 300 mL/h for 2–4 hours requires blood transfusion and operative control of hemorrhage.
- Cardiac tamponade: Penetrating or blunt injuries resulting in blood accumulation within the pericardial space and obstructive shock; can result in Beck's triad of jugular vein distension, hypotension, and muffled/distant heart tones; can mimic left-side tension pneumothorax; Kussmaul sign (rise in venous pressure with inspiration when breathing spontaneously) suggestive but tamponade can be present without elevated jugular venous pressure; confirm with ECHO portion of FAST; different treatments depending on injury pattern.
- Pulmonary contusion: Blunt or penetrating injury to the lung (usually high-force blunt mechanism) results in infiltrative and inflammatory process that typically worsens for several days before improvement; can be exacerbated by underlying medical conditions (e.g., chronic obstructive pulmonary disease, renal failure); limiting fluid administration is integral in not worsening condition.
- Tracheobronchial tree injury: Injury to the trachea or bronchus; patients demonstrate hemoptysis, emphysema, or tension pneumothorax; can be suggested with incomplete lung expansion after chest tube placement or ongoing large air leak from chest tube, high suspicion is key, immediate treatment involves passing ET tube past injury or main-stemming the unaffected lung.
- Blunt cardiac injury: Myocardial contusion, ventricular rupture, coronary artery dissection or thrombosis, valvular disruption; must suspect with high-energy thoracic trauma. Signs typically include arrhythmia with electrocardiogram and can be further evaluated with echocardiogram.
- Traumatic aortic rupture: Can cause sudden death at the scene within minutes if uncontained; incomplete laceration near ligamentum arteriosum can cause partial tears with blood contained by adventitial or soft tissue; can cause widened mediastinum, obliteration of the aortic knob, deviation of the trachea to the right, depressed left mainstem bronchus, elevated right mainstem bronchus, obliteration of the aorticopulmonary window, deviation of the esophagus to the right, widened paratracheal stripe, widened paraspinal spaces, presence of a pleural or apical cap, left hemothorax, fractures of the first or second rib or scapula. In presence of polytrauma, leave this injury alone and fix other problems first as survival with this injury suggests containment of rupture.
- Traumatic diaphragmatic injury: Blunt trauma resulting in tears, can develop over time ultimately resulting in abdominal contents herniating into chest cavity; more common on left side because of liver protection on the right; can be missed or misinterpreted chest X-rays and also low sensitivity on CT scan for diagnosing this injury; perform diagnostic laparoscopy if suspicious.
- Blunt esophageal rupture: Penetrating and rarely blunt trauma resulting in disruption of the esophagus allowing gastric contents in the mediastinum cavity resulting in mediastinitis; seen with left pneumothorax, hemothorax without rib fracture, blunt injury to the sternum or epigastric area, or with pain out of proportion to injury; must suspect with mediastinal air on computed tomography (CT) imaging; management depends on whether or not the rupture is contained and time from injury.
- Rib, sternum, and scapular fractures:
  - Rib 1–3 fractures: Protected by other bony structures; suggest high-magnitude injury with associated pulmonary and neurovascular injuries (blunt cerebrovascular injury); mortality up to 35%.
  - Sternal and scapular fractures: Direct blows, associated with pulmonary contusion, blunt cardiac injury; rarely surgically treated; sternoclavicular dislocation can cause superior vena cava obstruction.

- Middle rib 4–9 fractures: Majority of injuries; multiple rib fractures in younger patients suggest greater force than older patients; pain control needed to improve ventilation.
  - Lower rib 10–12 fractures: Suspicion for hepatosplenic injury.
  - Rib plating may be undertaken with severely displaced or multiple rib fractures leading to respiratory insufficiency and severe pain. Data suggests no changes in morbidity and mortality, but shorter hospital stays and time on the ventilator.
  - Rib fractures have an extremely high mortality in elderly patients and appropriate multimodal pain control with frequent assessment using incentive spirometry must be undertaken to prevent atelectasis and pneumonia leading to death.
- Abdominopelvic injuries:
  - Exploratory laparotomy (Ex-lap):
    - Performed with gunshot wounds because of high association with intra-abdominal injury.
    - Performed in any hemodynamically unstable patient with evidence or suspicion of intra-abdominal bleeding, which may include peritonitis, fascial penetration, positive FAST or diagnostic peritoneal lavage, evisceration, free air or fluid in the abdomen concerning for a ruptured hollow viscus, intraperitoneal bladder injury.
    - Treatment for solid organ injury depends on level of instability, surgical experience, and interventional capabilities.
  - Blunt injuries:
    - Direct blows or deceleration injuries mechanisms, type of trauma considered, external signs of trauma can suggest internal injury (e.g., seat-belt sign).
  - Penetrating injuries:
    - Most common injury to liver (40%), small bowel (30%), diaphragm (20%), and colon (15%).
    - Gunshot wounds can create cavitation and fragmentation effects.
    - Penetrating injuries can involve both the thorax and abdomen.
    - Penetrating bowel injury can be missed in low-velocity stab wounds because of limited fluid assessed by FAST and limited injury seen on CT.
    - Concomitant penetrating and blunt injuries may be present.
  - Diaphragm injury: Blunt trauma tears; most commonly 5–10 cm in length and on the left.
  - Duodenal rupture: Seen in high-energy blunt mechanisms to the abdomen.
  - Pancreatic injury: Seen in direct blows; serum amylase can be normal or elevated.
  - Genitourinary injuries: Seen with direct back or flank trauma; associated with contusions or hematomas and renal injuries; divided into above/posterior or below/anterior injuries of the urogenital diaphragm; posterior injuries associated with polytrauma and pelvic fracture, anterior injuries associated with straddle injury and can be isolated; evaluated by urethrography, cystography, or intravenous pyelogram.
  - Solid organ injuries: Direct-force injuries; most common injured organs are spleen (40–55%), liver (35–45%), and kidney (15%); multiple injury scoring scales from the American Association for Surgery of Trauma (AAST) involved in predicting mortality, operative rate, and cost (▶ Table 3.3); 5% associated with hollow viscus injuries; higher-grade injuries require more advanced surgical treatments and management of hemorrhage.
  - Hollow viscus injuries (5–10%): Blunt force to intestines from deceleration; associated with seat-belt sign and lumbar vertebral Chance fractures; AAST grading (▶ Table 3.4) predicts primary repair vs. resection/bypass.
  - Abdominal compartment syndrome:
    - Pressure > 25 mm Hg.
    - Risk factors: Packing abdomen after laparotomy, bowel edema from crystalloid resuscitation, reperfusion injury, ongoing intra-abdominal bleeding, primary fascial closure.
    - Diagnosed: Hypotension from impaired venous return and cardiac output, hypoxia from increased airway pressures and elevated diaphragm, oliguria from renal vein compression.
  - Retroperitoneal injury zones:
    - I: Midline along aorta, risk of injury to aorta, left gastric, splenic, common hepatic arteries, superior mesenteric artery, proximal renal artery, superior mesenteric vein, transverse colon.
    - II: Lateral, risk of injury to kidneys and renal vessels.
    - III: Pelvis, risk of injury to aorta and inferior vena cava.

Table 3.3 Grading schemes for solid abdominal organ injuries

	Liver[a]	Renal[d]	Spleen[b]	Pancreas[c]
I	<10% subcapsular hematoma <1-cm capsular laceration	Contusion Subcapsular perirenal hematoma No laceration	<10% subcapsular hematoma <1-cm capsular laceration	Minor contusion/laceration, no ductal injury
II	10–50% subcapsular hematoma <10-cm intraparenchymal hematoma 1–3 cm capsular tear, <10 cm length	<1-cm superficial laceration not involving collecting duct Nonexpanding perirenal hematoma in retroperitoneum	10–50% subcapsular hematoma <5-cm intraparenchymal hematoma 1–3 cm laceration not involving trabecular vessels	Major contusion/laceration without ductal injury
III	>50% subcapsular or parenchymal hematoma >10-cm intraparenchymal hematoma >3-cm capsular tear	>1-cm laceration not involving collecting duct Bilateral injuries	>50% subcapsular hematoma >5-cm intraparenchymal hematoma >3-cm laceration or involving trabecular vessels Ruptured hematoma	Distal laceration or parenchymal injury with ductal injury
IV	25–75% hepatic lobe or 1–3 Couinaud segments disrupted	Laceration into renal pelvis or urinary extravasation Injury to renal artery or vein with contained hemorrhage Segmental infarction Expanding subcapsular hematoma with renal compression	Segmental laceration, hilar vessel laceration with devascularization >25% spleen	Proximal laceration to the right of the superior mesenteric vein Parenchymal injury with injury to the bile duct/ampulla
V	>75% hepatic lobe or >3 Couinaud segments disrupted	Shattered kidney Renal hilum avulsion Laceration or thrombosis of main renal artery/vein Uretopelvic avulsion	Shattered spleen Hilar vascular injury with devascularization	Massive disruption of pancreatic head
VI	Hepatic avulsion			

[a,b,c] Advance 1 grade up to grade III for multiple injuries.

[d] Advance 1 grade up to grade III for bilateral injuries.

- Pelvic fractures and instability:
  - High-force injuries, 5–30% mortality with higher mortality in open fractures; assumed in patients with presumed hemorrhagic shock and no other source; stability conferred by bone, muscle, and ligaments.
  - Four mechanisms: (1) anteroposterior compression (15–20% injuries); (2) lateral compression (60–70% injuries); (3) vertical shear (5–15% injuries); or (4) combination injuries.
  - Associated with ruptured urethra (high-riding prostate, scrotal hematoma, blood at the urethral meatus), bladder injury, limb length discrepancy, rotational deformity of the leg without obvious fracture.
  - Rocking of the pelvis by pushing on the iliac crests should be performed only once as dislodged blood clots can worsen hemorrhage.

Table 3.4 Grading schemes for hollow abdominal organ injuries

	Stomach	Duodenum	Jejunum/ileum/colon/rectum
I	Hematoma < 3 cm	Hematoma in 1 segment	Small hematoma
	Partial-thickness laceration	Partial-thickness laceration	Partial-thickness laceration
II	Hematoma > 3 cm	Hemorrhage in multiple segments	Laceration < 50% circumference
	Laceration > 3 cm	Laceration < 50% circumference	
III	Laceration > 3 cm	Laceration 50–75% circumference in second segment, 50–100% in other segments	Laceration > 50% circumference
IV	Laceration of greater or lesser curvature vessels	Laceration 75–100% circumference in second segment	Transection
		Rupture of ampulla or common bile duct	
V	> 50% rupture	Massive duodenopancreatic injury and devascularization	Segmental tissue loss and devascularization

- – Open-book pelvic fractures should be stabilized by pelvic binder or sheet to reduce worsening of hemorrhage.
  - – Intraperitoneal gross blood warrants laparotomy whereas injury without immediate hemorrhage may be managed by angiography and embolization.
  - – Newer techniques include preperitoneal pelvic packing (PPP), resuscitative endovascular balloon occlusion of the aorta (REBOA); may prove to be more timely and efficacious, but more studies need to be conducted.
- Head and neck injuries: See Chapter 14.1 Traumatic Brain Injury and Chapter 14.2 Spinal Injury.
- Face trauma: See Chapter 7.3 Facial Trauma and Chapter 8.1 Ophthalmological Trauma and Other Emergencies.
  - ○ Lacerations: Irrigated, debrided of nonviable tissue and foreign objects, repaired primarily; injury to salivary glands, lacrimal duct, and facial nerve require operative repair.
  - ○ Fractures divided into superior 1/3 of face (naso-orbitoethmoid, frontal sinus), middle 1/3 (maxilla, zygoma, orbit, nose), and lower 1/3 (mandible); divided into LeFort classification: I (transverse across maxilla), II (pyramidal across maxilla and nasal bone), III (craniofacial disjunction).
  - ○ Superior 1/3 and maxilla repaired with fixation within 1–2 weeks.
  - ○ Nose undergoes closed reduction, splinting, and evaluation for septal hematomas.
  - ○ Zygoma reduced or displaced or treated with open repair of comminuted.
  - ○ Orbit treated with fixation depending on degree and type of fracture.
  - ○ Mandible treated with closed reduction, maxillomandibular fixation/wiring, or open fixation depending on type and degree of fracture.
- Neck trauma: See Chapter 7.3 Facial Trauma.
  - ○ Penetrating injuries divided into zones: Zone I (suprasternal notch to cricoid); zone II (cricoid to angle of mandible); zone III (angle of mandible to base of skull).
  - ○ All evaluated with CT and CT angiography for vessel injury; possible evaluation with laryngoscopy, bronchoscopy, and esophagoscopy.
  - ○ Operative exploration highly considered: Penetration in zone II (controversial), subcutaneous or retropharyngeal emphysema, hoarseness or stridor, active bleeding, absent carotid pulse, bruit/thrill, neurologic deficit.
- Musculoskeletal injuries: See Chapter 15.1 Fracture Basics and Compartment Syndrome.
  - ○ Hemorrhage from long-bone fractures can be significant; associated injuries should be suspected.
  - ○ Fracture immobilization using traction and splinting helps control blood loss, reduces pain, and reduces soft tissue injury.
  - ○ Joint dislocation deformities can be suspected on clinical examination (▶ Table 3.5); should be either repositioned or immobilized.
  - ○ Extremity areas with tenderness or deformity require X-ray evaluation; occult injuries may be identified during tertiary surveys.

Table 3.5 Joint dislocation deformities

Joint	Direction of dislocation	Deformity
Shoulder	Anterior	Squared off
	Posterior	Locked-in, internal rotation
Elbow	Posterior	Olecranon posteriorly displaced
Hip	Anterior	Flexed, abducted, externally rotated
	Posterior	Flexed, adducted, internally rotated
Knee	Any	Loss of normal contour, extended, may spontaneously reduce
Ankle	Lateral	Externally rotated, prominent medial malleolus
Subtalar	Lateral	Laterally displaced os calcis

Table 3.6 Gustilo-Anderson classification of soft tissue injuries

Grade	Wound	Management
I	<1-cm laceration, clean	Gram-positive coverage (first-generation cephalosporin), 3–6 L irrigation
II	1- to 10-cm laceration, limited soft tissue damage	
III	>10-cm laceration, amputation, gunshot, farm injury, crush >6 h, marked contamination	Gram-positive and -negative coverage (first-generation cephalosporin with aminoglycoside), 9 L irrigation, tissue flaps if possible
IIIa	Soft tissue with adequate tissue for coverage	
IIIb	Soft tissue without adequate tissue for coverage	
IIIc	Open injury with arterial injury	

- Soft tissue injuries treated with washout, antibiotics, and tissue flaps depending on degree of injury (▶ Table 3.6); wounds should be covered with saline-soaked gauze until operative treatment; washout and debridement performed <6 hours if possible.
- Avascular extremities: Circulatory evaluation should be performed in injured vessels; muscles with >6 hours of blood disruption undergo necrosis; assessment including pulses, capillary refill, and Doppler triphasic wave; extremities with coolness, pallor, paresthesias, and motor function abnormalities suggest arterial injury; arterial-brachial index (ABI), CT angiography, and arteriography used for assessment; urgent surgical consultation is warranted.
- Traumatic amputated extremities: Open fractures with prolonged ischemia and neurologic injury and muscle damage may require amputation; patients with clean, isolated extremity amputations below the knee or elbow can be candidates for reimplantation; amputated parts are washed with isotonic solution, wrapped in sterile gauze with antibiotic-containing isotonic solution, and transported on ice but not frozen; decisions to amputate limbs are multifactorial and depend on limb function, injury, and patient handicap (▶ Table 3.7).
- Crush injury/traumatic rhabdomyolysis: Multiple or large-extremity fractures resulting in elevated myoglobin resulting in metabolic acidosis, hyperkalemia, hypocalcemia, and disseminated intravascular coagulopathy; identified by dark amber urine, elevated urine myoglobin; treated with fluids to maintain urine output 100 mL/h.
- Open fractures and joint injuries: Risk of bacterial contamination, requires surgical washout and exploration; tetanus prophylaxis and antibiotic prophylaxis should be used.
- Peripheral nerve injury: See Chapter 14.5 Peripheral Nerve Injury.
- Compartment syndrome: Pressure within a musculofascial compartment causes failure of perfusion resulting in necrosis; most common in lower leg, forearm, foot, hand, gluteal region, and thigh; presents with pain out of proportion to stimulus, tenseness of compartment, asymmetry of the limb, pain on passive stretch, altered sensation, and high degree of clinical suspicion; absence of palpable distal pulse is an uncommon or late finding; intracompartmental pressure of 30–45 mm Hg or ompartment diastolic pressure ≤30 mm Hg are abnormal.
- Burn injuries: See Chapter 3.4 Burn Evaluation and Management.

Table 3.7 Mangled extremity severity score (MESS)

Skeletal/Soft tissue injury	
1	Low energy (stab, simple fracture, pistol gunshot wound)
2	Medium energy (open or multiple fractures, dislocation)
3	High energy (high-speed motor vehicle accident, rifle gunshot wound)
4	Very high energy (high-speed trauma and gross contamination)
Limb ischemia	
1	Pulse reduced/absent, normal perfusion
2	Pulseless, paresthesias, diminished capillary refill
3	Cool, paralyzed, insensate, numb
Shock	
0	Systolic > 90 mm Hg
1	Transient hypotension
2	Persistent hypotension
Age	
0	< 30 y
1	30–50 y
2	> 50 y

Note: MESS scores ≥ 7 predicted amputation with 100% accuracy; scores doubled for ischemia > 6 h.

- Genitourinary trauma:
  - Renal injury (▶ Table 3.3) grades I–III managed nonoperatively, grade IV managed depending on contralateral renal function, grade V treated with expanding hematoma by exploration with renorrhaphy or partial nephrectomy.
  - Ureter injury: Caused by penetrating injury and pelvic fracture; lower 1/3 treated with bladder reimplantation with or without psoas hitch, middle 1/3 treated with ureteroureterostomy, proximal 1/3 treated with nephrostomy tube.
  - Bladder injury: Caused by blunt or penetrating injury; extraperitoneal treated nonoperatively with follow-up cystography, intraperitoneal treated with exploration and repair.
  - Urethra injury: Caused by pelvic fracture or penetrating trauma; suspected with urethral blood, high-riding prostate, scrotal edema, and ecchymosis; Foley catheter not placed until retrograde urethrography completed; partial disruptions treated with Foley for 14–21 days, complete disruptions treated with endoscopic repair or bladder diversion.
- Ophthalmological trauma: See Chapter 8.1 Ophthalmological Trauma and Other Emergencies.
- Restraint device injuries:
  - Seat-belt sign: Linear contusion of abdominal wall, mesentery tear with bucket handle injury involving mesenteric vessels, rupture of small bowel or colon, injury to iliac artery or abdominal aorta, Chance fracture, pancreatic or duodenal injury.
  - Shoulder harness: Injury to the great vessels of the neck (blunt cerebrovascular injury), cervical spine fracture, rib fracture, pulmonary contusions, upper abdominal viscera injury.
  - Air bag: Corneal abrasion, head-and-neck trauma, thermal injury, cardiac contusion, cervical and thoracic spine fractures.

3.3 Specific Injury Patient Groups in Trauma

Michael Karsy, Austin Cannon, Andrea Weitz, and Milos Buhavac

- Pediatric trauma:
  - Strong hemodynamic functional reserve but with rapid changes during decompensation; smaller body mass confers greater force per body area, less protective structural tissue; internal organ injury

can occur without bony fracture; hypothermia develops completely and complicates resuscitation and coagulopathy; history taking and cooperation are difficult.

○ Polytrauma impacts in pediatric patients: 50% show cognitive and physical handicaps, 60% show personality change.

○ Physiology estimates:
   – Estimated pediatric weight $(kg) = (2 \times age) + 10$.
   – Normal systolic blood pressure $(mm\ Hg) = 70–90 + (2 \times age)$.
   – Normal diastolic blood pressure $(mm\ Hg) = 2/3rd \times systolic$.
   – Endotracheal tube length $(cm) = 3 \times width$.
   – Urine output: < 1 years old (>2 mL/kg/h), young children (>1.5 mL/kg/h), older children (>1 mL/kg/h); lower limit does not reach 0.5 mL/kg/h until child is a nongrowing adolescent.

○ Broselow tape measures height and infers patient weight and drug doses.

○ ABCDE trauma assessment used with some differences than adults:
   – Airway: Shorter necks and trachea, larger tongue, floppy epiglottis.
   – Breathing: Primarily diaphragmatic breathers, gastric distension performed early.
   – Circulation: Tachycardia first sign of hypovolemia.
   – Disability.
   – Exposure.

○ 1-inch padding beneath infant or toddler shoulder blades creates proper neutral alignment.

○ Shock may not show hemodynamic changes until severe volume depletion is seen; tachycardia, poor skin perfusion, weakened pulses, narrowed pulse pressure < 20 mm Hg, skin mottling, cool extremities, and decreased level of consciousness are early signs of hypovolemia.

○ Vascular access can be obtained via an interosseous bone marrow needle, 18 gauge in infants, 15 gauge in young children; access to the distal lateral femur or anterior tibial prominence can be performed, saphenous cut-down is an option, scalp veins can be accessed but have risk of superior sagittal sinus injury.

○ Fluid boluses are 20 mL/kg up to 50 mL/kg to replace 25% of lost volume, third bolus of 10 mL/kg of packed red blood cell should be considered.

○ Thoracic trauma: 8% of injuries, 2/3 of patients will have multiple injuries; commonly blunt injuries (e.g., pulmonary contusion, rib fracture, mediastinal trauma, pneumothorax).

○ Abdominal trauma: 1/3 of injuries are solid organ; lap-belt injuries (e.g., enteric disruption, Chance fracture) are common; small bowel injuries at the ligament of Treitz, blunt pancreatic injuries, mesenteric avulsion, small bowel injuries, bladder rupture; penetrating injuries of the perineum or straddle injuries are more likely to cause intraperitoneal injuries; FAST shows modest sensitivity for hemoperitoneum in young children.

○ Head trauma: See Chapter 14.1 Traumatic Brain Injury; better prognosis than adults except in children < 3 years; fontanelle and cranial sutures can assess intracerebral pressure; vomiting and amnesia are common after head injury but do not necessarily reflect worsening hemorrhage; impact seizures are more common; elevation of intracranial pressure can occur more quickly than in adults because of tighter intracranial spaces.

○ Spinal cord injury: See Chapter 14.2 Spinal Injury; uncommon and mostly caused by motor vehicle crashes (< 10 years) or vehicles and sports (10–14 years); pseudosubluxation more common in younger children (40% children < 7 years show C2 on C3 displacement vs. 20% children up to 16 years); skeletal growth centers can resemble fracture; spinal cord injury without radiographic abnormality (SCIWORA) more common.

○ Musculoskeletal trauma: Lower blood loss with long-bone and pelvic fractures, hemodynamic instability with isolated femur fractures should warrant evaluation of additional areas; incomplete/greenstick fractures are more common; supracondylar fractures of the elbow or knee have a higher likelihood for vascular and growth plate injury; multiple healing fractures, bilateral rib fractures, fractures of long bones in children < 3 years, and fractures inconsistent with history or trauma severity should warrant evaluation of nonaccidental trauma.

• Geriatric trauma:

○ Less likely to be injured, but higher mortality rate (9.2% with preexisting disease vs. 3.2% for younger patients with preexisting disease), 33% die from sequential organ failure rather than initial trauma.

- ○ Decreased physiological reserve, impact of multiple medications, altered adjustment and ability to avoid injury, higher risk of pulmonary complications (atelectasis, pneumonia, pulmonary edema), decreased cardiac index, decline in renal function, decline in neurological plasticity, stiffening of the spine with increased risk of injury, increased osteoporosis, decreased resistance to hypothermia, decreased muscle tone musculoskeletal stabilization, decreased immune function.
- ○ Most commonly caused by falls (40% of deaths in the elderly).
- ○ ABC trauma assessment complicated by macroglossia, microstomia (smaller mouth), arthritis of the temporomandibular joints and cervical spine, calcification of the laryngeal cartilage, loss of respiratory reserve.
- ○ Normal blood pressure can signify volume depletion due to normal higher baseline pressures.
- ○ Ribs, proximal femur, hips, humerus, and wrist are highest fracture sites.
- ○ Elder abuse should be suspected with injuries or neglect not fitting clinical picture.
- • Pregnant women and fetal trauma[14]:
  - ○ Uterus rises out of pelvis at 12 weeks, uterus at umbilicus at 20 weeks, uterus at costal margin by 34–36 weeks; organs pushed cephalad and somewhat protected from blunt trauma.
  - ○ Injuries caused by motor vehicle collisions (59.6%), falls (22.3%), direct assaults (16.7%), and other (0.1%).
  - ○ Affects 1:12 pregnancies; minor trauma involved in 90% of cases, 60–70% rate of fetal loss from minor trauma.
  - ○ Main cause of fetal death is maternal shock and death, second cause of fetal death is abruption placentae.
  - ○ Decreased maternal intravascular volume results in increased uterine vascular resistance and fetal oxygenation compromise.
  - ○ Plasma volume expands during pregnancy and hematocrit of 31–35% is normal in late pregnancy; healthy women can lose 1.2–1.5 L of blood before showing hypovolemia; fibrinogen, and coagulation factors mildly elevated where decreases may include disseminated intravascular coagulation.
  - ○ Cardiac output increases by 1.0–1.5 L/min by 10th week of pregnancy; uterus and placenta receive 20% of cardiac output; vena cava compression in supine position decreases cardiac output by up to 30%; heart rate increases 10–15 beats/min; systolic and diastolic blood pressure decline 5–15 mm Hg in second trimester and returns at third trimester; flattened or inverted T-wave with increased ectopia can be normal; minute ventilation increases and $PaCO_2$ of 25–30 can be normal while elevated values can suggest respiratory failure;
  - ○ Gastric emptying is reduced, renal perfusion increases, loosening of joints and enlargement of pelvic vessels occur; elevated blood pressure with neurological change resembling head injury can be due to eclampsia.
  - ○ Blunt injury can cause uterine rupture and fetal death; shoulder restraint reduces impact on uterus.
  - ○ Penetrating injuries can cause damage to uterus and displaced organs.
  - ○ Uterus position on the left and left lateral decubitus position can improve venous return and cardiac output; fluid resuscitation is important to restore blood flow to the uterus; vasopressors are used as last resort.
  - ○ All standard medications and defibrillation regimens can be used during pregnancy; this avoids delays in care to account for dosages or pregnancy drug risk categorization in the setting of a trauma scenario.
  - ○ Early intubation, removal of uterine/fetal monitors, or perimortem cesarean delivery can all be utilized to protect the mother's life.
  - ○ Fetal tocodynamometer is used with fetus > 20 weeks gestation.
  - ○ Fetomaternal hemorrhage as detected by the Kleihauer-Betke test in an Rh-negative mother should warrant Rh immunoglobulin therapy for 72 hours; Kleihauer-Betke test measures amount of fetal hemoglobin transmitted to mother's bloodstream.
  - ○ Minor and major traumas undergo fetal monitoring for at least 24 hours (▶ Table 3.8).
  - ○ Uterus is thin walled and protected by pelvic girdle in first trimester, thick-walled and easily injured in third trimester.
  - ○ Intimate partner violence should be considered when clinical presentation does not fit injury pattern.

Table 3.8 Management of blunt trauma in pregnancy

Evaluation	Discharge criteria
Primary maternal and fetal survey	Resolution of contractions
Lab: blood type, Rh factor test, hemoglobin/hematocrit, Kleihauer-Betke test, coagulation tests	Reassuring fetal heart tracing
Obstetric ultrasound	Intact membranes
If > 20 wk, monitor for contractions	No vaginal bleeding
If < 3 contractions/h, monitor for 4 h, then discharge	No uterine tenderness
If 3–7 contractions/h, monitor for 24 h, then discharge	All Rh-negative patients should receive Rh immune globulin therapy if injury effect the uterus or close to it

- Perimortem cesarean delivery considered after 23–24 weeks if no return of spontaneous circulation within 4–5 minutes of cardiac arrest; can increase venous return and cardiac output potentially improving maternal survival.
- Postmortem cesarean section can be successful if within 4–5 minutes of arrest.

3.4 Burn Evaluation and Management

Michael Karsy, Austin Cannon, Andrea Weitz, and Milos Buhavac

- Types:
  - Scalds: Most common, from hot liquids, common burn injury in child abuse (dip line pattern).
  - Flame: Second most common, usually full-thickness burns.
  - Flash: Explosion of flammable liquids or gases.
  - Contact: Skin contact with hot or cold objects, seen in industrial accidents and trauma.
  - Electrical: Worse injury at entry and exit sites, deep tissue damage greater than skin injury, cardiopulmonary resuscitation can be necessary, fractures of spine and long bones can be due to muscle contraction.
  - Chemical: Initially treated with irrigation but depends on the type of chemical.
- Burn depth:
  - First degree: Epidermal injury, painful to palpation, pink, no blisters.
  - Second degree/partial thickness: partial dermal injury, painful to palpation, white-pink, blisters present; epithelialization progresses from follicles, sweat glands, and skin edges.
  - Third degree/full thickness: Entire dermal injury, insensate to palpation, white-black-red.
  - Fourth degree: Fascia, muscle, or bone involvement.
- Associated injuries:
  - Airway injury: Can result in airway obstruction due to edema up to 72 hours postinjury, mucosal and tracheobronchial injury can lead to chemical pneumonitis, pneumonia, pulmonary edema, and acute respiratory distress syndrome.
  - Gastrointestinal: Adynamic ileus common; gastric (Curling) ulcer of stomach, duodenum, jejunum; acalculous cholecystitis.
  - Ocular: Corneal abrasions, cataracts.
- Workup: History of burn type and location, removal of all burned clothing and constricting jewelry, calculation of total body surface area (TBSA) for burn by rule of nines (▶ Table 3.9).
- Treatment location:
  - Outpatient: < 5% TBSA partial-thickness injury, close follow-up and ability for outpatient wound care, 5–10% TBSA partial-thickness injuries require burn center follow-up.
  - Inpatient: > 10% TBSA partial-thickness injury; burns of face, hands, feet, genitalia, or major joints; any full-thickness burns; inhalational injury; chemical or electrical burns; preexisting medical conditions; polytrauma; patients with social situations warranting close observation.

Table 3.9 Wallace rule of nines for estimating body surface area of burns

Part	Adults	Children
Entire arm (per each arm)	9%	9%
Entire head	9%	18%
Entire chest	9%	9%
Entire abdomen	9%	9%
Entire back	18%	18%
Entire leg (per each leg)	18%	13.5%
Groin	1%	1%

- Treatment:
  - Stabilization of airway with preemptive tracheostomy with airway injury, 100% oxygenation and monitoring of carboxyhemoglobin levels (> 10–20% abnormal) with inhalational injury, endoscopic or bronchoscopic evaluation of airway.
  - Monitoring of acid/base status to evaluate CO injury, hourly fluid monitoring, electrolyte repletion, evaluation of myoglobinuria, tetanus prophylaxis, prophylactic antibiotics not used.
  - Early enteral feeding cam improve outcome, caloric needs increase up to 2 × after injury, proton pump or H2 inhibitor stress prophylaxis.
  - Wound care: Cover wound, followed by excision and grafting if wound does not heal by 2–3 weeks; topical antimicrobials (e.g., bacitracin, mupirocin, silver sulfadiazine) reduce risk of wound infection; escharotomies (decompression of extremities at risk of compartment syndrome, decompression of chest to improve respiratory function).
  - Graft types: Autograft sheet vs. mesh, allograft, xenograft, dermal substitutes.
  - Graft priority: Hands, feet, joints, extremities, face, trunk.
  - Fluid resuscitation: Multiple formulas, Parkland (Lactated ringer 3–4 mL/kg/%TBSA injury with half given within 8 hours and other half over 16 hours), continued resuscitation of 1–2 mL/kg/%TBSA injury with adjustment based on vitals.
  - Resuscitation end points: Urine output (30 mL/h adults, 1–1.5 mL/kg/h pediatrics), mean arterial pressure ≥ 60 mm Hg, normal mentation, extremity perfusion, acid/base normalization, mixed venous O_2 > 70%.
- Complications:
  - Pneumonia: Early infection due to gram-positive organisms, late infection due to gram-negative organisms, can occur in 50% of patients.
  - Wound sepsis: Worsening of partial- to full-thickness injury or formation of ischemic necrosis, wound cultures not accurate, skin biopsies monitor bacterial growth, most common infections (S. aureus, Pseudomonas, Acinetobacter, Enterococcus spp, Candida).
  - Wound contractures can be treated with grafting or Z-plasty; hypertrophic scar occurs with deep wounds that take > 2 weeks to heal and are treated with pressure reduction, massage, steroid injections, and laser resurfacing.

References

[1] Minei JP, Schmicker RH, Kerby JD, et al. Resuscitation Outcome Consortium Investigators. Severe traumatic injury: regional variation in incidence and outcome. Ann Surg. 2010; 252(1):149–157

[2] Haagsma JA, Graetz N, Bolliger I, et al. The global burden of injury: incidence, mortality, disability-adjusted life years and time trends from the Global Burden of Disease study 2013. Inj Prev. 2016; 22(1):3–18

[3] Newgard CD, Schmicker RH, Hedges JR, et al. Emergency medical services intervals and survival in trauma: assessment of the "golden hour" in a North American prospective cohort. Ann Emerg Med. 2010; 55(3):235–246.e4

[4] ATLS, Subcommittee; American College of Surgeons' Committee on Trauma; International ATLS Working Group. Advanced trauma life support (ATLS(R)): the ninth edition. J Trauma Acute Care Surg. 2013; 74(5):1363–1366

[5] Sperry JL, Guyette FX, Brown JB, et al. PAMPer Study Group. Prehospital plasma during air medical transport in trauma patients at risk for hemorrhagic shock. N Engl J Med. 2018; 379(4):315–326

[6] Holcomb JB, Tilley BC, Baraniuk S, et al. PROPPR Study Group. Transfusion of plasma, platelets, and red blood cells in a 1:1:1 vs a 1:1:2 ratio and mortality in patients with severe trauma: the PROPPR randomized clinical trial. JAMA. 2015; 313(5):471–482

[7] Roberts I, Shakur H, Coats T, et al. The CRASH-2 trial: a randomised controlled trial and economic evaluation of the effects of tranexamic acid on death, vascular occlusive events and transfusion requirement in bleeding trauma patients. Health Technol Assess. 2013; 17(10):1–79

[8] Steenburg SD, Sliker CW, Shanmuganathan K, Siegel EL. Imaging evaluation of penetrating neck injuries. Radiographics. 2010; 30(4): 869–886

[9] Soto JA, Anderson SW. Multidetector CT of blunt abdominal trauma. Radiology. 2012; 265(3):678–693

[10] Provenzale JM. Imaging of traumatic brain injury: a review of the recent medical literature. AJR Am J Roentgenol. 2010; 194(1):16–19

[11] Oikonomou A, Prassopoulos P. CT imaging of blunt chest trauma. Insights Imaging. 2011; 2(3):281–295

[12] Kaewlai R, Avery LL, Asrani AV, Novelline RA. Multidetector CT of blunt thoracic trauma. Radiographics. 2008; 28(6):1555–1570

[13] Betts AM, O'Brien WT, Davies BW, Youssef OH. A systematic approach to CT evaluation of orbital trauma. Emerg Radiol. 2014; 21(5): 511–531

[14] Murphy NJ, Quinlan JD. Trauma in pregnancy: assessment, management, and prevention. Am Fam Physician. 2014; 90(10):717–722

4 General Surgery

Edited by Rebecca Kim and Milos Buhavac

4.1 Acute Abdomen

Milos Buhavac, Ronald Buczek, Austin Cannon, Bao Nguyen, and Andrea Weitz

4.1.1 Overview and Principle

- Acute abdomen refers to a constellation of signs and symptoms that include sudden-onset abdominal pain and associated tenderness on examination that requires immediate surgical evaluation and possible intervention.
- Approximately 10% of emergency room visits are for abdominal pain, so rapid assessment by surgical specialists is imperative to rule out an acute abdomen.
- History and physical examination are the mainstay of diagnosis (site, onset, character, radiation, associated symptoms, timing, exacerbating/relieving factors, severity):
  - Past medical history: To evaluate risk factors and narrow down a differential diagnosis.
  - Most important thing to ascertain: "Is the patient sick?" and "Does the patient need an operation?" and Do not delay treatment in an attempt to obtain a diagnosis.
  - Physical examination: Can be very important in narrowing down the cause, although physicians must be aware of localized and referred pain.
- All patients with a suspected acute abdomen require two intravenous (IV) lines in case of need for large volume resuscitation and a full set of laboratory tests including a blood type and red blood cell (RBC) antibody screen and when appropriate blood type and cross-match.
- If acute abdomen is suspected, general surgical consultation should be made immediately so as not to carry out unwarranted tests.
- In a hemodynamically stable patient, imaging should be obtained to confirm cause of disease and rule out nonsurgical causes.
  - Imaging includes ultrasound, computed tomography (CT) imaging with oral and IV contrast, and CT angiography.
- In a hemodynamically unstable patient, aggressive fluid resuscitation and antibiotic administration should be started immediately, before a diagnosis is made.
- Several disease entities exist that mimic an acute abdomen but do not require surgical evaluation and intervention:
  - Drugs and toxins
  - Hematologic
  - Endocrine and metabolic
- Many of the diseases that present with an acute abdomen can be managed in various ways. Early involvement of a surgical specialist to evaluate the patient, perform a history and physical examination, order appropriate laboratory tests and images, and decide on the optimal type of intervention necessary often dictates how well the patient will do and the associated morbidity and mortality they will experience.

4.1.2 Hollow Viscous Injuries Causing Acute Abdomen

- See ▶ Fig. 4.1 and ▶ Fig. 4.2.
- Hollow viscus injuries: Esophagus, stomach, small bowel, and colon.
- Esophagus:
  - Although thought of as mediastinal, if the esophagus is diseased/damaged in the peritoneal cavity, an acute abdomen can ensue.
  - Perforation: Can be secondary to Boerhaave syndrome, malignancy, caustic ingestion, foreign body ingestion; infectious and iatrogenic.
  - Rapid evaluation including physical examination (pain in the chest/epigastrium, neck, back or shoulders; vomiting, hematemesis; dysphagia; tachypnea; cough and fever), laboratory tests, imaging

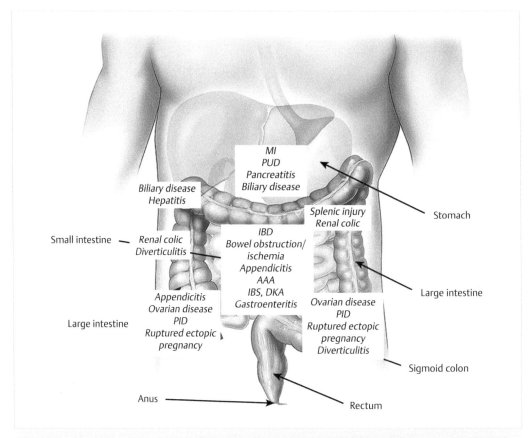

Fig. 4.1 Summary of surgical and non-surgical causes of acute abdomen. AAA, abdominal aortic aneurysm; DKA, diabetic ketoacidosis; IBD, inflammatory bowel disease; IBS, irritable bowel syndrome; MI, myocardial infarction; PID, pelvic inflammatory disease; PUD, peptic ulcer disease.

   either in the form of gastrografin swallow and thin barium swallow (full-strength barium can cause mediastinal and peritoneal fibrosis if a free perforation is present and worsen patient pain and inflammatory response) or CT esophagram (imaging may show contrast outside gastrointestinal (GI) tract, pneumomediastinum, pneumothorax, pneumoperitoneum to determine the extent of the perforation (chest, abdomen, or both) and if it is free or contained.

- Timing of presentation is key as those who present early before frank mediastinitis or peritonitis have lower associated morbidity and mortality; 10% mortality if within 24 hours but up to 50% thereafter.
- If within 24 hours, surgical intervention is warranted if the perforation is present and free in the abdomen. The decision for thoracic intervention is more nuanced and beyond the scope of this chapter.
- Aggressive resuscitation, antibiotics, and either surgical intervention, draining, or endoscopy are warranted.
- Free perforations may be closed primarily in 2 layers after adequate debridement, or if the tissue is very poor just with a pedicled flap after adequate debridement. If the tissue is too unhealthy, it can be drained widely or resected more extensively with a plan for immediate or delayed reconstruction. Finally, if resection is warranted, esophagostomy with a spit fistula in the neck is acceptable to stop further soilage.
- In the setting of a perforated esophageal malignancy, esophagectomy with diversion is warranted.

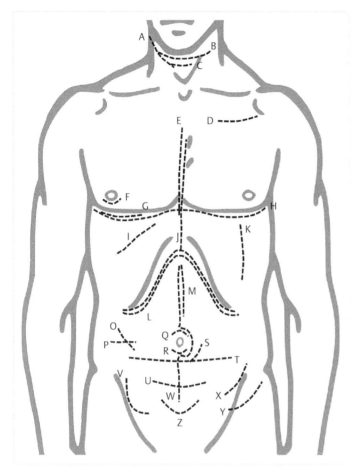

Fig. 4.2 Summary of neck, chest, and abdominal surgical incisions. A, carotid incision; B, thyroidectomy incision; C, tracheotomy incision; D, subclavicular incision; E, sternotomy incision; F, infra-areolar incision (either side); G, inframammary incision (either side); H, clamshell incision; I, Kocher/subcostal incision; J, Mercedes Benz incision; K, paramedian incision (either side); L, chevron incision; M, epigastrin/upper midline incision; O, McBurney's/ Gridiron incision (right side only, for appendectomy); P, Rockey-Davis/Lanz incision (right side only, for appendectomy); Q, supraumbilical incision; R, infraumbilical incision; S, pararectus incision; T, Maylard incision; U, Pfannenstiel/Kerr/pubic incision; V, Gibson incision (either side, but conventionally left); W, midline incision; X, inguinal incision; Y, femoral incision; Z, Turner-Warwick incision. Source: Marielle Volz (Mvolz [Public Domain]).

- ○ If a caustic injury is suspected, esophagogastroduodenoscopy (EGD) is warranted to determine the extent of the mucosal injury. Extending the myotomy and repairing the mucosal layer separately is warranted.
- ○ If surgery is chosen as the form of treatment, feeding gastrostomy or jejunostomy tubes are indicated for long-term enteral access while any repair heals.
- ○ If a contained perforation is present, then nonoperative management may be appropriate, with drains placed by interventional radiology.
- ○ Boerhaave syndrome is a rare but potentially lethal entity that results from effort-induced spontaneous rupture of the esophagus.
- ○ Hemorrhage: most esophageal-related bleeding is usually managed medically and endoscopically; Mallory Weiss syndrome (upper GI bleeding secondary to longitudinal mucosal tears) can be managed in this way, but if hemorrhage is uncontrollable and no portal hypertension is present, surgical evaluation may be necessary.
- Stomach perforation:
  - ○ Although far less common now because of the abundance of proton-pump inhibitors, gastric ulcers still are the most common cause of gastric perforation. Other causes include malignancy, caustic ingestion, foreign body ingestion, infectious, and iatrogenic.
  - ○ Five different types of gastric ulcer exist (Johnson classification):
    - – Type 1: Body/antrum of the stomach along the lesser curve. Most common, not associated with acid hypersecretion.
    - – Type 2: Type 1 ulcer + duodenal ulcer. Second most common, associated with acid hypersecretion.

- Type 3: Ulcer located in the prepyloric area. Third most common, associated with acid hypersecretion.
- Type 4: Close to the gastroesophageal junction (GEJ). Not associated with acid hypersecretion.
- Type 5: Diffuse ulceration associated with drug, most commonly nonsteroidal anti-inflammatory drug use, not associated with acid hypersecretion.

  ○ It is important to distinguish between a contained perforation and a free perforation; history and physical examination as well as imaging can help differentiate these two entities.
  ○ For patients with free perforation, there are several surgical options. If the defect is small after debridement, then a Graham patch or modified Graham patch can be attempted. If no omentum is present, then other flaps such as a jejunal serosal or falciform ligament patch can be applied.
  ○ More extensive resections include Bilroth 1 and 2 and subtotal gastrectomies with Roux-en-Y gastrojejunostomies.
  ○ If acid hypersecretion is suspected, vagotomy is indicated as part of the surgery, because of the high risk of recurrence.
  ○ All patients should be tested for *Helicobacter pylori*, and all suspicious ulcers biopsied and sent for analysis; 2-week course of eradication therapy.
  ○ Hemorrhage:
    - Most common complication of gastric ulcers.
    - If ulcer present, same classification system as above.
    - If ulcer is not present, other causes of upper intestinal hemorrhage include Dieulafoy lesion, arteriovenous malformation, esophageal varices, isolated gastric varices, and gastric cancer.
  ○ Involves the usual management algorithm for critically ill patients:
    - A: Secure the airway.
    - B: Place patient on ventilator and evaluate them for degree of aspiration that may affect ventilation.
    - C: Place two large-bore IVs or a central line for resuscitation. Obtain laboratory tests including complete blood count (CBC), coagulation panel, comprehensive metabolic panel, and ROTEM clotting analysis, and correct any coagulopathy that may be present. Transfusion should be used if appropriate.
    - Nasogastric (NG) tubes should be placed in all patients with hematemesis.
    - Resuscitation is the first step in management.
    - Patients are risk stratified according to hemodynamic status, comorbidities, age, and laboratory test results.
    - In patients who are hemodynamically stable, the first intervention should be EGD to localize the area of bleeding. Multiple risk classification systems, such as the Forrest classification, Rockall score, and Glasgow-Blatchford bleeding score, can predict mortality, risk of rebleeding, and planning of endoscopic treatment.
    - IV erythromycin should be strongly considered before EGD to improve gastric emptying and visualization.
    - In patients who have had two attempts at endoscopy and require ongoing blood transfusion but are hemodynamically stable, IR embolization is an appropriate next step in the treatment algorithm.
    - Patients who require ongoing large-volume resuscitation or are hemodynamically unstable and have had a source of bleeding identified should be taken to the operating room if appropriate for stabilization.
    - Duodenal ulcers should be approached from an anterior duodenotomy with the placement of three stitches: Figure-of-eight stitches above and below the ulcer to control bleeding from the gastroduodenal artery; a U-stitch medial to the ulcer to gain control of the transverse pancreatic branch. The medial stitch should be an absorbable suture such as Vicryl to avoid damaging the retroduodenal bile duct at this location. Bleeding duodenal ulcers are usually from a posterior wall ulcer due to the gastroduodenal artery.
    - Bleeding ulcers in other locations can be accessed through anterior gastrotomies, oversewn, and biopsied. If there is extensive devitalized tissue, resections can be performed as mentioned above.
    - After any intervention, patients should be started on a proton-pump inhibitor drip and treated for *H. pylori* if testing is positive.
  ○ Ischemia:
    - Although exceedingly rare, there are pathologies that can cause partial or total gastric ischemia.

- Gastric volvulus secondary to paraesophageal/diaphragmatic hernias; organo-axial (most common) or mesentery-axial.
- Strangulation and necrosis can occur.
- CT findings of the upper GI tract can raise concern for diagnosis, but if uncertain, can perform EGD to directly visualize ischemic mucosa.
- Ischemia after foregut surgery (gastric sleeve/bypass) due to small- and large-vessel injury can lead to leaks. Bariatric patients do not present in the usual fashion, and tachycardia is often the first sign of a staple line leak. If there is not frank peritonitis and the leak is contained, patients may be managed with drains and bowel rest.

- Small bowel:
  - Diseases of the small bowel that may lead to an acute abdomen are most commonly caused by obstructions.
  - Obstruction can be classified as intraluminal, mural, or extramural.
  - The most common causes of small-bowel obstruction in the developed world are adhesions from previous surgeries. Other causes include hernias, cancer, inflammatory bowel disease (IBD).
  - Irrespective of the cause of obstruction, the progression of the disease is usually the same.
  - Obstruction initially leads to increased peristalsis, which is why most patients describe colicky abdominal pain. When the bowel is no longer able to perform peristalsis, it distends, and water and electrolytes collect within the wall and the lumen of the bowel. Once the distention is large enough, venous outflow is halted. Once venous outflow pressures become large enough, arterial inflow is also halted. The bowel undergoes ischemia and necrosis and ultimately perforates, causing peritonitis.
  - Patients with small-bowel obstructions should undergo NG tube placement and resuscitation with appropriate fluids.
  - Intraluminal small-bowel disease:
    - Disease within the lumen of the small bowel includes foreign bodies, gallstones, infections, bezoars, enteroliths, foreign bodies, meconium, intussusception, congenital anomalies.
    - Although these can cause physical obstruction, sometimes the small bowel itself can be directly injured and cause perforation without obstruction.
    - Depending on the type of foreign body ingested, management options include endoscopic removal, surgical exploration or serial abdominal examinations and expectant management until the object is passed in the stool.
    - Depending on the degree of injury to the bowel, either segments can be resected or an enterotomy made and the offending object removed.
  - Mural small-bowel disease:
    - Many diseases can affect the wall of the small intestine including cancer—both primary neoplasms and metastasis, inflammatory conditions such as Crohn and infections, and even hematomas secondary to trauma or iatrogenic injury.
    - Benign neoplasms include adenomas, lipomas, hamartomas, and hemangiomas.
    - Benign lesions very rarely cause symptoms and are usually found incidentally during a work-up for something else or as the lead point of an intussusception.
    - Malignant lesions include neuroendocrine tumors (most common), adenocarcinomas, lymphoma, and stromal cell tumors.
    - Although the management of these tumors is beyond the scope of this chapter, some degree of resection is usually indicated in the presence of perforation or obstruction.
    - Inflammatory disease such as Crohn's disease should be managed nonoperatively because of the chronic nature of the disease and the potential for short-gut syndrome if serial resections are performed. Indications for surgery include perforation, obstruction, peritonitis, excessive bleeding, and toxic megacolon. Other nonurgent indications for surgery include stricturing disease that is not completely responsive to medical therapy.
    - Infections such as tuberculosis and actinomycosis, although rare, can also lead to inflammation and the development of an acute abdomen secondary to perforation.
  - Extramural small-bowel disease:
    - The most common cause of small-bowel obstruction is adhesions secondary to previous surgeries.

- Other causes: Adjacent tumor, abscess or infection, hematoma, malrotation, annular pancreas, endometriosis, superior mesenteric artery syndrome, volvulus.
- Good surgical acumen is necessary to distinguish patients with a partial small-bowel obstruction from those with a complete obstruction, as complete obstructions are unlikely to respond to nonoperative management. Any patient with signs of peritonitis on physical examination, laboratory data to suggest ischemia or sepsis (noncorrecting lactate despite adequate resuscitation), or imaging consistent with ischemia/necrosis or a closed-loop obstruction should be taken immediately to the operating room for surgical exploration and possible bowel resection.
- Other causes of extramural obstruction include hernias, which we will mention separately, and cancer.
- Extramural compression from benign or malignant en-bloc resection, radiation, and venting gastrostomy tubes to provide continuous decompression in palliative settings.
- Closed-loop small-bowel obstruction involves obstruction at two points along the small bowel. This can be secondary to multiple adhesions or an internal hernia. Closed-loop small-bowel obstructions can have mesenteric swirling on CT scan, suggesting volvulus of the affected bowel and impending ischemia and necrosis due to lack of blood flow. This is a surgical emergency that requires immediate operative intervention: "time is tissue," and surgery should not be delayed even if there is no evidence of peritonitis on physical examination or evidence of an immune response or elevated lactate on laboratory tests.

○ Diagnosis of small-bowel disease:
- Abdominal X-ray series.
- Includes Upright, supine, and left lateral decubitus to evaluate bowel size and free air.
- Distal gas suggests ileus rather than obstruction; air-fluid levels in small vs. large bowel suggest obstruction and can help localize site; focal closed loops of bowel suggest strangulation; bowel gas can still be seen with varying levels of obstruction.
- Sigmoid volvulus shows coffee-bean sign with apex in left lower quadrant; cecal volvulus shows large air-filled cecum in right lower quadrant.
- Enema with water-soluble contrast agent used for identifying obstruction; upper GI series with small-bowel follow-through used for uncertain lesions, partially obstructed lesions, or malrotation.
- CT imaging with oral and IV contrast used to identify transition point of obstruction, first-line imaging with suspected obstruction.

○ Treatment:
- Early postoperative obstruction usually self-resolves with bowel rest, IV fluids, correction of electrolytes, large bore nasogastric tube decompression, and treatment of primary cause (e.g., IBD).
- True complete bowel obstruction is a surgical emergency except for debilitated patients or those with a hostile abdomen.
- Early surgical consultation is advised to aid in monitoring and management.
- Gastrografin administration can be used in patients with abdominal surgery to aid in clearing obstruction and monitoring resolution.
- Contrast or air enema can aid with reduction of intussusception in children but should be used with caution in adults because of high likelihood of neoplasm.
- Flexible sigmoidoscopy with placement of rectal tube is used initially for sigmoid volvulus; recommendation for sigmoid resection because of 50% recurrence rate.
- Exploratory laparotomy is used with worsening patients, signs of peritonitis or infection, complete obstruction, ischemic bowel, nonreducible hernia; bowel diversion (e.g., colostomy with Hartmann pouch, diverting ileostomy) is used for large-bowel obstruction; colonic stenting for palliation or bridge to surgery.

• Large bowel:
○ The large bowel causes of an acute abdomen are different from those in the small bowel. Although obstruction is an important part of the differential diagnosis, infectious/inflammatory diseases are increasingly common.
○ Obstruction of the large intestine is caused by diseases similar to those of the small intestine.
○ Large-bowel obstruction is most commonly from colon cancer (60% cases).

- If encountered during a laparotomy for perforation, the affected segment of bowel should be resected along with its feeding arterial supply. Anastomosis with diversion is then a reasonable way to reconstruct. Alternatively, an end colostomy can be performed.
- Appendicitis:
  - Occurs secondary to some sort of obstructive process, either lymphoid hyperplasia or obstruction from a fecolith.
  - 6–7% of the population will develop appendicitis during their lifetime.
  - Peak in second decade of life.
  - Spectrum of disease ranges from acute uncomplicated appendicitis to perforated appendicitis.
  - Nonoperative management of acute uncomplicated appendicitis may be managed safely with antibiotics if there is absence of a fecolith.
  - Options for operative intervention include open and laparoscopic surgery.
  - Alternate pathologies found during routine appendectomy may warrant deviation from the usual protocol of removing the appendix.
    – IBD can sometimes mimic the signs and symptoms of appendicitis. If the cecum or the base of the appendix is involved and there is significant inflammation, the appendix should be left alone because of the risk of staple line leak and fistula formation. If the cecum is not involved, the appendix may be taken out so as not to confound a possible inflammatory disease diagnosis at a later date.
    – Mass on the appendix: Classic teaching tells us that if a tumor is over 2 cm or the base of the appendix is involved, a right hemicolectomy should be performed. In reality, if this is encountered and there is no evidence of perforation, the safest way to proceed may be to abort the procedure and have the patient follow up with a surgical oncologist who will be able to coordinate all further care.
  - Special mention should be given to elderly and pregnant patients. In pregnancy, the increased morbidity and mortality of ruptured appendicitis means that nonoperative management is not recommended. In elderly patients, one must exclude a malignant cause for appendicitis once an appropriate time interval has elapsed so that colonoscopy can be performed safely.
- Colonic volvulus:
  - Occurs when a segment of large intestine, usually the sigmoid colon, twists on its mesenteric axis, causing obstruction and potentially occlusion of the blood supply.
  - Sigmoid volvulus is associated with increased age, chronic constipation, and psychiatric conditions.
  - The first step in management should be correction of fluid and electrolyte abnormalities and proximal decompression with an NG tube if there is evidence of proximal bowel dilation.
  - If there are signs of peritonitis on physical examination or evidence of nonviable bowel on imaging and laboratory studies, patient should proceed immediately to the operating room for exploration and possible bowel resection.
  - If peritonitis or nonviable bowel are absent, then endoscopic detorsion should be attempted with elective resection planned because 50% of sigmoid volvulus will recur.
- Cecal or cecocolic volvulus
  - Cecal or cecocolic volvulus occurs when there is axial rotation of the terminal ileum, cecum, and ascending colon.
  - Affects women more than men and occurs most commonly in the fifth decade of life.
  - Unlike sigmoid volvulus, detorsion is not an option and resection is the procedure of choice even if there is no evidence of compromised bowel. A right hemicolectomy is the surgery of choice, and as long as patient physiology allows, an ileocolic anastomosis can be performed.
- Pseudo-obstruction:
  - Not a mechanical obstruction but rather a functional failure of bowel motility that result in massive dilation and perforation if not managed appropriately.
  - Associated with medications such as opiates and neuroleptics, metallic derangements, and a host of autoimmune disease.
  - Thought to be due to sympathetic overactivity and metabolic derangements.
  - Stepwise approach to care is based on size of cecum, which is most likely to perforate.
  - As long as there is no evidence of perforation and no distal obstructing mass, patients with cecum < 12 cm should undergo an aggressive bowel regimen, cessation of all opioids, and correction of electrolyte and metallic abnormalities.

- For patients with cecum > 12 cm, neostigmine can be attempted as well as an epidural. If this fails, colonoscopic decompression is immediately warranted.
- If all the above maneuvers fail to resolve the cecal dilation, laparotomy is indicated because of the high likelihood of perforation.

4.1.3 Inflammatory Causes of Acute Abdomen

- See ▶ Fig. 4.1 and ▶ Fig. 4.2.
- Diverticulitis:
  - This disease entity occurs when preexisting diverticula, formed by outpouchings in the colon—most commonly the descending and sigmoid colon, become inflamed.
  - Further classified as uncomplicated or complicated.
    - Uncomplicated diverticulitis can be managed in either the inpatient or outpatient setting with oral antibiotics and a short course of bowel rest. There is usually inflammation of a short segment of the colon with no evidence of abscess, stricture/obstruction, or perforation. Failure for symptoms to resolve in 24–48 hours warrants further evaluation for progression of disease.
    - Complicated diverticulitis is further subclassified into perforation, hemorrhage, obstruction, and in chronic settings, fistula formation.
  - Perforated diverticulitis follows the Hinchey classification:
    - Stage 1: Pericolonic or mesenteric abscess.
    - Stage 2: Pelvic abscess.
    - Stage 3: Purulent peritonitis.
    - Stage 4: Feculent peritonitis.
    - Stages 1 and 2 can usually be managed with IV antibiotics and, depending on the abscess size, either needle aspiration or drain placement.
    - Stages 3 and 4 are usually associated with sepsis and septic shock; after initial resuscitation patients should undergo exploratory laparotomy, washout, and resection of the affected portion of bowel. Evidence suggests that performing a primary anastomosis and diverting-loop ileostomy for stage 3 disease may be safe but that a colectomy and end colostomy should be performed for stage 4 disease.
    - There is literature that argues in favor of doing laparoscopic lavage for stage 3 disease; however, this has not been studied in any prospective trials.
  - IBD comprises a spectrum of diseases from Crohn's disease to ulcerative colitis.
  - An acute abdomen can occur when fulminant colitis, toxic megacolon, perforation, or massive bleeding occur.
  - Although uncommon, massive life-threatening hemorrhage can occur with IBD.
  - Fulminant colitis:
    - Fulminant colitis is characterized by fever, abdominal pain and tenderness, elevated white blood cell (WBC) count, and tachycardia as part of the systemic inflammatory immune response.
    - Initial treatment involves resuscitation with IV fluids, NG tube, IV antibiotics, and steroids.
    - If patients fail to respond in a timely fashion, no more than 2–3 days, laparotomy is indicated because mortality increases substantially in the presence of perforation.
  - Toxic megacolon:
    - Toxic megacolon is a separate entity to fulminant colitis and is characterized by bacterial invasion of the colon wall, dilation, and necrosis. CT imaging shows a distended colon that may have evidence of ischemia/necrosis such as pneumatosis or free air.
    - By definition, these patients present with sepsis and septic shock and should receive aggressive management to resuscitate them and prepare them for emergency surgery including IV fluids, IV antibiotics, stress dose steroids, and vaso pressor medication if necessary.
  - Surgical management in all three instances should be aimed at removing all of the potentially diseased colon without putting the patient at undue risk from an extensive surgery.
  - Total abdominal colectomy with end ileostomy in the acute setting is the safest procedure of choice. Attempting anastomosis in an acutely ill patient, especially one who is acidotic and hemodynamically unstable, will put the patient at undue risk of anastomotic leak and further complications.

- Infectious colitis:
  - There are several causes of infectious colitis, but we will focus primarily on *Clostridium difficile*.
  - It is commonly associated with antibiotic administration, with clinical presentation of disease occurring approximately 1 week after administration, although this is fairly variable.
  - Patients classically present with watery stool and, depending on the severity of disease, abdominal pain, distention, fever, and even peritonitis and cardiovascular instability in severe cases. Diarrhea may be absent in 20–30% of patients.
  - Diagnosis is made by enzyme-linked immunosorbent assay of *C. difficile* toxin in stool, polymerase chain reaction for DNA, or if uncertain via direct visualization of pseudomembranes/yellow plaques via colonoscopy/sigmoidoscopy/proctoscopy.
  - Management depends on severity of disease:
    - For initial nonsevere disease (WBCs < 15, Cr < 1.5), treatment with 125 mg of oral vancomycin four times daily for 10 days, 200 mg of fidaxomicin twice a day for 10 days, or oral 500 mg of metronidazole three times a day for 10 days if the first two options are not available.
    - For initial severe disease (WBCs > 15, Cr > 1.5), treatment should be with 125 mg of oral vancomycin four times a day for 10 days or 200 mg of fidaxomicin twice a day for 10 days.
    - For fulminant *C. difficile* colitis or *C. difficile* with septic shock or megacolon, 500 mg of enteral vancomycin four times a day (rectal vancomycin may be added in the setting of ileus) plus 500 mg of IV metronidazole three times a day.
    - Similar to fulminant colitis secondary to IBD, nonoperative management should only be trialed for 2–3 days before laparotomy is indicated. Patients with toxic megacolon should proceed immediately to the OR for exploration and possible bowel resection once they have been resuscitated and adequately prepared.
    - Total abdominal colectomy and end ileostomy is once again the procedure of choice.

4.1.4 Other Causes of Acute Abdomen

Hernia

- Protrusion of tissue through normally containing tissues; reducible if can be returned to normal location, incarcerated if nonreducible, strangulated if vascular compromise is present.
- 5% lifetime risk, 1–3% risk of strangulation that increases with age and femoral location.
- Hernias that can cause an acute abdomen are either incarcerated or strangulated. With < 4–6 hours of incarceration, it is reasonable to try to reduce most simple hernias by placing pressure onto the hernia and directing the contents back down into the peritoneal cavity through the neck of the hernia. Useful adjuncts are adequate pain medication, patient positioning in the Trendelenburg position, and ice packs to cause vasoconstriction and reduce associated edema.
- Hernias with small-diameter necks are far more likely to incarcerate and strangulate than ones with wide necks.
- Patients with incarcerated hernias should undergo reduction and evaluation for compromised bowel because of the risk of strangulation.
- Strangulated hernias already have compromised bowel within them, and patients often present with signs and symptoms of sepsis as well as evidence on imaging of ischemia and necrosis.
- Anatomy:
  - Lateral abdominal wall layers: Skin, subcutaneous fat/Camper fascia, Scarpa fascia, external oblique, internal oblique, transversus abdominis, transversalis fascia, peritoneum.
  - Inguinal canal: Contains spermatic cord, ilioinguinal nerve, genital branch of genitofemoral nerve; bordered inferiorly by inguinal ligament, superiorly by conjoint tendon.
- Locations:
  - Paraesophageal hernias: Usually are repaired electively but in rare cases can lead to gastric volvulus.
  - Diaphragmatic hernias: Either congenital or acquired through trauma or secondary to iatrogenic injury, these hernias can often be missed on CT scan. If there is suspicion, it should be evaluated via diagnostic laparoscopy.

- Internal hernia: Secondary to surgery where mesenteric defects after bowel resection do not close properly, allowing contents to herniate. Can be seen in three locations after Roux-en-Y gastric bypass surgery:
  - Petersen's defect between the Roux limb and the transverse colon mesentery.
  - Between the biliopancreatic limb and the Roux limb at the jejunojejunostomy.
  - Through the defect in the transverse mesocolon itself if a retrocolic Roux limb is used.
- Abdominal wall hernia types:
  - Ventral hernia: These can be primary hernias like umbilical hernias or secondary to trauma or previous surgery.
  - Indirect inguinal: Sac through internal ring lateral to inferior epigastric vessels, more common than direct hernia.
  - Direct inguinal: Sac through Hesselback triangle (medially bound by rectus, laterally bound by inferior epigastric vessels, inferiorly bound by inguinal ligament), medial to inferior epigastric vessels.
  - Pantaloon: Combined direct and indirect hernia.
  - Femoral: Sac exit through femoral canal (medially bound by lacunar ligament, laterally bound by femoral vessels, anteriorly bound by inguinal ligament, posteriorly bound by Cooper ligament), high risk of incarceration and strangulation, should always be taken to operating room for emergent repair.
  - Umbilical: Congenital or acquired sac exit through ventral naval.
  - Epigastric: Sac exit through linea alba above umbilicus.
  - Incisional: Sac exit through fascial defect from a prior fascial repair.
  - Rectus diastasis: Weakening of linea alba, not a true hernia.
  - Amyand: Inguinal hernia containing appendix.
  - Grynfeltt: Sac exit through superior lumbar triangle, high risk of incarceration.
  - Littre: Inguinal sac exit containing Meckel diverticulum; high risk of incarceration.
  - Obturator: Sac exit through obturator foramen; rare type of hernia in elderly women, usually multiparous; usually associated with recent weight loss.
  - Parastomal: Hernia at ostomy site.
  - Petit: Sac exit through inferior lumbar triangle.
  - Richter: Sidewall of viscus incorporated into hernia sac; incarceration can cause bowel obstruction.
  - Sciatic: Sac exit through greater or lesser sciatic foramen.
  - Sliding: Hernia composed of viscus.
  - Spigelian: Sac exit through semilunar line lateral to rectus abdominis at semicircular line.
  - De Garengeot: Appendix in a femoral hernia.
- Diagnosis: Examination through scrotum with palpation of inguinal ring to identify location, bowel obstruction, and other masses considered; CT can evaluate hernia location and hernia contents.
- Treatment: Reduction of hernia attempted; painful or indurated sac prompts urgent treatment.
- Ventral, umbilical, or incisional hernias: 3–4 cm treated open, larger treated laparoscopically; various strategies (e.g., onlay, inlay, intraperitoneal underlay, retro-rectus with or without transversus abdominis release).
- Inguinal and femoral: No consensus regarding open vs. laparoscopic repair; 1–2% recurrence rate; open repair strategies vary for inguinal hernias (e.g., Bassini, McVay, Shouldice, Lichtenstein, plug-and-patch), transabdominal preperitoneal (TAPP), total extraperitoneal preperitoneal (TEPP) approaches for laparoscopic repair, and other minimally invasive or robotic approaches.
- Complications: Eventual repair failure because of technical errors, infection similar between mesh and nonmesh approaches, preperitoneal bleeding can result in hypotension, dysejaculation (0.25%), testicular atrophy, urinary retention, ilioinguinal neuroma, or chronic pain.
- In the setting of compromised or dead bowel, mesh should be avoided, but if absolutely necessary, bioabsorbable meshes should be used to lower the risk of infection. Definitive repair can be scheduled for a later date.

Solid Organs

- Bleeding or inflammation of solid organs are common causes of acute abdomen.
- Pancreatitis is the main cause of abdominal pain that requires evaluation by a surgeon.

○ The revised Atlanta classification requires two or more of the following criteria to be present to diagnose acute pancreatitis: Abdominal pain; serum amylase or lipase three times the upper limit of normal; characteristic CT findings.

○ Gallstone and alcohol are the first and second most common causes of acute pancreatitis.

○ Classified as early phase (characterized by the systemic inflammatory response) and a late phase (occurs only in patients with moderate-to-severe pancreatitis) that is characterized by local complications and persistent organ failure.

○ Mild, moderately severe (where patients experience morbidity from local complications but little mortality), and severe pancreatitis.

○ Modified Marshall score (includes PaO_2/FiO_2, serum creatinine, systolic blood pressure, and responsiveness to fluid resuscitation) helps indicate if organ failure is present. Organ failure can further be classified as transient, lasting less than 48 hours, or persistent, lasting more than 48 hours.

○ Acute pancreatitis can also be classified as interstitial edematous pancreatitis (IEP) or necrotizing pancreatitis. Both diagnoses are made on imaging: IEP is more common vs. necrotizing pancreatitis, can involve the pancreas only, the peripancreatic space only, or both spaces.

○ Fluid collections can also be placed in one of four classifications: acute pancreatic fluid collection; acute necrotic collection; pseudocyst; walled-off necrosis.

○ Depending on the severity of disease, initial management should follow the usual airway–breathing–circulation (ABC) algorithm.

○ In patients with severe disease, placing a definitive airway may be necessary to manage the development of pleural effusions, pulmonary edema, and even acute respiratory distress syndrome. Patients who require a large-volume resuscitation are also at risk of requiring a definitive airway.

○ Mechanical noninvasive positive pressure ventilation may be necessary in patients with a reduced PaO_2/FiO_2 ratio.

○ Because of the systemic inflammatory response associated with pancreatitis, all patients should have adequate access and be receiving IV fluids. Fluids should be adjusted to ensure adequate perfusion of vital organs (e.g., monitoring urine output).

○ Infection:
  – Major source of morbidity and mortality, especially when occurring within a week of pancreatitis onset.
  – Unless there is presence of gas on scans, antibiotic therapy should not be initiated.
  – The only way to confirm the presence of infection is to sample the suspected fluid but not without risk of biopsy.
  – Recent literature supports the delay of surgical management and the placement of drains through the retroperitoneum, which can then be used as port sites for eventual debridement (i.e., the step-up approach).

○ Other life-threatening complications include hemorrhagic pancreatitis, pseudoaneurysm formation, splenic vein thrombosis, and abdominal compartment syndrome.

○ Fluid collections adjacent to major vessels can erode through vessels and form a pseudoaneurysm. Patients develop life-threatening bleeding and require emergent IR angioembolization.

○ Inflammation can cause splenic vein thrombosis, leading to isolated gastric varices, which can cause life-threatening hemorrhage. Control of these varices should first be attempted by endoscopic therapy; if that fails, a splenectomy is often necessary to prevent ongoing bleeding.

○ Abdominal compartment syndrome is a complication of a large-volume resuscitation. Associated signs are increased peak airway pressures, difficulty with ventilation, increased central venous pressure, evidence of end-organ hypoperfusion in the setting of intra-abdominal hypertension, which can be measured by bladder pressures in a paralyzed patient.

• Vasculature:

○ GI bleeding: See Chapter 14.2, Abdominal Pathology.

○ Abdominal vascular causes: See Chapter 5.1.3, Vascular Occlusion and Ischemia and Ischemia and 5.3 Vascular Aneurysms and Dissections.

○ Abdominal vasculature can itself lead to an acute abdomen in the form of an abdominal aortic aneurysm (AAA) or cause ischemia of the bowel secondary to dissection, low-flow states, or occlusion of blood vessels from an embolic or thrombotic source.

○ Patients can present with an acute abdomen and then rapidly decline in the setting of rupture.
○ 50% of patients with a ruptured AAA die before arrival to the hospital.
○ Patients that are symptomatic or have evidence of rupture on scan require emergent surgery.
○ Once again, management proceeds in an algorithmic order. In stable patients, intubation and mechanical ventilation can wait. Placement of large-bore IVs for fluid resuscitation is imperative as is doing laboratory tests to obtain a blood type and crossmatch.
○ Alerting vascular surgery early is key to optimizing outcomes for these patients.
○ Compromising blood flow to the bowels is a surefire way to ensure ischemia and potentially necrosis and perforation.
○ Shock from sepsis, hypotension, cardiogenic shock, or other types of malperfusion can lead to reversible or irreversible tissue ischemia. In disease states, blood flow to the intestines is often one of the first things to be sacrificed. By ensuring adequate resuscitation, blood flow can be restored and bowel ischemia, necrosis, and perforation avoided. The use of vasopressors may increase mean arterial pressure at the expense of splanchnic flow.
○ Mesenteric emboli are most often due to cardiac arrhythmias, specifically atrial fibrillation. Other etiologies include myocardial infarction, more proximal thrombus, and clotting disorders. Emboli tend to lodge in the distal mesenteric arterial vessels and cause segmental bowel infarction. These areas should be resected and the bowel observed for further ischemia while the patient is receiving anticoagulation medications.
○ Mesenteric thrombosis tends to occur in the setting of chronic mesenteric ischemia and is located more proximally in the mesenteric arterial tree. The amount of bowel that is affected can be more substantial. Areas of nonviable bowel should be resected and the patient left in discontinuity with an open abdomen until an appropriate vascular intervention is performed.
○ Watershed areas can be at particular risk as the boundary between major vascular blood supplies is treated. Griffith's point at the splenic flexure and Sudek's point at the rectosigmoid junction are at particular risk.

4.2 Abdominal Pathology

Milos Buhavac, Austin Cannon, Bao Nguyen, and Andrea Weitz

4.2.1 Gastrointestinal Bleeding

• Definition:
  ○ Hematemesis: Bright red or coffee ground emesis, upper GI bleed.
  ○ Hematochezia: Bright red blood per rectum, lower GI bleed, or large upper GI bleed.
  ○ Melena: Black tarry stool, gradual upper GI bleed.
• Differential diagnosis: Gastric or duodenal ulcer, hemorrhoids, GI instrumentation, antiplatelet medication, blunt/penetrating trauma, varices, angiodysplasia, diverticulosis, neoplasms, esophagitis/gastritis/colitis, IBD, chronic alcohol or drug use.
• Diagnosis: Evaluation of vital signs for shock; CBC and basic metabolic panel (BMP) used to assess status; history and physical examination used to evaluate for cirrhosis; digital rectal examination to assess hemorrhoids, anal fissure/fistula, or rectal mass; CT is helpful in select cases.
• Treatment:
  ○ Two large-bore IV lines; initial resuscitation with crystalloid then 1:1:1 packed RBCs/platelets/fresh-frozen protein; Foley catheter to monitor volume status and adequacy of resuscitation; transfer to intensive care unit depending on hemodynamic instability.
  ○ Nasogastric tube to reduce aspiration risk; gross blood indicates upper GI.
  ○ EGD vs. colonoscopy with intervention performed depending on ability to localize bleed source and type.
  ○ Angiography with embolization useful for bleeds > 1 mL/min.
  ○ Tagged RBC scan can be used for nonurgent bleed localization.

- Gastritis and peptic ulcer disease:
  - Gastritis: Inflammation of intestinal mucosa; described by location and erosive vs. nonerosive; commonly found in antrum and body; chronic variant results in loss of mucosa or metaplastic changes; untreated can progress to ulcer disease.
  - Peptic ulcer disease: Disruption in lining of stomach or duodenum; 2% U.S. incidence.
  - Duodenal ulcer is more common in younger patients, and gastric ulcer in elderly.
  - Causes: Chronic nonsteroidal anti-inflammatory drug (NSAID) use, cigarette smoke, burn injury (e.g., Curling ulcer), traumatic brain injury (e.g., Cushing ulcer), massive transfusion, sepsis, trauma.
  - Presents: Epigastric abdominal burning with eating (gastric) or postprandial (duodenal).
  - *Helicobacter pylori* found with 90% of duodenal ulcers and 70–90% of gastric ulcers; 33% U.S. incidence; diagnosed with biopsy or fecal antigen test; confirmed cured with urea breath test; treated with triple therapy (proton pump inhibitor [PPI], clarithromycin AND amoxicillin OR metronidazole); cultured with antibiotic resistance or concerning ulcer features.
  - Classified by modified Johnson classification based on ulcer location.
  - Complicated disease is associated with hemodynamic instability, peritonitis, jaundice, or mass.
  - Diagnosis: Physical examination, CBC, BMP, *H. pylori* testing, EGD, or upper GI series if warranted.
  - Zollinger-Ellison syndrome:
    - Pancreatic, duodenal, or nodal gastrinoma resulting in diarrhea.
    - Multiple concurrent duodenal and gastric ulcers.
    - Diagnosed with elevated gastrin levels, CT, ultrasound, octreotide, and rarely angiography with venous sampling.
    - Treatment: Surgical resection curative in 60% patients but 50% of lesions are malignant.
  - Treatment:
    - Nasogastric decompression, proton-pump inhibitor or H2 blocker, treatment of *H. pylori*, smoking cessation, modification of medications (e.g., NSAIDs).
    - EGD for biopsy of gastric ulcers and control of bleeding with cauterization, epinephrine injection or clipping, surgical.
    - Surgical options for large duodenal ulcers: Highly selective vagotomy; omental patch over perforated duodenum; truncal vagotomy with pyloroplasty or gastrojejunostomy; vagotomy with antrectomy and gastroduodenostomy (Billroth I), loop gastrojejunostomy (Billroth II), or Roux-en-Y gastrojejunostomy; distal gastrectomy with Billroth I, Billroth II, or Roux-en-Y reconstruction.
  - Complications of surgical treatment: Early or late dumping after pyloroplasty or gastrojejunostomy (5–10%); diarrhea (5–10%); delayed gastric emptying; afferent or efferent loop syndrome; Roux stasis syndrome; marginal ulcer; bile reflux gastritis; cholelithiasis; nutritional deficiencies.
- Esophageal varices:
  - Dilation of distal esophageal vessels due to portal hypertension.
  - Treatment: Initial treatment with vasopressin; β-blockers; EGD with treatment; Sengstaken-Blakemore tube or four-port Minnesota tube used for balloon tamponade; various transjugular intrahepatic portosystemic shunt (TIPS) used for nontransplant candidates, increased risk of encephalopathy.
- Mallory-Weiss tear:
  - Mucosal tear at GEJ due to retching or vomiting.
  - Treatment: Observation; antiemetic; endoscopic stenting vs. surgical repair can be used.
- Dieulafoy lesion:
  - Enlarged artery with in gastric mucosa; usually on lesser stomach curvature but can occur elsewhere; congenital.
  - Treatment: EGD treatment (injection, coagulation, clips); treated surgically or with embolization in refractory cases.
- Diverticulosis:
  - Outpouching of bowel; 30% incidence in patients by age 60 years, 25% lifetime risk of bleeding; 25% risk of complications (e.g., abscess, bowel obstruction, colovesical fistula, peritonitis).
  - Associated with aging, obesity, smoking, poor exercise, low-fiber diets, steroids, NSAIDs.

- Treatment: Observation, colonoscopy with coiling, vasopressin injection, rarely requires surgical treatment.
- Arteriovenous malformations:
  - Vascular abnormality with increased incidence in elderly.
  - Diagnosed with angiography or colonoscopy.
  - Treatment: Observation; segmental resection with chronic bleeding.
- Meckel diverticulum:
  - Most common congenital lesion of small bowel; ectopic gastric and pancreatic tissue; results in ileal ulceration; localized with nuclear medicine scan (Meckel's scan).
  - Associated with intussusception in children.
  - Treatment: Segmental resection with end-to-end anastomosis.
- Benign anorectal disease:
  - 11% of lower GI bleeding; commonly includes hemorrhoids, anorectal varices, fissures, and fistulas.
  - Treatment: Observation with conservative management; diet modification; surgical treatment used for refractory conditions.
- Aortoenteric fistula:
  - Abnormal connection between aorta and bowel after aortic aneurysm repair; presents > 6 months after aneurysm repair; usually 3rd or 4th portion of duodenum; diagnosed with CT.
  - Treatment: Resection and reconstruction.

4.2.2 Esophageal Diseases

- Achalasia:
  - Poor esophageal peristalsis with incomplete relaxation of lower esophageal sphincter; idiopathic degeneration or infectious degeneration of Auerbach plexus.
  - 1–10% risk of squamous cell carcinoma (SCC) after 15–25 years.
  - Presents: Dysphagia progressive from liquids to solids, regurgitation, pain, nocturnal coughing, recurrent pulmonary infections.
  - Diagnosis: Barium swallow study shows bird's beak narrowing of distal esophagus with proximal dilation; esophageal manometry gold standard of testing and usually shows aperistaltic esophagus with non relaxing LES.
  - Treatment: Nitrates (e.g., isosorbide), calcium channel blockers (e.g., nifedpine), and Botox injection (poor surgical candidates); pneumatic balloon esophageal dilation (70% effective); laparoscopic Heller myotomy with partial fundoplication (gold standard); esophagectomy for refractory cases, per-oral endoscopic myotomy (POEM).
- Diffuse esophageal spasm:
  - Repetitive, uncoordinated esophageal spasm worse during periods of stress.
  - Presents: Chest pain, dysphagia, reflux.
  - Diagnosis: Barium swallow study shows a corkscrew esophagus, manometry shows simultaneous, multipeak, or > 2.5-second contractions.
  - Treatment: Avoiding triggers; nitrates; calcium channel blockers; anticholinergic agents; Botox injections; esophagomyotomy and partial fundoplication for medically refractory cases.
- Nutcracker esophagus:
  - Hypermotile peristalsis of unknown etiology.
  - Presents: Chest pain, dysphagia, reflux (50%).
  - Diagnosis: Manometry showing contractions 2 standard deviations above normal, particularly at the lower esophageal sphincter.
  - Treatment: Treatment of reflux; nitrates; calcium channel blockers; antispasmotics; laparoscopic Heller myotomy with partial fundoplication.
- Hypertensive lower esophageal sphincter:
  - Diagnosis: Manometry showing sphincter pressure > 35 mm Hg with normal relaxation; usually normal peristalsis.
  - Treatment: Botox injection; balloon esophageal dilation; laparoscopic Heller myotomy with partial fundoplication.

- Scleroderma:
  - Fibrosis of esophageal smooth muscle, loss of lower esophageal sphincter tone, poor peristalsis resulting in reflux and esophagitis.
  - Diagnosis: Manometry showing poor lower esophageal sphincter tone with normal relaxation.
  - Treatment: Reflux treatment; partial fundoplication.
- Esophageal diverticula:
  - Abnormal outpouchings of epithelial-line mucosa.
  - True diverticula involve all three layers, false diverticula involve mucosa and submucosa, traction diverticula result from inflammatory lymph nodes pulling esophageal tissue, pulsion diverticula result from elevated intraluminal pressure.
  - Zenker diverticulum: Most common type; more often in older patients; false diverticulum; herniation between thyropharyngeus and cricopharyngeus muscles in Killian triangle; presents with aspiration, halitosis, regurgitation of undigested food; diagnosed with barium esophagram; treated with diverticulectomy with possible myotomy of cricopharyngeus muscle, endoscopic transoral stapling.
  - Midesophagus: Usually traction diverticulum from infection; most often asymptomatic; diagnosed with barium enema or chest CT.
  - Epiphrenic: False diverticula; associated with motility disorder due to thickened musculature or increased intraluminal pressure; treated with diverticulectomy.
- Gastroesophageal reflux:
  - Decreased lower esophageal tone, shortening of the intra-abdominal esophageal segment, hiatal hernia, increased intra-abdominal pressure, and poor esophageal motility result in gastric acid reflux.
  - Presents with heart burn (80%), regurgitation (50%), dysphagia, pain, bloating, wheezing.
  - Diagnosis: Upper endoscopy used to rule out other diseases, including esophagitis, Barrett esophagus, and cancer; manometry used to rule out motility disorders; esophagogram used to evaluate gastroesophageal pathology.
  - Barrett esophagus: Prolonged gastric juice reflux resulting in metaplasia of the distal esophagus, 50 × increased risk of adenocarcinoma.
  - Treatment: 6 weeks of PPIs or H2 blockers initiated based on history; dietary modifications (avoiding smoking, alcohol, fatty foods, eating within 2 hours of bedtime, weight loss, elevating head of bed); fundoplication (e.g., Nissen, Dor, or Toupet types) used for inadequate symptom control or esophageal metaplasia; Collis gastroplasty may be indicated for a short esophagus (to lengthen the intra-abdominal portion).
  - Surgical complications: Pneumothorax, gastroesophageal injury, delayed gastric emptying, hiatal hernia; dysphagia, increased flatulence, bloating, or vomiting from fundoplication.
- Hiatal hernia:
  - Abnormal esophageal migration above the diaphragm.
  - Type I/sliding: GEJ above diaphragm; 90% cases; results from weakness of the esophageal hiatus and increased intra-abdominal pressure; reflux common; surgically treated if symptomatic or reflux.
  - Type II/paraesophageal/rolling: Rare type of herniation; surgery recommended.
  - Type III: Combination of types I and II; stomach cardia and fundus herniate into thorax.
  - Type IV: Stomach and other intra-abdominal organs herniate into thorax.

4.2.3 Intestinal Obstruction

- Adynamic ileus/acute paralytic ileus:
  - Functional obstruction of the bowels due to poor motility.
  - Causes:
    - Metabolic: Electrolyte derangement, ketoacidosis.
    - Medications: Narcotics, anticholinergics, polypharmacy, dopaminergics, antipsychotics, tricyclic antidepressants.
    - Infection: Sepsis, peritonitis, focal abdominal infections.
    - Other: Pancreatitis, hematoma, vertebral fracture.
    - Neuropathy: Diabetes, multiple sclerosis, Hirschsprung disease.
  - Ogilvie syndrome: Colonic pseudo-obstruction secondary to surgery or severe illness; typically older adults.

- ○ Cecal dilation > 12 cm concerning for risk of perforation, risk of bowel necrosis regardless of decompression.
- ○ Presentation: Nausea, vomiting, decreased flatus, constipation, abdominal pain, abdominal fullness, decreased abdominal sounds.
- ○ Diagnosis: History and examination, BMP with evaluation of electrolytes, acidosis/alkalosis, urinalysis, amylase in select cases; abdominal X-rays used to evaluate and monitor ileus.
- ○ Treatment: 2–5 days bowel rest if mild; electrolyte repletion; revaluation of medications; digital rectal exam to rule out obstruction; enema; colonoscopic decompression; IV neostigmine in monitored setting due to risk of bradycardia; partial colectomy.
- Dynamic ileus:
  - ○ Functional obstruction of bowels due to prolonged muscular contraction.
  - ○ Causes: Heavy metal poisoning, porphyria, uremia, intestinal ulceration.
- Bowel obstruction: See Chapter 4.1 Acute Abdomen.

4.2.4 Inflammatory Bowel Disease (IBD)

- Inflammatory conditions of the bowel resulting in fibrosis, strictures, and fistulas.
- Risk factors: Family history of IBD, smoking, infection, diet, alcohol, oral contraceptives, immunological diseases.
- Extraintestinal findings in IBD: Erythema nodosum (5–15%; red, raised rash on lower legs; more often in women), pyoderm gangrenosum (erythematous lesion on leg that can form a painful ulcer), ocular inflammation (10%; includes uveitis, iritis, conjunctivitis, and episcleritis), arthritis, sacroilitis/ankylosing spondylitis, fatty liver infiltration (40–50%), cirrhosis (2–5%), primary sclerosing cholangitis (40–60%), pericholangitis, cholangiocarcinoma.
- Ulcerative colitis (UC):
  - ○ Diffuse inflammatory disease of colorectal mucosa, not transmural; rectum involved in 95% of cases and inflammation spreads contiguously from distal to proximal; crypt abscesses with inflammatory pseudopolyps may be present.
  - ○ Presents: Bloody diarrhea, rectal bleeding, rectal cramping (tenesmus).
  - ○ Incidence 8–15:100,000 in the United States.
  - ○ Diagnosis: CBC, BMP, stool culture for infection, nutritional status evaluation, abdominal X-ray to evaluate colonic distension and exclude toxic megacolon or pneumoperitoneum, barium enema useful to evaluate bowel pathology, endoscopy used to identify disease extent and biopsy sites.
  - ○ Toxic megacolon: Seen in 10% of cases; high risk of perforation with high mortality (40%); significant pain; colon > 6 cm; treated with bowel rest, decompression, IV steroids, evaluation of infection and antibiotics, total colectomy if patient perforation, peritonitis, or hemorrhage develops.
  - ○ Colorectal cancer risk increases 1–2% after 8–10 years of disease; carcinoma ruled out with strictures; surveillance colonoscopy required.
  - ○ Treatment: First-line treatment aims to reduce inflammation (sulfasalazine, mesalamine), antibiotics used to treat colitis or toxic megacolon, corticosteroids, immunosuppression (e.g., azathioprine, cyclosporine, methotrexate, vedolizumab); surgical treatments: proctocolectomy with ileal pouch to anal anastomosis and diverting loop ileostomy, proctocolectomy with end ileostomy, total abdominal colectomy with ileorectal anastomosis. Depending on the severity of the disease, the operations are typically performed in a 2- or 3-stage manner that allows the inflammation to settle prior to proctectomy. If rectum is left behind, this needs close surveillance given cancer risk.
- Crohn's disease (CD):
  - ○ Chronic, transmural, granuloma-forming, segmental/skip lesions, intermittent inflammation of any portion of the GI tract (mouth to anus).
  - ○ Most commonly affects terminal ileum and cecum (55%), followed by distal rectum and anal canal (35%), small bowel (30%), and colon (15%).
  - ○ Presents: Diarrhea (90%), recurrent abdominal pain, obstructive symptoms, recurrent anal fissures/fistulas/abscesses, malnutrition, extraintestinal symptoms (30%), toxic megacolon (5%).

- ○ Diagnosis: CBC, albumin, bowel function tests, anti-*Saccharomyces cerevisiae* serological markers (60%); upper GI series with small-bowel follow-through, barium enema and CT can evaluate bowel; EGD or colonoscopy used for biopsy and surveillance follow-up.
- ○ Less common risk of colorectal carcinoma than UC except for pancolitis.
- ○ Treatment: Oral aminosalicylate (e.g., mesalamine); antibiotics (e.g., metronidazole, fluoroquinolones); corticosteroids for acute exacerbation; immunosuppression (e.g., azathioprine, 6-mercaptopurine, cyclosporine, infliximab, vedolizumab); drainage of intra-abdominal abscesses; resection after stabilization of acute flares; total colectomy or proctectomy with end ileostomy used for medically refractory cases; stricturoplasty or repair of fistulas depends on cases; goal to preserve bowel and avoid short bowel syndrome.
- ○ Recurrence rate of 40–50% after 10 years from an initial operation, 75% of patients undergo some surgical treatment, 15% mortality at 30 years otherwise patients live normal lives.
- Indeterminate colitis: 10–15% of cases of unclear UC or CD; mimics infectious colitis.

4.2.5 Colorectal Disease

- Hemorrhoids:
  - ○ Abnormal dilation of a fibrovascular cushion; internal vs. external type in relation to dentate line.
  - ○ Internal hemorrhoids:
    - – First degree: Painless bleeding without prolapse.
    - – Second degree: Prolapse with defecation but spontaneously reduces.
    - – Third degree: Prolapse with defecation requiring manual reduction.
    - – Fourth degree: permanently prolapsed.
  - ○ Presentation: Bright red painless bleeding (low-grade internal type or external type without thrombosed veins) or painful bleeding (incarcerated or prolapsed internal type with or without manual reduction), pruritus, does not show incontinence.
  - ○ Diagnosis: Physical examination and rule out of other external conditions; endoscopy, anoscopy, or colonoscopy used for concerning patients.
  - ○ Treatment: Increased fiber and fluid intake, improved anal hygiene, avoidance of straining with bowel movements, topical steroids or vasoconstricting agents used for all hemorrhoids initially; rubber band ligation used for persistent internal hemorrhoids, sclerotherapy used for patients with anticoagulation or immunocompromise, cryo- or thermoablation can be used as options; surgical treatment involves Ferguson hemorrhoidectomy, circumferential staple hemorrhoidectomy, or hemorrhoidal artery ligation.
  - ○ Thrombosed external hemorrhoids with pain presenting within 48 hours can be excised.
- Anal fissure:
  - ○ Tear in dermal skin of anus distal to the dentate line; commonly posterior midline due to strained defecation and elevated internal anal sphincter pressure causing tissue ischemia.
  - ○ Lateral or multiple tears raise concern for trauma, IBD, neoplasm, or infection.
  - ○ Treatment: Stool softeners, laxatives, sitz baths, topical calcium channel blockers, anesthetic suppositories, nitrates, Botox of internal anal sphincter; surgically treated with lateral internal sphincterotomy or fissurectomy with flap.
- Anorectal abscess:
  - ○ Infection of the anus; simple if superficial vs. complex and extends deeply; 50% become chronic and can result in fistula formation; associated with trauma, constipation, infection, IBD, or idiopathic (most cases).
  - ○ Classification by location: Ischiorectal, interspincteric, transphincteric, perianal/subcutaneous (most common), supralevator (least common), horseshoe abscess (circumferential around anus or rectum).
  - ○ Presents: Significant perianal pain and tenderness.
  - ○ Diagnosis: Physical exam usually sufficient, proctosigmoidoscopy used to rule out other conditions, CT used to evaluate deep abscesses, abscesses with intra-abdominal sources, or obese patients.
  - ○ Treatment: Superficial abscesses drained and packed in emergency department; antibiotics used for cellulitis, fasciitis, immunocompromised patients, or patients who fail to improve; complex abscesses drained in operating room with debridement of necrotizing fasciitis or Fournier gangrene if needed and repair of fistulas.

- Fistula:
  - Abnormal communication between skin and anal canal.
  - Classification by location: Superficial, intersphincteric, transsphincteric, suprasphincteric, extrasphincteric.
  - Presents: Anal drainage, history of abscess, granulation tissue at opening, probing with or without magnetic resonance imaging (MRI) used to delineate anatomy.
  - Treatment: Fistulotomy used for simple fistulas by opening tract allowing healing by secondary intention; complex fistulas ligated with seton (e.g., heavy suture, or vessel loop) used to induce tract fibrosis or occlusion with plug/fibrin.
- Pilonidal disease:
  - Obstructed hair follicle at top of intergluteal cleft resulting in abscess or chronic drainage; must rule out fistula and deeper infections.
  - Treatment: Weekly hair shaving, sitz bath, phenol injections, abscess drainage, or resection of chronic lesions.
- Pruritus ani:
  - Chronic itching of anal skin; 1–5% incidence mostly in males age 40–70 years; 100 different causes most commonly due to anorectal issues (e.g., hemorrhoids, fissures); other causes include infection, contact dermatitis, food allergies, dermatological conditions, steroid-induced dermatitis.
  - Treatment: Maintaining hygiene, treatment of secondary causes, sitz bath, warm tap water enema, removal of irritants, corticosteroid cream, zinc oxide barrier cream, capsaicin cream, anal tattooing/nerve denervation with methylene blue.
- Rectal prolapse:
  - Redundant protrusion of rectal mucosa or rectal intussusception (false/incomplete), complete protrusion of rectal wall through anal orifice (true/complete type).
  - More common in elderly women with multiparity and chronic constipation and straining.
  - Presents: Fecal incontinence, physical findings.
  - Diagnosis: Sigmoidoscopy to evaluate bowel condition and lesions; manometry, electromyography, and defecography used for further investigation MRI and CT to evaluate causes.
  - Treatment:
    - False prolapse: Conservative treatment in children with reduction of rectum after defecation; hemorrhoidectomy with mucosal resection, stool bulking, biofeedback, and pelvic floor exercises used in adults.
    - True prolapse: Abdominal rectopexy with sigmoid resection, rectopexy with mesh, perineal rectosigmoidectomy/Altemeir procedure, mucosal stripping/Delorme procedure.

4.2.6 Bariatric Surgery

- Adult weight classes defined by body mass index (BMI): overweight (25–29.9); Class I obesity (30–34.9); Class II (severe) obesity (35–39.9), Class III (morbid) obesity (≥40.0).
- Pediatric weight classes (BMI): overweight (85–95th percentile), obese (>95th percentile), severe obesity (99th percentile).
- 1/3 population in U.S. obese.
- Obesity increases risk of certain cancer (e.g., endometrial, breast, colorectal), hypertension, myocardial infarction risk, obstructive sleep apnea, type 2 diabetes, nonalcoholic steatohepatitis, gastroesophageal reflux, cholelithiasis, acute pancreatitis, preeclampsia, musculoskeletal pain, and osteoarthritis.
- Obesity promotes prothombosis because of high intra-abdominal pressures resulting in venous compression, reduced activity, and higher peripheral estrogen from fat cells.
- Medical treatment:
  - Physical activity, diet modification, behavioral modification.
  - Lorcaserin (appetite suppressant), orlistat (lipase binder) with limited long-term benefit.
- Surgical treatments:
  - Selection: BMI ≥ 40, BMI ≥ 35 with associated comorbidities, failure of nonsurgical weight loss, absence of severe comorbidities (e.g., cardiac disease, drug/alcohol use, psychiatric conditions, coagulopathy).
  - Work-up: Nutritional, psychological, sleep apnea, and cardiovascular assessment.

○ Strategies: malabsorptive, restrictive, or combined operations.

○ Range of 40–66% weight loss depending on procedure and patient, maximized weight loss at 18–24 months.

○ Laparoscopic sleeve gastrectomy (stomach stapling), laparoscopic roux-en-y gastric bypass (stomach shrinking, gastrojejunostomy, jejunojejunostomy), laparoscopic gastric banding (balloon around gastric cardia), biliopancreatic diversion.

○ Complications: Gastric leak with fistulization, internal hernia, dumping syndrome, stricture formation, marginal ulcer.

• Bariatric surgery decreases mortality risk; can resolve type 2 diabetes, hypertension, gastroesophageal reflux, sleep apnea, joint pain.

4.3 Pancreas and Hepatobiliary Pathology

Michael Karsy and Milos Buhavac

4.3.1 Pancreatic Disease

• Physiology[1,2]:

○ Endocrine function: Islets of Langerhans form endocrine cells within exocrine tissue (alpha cell: glucagon; β cell: insulin; gamma cell: pancreatic polypeptide; delta cell: somatostatin).

○ Exocrine function: Endopeptidase, exopeptidases, and other enzymes.

○ Pancreas divisum: Failure of duct of Wirsung and duct of Santorini to fuse.

○ Annular pancreas: Ring of pancreatic tissue encircling duodenum and rarely causing obstruction.

○ Heterotopic pancreatic tissue: Common around duodenum, gastric mucosa, and Meckel diverticulum.

○ Accessory duct: Secondary duct entering duodenum, main pancreatic duct joins common bile duct to empty in medial second portion of duodenum at ampulla of Vater.

• Acute pancreatitis:

○ Heterogeneous, multifactorial inflammation of the pancreas.

○ Mostly self-limited (90%); most common cause of hospitalization for GI disease; 50% risk of infection; 2% mortality in acute pancreatitis vs. 50% mortality in pancreatitis with infection/necrosis.

○ Type and severity distinguished by Atlanta Classification[3]:
  – Type: Edematous interstitial vs. necrotizing.
  – Severity: Mild (no organ or systemic complications), moderate (transient organ failure or systemic complications), severe (persistent multiorgan failure).

○ Causes: Toxic metabolites (e.g., alcohol), oxidative stress (e.g., fats, alcohol), stone/ductal obstruction, necrotizing fibrosis (e.g., disruption of pancreas architecture), immune destruction of duct.

○ Risk factors: Cholelithiasis (40%), alcohol (40%), idiopathic (15%), obstruction, neoplasms, infection/ parasites, pancreas divisum (rare), hypercalcemia, hyperlipidemia, trauma, hereditary (e.g., hyperlipoproteinemia, cystic fibrosis), iatrogenic from surgery or procedures, medications.

○ Prognostic tools: Ranson criteria, Acute Physiology and Chronic Health Evaluation II (APACHE II) score, Bedside Index of Severity in Acute Pancreatitis (BISAP), modified Marshall scoring system.

○ Diagnosis: Turner sign (left flank ecchymosis), Cullen sign (periumbilical ecchymosis), CBC, BMP, coagulation factors, amylase (elevated in 90% of cases, sensitive but not specific for pancreatitis, useful to follow disease), lipase (specific but not sensitive, diagnostic), hepatic function panel, abdominal X-ray can show dilated bowel loop near pancreas, ultrasound (used to evaluate cholelithiasis), CT imaging with IV contrast (most common imaging modality), endoscopic retrograde cholangiopancreatography/magnetic resonance cholangiopancreatography (used to diagnose and/or treat gallstone pancreatitis), fine-needle aspiration to evaluate infection.

○ Treatment: Monitoring in intensive care unit, restricted oral intake, IV hydration, nasogastric decompression, Foley catheter to monitor urine output, broad-spectrum antibiotics (e.g., imipenem) for infected pancreatitis, meperidine > morphine for pain control, treatment of alcohol withdrawal, nasojejunal feeding after stabilization, octreotide for bowel rest; surgical treatment based on step-up approach used for infected pancreatic necrosis, secondary conditions, or repair of ascites.

- ○ Pseudocyst: Fluid-filled space near pancreas that communicates with ductal system; usually self-resolve but if > 6 cm unlikely to resolve; can result in erosion into vessels, gastric obstruction, or perforation with peritonitis; treated after 4–6 weeks by endoscopic, surgical, or percutaneous drainage.
  - ○ Complications: Pseudocyst, hemorrhage, splenic vein thrombosis, pancreatic ascites, pancreaticoenteric fistula.
- Chronic pancreatitis:
  - ○ Recurrent abdominal pain with pancreatic insufficiency and destruction.
  - ○ Causes: Alcohol, recurrent cholelithiasis, smoking, autoimmune disease, hypercalcemia, diabetes, hereditary causes, pancreas divisum, idiopathic, tropical pancreatitis.
  - ○ Presents: Abdominal pain, weight loss, steatorrhea.
  - ○ Work-up: Similar to acute pancreatitis; fecal elastase can be more useful.
  - ○ Treatment: Pain control, behavioral modification, antacid, pancreatic enzyme supplementation, steroids for autoimmune pancreatitis, surgical management of pancreatitis-related issues (e.g., pseudocysts, bowel obstruction), pancreatic resection for refractory cases (e.g., Beger, Berne, Duval, Frey, Puestow, or Whipple procedures; pancreatectomy), autologous islet cell transplantation, celiac plexus blockade for pain control.

4.3.2 Hepatobiliary Disease

- Gallbladder anatomy: 30- to 50-mL capacity, 300-mL capacity when obstructed; located between right and left hepatic lobes; left and right hepatic ducts form common duct, cystic duct connects to common duct, common duct empties into duodenum; Calot triangle (defined by the common hepatic duct, liver, and cystic duct); significant anatomical and blood supply variability; intraoperative visualization of "critical view" of hepatocystic triangle (borders of cystic duct, gallbladder edge, liver edge) cleared of fat and fibrous tissue necessary for safe resection; lower 1/3 of gallbladder separated from the liver to expose the cystic plate; structures should be seen entering the gallbladder.[4]
- Cholelithiasis:
  - ○ Defines stones within gallbladder however disease may exist with or without stones.
  - ○ Cholesterol supersaturation most critical to gallstone formation.
  - ○ 12% of population with 80% asymptomatic.
  - ○ Risk factors: Female (2 × as common), older adults, obesity, pregnancy, rapid weight loss, total parenteral nutrition, pancreatitis, diabetes, malabsorption, hemolytic conditions, spinal cord injury, increased triglyceride levels, medications (e.g., estrogens).
  - ○ Gallstone types: Mixed (75%), pure cholesterol (10%), bilirubin pigmented (15%).
  - ○ Prophylactic cholecystectomy is controversial but is considered in American Indians because of higher rate of cancer, heart and lung transplant patients.
  - ○ Cholecystectomy can be safely performed during pregnancy.
  - ○ Medical treatments: Dissolution therapy with chenodeoxycholic acid for reducing cholesterol-to-bile salt ratio useful for small stones but high recurrence rate; extracorporeal shock wave lithotripsy similar to dissolution therapy.
  - ○ Biliary colic:
    - – Intermittent cystic duct obstruction by stone; 50–70% recur; 1–2% risk of complications.
    - – Presents: Steady pain in right upper quadrant (RUQ), follows fatty meal, 1–6 hours, steady pain, mild tenderness to palpation, negative Murphy sign.
    - – Diagnosis: Ultrasound (95% sensitive, 90% specific), X-rays only helpful for some stones.
    - – Treatment: Colic with gallstones treated with elective laparoscopic cholecystectomy.
  - ○ Acute calculus cholecystitis:
    - – Stone obstruction of cystic duct; 75% recur; 17% complication rate.
    - – Presents: Acute, RUQ pain, pain lasts > 6 hours, fevers, Murphy sign, palpable gallbladder (30% of cases).
    - – Diagnosis: Elevated leukocytes, alkaline phosphatase, serum aminotransferase, bilirubin; ultrasound (primary imaging); CT scan used to evaluate cholecystitis complications; hepatobiliary iminodiacetic acid (HIDA) scan (95% sensitive but takes time).
    - – Complications: Hydrops of gallbladder, gangrenous cholecystitis, gallbladder empyema, perforation, emphysematous cholecystitis.

- Treatment: IV hydration, antibiotics if severe or complicated cholecystitis, elective laparoscopic chole-cystectomy within 72 hours or sooner if immunocompromised, percutaneous drain placement can be used as temporizing measure, intraoperative cholangiography is used to evaluate ductal obstruction.
○ Choledocholithiasis
  - Stone in bile ducts; commonly cholesterol and black pigment; may be asymptomatic.
  - Mirizzi syndrome: Stone in gallbladder neck or cystic duct resulting in bile duct obstruction and jaundice.
  - Complications: Acute gallstone pancreatitis, cholangitis.
  - Treatment: Laparoscopic cholecystectomy with transcystic duct or common bile duct exploration, endoscopic retrograde cholangiography with endoscopic papillotomy (endoscopic retrograde cholangiopancreatography [ERCP]), laparotomy for common bile duct exploration, multiple strategies for retained stones (placement of T-tube, delayed cholangiography, ERCP, percutaneous transhepatic stone extraction, reoperation).
○ Cholangitis:
  - Bacterial infection due to stone obstruction and bile stasis, can also be due to tumors, adhesions, or congenital abnormalities.
  - Common organisms: *Escherichia coli*, *Klebsiella*, *Pseudomonas*, *Enterococcus* spp., *Proteus*.
  - Emphysematous cholecystitis: Gallbladder wall infection with gas-forming bacteria; associated with diabetes; surgical emergency.
  - Diagnosis: Charcot triad (fever, RUQ pain, jaundice), Reynolds pentad (Charcot triad, altered mental status, hypotension), elevated WBCs or shift, bilirubin, alkaline phosphatase; ultrasound, CT used to evaluate abscess and pancreatitis.
  - Treatment: Blood cultures, immediate antibiotics, fluid resuscitation, surgical treatment if not improving (ERCP with stent placement, percutaneous transhepatic biliary drainage, emergent laparotomy).
○ Acalculous cholecystitis:
  - Bile stasis due to prolonged fasting, immobility, or hemodynamic instability that can progress to cholecystitis; secondary infection, gangrene, or perforation is common and often found at time of diagnosis; persistent stasis can result in formation of biliary sludge.
  - Diagnosis: Patients in intensive care with comorbidities, RUQ pain, fever, elevated amylase; ultrasound or CT of abdomen show thickened gallbladder wall and pericholecystic fluid.
  - Treatment: Laparoscopic or open cholecystectomy once stable, percutaneous cholecystostomy.
○ Biliary dyskinesia: Delayed gallbladder emptying identified on HIDA scan in absence of stones or sludge; symptom
  improvement with cholecystectomy.
○ Gallstone ileus:
  - Bowel obstruction from > 2.5 cm gallstone in intestine; can create cholecystoenteric fistula.
  - Presents: Tumbling ileus (intermittent obstruction) or complete obstruction at terminal ileum, Bouveret syndrome (obstruction at pylorus or duodenum), treated with stone excision.
○ Porcelain gallbladder: Calcification of gallbladder wall, associated with gallbladder carcinoma and thus prophylactically resected.

4.3.3 Cirrhosis

- End-stage chronic liver disease with fibrosis of normal hepatic architecture; loss of hepatocyte function; increased transmural flow results in portal hypertension.[5,6]
- Fibrosis types: Micronodular (< 3 mm), macronodular (≥ 3 mm), mixed.
- Cause: Alcohol abuse (30%, mostly micronodular type), hepatitis B (15%), hepatitis C (33%), hepatitis D, nonalcoholic fatty liver disease (NAFLD, 18%), cholecystitis (intrahepatic or extrahepatic), autoimmune hepatitis, genetic conditions (e.g., cystic fibrosis, Wilson disease), toxic exposure, other infections, venoocclusive disease.
- Cause in children commonly includes biliary atresia and portal vein thrombosis.
- Presents: Weight gain/loss, fatigue, clinical history of common cause, physical findings (jaundice, dark urine, muscle wasting, purpura, encephalopathy, spider angiomata, asterixis, gynecomastia, ascites, caput medusa, splenomegaly, gastroesophageal varices).

- Diagnosis: Elevated direct or indirect bilirubin, elevated alkaline phosphatase, transaminases, low albumin or coagulation factors; ultrasound (90% sensitive, primary diagnostic modality), CT imaging of varices, CT angiography to evaluate hepatic vasculature, angiography to evaluate vasculature, liver biopsy used to evaluate fibrosis, paracentesis can evaluate cancer and bacterial peritonitis.
- Disease severity:
  - Child-Turcotte-Pugh score calculates mortality risk after major surgery (class A: 5–7 points, 2% mortality; class B: 8–10 points, 10% mortality; class C: ≥ 11 points, > 50% mortality); factors creatinine, bilirubin, sodium, ascites, and encephalopathy; correlates with disease severity.
  - Model for end-stage liver disease (MELD) predicts 3-month mortality following surgery in patients who had undergone a TIPS procedure; uses bilirubin, creatinine, and international normalized ratio. More objective than Child-Turcotte-Pugh score.
- Complications:
  - Portal hypertension:
    - Portal vein obstruction preventing normal fluid flow, defined as hepatic venous pressure gradient > 5–10 mm Hg.
    - Classification: Prehepatic/presinusoidal, intrahepatic/sinusoidal, posthepatic/postsinusoidal, high-flow states.
    - Diagnosis: Portal venography, hepatic vein angiography, hepatic vein wedge pressure measurement.
  - Varices:
    - Dilation of extrahepatic veins in the lower esophagus, abdominal wall, rectal wall, or diaphragm to improve venous return to systemic circulation.
    - Found in 20–70% of patient with cirrhosis; annual bleed rate of 15% with high risk of rehemorrhage; 7–15% mortality rate.
    - Screening performed every 1–3 years.
  - Ascites: Peritoneal fluid accumulation due to increased hydrostatic pressure and lymphatic outflow.
  - Encephalopathy:
    - Altered consciousness, asterixis, rigidity, or hyperreflexia due to elevated systemic ammonia and other factors.
    - Worsened by GI hemorrhage, shunting procedures, bacterial peritonitis, high protein in diet, narcotics/sedatives.
  - Hepatorenal syndrome: Oliguria and increased BUN or creatinine due to liver dysfunction; can show rapid onset or slow progression; defined as type I (acute renal failure) and type II (slower renal failure).
  - Hepatopulmonary syndrome: Elevated alveolar:arterial gradient > 20 mm Hg with intrapulmonary vasodilation; results in dyspnea; treated with oxygen until transplantation.
- Treatment:
  - Medical:
    - Prophylaxis of small varies: β-blockers, H2 blockers, proton-pump inhibitors, antibiotics when patients admitted.
    - Somatostatin, octreotide, vasopressin, or terlipressin used for acute variceal bleeding.
    - Low-sodium diet and diuretics to reduce ascites risk.
    - Antibiotics (e.g., neomycin) used to temporarily reduce intestinal ammonia-producing flora.
    - Low-nitrogen diet.
  - Surgical:
    - All patients with new cirrhosis diagnosis undergo esophagogastric endoscopy to evaluate for varices, treatment includes esophageal variceal ligation, rubber bands, or sclerotherapy.
    - Sengstaken-Blakemore gastric tube for acute variceal bleeding.
    - TIPS used to relieve portal hypertension but increase risk of hepatic failure and encephalopathy; not used in setting of heart failure, pulmonary hypertension, hepatic cysts, infections, or biliary obstruction.
    - Extrahepatic portosystemic shunts can be used but these increase risk of hepatic failure and encephalopathy.
    - Selective distal splenorenal shunts can improve varices with lower incidence of hepatic failure and encephalopathy.
    - Liver transplantation can be a definitive therapy.
    - High-volume paracentesis can temporarily aid symptoms of ascites.

– Surgical peritoneal-venous shunts (e.g., LeVeen, Denver shunt) can improve drainage of peritoneal fluid to systemic circulation.

4.4 Spleen Pathology

Andrea Weitz

4.4.1 Anatomy

- 10 cm in length.
- Protected posteriorly by the 9th to 12th ribs.
- Intimately related to the splenic flexure of the colon, greater curvature of the stomach, the left kidney, and the pancreatic tail.
- Held in place by ligaments: Splenogastric, splenocolic, splenophrenic, and splenorenal.
  - Splenogastric ligament contains numerous short gastric vessels that originate from the splenic artery to supply the greater curvature of the stomach.
  - Other ligaments attach the spleen to the splenic flexure of the colon, Gerotas fascia of the kidney, and the diaphragm, respectively, and contain very few vessels, making it safe to take down with electrocautery and/or sharp dissection.
- The splenic hilum and/or the inferior pole is attached to the omentum.
- Splenic artery is a branch off the celiac artery and travels along the superior aspect of the pancreas leading to the hilum.
- It branches into the upper and lower pole arteries, which travel in a radial manner, making dissection in a parallel fashion and a partial splenectomy possible.
- Note that the splenic artery can branch in the hilum or 5–10 cm away from it.
- Splenic vein travels more posteriorly and inferiorly to the artery and drains into the portal vein. The inferior mesenteric vein can be found to drain into the splenic vein or the superior mesenteric vein. after receiving the inferior mesenteric vein and joining the superior mesenteric vein.
- Accessory spleens can be found in 10–20% of patients and are usually in the hilum, splenic ligaments, or greater omentum but can be found throughout the abdomen.

4.4.2 Physiology

- Immunological function includes production of immunoglobulin M (IgM), tuftsin, properdin, and interferon.
- Red blood cell (RBC) morphology and therefore RBC function is maintained by splenic filtration (▶ Table 4.1).
- Aged RBCs (< 120 days) have decreased plasticity and become trapped and destroyed by the spleen.
- Removes viruses and encapsulated bacteria, including *Streptococcus, Hemophilus influenza, Neisseria meningitis,* and *Salmonella*
- Receives 5% of cardiac output and removes old or abnormal erythrocytes, platelets, and neutrophils from the circulation.
- Serves as a reservoir for platelets.

Table 4.1 Biological substances removed by the spleen

Healthy individuals	Patients with disease
Red blood cell membrane	Spherocytes
Red blood cell surface pits and craters	Sickle cells, hemoglobin C cells
Howell-Jolly bodies (nuclear remnants)	Antibody-coated red blood cells
Heinz bodies (denatured hemoglobin)	Antibody-coated platelets
Pappenheimer bodies (iron granules)	Antibody-coated white blood cells
Acanthocytes (spur cells)	
Senescent red blood cells	
Particular antigens	

4.4.3 Nontrauma Pathologies

- This includes hematologic disorders, neoplasm, and benign conditions.[7,8,9,10,11,12,13]
- Initial therapy for hematologic disorders of the spleen is usually medical and surgery is warranted only after medical attempts fail.

4.4.4 Hematological Conditions

- Idiopathic thrombocytopenic purpura (ITP):
  - Most common indication for an elective splenectomy.
  - Acquired condition in which antibodies are produced against a platelet glycoprotein where the spleen is the major site of production for these antibodies.
  - Adults with platelet counts of > 50,000/microL can be monitored.
  - Adults who are symptomatic or have platelet counts < 30,000/microL should be treated with glucocorticoids; > 50% of patients will respond.
  - In refractory cases or in patients with bleeding, intravenous immunoglobulin (IVIG) can be used, but results are transient.
  - If splenectomy is refused, rituximab (anti CD-20 monoclonal antibody) has demonstrated short-term effectiveness.
  - Indications for splenectomy are failure to respond to medical treatment, intolerable side effects from steroids, or a life-threatening, progressive hemorrhage such as in the central nervous system.
  - Complete response is achieving platelet count of at least 100,000/microL whereas a partial response is at least 30,000/microL.
  - Most patients will show a partial response after about 10 days.
  - If patients fail after a splenectomy, such as with continued thrombocytopenia, they should be investigated for accessory splenic tissue with a peripheral smear. Nuclear studies with Tc-99m-labeled heat-damaged RBCs are indicated.
  - Can use rituximab in those who fail to respond to splenectomy.
- Thrombocytopenic purpura (TTP):
  - Pentad of hemolytic anemia, consumptive thrombocytopenia, mental status changes, renal failure, fever; antibodies to ADAMTS13 enzyme; decreases breakdown of von Willebrand factor multimers.
  - Only hemolytic anemia and thrombocytopenia are required to initiate therapy.
  - Symptoms are due to multiorgan microvascular thrombosis.
  - First-line therapy is plasmapheresis.
  - If first-line therapy fails, then rituximab, cyclosporin, or increased plasma exchange frequency can be.
  - Splenectomy has limited indication in patients who do not respond to medical therapy.
- Anemias:
  - Hemolytic anemias are a group of disorders where splenectomy is almost always curative.
  - Hereditary spherocytosis:
    - Autosomal-dominant disorder characterized by a defect in spectrin (RBC membrane protein).
    - RBCs are small, spherical, and rigid and fail to deform to traverse the splenic microcirculation, leading to sequestration and destruction of RBCs in the spleen.
    - Causes anemia, jaundice, splenomegaly, fatigue, and pigmented gallstones.
    - Splenectomy is indicated in almost all cases (should wait until age 6 years to avoid overwhelming postsplenectomy infection [OPSI] unless child is transfusion dependent).
    - Before splenectomy, should check for gallstones and perform cholecystectomy if indicated.
  - Hereditary elliptocystosis:
    - Autosomaldominant condition with an intrinsic cytoskeleton defect of the RBC.
    - If mild or asymptomatic anemia, patients do not require specific treatment.
    - Patients with symptomatic anemia can undergo splenectomy to prolong RBC survival.
  - Pyruvate kinase deficiency:
    - More commonly an autosomal recessive disease leading to enzyme-deficiency hemolytic anemia. Autosomal recessive disease.
    - Results in decreased RBC deformability and the creation of echinocytes.

- Increases the likelihood that the cell will be trapped and destroyed by the spleen.
- Results in splenomegaly, hemolytic anemia, and transfusion requirements.
- Can be mitigated with splenectomy
  - Glucose-6-phosphate dehydrogenase deficiency:
    - X-linked deficiency.
    - Hemolytic anemia often occurs after infection or exposure to certain foods, chemicals, or medications.
    - Splenectomy is rarely indicated.
  - Warm autoimmune hemolytic anemias (acquired autoimmune hemolytic anemia):
    - RBCs coated with autoantibodies (IgG) that interact with their antigens at 37 °C.
    - Anti-immunoglobin IgG antiserum causes agglutination of the patient's RBCs and has a positive direct Coombs test.
    - Treatment is directed against the underlying disease (chronic lymphocytic leukemia, non-Hodgkin lymphoma, collagen vascular disease).
    - Splenectomy is effective in 60–80% of cases that are nonresponders to treatment or are requiring high doses of steroids.
  - Cold autoimmune hemolytic anemia (acquired autoimmune hemolytic anemia):
    - Characterized by IgM antibodies that fixate on C3 and cause RBCs to bind at temperatures approaching 0 °C.
    - Treatment is medical and includes alkylating agents, rituximab, or interferon.
    - Splenectomy has no therapeutic benefit.
- Congenital hemoglobinopathies:
  - Sickle cell anemia:
    - Splenectomy may be required in those who have acute splenic sequestration crisis and require multiple transfusions.
  - Thalassemias:
    - Autosomal dominant.
    - Result from a defect in the hemoglobin synthesis that causes varying degrees of hemolytic anemia.
    - Splenectomy can be required in those who have acute splenic sequestration crisis and require multiple transfusions.

Malignant Disease

- Hodgkin disease:
  - Malignant lymphoma that affects adults in their 20 s and 30 s.
    - Once a part of diagnosis and staging, splenectomy for lymphoma or leukemia is rare.
    - Splenectomy may be indicated for palliation of splenomegaly or hypersplenism.
  - Typically presents with cervical lymphadenopathy, rarely presents with weight loss, night sweats, and pruritus.
  - Characterized as lymphocyte predominant, nodular sclerosing, mixed cellularity, or lymphocyte depleted.
  - Uses Ann Arbor staging classification (divides tumors by location and extent of spread).
  - Often cured with radiation therapy alone.
  - Laparotomy is no longer indicated and those that are likely to relapse, with evidence of intra-abdominal involvement, or with B symptoms (constitutional symptoms) should receive systemic chemotherapy.
- Non-Hodgkin lymphoma:
  - Most common primary splenic neoplasm.
  - 50–80% of patients have involvement of the spleen.
  - 75% of these patients have clinically apparent hypersplenism.
  - Splenectomy is indicated in those with splenomegaly and abdominal pain, early satiety, and fullness.
  - Splenectomy is also indicated for hypersplenism and anemia, neutropenia, and thrombocytopenia.
- Hairy cell leukemia:
  - Accounts for 2% of adult leukemia.
  - Characterized by splenomegaly, pancytopenia, and neoplastic mononuclear cells in peripheral blood and bone marrow.

- B lymphocytes are affected.
- Found in older men with palpable splenomegaly.
- Treatment is generally with chemotherapy or with immunotherapy for refractory cases.
- Splenectomy is indicated if patients have symptomatic anemia, infections secondary to neutropenia, or hemorrhage from thrombocytopenia.
- Chronic lymphocytic leukemia:
  - Disease of B lymphocytes.
  - Predominantly men > 50 years old.
  - Treatment consists of chemotherapy or monoclonal antibodies.
  - Splenectomy indicated with refractory splenomegaly and pancytopenia.
- Chronic myelogenous leukemia:
  - Progressive replacement of normal diploid cells in bone marrow with neoplastic myeloid cells.
  - Characterized by the fusion of the fragments of chromosomes 9 and 22 resulting in the BCL-ABL gene product (tyrosine kinase) that accelerates cells division and inhibits DNA repair.
  - Therapy can include a tyrosine kinase inhibitor and other chemotherapeutic modalities.
  - Symptomatic splenomegaly and hypersplenism can be treated with splenectomy but has no survival benefit when performed in the early chronic phase.
- Metastasis:
  - Metastases to the spleen are rare, but have been reported in lung, colorectal, ovarian, and breast cancer.
  - Splenectomy may be indicated for palliation of symptoms, but there is little data to suggest survival benefit.
- Primary tumors:
  - Benign (hemangiomas, lymphangiomas, sclerosing angiomatoid nodular transformation).
  - Malignant (angiosarcomas, lymphangiosarcomas, hematopoietic neoplasms).
  - Splenectomy may be needed for diagnosis if biopsy not possible.

Splenic Cysts

- True cysts (parasitic or nonparasitic):
  - Nonparasitic:
    - Congenital, benign.
    - Lined with squamous epithelium.
    - Can cause early satiety, abdominal fullness, shortness of breath, pleuritic chest pain, left shoulder pain.
    - Partial splenectomy can preserve splenic function (need 25% of spleen to protect against pneumococcal pneumonia).
  - Parasitic:
    - Occur in areas of endemic hydatid disease (*Echinococcus* spp.).
    - Radiographic imaging will demonstrate cyst wall calcifications and daughter cysts.
    - Serological testing is helpful for diagnosis.
    - Splenectomy is treatment of choice; careful not to spill cystic contents that can cause anaphylactic shock or intraperitoneal dissemination and infection.
- Pseudocysts:
  - Not lined with epithelium, usually as a result of trauma.
  - Small cysts (< 4 cm) do not require treatment.
  - Symptomatic cysts can be treated with total or partial splenectomy.
- Splenic abscess:
  - Mortality rate for a splenic abscess ranges from 15 to 20% for unilocular lesions to 80% for multiple abscesses in immunocompromised patients.
  - Malignant neoplasms, polycythemia vera, endocarditis, prior trauma, hemoglobinopathies, urinary tract infection, IV drug use, or acquired immune deficiency syndrome are all factors that predispose patients to splenic abscesses.
  - Usually hematogenous spread.
  - Gram-positive (*Staphylococcus*, *Streptococcus*, or *Enterococcus* spp.) or gram-negative enterics are often involved.

○ *Mycobacterium tuberculosis*, *M. avium*, *Actinomyces*, and fungal spp. can be involved (immunocompromised patients).
○ Diagnose with computed tomography (CT) scan or ultrasound.
○ Treatment differs for unilocular abscess (treat with percutaneous drainage and antibiotics) and multilocular lesions (treat with splenectomy [laparoscopic or open], drainage of left upper quadrant, and antibiotics).

Operative Techniques

• Open (discussed in Operative management in Chapter 4.4.5 Trauma Splenectomy).
• Laparoscopic splenectomy contraindications:
  ○ Absolute includes massive splenomegaly (> 30 cm in length), portal hypertension, splenic trauma.
  ○ Relative includes moderate splenomegaly (> 20–25 cm in length), severe uncorrectable cytopenia, splenic vein thrombosis, bulky hilar adenopathy, morbid obesity.
  ○ Vaccines should be given 15 days before elective splenectomy or within 30 days of an emergent splenectomy to reduce risk of OPSI.

4.4.5 Trauma Splenectomy

• Incidence and mechanism of injury:
  ○ First or second most commonly injured solid viscus in the abdomen after blunt trauma.
  ○ Splenic injury occurred in 2.6% of all patients evaluated for trauma.
  ○ Splenic injuries occur via three mechanisms: penetrating, blunt, or indirect trauma (i.e., iatrogenic).
  ○ Blunt splenic injuries can bleed either immediately or on a delayed basis.
  ○ Delayed bleeding can occur as a subcapsular clot breaks down several days after injury, leading to capsular rupture.
• Diagnosis:
  ○ Assess airway, breathing, and circulation.
  ○ Initial history should include previous splenectomy, direct blows to lower left chest or left upper abdomen, or preexisting conditions that may cause splenomegaly, nonsteroidal anti-inflammatory use, anticoagulation use, portal venous disease, or bleeding propensity.
  ○ Physical exam should assess left lower rib pain or tenderness but may not demonstrate any significant findings.
  ○ Choice of imaging must be based on hemodynamic status of patient.
  ○ Extended focused assessment with sonography in trauma (E-FAST) (replaced diagnostic peritoneal lavage) is effective and rapid to detect free fluid, but it can have a 42% false-negative rate.
  ○ CT scan with IV contrast is the gold standard in a hemodynamically stable or stabilized patient.
  ○ CT scan with IV contrast has a specificity and sensitivity for splenic injuries near to 96–100%.
  ○ CT scan may demonstrate a hematoma, laceration, or the presence of a "blush."
  ○ A blush is a hyperdense area with a collection of contrast agent in it, concerning for ongoing bleeding.
• Nonoperative management:
  ○ Appropriate patient selection is essential.
  ○ Must be hemodynamically stable (systolic blood pressure > 90 mm Hg).
  ○ Must not have persistent peritonitis (concern for a concomitant intestinal injury).
  ○ Must be able to closely follow the patient with serial abdominal exams and hemodynamic status (i.e., patient should not be intubated and sedated, severe head trauma, or other).
  ○ If the patient is stable enough to go to the CT scanner and a ruptured spleen is seen, nonoperative management is reasonable if they continue to remain stable.
  ○ If patient is stable with a grade I, II, or III injury, nonoperative management is reasonable with possible assistance of angioembolization.
  ○ There is some evidence that older patients (> 55 years old) may have a worse outcome with nonoperative management than younger patients, making age a relative contraindication.
  ○ The presence of a severe head injury has been suggested to be another relative contraindication to nonoperative management.

- Management includes admission to an intensive care unit (grade II injury or above), kept with nothing by mouth, follow hemodynamic status including urine output, serial blood counts and serial abdominal exams.
    - Criteria for failure of non-operative management varies across institutions but typically relies on thresholds of hemodynamic monitoring, blood count drop, or need for transfusion over a set time period.
- Some studies have suggested to keep a patient on bedrest, but early mobilization has not demonstrated a failure in nonoperative management.
- If stable for 24–72 hours, the patient can be transferred to the ward.
- Length of hospital stay is not clearly defined, but studies have shown that most failures of nonoperative management will occur within the first 6–8 days after injury.
- Vaccines for *Haemophilus influenzae*, meningococcal, and streptococcal infection should be given before discharge.
- Once discharged, patients should be counseled not to engage in contact sports for 2–6 months.
- Most common complications of nonoperative management include continued bleeding and delayed diagnosis of an associated intra-abdominal injury (i.e., bowel or pancreas) which can occur 5–10% of the time.
- Transcatheter embolization:
    - Embolization of a ruptured spleen can be an important adjunct to nonoperative management.
    - There are no consensus guidelines for when angiography and embolization are indicated.
    - Current trends suggest embolization for higher-grade injuries, CT evidence of active extravasation, pseudoaneurysm, or arteriovenous fistula.
- Operative management:
    - Indicated if patient has an ultrasound or diagnostic peritoneal lavage that shows signs of intraperitoneal hemorrhage as well as hemodynamic instability (i.e., heart rate > 120 bpm, systolic blood pressure < 90 mm Hg or > 90 mm Hg but requiring blood products/boluses or vasopressors or base excess of > –5 mmol/L or shock index of > 1 or transfusion products of 4–6 units of packed RBCs within the first 24 hours), evidence of skin vasoconstriction, altered level of consciousness, and/or shortness of breath.
    - Create a midline incision and can extend incision superiorly and to the left of the xiphoid process to improve exposure to the left upper quadrant.
    - Vaccines should be given before discharge.
    - Complications include postoperative bleeding (splenic bed, short gastric vessels, hilum), necrosis of stomach after division of short gastric vessels leading to a gastric leak, pancreatic injury, thromboembolism, and OPSI.
    - Consider anticoagulation after patients have been stable for 24 hours.
    - OPSI is very rare (3.2–3.5% lifetime risk), but given its high mortality rate (40–50%), vaccines for encapsulated bacteria (Haemophilus influenza type B, Streptococcus pneumoniae, and Neisseria meningitidis) are required after splenectomy and should be given prior to discharge (and ideally after post-operative day 5) for those patients at risk of being lost to follow-up.

4.5 Breast Diseases

Michael Karsy

4.5.1 Fibroadenoma

- Rubbery, well-circumscribed, rubbery, nontender mass; can be hormonally dependent.
- Most common breast lesion in women < 30 years.
- Work-up: Ultrasound and biopsy.
- Excisional biopsy of lesions > 2 cm, rapidly increased size, or patient anxiety.

4.5.2 Fibrocystic Changes

- Range of diffuse, hormonally related fibrous and cystic changes of normal breast structure; can be cyclical with menstrual cycle.
- Three types: Nonproliferative, proliferative, atypia.
- Presents: Cyclical pain, tenderness, bilateral cysts in young adults.
- Slight risk of breast cancer.
- Work-up: Core or excisional biopsy for diagnosis or symptom control, repeated breast examinations, baseline mammography, danazol, tamoxifen.

4.5.3 Phyllodes Tumor, Cystosarcoma Phyllodes

- Round, mobile, painless mass containing mesenchymal and stromal elements (sarcomatous lesion).
- Differentiated as malignant depending on number of mitoses/high-power field.
- Treatment: Wide local excision with negative margin because of high recurrence rate.

4.5.4 Intraductal Papilloma

- Benign, solitary epithelial lesion of subareolar duct; can be multiple with diffuse papillomatosis.
- Presents: Bloody or clear nipple discharge.
- Treatment: Excision of duct to rule out invasive carcinoma.

4.5.5 Fat Necrosis

- Breast fat necrosis due to trauma, surgery, infection, duct ectasia, or aseptic saponification; usually superficial with overlying skin changes and < 2 cm in size.
- Treatment: Observation if clear history of trauma or excisional biopsy to rule out malignancy.

4.5.6 Plasma Cell/Periductal Mastitis

- Inflammation of ductal system with plasma cell infiltration at time of menopause.
- Presents: Noncyclical, focal breast pain, nipple retraction, nipple discharge, subareolar masses.
- Treatment: Excisional biopsy to rule out malignancy.

4.5.7 Galactocele

- Obstructed lactiferous duct with yellow or greenish-yellow nipple discharge.
- Treatment: Needle aspiration or excision.

4.5.8 Mastitis

- Painful infection of breast; common in lactating women; due to skin or oral flora.
- Treatment: Culture of breast milk and antibiotic treatment (dicloxacillin, amoxicillin/clavulanate with addition of metronidazole if abscess), breast pumping/feeding/massage blocked duct to fully empty breast, warm compresses, NSAIDS, aspiration, incision and drainage with samples sent to rule out inflammatory carcinoma, excision of subareolar tissue for recurrent infection.

4.5.9 Mondor Disease

- Superficial thrombophlebitis of thoracoepigastric vein due to trauma or surgery; presents with tender area of linear skin dimpling.
- Treatment: nonsteroidal anti-inflammatories, warm compresses, mammography if > 35 years.

4.5.10 Gynecomastia

- Male breast gland proliferation, > 2 cm in diameter.
- Types:
  - Pubertal: Starts at age 10–12 years and regresses at age 16–17 years; treated with reassurance.
  - Senescent: Starts at age > 50 years and regresses within 6–12 months.
  - Drug-induced: Can involve use of a wide variety of agents.
  - Pathologic: Due to obesity, cirrhosis, renal failure, malnutrition, hyperthyroidism, adrenal dysfunction, hypogonadism, testicular tumors.
- Treatment: Biopsy if unclear etiology or senescent type, resection for social issues.

4.5.11 Poland Syndrome

- Hypoplasia of chest well with absence of breast and pectoralis major.

4.5.12 Nipple Discharge

- Red flags: Unilateral, bloody, single duct/quadrant; spontaneous, occult blood; palpable mass.
- Galactorrhea: Due to pregnancy, pituitary adenoma, hypothyroidism, nipple stimulation, stress, oral contraceptives, tricyclic antidepressants.
- Bloody: Benign intraductal papilloma most common; must rule out invasive papillary cancer.
- Other types: Galactorrhea, serous.
- Serous: Due to normal menses, oral contraceptives, fibrocystic changes, pregnancy.
- Yellow/green: Due to fibrocystic changes, galactocele.
- Purulent: Breast abscess.

4.5.13 Cancer

- Most common cancer in women (30% all cancers), develops in 12% of women and results in death of 3.5% of women.
- Risk factors: Older age (average age at diagnosis is 62 years), developed countries, familial history of breast cancer, genetic mutations (10% of breast cancer, atypical ductal or lobular hyperplasia), noninvasive carcinoma (ductal carcinoma in situ, lobular carcinoma in situ), early menarche, late menopause, nulliparity, age > 30 at 1st delivery, exogenous hormone replacement, radiation exposure, alcohol.
- Screening:
  - Between ACS, ACOG, NCCN, USPSTF
  - In general, women of average risk between the ages of 50-70 should be screened with mammography every 1-2 years. Screening for women 40-49 will need to be individualized.
  - High-risk women (20% lifetime cancer risk) should have clinical exams every 6 months, screening 5–10 years before age of youngest diagnosed relative or age 25 years in BRCA mutation carriers.
- Presents: Nonpalpable or palpable mass, skin changes (dimpling, nipple retraction, erythema, edema, peau d'orange, ulceration, eczema, nipple excoriation), bloody discharge, less likely to present with pain, pain from metastatic lesions.
- Diagnosis: Mammography (irregular margins or masses, architectural distortion, asymmetric thickening, pleomorphic calcification, increased vascularity, utilizes breast imaging reporting and data system [BI-RADS] classification [▶ Table 4.2]), ultrasound (visualizes lesions > 0.5 cm), magnetic resonance imaging (useful in women with high lifetime risk), digital breast tomosynthesis.
- Work-up (for any breast lesion including cancer):
  - Nipple discharge: Ultrasound, mammogram, occult blood, galactogram.
  - Cystic lesions: Asymptomatic simple cysts require reassurance, symptomatic cysts or atypical imaging findings require fine-needle aspiration and cytological work-up.
  - Solid lesions: Close monitoring with serial breast examinations, mammography, and fine-needle aspiration; diagnostic mammography and biopsy used if concern for malignancy.

Table 4.2 Breast imaging reporting and data system (BI-RADS) classification

BI-RADS classification	Findings	Cancer risk
0	Incomplete imaging	
I	Negative; symmetrical; no masses, architectural disturbances, or suspicious calcification	
II	Benign findings (e.g., calcified fibroadenoma, fibrocystic changes, lipoma, galactocele, simple cysts)	
III	Probably benign; short-interval follow-up suggested	~2%
IV	Suspicious; biopsy suggested; divided into IVa (low suspicion), IVb (intermediate suspicion), IVc (moderate suspicion)	~30%
V	Highly suggestive of malignancy	95%
VI	Biopsy-proven malignancy	

- ○ Biopsy: Fine-needle aspiration (90–94% accuracy), image-guided core needle biopsy, excisional biopsy (definitive diagnosis, used for nonpalpable lesions).
- ○ Tumor, node, malignancy (TNM) classification (▶ Table 4.3) used to stage tumor for prognosis and treatment; staging more important than histology for prognosis.
- Histology:
  - ○ Ductal carcinoma in situ (DCIS): Pre-malignant cancer originating from the breast duct epithelium (Stage 0).
  - ○ Lobular carcinoma in situ (LCIS): Malignant stroma cells with high likelihood of malignant progression.
  - ○ Invasive ductal carcinoma: Most common breast malignancy (80% cases), originates from the breast duct epithelium, multiple histological variants.
  - ○ Invasive lobular carcinoma: Less common (5–10% cases).
  - ○ Paget disease: 1–3% malignancies, associated with DCIS and eczematous changes of the nipple–areola complex. Diagnosis is based on biopsy showing Paget cells (large cells with clear cytoplasm and eccentric, hyperchromic nuclei). Paget's disease of the breast is a red flag for breast cancer. It is imperative to work-up an underlying breast cancer in women diagnosed with Paget's disease of the breast. If a breast cancer is identified, patient will require at minimum central lumpectomy including the nipple–areola complex.
  - ○ Inflammatory breast carcinoma: 1–4% cases, associated with peau d'orange of the skin, commonly presents with metastases and in aggressive form.
- Treatment:
  - ○ Lymph nodes:
    - – Axillary nodes drain 75–95% of ipsilateral breast.
    - – Node level: I (lateral to pectoralis minor), II (deep to pectoralis minor), III (medial to pectoralis minor).
  - ○ Large variety of surgical treatments depending on tumor stage, type, and oncological plan; neoadjuvant therapy can be used before surgery for large lesions; multidisciplinary care.
  - ○ Breast-conserving surgical resection (includes lumpectomy, partial mastectomy, sentinel lymph node biopsy), subcutaneous mastectomy (experimental), skin-sparing simple mastectomy, simple/total mastectomy (DCIS, LCIS), modified radical mastectomy, radical Halsted mastectomy (rarely used), axillary lymph node dissection (level I and II nodes).
  - ○ Breast-conserving resections with adjuvant therapy can be equivalent to mastectomy.
  - ○ Combinations of radiotherapy, chemotherapy, hormonal therapy (tamoxifen for premenopausal patients, aromatase inhibitors for postmenopausal patients), and immunotherapy may be used.
  - ○ Oncotype diagnostic testing for genomic profile can be used to stratify risk.
  - ○ Breast reconstruction:
    - – Can be performed immediately or delayed after radiation; does not delay treatment or reduce surveillance.

– Prosthetic breast implant, myocutaneous flap, deep inferior epigastric perforator flap, nipple-areolar reconstruction.
• Breast cancer during pregnancy:

Table 4.3 TNM (tumor, node, malignancy) staging for breast cancer

TNM staging	Findings
T0	T0: no primary tumor
	Tis: carcinoma in situ (Ductal carcinoma in situ or Paget disease)
T1	≤2 cm
	T1mi: ≤1 mm
	T1a: 1–5 mm
	T1b: 5–10 mm
	T1c: 1–2 cm
T2	>2 but ≤5 cm
T3	>5 cm
T4	Invasion of any adjacent or distant structure
	T4a: tumor into chest wall
	T4b: tumor into skin
	T4c: tumor into chest wall and skin
	T4: inflammatory breast cancer
N	N0: no regional nodes
	N1mi: micrometastasis 0.2–2mm
	N1a: 1–3 lymph nodes with 1 area > 2 mm
	N1b: ipsilateral internal mammary lymph node or sentinal node
	N1c: N1a or N1b
	N2a: 4–9 lymph nodes with 1 area > 2 mm
	N2b: > 1 internal mammary lymph node
	N3a: ≥ 10 lymph nodes with 1 area > 2 mm or infraclavicular spread with 1 area > 2 mm
	N3b: 1 axillary lymph node and enlarged internal mammary lymph node OR ≥ 4 axillary lymph nodes
	N3c: supraclavicular spread
M	Distant metastasis
Stage	
0	Tis, N0, M0 (cancer in ducts and lobules)
IA	T1, N0, M0 (cancer small and noninvasive)
IB	T0 or T1, N1, M0 (small, noninvasive, spread to lymph nodes)
IIA	T0, N1, M0 (spread to 1–3 axillary lymph nodes)
	T1, N1, M0 (≤2 cm and not spread)
	T2, N0, M0 (2–5 cm and not spread)
IIB	T2, N1, M0 (2–5 cm and spread to 1–3 axillary lymph nodes)
	T3, N0, M0 (≥5 cm and not spread)
IIIA	N2, M0 (any size, spread to 4–9 lymph nodes or internal mammary lymph nodes)
	T3 (≥5 cm and spread to 1–3 axillary lymph nodes)
IIIB	T4 (spread to chest wall, inflammatory breast cancer, ≤9 axillary lymph nodes)
IIIC	Any T, N3, M0 (any size, ≥10 axillary lymph nodes, internal mammary lymph nodes, collar bone lymph nodes)
IV	Any T, any N, M1

- Pregnancy termination does not decrease tumor stimulation; modified radical mastectomy used during 1st and 2nd trimester.
  - Preoperative adjuvant therapy with breast-conserving resection used during 2nd and 3rd trimester.
  - Axillary node dissection performed during 3rd trimester.
  - Radiation deferred until after delivery.
- Male breast cancer: 1% of breast cancers; presents late and in more advanced stages; infiltrating ductal is most common type; node-positive disease has worse prognosis than women.

4.6 Surgical Oncology

Austin Cannon and Milos Buhavac

4.6.1 Overview and Principles

- Second leading cause of death in the United States, closely following heart disease.
- Since 1999 most cancer mortalities have declined; notable exceptions include liver cancers due to the prevalence of hepatitis C among baby boomers, pancreatic cancer thought to be related to increasing rates of obesity, and melanoma.
- Most common anatomic sites (in the United States) in order of decreasing prevalence:
  - Female breast cancer.
  - Lung and bronchus malignancies.
  - Male prostate cancer.
  - Colorectal cancer.
  - Melanoma.
- Mortality from malignancies differ by sex:
  - Female cancer mortalities in decreasing numerical order: lung, breast, colon.
  - Male cancer mortalities in decreasing numerical order: lung, colon, prostate.
- Staging:
  - Multiple staging systems exist for some malignancies.
  - Most widely applicable system is the American Joint Committee on Cancer (AJCC) system: tumor (T), node (N), and metastasis (M) scoring system to describe progression of disease.
  - National Comprehensive Cancer Network (NCCN) guidelines provide an excellent resource for the diagnosis, staging, and surgical/medical treatment algorithms of most malignancies.
  - Performed at various periods throughout the course of disease to detect progression of disease and to determine the T, N, and M stage of the malignancy as accurately as possible in order to assign an overall stage.
    - Accurate initial staging is paramount to facilitating proper diagnosis and to initiating correct treatment.
    - Incomplete or inaccurate staging can result in unnecessary chemotherapy, radiation, surgery, or undertreatment of disease by withholding these modalities.
    - Improper staging also creates confusion between different treatment providers as well as the patient.
    - Staging can be described as clinical, pathologic, post-neoadjuvant therapy, or restaging after treatment.
    - Different malignancies have different staging guidelines regarding the use of serum cancer markers, imaging studies, and the use of other diagnostic modalities such as endoscopic ultrasound (EUS) in an attempt to accurately determine the extent of disease.
- The goal of nonpalliative oncologic surgery is generally resection with a margin free of tumor involvement. Acceptable margin sizes depend on the type of malignancy being treated. Postsurgical margins are described pathologically:
  - R0—Margin that is clear of macroscopic and microscopic tumor involvement.
  - R1—Margin that has microscopic residual tumor at the margin.
  - R2—Margin with gross/macroscopic tumor involvement.

4.6.2 Esophageal Cancer

- Epidemiology and risk factors:
  - Approximately 17,000 new cases of esophageal cancer each year in the United States and 480,000 across the world. Of the 17,000 U.S. cases, 16,000 are expected to die because of the disease.
  - Eighth most common solid organ tumor and sixth leading cause of death due to cancer worldwide.
  - Male predominance.
  - Two histologic types: Adenocarcinoma and squamous cell carcinoma (SCC).
  - Adenocarcinoma:
    – More prevalent in the United States and has increasing incidence.
    – Risk factors: Barrett esophagus secondary to long-standing gastroesophageal reflux disease (GERD); obesity leading to GERD; smoking.
  - SCC:
    – More common worldwide but decreasing incidence in the United States.
    – Risk factors: Tobacco and alcohol are strongest risk factors for SCC and have synergy to increase risk more when combined than each separately; African Americans have higher risk in the United States; prior caustic ingestion.
    – Highest rates in Middle East and Asia.
    – Human papilloma virus infection represents very small subset of esophageal SCCs.
- Presentation, diagnosis, and staging:
  - Most are advanced by the time of diagnosis and most patients ultimately succumb to the disease.
  - May arise at any level of the esophagus (proximal, middle, distal), but SCCs typically occur proximally and adenocarcinomas distally or at the GEJ.
  - Most are symptomatic and advanced at time of diagnosis:
    – Dysphagia most common symptom; progresses from solids to liquids over time.
    – Weight loss secondary to dysphagia.
    – History of reflux.
    – Odynophagia.
    – Regurgitation.
    – Retrosternal pain.
    – Hoarseness if laryngeal nerve involvement.
  - Diagnosis:
    – Endoscopic examination with multiple biopsy performed to make the diagnosis.
    – Endoscopic evaluation should be performed in any patient with dysphagia to detect a neoplastic process even when an esophageal motility disorder, such as achalasia, is suspected.
    – Barium swallow may be used to determine degree of esophageal obstruction and function, but endoscopic evaluation with EGD is still mandatory.
    – Tumor distance relative to incisors and GEJ should be documented.
  - Staging:
    – Staging work-up for esophageal cancer must include biopsy to determine histologic type, distance from GEJ and incisors.
    – Endoscopic ultrasound (EUS) to assess depth of invasion and paraesophageal lymph node status and EUS-guided biopsy when suspicious nodes are encountered.
    – Chest/abdomen/pelvis CT scan with oral and IV contrast to identify locoregional extent of disease and any metastatic lesions.
    – Positron emission tomography (PET)-CT has higher sensitivity for detecting metastatic disease and is also recommended. PET can detect distant disease in up to 20% of patients where no metastatic disease was observed on conventional CT.
- Stage-based treatment:
  - Adenocarcinoma and SCC are treated similarly, although the staging systems differ slightly, with SCC staging taking into account esophageal location. Tumors of the cervical esophagus are typically treated with definitive chemoradiation because of the higher operative morbidity rates at this location.

- Barrett's esophagus/low-grade dysplasia:
  - Controversy concerning management exists in the setting of Barrett's esophagus or low-grade dysplasia.
  - Ensure adequate biopsies to exclude a missed adenocarcinoma.
  - Initiate acid-reducing medications (PPIs) if not already taking.
  - Aggressive endoscopic surveillance; time period debated but initially every 3–6 months with biopsies, and yearly thereafter.
  - Consider acid-reducing surgery if noncompliant with PPI therapy or PPI fails to suppress acid reflux; however, surgery has not been shown to decrease dysplasia or improve outcomes.
- High-grade dysplasia (Tis, N0, M0) and T1a, N0, M0 disease:
  - Malignant changes are confined to mucosa (high-grade dysplasia) or muscularis mucosa (T1a) without penetration of basement membrane, indicating very low/no risk of disease spread to lymphatics (< 2%).
  - Options for management include continued surveillance, endoscopic mucosal ablation/resection, or esophagectomy.
  - Historical standard was esophagectomy, but not all dysplasia will progress to invasive disease.
  - Endoscopic ablation/resection is currently favored with ongoing surveillance if disease has favorable features (low grade, no lymphovascular invasion, noncircumferential).
- T1b, M0, N0 disease:
  - T1b disease is classified by tumors that invade the lymphatic containing submucosa.
  - Treat with esophagectomy and regional lymphadenectomy.
- T2–T4a, any N, M0:
  - Locally advanced resectable cancer (4b nonresectable because of invasion of vital structures).
  - CROSS and MAGIC trials demonstrated increase in R0 resection rates with neoadjuvant chemotherapy and radiation, and longer survival (49 mo vs. 24 mo).
  - Esophagectomy with regional lymphadenectomy after neoadjuvant chemotherapy and radiation.
  - Adjuvant therapy with chemoradiation is recommended for patients with T3/4 disease, positive nodal disease, R1 or R2 resection, or high risk of local/systemic recurrence.
- T4b or M1 disease:
  - T4b tumors invade nonresectable structures (aorta, left atrium, spine).
  - M1 disease indicates systemic metastasis of the malignancy.
  - These patients are not candidates for curative therapy.
  - Palliative therapies can be pursued and may include chemoradiation, endoscopic stent placement, or enteral feeding tube placement.
- Esophagectomy:
  - Common operative approaches:
    - Open, minimally invasive, or hybrid Ivor Lewis esophagectomy: Upper midline laparotomy/laparoscopy combined with right posterolateral thoracotomy/Video assisted thoracoscopic surgery.
    - Open or minimally invasive transhiatal esophagectomy: Upper midline laparotomy/laparoscopy combined with left neck incision.
    - McKeown or 3-incision esophagectomy: Right posterolateral thoracotomy, upper midline laparotomy, left neck incision.
    - Left thoracoabdominal esophagectomy (less common): Left posterolateral approach; may add left neck incision.
  - Complications of esophagectomy:
    - Better outcomes in high-volume centers.
    - High complication rate (~50%).
    - Historically high mortality rates, but these are improving and now < 5%.
    - Respiratory complications are most common complication; pneumonia, respiratory failure; reduced by smoking cessation, appropriate analgesia, pulmonary toilet.
    - Anastomotic leak: Suspect if change in chest tube/drain output character or amount; evaluate with esophagogram with water-soluble contrast followed by thin barium if negative, or CT with contrast; manage expectantly if leak is small and contained; free leaks require intervention with either repair or revision of anastomosis; may consider esophageal stent if diagnosis is delayed.

– Chyle leak: Diagnose with increased output from chest tubes with initiation of enteral feeding, high chylomicrons, and triglycerides in fluid; output can exceed 2 L per day; initial management by low-fat diet. If this is inadequate, patient may need to be nothing by mouth with total parenteral nutrition; either interventional radiology (IR) embolization if feasible or operative ligation used if leak persists.

– Other acute complications include atrial fibrillation, recurrent laryngeal nerve injury.

– Esophageal stricture and dysmotility are late complications and can be diagnosed by endoscopy or barium swallow. Treat strictures via endoscopic dilations.

- Outcomes:
  - High mortality rates due to advanced stage at initial presentation.
  - Survival is dependent on stage at presentation, with 5-year survival rates of 90% and 75% for Tis and T1 disease, respectively, but only 20% with node-positive disease.

4.6.3 Gastric Cancer

Epidemiology and Risk Factors

- Epidemiology:
  - Rates of gastric cancer have been decreasing over the past century in the United States; now 14th most common cancer and cause of cancer mortality.
  - Worldwide gastric cancer is much more prevalent than in the United States.
  - Fourth most common cancer and 2nd leading cause of cancer mortality worldwide.
  - Common in East Asia and South America.
  - Rates highest in Japan and Korea.
  - Japan has instituted screening for gastric cancer with associated decrease in mortalities.
- Risk factors:
  - *Helicobacter pylori* increases the risk of distal gastric cancer thought to be secondary from chronic inflammation and gastritis.
  - Some types of gastric polyps.
  - Nitrosamines from high-salt foods or smoked meats.
  - Pernicious anemia.
  - Hereditary syndromes: CDH1 mutation, familial adenomatous polyposis (FAP), and Lynch syndrome.
- Types of gastric cancer:
  - Over 90% of gastric tumors are adenocarcinomas, rarer types include GI stromal tumors (GISTs), mucosa-associated lymphoid tissue lymphomas (MALTomas), and carcinoid tumors.
  - Two subtypes of adenocarcinoma: intestinal and diffuse.
    - Intestinal: Well differentiated; observed in older patients, high-risk populations, and associated with *H. pylori*.
    - Diffuse: Poorly differentiated; observed in inherited syndromes and is more aggressive.

Presentation, Diagnosis, and Staging

- Symptoms are typically vague and nonspecific:
  - Early stages: Include nausea, epigastric pain, early satiety, and weight loss that are easily attributed to peptic ulcer disease or gastritis.
  - More advanced tumors: May present with dysphagia, regurgitation, gastric outlet obstruction, or upper GI bleeding with associated anemia.
- Physical examination typically unremarkable, but special attention should be paid to examining nodal basins.
  - Periumbilical (Sister Mary Joseph node).
  - Left supraclavicular (Virchow node).
  - Prerectal metastases appreciated on rectal examination (Blumer shelf).
- Diagnosis is made with endoscopic examination (EGD) and biopsy:
  - EUS is used to detect depth of tumor invasion and lymph node involvement (T and N stages).
- Staging:
  - EGD with EUS is used to assess T and N stages of disease.

○ Chest/abdomen/pelvis CT to assess for metastatic disease as well as to complement EUS in assessing nodal disease.
○ PET-CT has limited use because only half of gastric cancers are PET avid.
○ Staging laparoscopy used because of high rates of occult metastatic disease not appreciated on CT; patients with presumed M0 gastric adenocarcinoma undergo a staging laparoscopy with peritoneal washings; sensitivity for peritoneal metastases > 95%; patients with positive peritoneal washings are classified as having M1 disease.
○ Siewert classification used to determine treatment because cancers at the GEJ and proximal stomach behave more aggressively and similarly to esophageal cancers; Siewert I: 1–5 cm above GEJ, treat as esophageal; Siewert II: 1 cm above to 2 cm below GEJ, treat as esophageal; Siewert III: 2–5 cm below GEJ, treat as gastric.

Stage-Based Treatment

- The goal of surgical management for gastric adenocarcinoma is a R0 resection because R1 resection portends a poor prognosis.
- Unresectable disease includes distant metastases, peritoneal disease, infiltration to the root of the mesentery, metastatic para-aortic lymph nodes, or invasion/encasement of major vascular structures (does not include splenic vessels).
- Tis (carcinoma in situ), T1a (tumor invades lamina propria or muscularis mucosa) disease:
  ○ For these early cancers with favorable characteristics and no nodal disease, endoscopic mucosal resection can be employed in high-volume centers.
- T1b (tumor invades submucosa):
  ○ Submucosa contains lymphatics, and T1b gastric tumors have higher risk of lymphatic disease.
  ○ Recommendation for T1b tumors is subtotal or total gastrectomy depending on location.
- T2–T4, any N, M0, and surgically resectable disease:
  ○ Neoadjuvant therapy with chemotherapy and/or radiation recommended, followed by repeat staging with chest/abdomen/pelvis CT.
  ○ Subtotal or total gastrectomy with selective spleen/pancreas resection in appropriate patients with resectable T4 disease.
  ○ Adjuvant therapy if node positive or high risk of recurrence.
  ○ Management of R1 resection is controversial, and re-resection or adjuvant therapies may be used.
  ○ R2 resections receive adjuvant therapy or palliative management if appropriate.
- Unresectable or metastatic disease:
  ○ Represent nearly half of all gastric cancers at diagnosis.
  ○ Confers an approximate survival of 5 months from time of diagnosis.
  ○ Palliative chemotherapy may be pursued.
  ○ Patients with debilitating symptoms may be considered for surgical therapy despite their metastatic disease to alleviate pain/obstruction/hemorrhage.

Gastrectomy

- Goal is R0 resection for curative intent.
- Margins of 5 cm should be pursued because of high chance of submucosal tumor invasion.
- Distal gastrectomy can be employed to treat tumors of the body and antrum.
- Proximal lesions are typically treated with a total gastrectomy because of increased complications from proximal subtotal gastrectomy.
- Reconstruction is performed with a Billroth II or Roux-en-Y gastrojejunostomy or esophagojejunostomy if total gastrectomy is performed.
- Laparoscopic approaches have been shown to be safe with equivalent oncologic outcomes when performed by experienced surgeons.
- Lymph node dissection:
  ○ Sufficient nodal dissection must include at least 15 nodes.

○ Extent of nodal dissection is contentious and continues to be debated.
○ Lymphadenectomy defined as D1 (perigastric nodes), D2 (perigastric nodes and lymph nodes along the left gastric artery, common hepatic artery, celiac artery, and splenic artery.), and rarely performed D3 (all of the above plus periaortic nodes with or without splenectomy/pancreatectomy).
○ Japanese studies have demonstrated increased survival with D2 dissection, but non-Japanese studies have demonstrated that D2 lymphadenectomy results in higher morbidity and mortality without differences in disease recurrence or overall survival.
• Complications of gastrectomy:
  ○ Leak (either gastric or duodenal stump if Billroth II reconstruction): Treat with reoperation versus drain/covered stent and expectant management.
  ○ Rapid transit leading to diarrhea.
  ○ Billroth II complications (treat most with revision to Roux-en-Y):
    – Bile acid reflux leading to alkaline gastritis.
    – Afferent loop syndrome.
    – Efferent loop syndrome.
    – Dumping (early and late).
  ○ Roux-en-Y complications:
    – Internal hernia.
    – Marginal ulcers.
  ○ Vitamin and mineral deficiencies.
  ○ Weight loss.
  ○ Remnant or recurrent cancer.

Outcomes

• Overall 5-year survival < 25%.
• Many patients present with an advanced stage; > 60% present with either locally advanced or distant disease.
• 5-year survival for patients with potentially resectable tumor is 25–50%.
• Early gastric cancer cure rates are ~80%.
• Recurrence rates are high (40–80%) after gastrectomy and typically occur within 3 years of resection.

4.6.4 Cancers of the Small Intestine

• Epidemiology and risk factors:
  ○ Very rare:
    – < 3% of all gastrointestinal cancers.
    – Predisposing factors that increase risk are largely genetic and include FAP, Lynch syndrome, and Peutz-Jeghers syndrome.
    – Other risk factors include chronic inflammation (e.g., Crohn's or celiac disease) and Meckel diverticulum, but the absolute risk of small-bowel malignancy in these conditions remains extremely low overall.
  ○ Most common malignant small-bowel tumors:
    – Neuroendocrine tumors (NETs) (carcinoids): Most common small-bowel malignancy; may be functional and produce serotonin, gastrin, somatostatin; serotonin syndrome if metastatic (typically to liver); markers include chromogranin A, 5-HIAA.
    – Adenocarcinomas: Second most common malignancy of small bowel; highest risk on patients with Crohn's disease.
    – GISTs: GI stromal tumors derived from myofibroblast cells; *c-KIT* tyrosine kinase mutation present in most GISTs.
    – Lymphomas: From lymphoid follicles in submucosa; associated with bulky lymphadenopathy.
    – Metastatic disease: From melanoma, colon, or breast typically.
• Presentation and diagnosis:
  ○ Symptoms often delayed because of nonspecificity:
    – nausea.
    – vomiting.

- bloating.
  - ○ As lesion grows, patients will later present with more significant symptoms:
    - – Obstruction.
    - – GI bleeding.
    - – Intussusception.
    - – Perforation.
  - ○ Diagnosis:
    - – Push or double balloon endoscopy.
    - – Video capsule endoscopy.
    - – Abdomen/pelvis CT.
- Treatment:
  - ○ Assuming no metastatic disease, treatment includes segmental small-bowel resection with primary anastomosis, and regional lymphadenectomy.
  - ○ Other considerations include:
    - – For small-bowel NETs, octreotide therapy may be considered in both neoadjuvant and/or adjuvant settings.
    - – For GISTs, imatinib (Gleevac) may be administered in neoadjuvant and/or adjuvant settings (large tumor, high mitotic rate).
    - – For metastatic disease, palliative resection or bypass may be considered in cases of obstruction.
  - ○ Treatment of lymphomas should be made in a multidisciplinary fashion with a hematologist/ oncologist specialist to ensure that resection is advisable. Some may be adequately treated with chemotherapy/radiation alone.
- Outcomes:
  - ○ Because of extremely low incidence of these cancers, there have been no large studies examining outcomes for these diagnoses. Unresectable disease at time of presentation is known to carry very poor outcomes, with 5-year survival rate close to 0%.

4.6.5 Colorectal and Cancer

- Epidemiology and risk factors:
  - ○ Third most common cancer diagnoses and second leading cause of cancer-related deaths in men and women in the United States.
  - ○ Lifetime risk of colorectal cancer is ~5%.
  - ○ May develop in either hereditary or sporadic forms:
    - – Hereditary includes FAP and hereditary nonpolyposis colorectal cancer/Lynch syndrome among others; develops at younger age; may have multiple synchronous tumors; FAP associated with *APC* mutation and Lynch syndrome associated with *MMR*.
    - – Sporadic tumors occur in older populations; typically isolated tumors.
      Thought to develop with mutations in *APC, K-RAS, DCC,* and *p53* genes in an adenoma-to-carcinoma sequence.
  - ○ Screening:
    - – In the United States, screening is recommended beginning at age 40 years for men and women unless there is a known familial syndrome or if a close relative was diagnosed with colon cancer before age 50 years, in which cases screening should be initiated earlier.
    - – Methods include colonoscopy (favored), flexible sigmoidoscopy with fecal occult blood testing (FOBT), or FOBT alone. Newer methods include CT colonography, but use is limited.
    - – Follow-up screening is performed every 10 years or less if polyps or dysplasia are observed.
    - – Polyps may be endoscopically treated with resection during colonoscopy.
    - – Tumors observed should be biopsied and then tattooed so they can be easily located during the time of formal resection.
- Presentation, diagnosis, and staging:
  - ○ Signs and symptoms vary depending on tumor location, size, and presence of metastatic disease:

- Right-sided colon cancers are typically asymptomatic but may cause bleeding and anemia. Advanced lesions may result in obstruction.
- Left-sided colon cancers may present with a change in bowel habits, constipation, narrowed caliber of stools, obstructive symptoms, melena or hematochezia, and rarely fistulous disease.
- Rectal cancers may not only present similarly to left-sided colon cancers but also may have pelvic or inguinal nodal disease, or the ability to appreciate a mass on rectal examination.
  - Diagnosis and staging:
- Colonoscopy with biopsy remains the standard to diagnose colon cancer as well as to evaluate the entire colon and rectum to ensure there are no additional lesions.
- Staging is determined by depth of invasion (T), lymph node involvement (N), and the presence of metastases (M).
- Full history and physical examination including rectal exam.
- Tumor marker carcinoembryonic antigen (CEA) level for later monitoring.
- Chest/abdomen/pelvis CT to evaluate for metastatic disease.
- Patients with rectal cancers (< 12 cm from anal verge) should also undergo a rigid proctoscopy to determine accurate distance from anal verge in addition to either pelvic MRI or endorectal ultrasound to evaluate depth of invasion (T stage) and presence of nodal disease (N stage).
  - Treatment:
- Colon cancers that have not metastasized should be resected assuming acceptable patient comorbidities and life expectancy.
- Recommend resection with 4- to 5-cm margins.
- Resect > 12 lymph nodes with specimen to complete staging accurately.
- Ligate blood supply near take off to achieve adequate lymph node harvest.
- May be performed open/laparoscopic/robotic with similar patient outcomes.
- Colon cancers that have limited metastasis to liver or lung may still be resectable.
- Recommend multidisciplinary review at specialized high-volume centers.
- May include neoadjuvant treatment, concomitant liver/lung resection along with colon resection, or staged operative and nonoperative treatments.
- Widespread metastatic disease typically treated with palliative chemotherapy; may consider resection or ostomy creation in cases of obstruction.
- Rectal cancers are treated differently than colon cancers, which is why they must be distinguished as they tend to be more aggressive; T1–T2, N0, M0 disease may be treated with surgery (either low anterior resection [LAR] or abdominal perineal resection [APR]); T3–T4 or any N disease treated first with neoadjuvant chemoradiation followed by surgery.
- Adjuvant treatment with chemotherapy (FOLFOX) typically recommended for nodal disease or aggressive tumor characteristics on pathology review.
- Complications:
  - Colorectal surgery is typically tolerated well; however, special risks include the following:
- Leak: most feared complication; an anastomotic leak will manifest with signs of sepsis. If patient is stable, a small leak may potentially be treated with IR drainage but most patients must return to the operating room for either repair or redo anastomosis, usually with proximal diversion.
- Abscess: Deep organ-space infection diagnosed with CT; treat with antibiotics and IR drain unless unstable.
- Postoperative ileus: Common especially after open surgeries. Ensure adequate electrolytes, limitation of narcotics, and rule out infectious causes.
- Dehydration: Can develop after any resection of colon but most common in patients with ileostomy with high output. Ensure adequate rehydration and rule out infectious causes, then consider motility-slowing agents.
- Outcomes:
  - Colon and rectal cancers continue to constitute a large share of deaths due to cancer, but overall 5-year survival statistics have gradually improved over the past several decades and are now > 60%.

4.7 Transplantation

Michael Karsy and Austin Cannon

Also see Chapter 6.1.3 Cardiac Transplantation.

4.7.1 Liver Transplantation

- Terminology[14,15]:
  - Orthotopic liver transplant (OLT) replaces the removed liver with a transplanted allograft liver in the anatomically correct position; heterotopic liver transplant placed the liver in a nonanatomic position, but this technique is no longer in use because of poor outcomes.
  - Auxiliary liver transplant is placement of a donor liver in the presence of the native liver.
  - Segmental liver transplant is placement of a portion of donor liver into the recipient. Grafts may be either cadaveric or from a living donor.
- Indications:
  - Acute liver failure (e.g., drug toxicity, hepatitis, metabolic disease, Budd-Chiari syndrome, acetaminophen), complications of cirrhosis (e.g., ascites, spontaneous bacterial peritonitis, encephalopathy, portal hypertension, variceal hemorrhage, early stage hepatocellular carcinoma), fulminant viral hepatitis.
  - Risk of death in < 7 days without transplantation; suggested by severe jaundice and early hepatic encephalopathy.
  - Metabolic diseases (alpha 1 antitrypsin deficiency, glycogen storage disease, hemochromatosis, Wilson disease).
  - Chronic liver disease (hepatopulmonary syndrome, hepatorenal syndrome, portopulmonary hypertension).
  - Biliary disease (primary biliary cirrhosis, primary sclerosing cholangitis, extrahepatic biliary atresia).
  - Early, small hepatocellular carcinoma with multifocal disease, traditional criteria included 1 nodule ≤ 5 cm or ≤ 3 nodules of ≤ 3 cm (Milan criteria); however, more aggressive disease is now being treated with transplantation using the UCSF criteria (single tumor < 6.5 cm, 2–3 lesions none exceeding 4.5 cm and total tumor diameter < 8 cm without extrahepatic spread or vascular invasion).
  - See Chapter 10 Pediatrics for indications for liver transplantation in pediatric patients, e.g., hepatoblastoma.
  - In rare cases, liver transplantation may be undertaken for traumatic injury to the liver not amenable to damage control maneuvers or resection.
  - Variation in graft and patient survival, generally 80–90% graft survival at 1 year.
- Evaluation:
  - MELD score:
    - Values range from 6 to 40; estimates 3-month postoperative survival follows TIPS; 90% survival for score of 6, 7% survival for score of 40.
    - Incorporates dialysis, creatinine level, bilirubin, international normalized ratio, and sodium level.
    - Standard MELD exceptions with specific diagnostic criteria assigned score of 22, with 10% increase in score every 3 months: hepatocellular carcinoma, hepatopulmonary syndrome, portopulmonary hypertension, hepatic artery thrombosis, familial amyloid polyneuropathy, primary hyperoxaluria, cystic fibrosis, hilar cholangiocarcinoma.
  - Absolute contraindications: Unable to survive surgery, active sepsis, short life expectancy, active alcohol or substance abuse within last 3–6 months, surgery not possible for technical reasons (e.g., morbid obesity, multiple venous thrombi), elevated pulmonary artery pressures (> 45 mm Hg).
  - Relative contraindications: Advanced age, cholangiocarcinoma, previous malignancy, chronic or respiratory infections, poor social support.
  - ABO blood type compatibility but not human leukocyte antigen matching required.
  - High risk of cerebral edema and herniation with acute liver failure; requires monitoring before transplantation.

- Organ types:
  - Standard-criteria donor (SCD): Whole organ; brain-dead donor < 80 years old; harvested and stored in cold preservation fluid ideally < 12 hours.
  - Donation after cardiac death (DCD): Whole organ; harvested after life support withdrawn and heart stops, resulting in longer warm ischemia times.
  - Cadaveric reduced-size grafts: Partial grafts; used with donor–recipient mismatch to prevent hypoperfusion; less common.
  - Living donor liver transplantation (LDLT): Full left or right lobe for pediatric or adult recipients; higher complications, retransplantation, biliary, and vascular complications than SCD.
- Surgical technique:
  - Bilateral subcostal incisions with midline extension to xiphoid (e.g., Mercedes-Benz or inverted Y incision); suprahepatic veins and portal structures isolated and mobilized.
  - Temporary portal vein to inferior vena cava bypass selectively performed to decrease intestinal edema, reduce hypotension with vena cava clamping, or reduce portal hypertension and for difficult hepatectomies.
  - Alternatively, use of the piggyback technique where the donor suprahepatic inferior vena cava (IVC) is anastomosed to the common lumen of recipient hepatic veins entering the recipient IVC allows liver transplantation without having to cross clamp the IVC or create a temporary vascular bypass.
  - Vessel anastomosis: Suprahepatic vena cava, infrahepatic vena cava, hepatic artery, portal vein.
  - Biliary anastomosis: end-to-end bile duct anastomosis, choledochojejunostomy.
  - Piggyback technique: Portion of vena cava left on recipient liver, donor liver attached in end-to-side fashion.
- Postoperative care and complications:
  - Hemodynamic monitoring and resuscitation requirements; coagulopathy corrected; ventilation supported for 24–48 hours, although some patients may be successfully extubated immediately after the operation; electrolyte management; serial vascular ultrasounds to evaluate graft perfusion and flow through new anastomoses; infection prophylaxis with trimethoprim/sulfamethoxazole, fluconazole, and ganciclovir; liver function tests and biopsies used to evaluate graft function.
  - Primary nonfunction: Failure of organ to regain function within 24–48 hours; urgent retransplantation required; rare with modern storage solutions.
  - Rejection: Occurs in 60% patients at some point; acutely treated and responsive to corticosteroids; chronic ductopenic rejection/vanishing bile duct syndrome occurs after 2 months and requires retransplantation.
  - Small-for-size syndrome: Overperfusion; predictive from graft-to-recipient weight ratio < 0.8%.
  - Large-for-size syndrome: Poor organ perfusion; predictive from graft-to-recipient weight ratio > 4%.
  - Hepatic artery thrombosis: Can occur intraoperatively or postoperatively from vessel injury or intimal dissection.
  - Portal vein thrombosis: Early onset due to technical errors and treated with thrombectomy and systemic anticoagulation; late onset due to intimal hyperplasia and may require selective shunting.
  - Vena cava obstruction: Rare.
  - Biliary leak or stricture: Diagnosed with cholangiogram or endoscopic retrograde cholangiopancreatography; typically treated with stents or percutaneous drains but reoperation is sometimes required.
  - Renal dysfunction: Hypoperfusion with increased risk from calcineurin inhibitors.
  - Infection: Bacterial infections most common compared with viral and fungal infections.
  - Post-transplantational lymphoproliferative disorders: Epstein-Barr virus and cytomegalovirus infection; decreases with immune suppression and antiviral therapies.
  - Recurrence of native disease.
  - Hypertension and hyperlipidemia: Delayed, common findings after transplantation.
  - Distinct immunosuppression protocols used by institution to manage organ rejection (▶ Table 4.4 and ▶ Table 4.5).

Table 4.4 List of immunosuppressant medications[16]

Induction	
Corticosteroids	• Methylprednisolone and prednisone are most commonly used
T-cell-depleting monoclonal antibodies	• Muromonab-CD3 • Alemtuzumab
T-cell-depleting polyclonal antibody	• Thymoglobulin
Cytotoxic T lymphocyte-associated protein 4 inhibitor	• Belatacept
Interleukin-2 subunit	• Daclizumab, basiliximab; anti-CD25 inhibitor of interleukin-2 receptors on T-cells
Maintenance	
Calcineurin inhibitors	• Tacrolimus (Prograft) • Cyclosporine • Inhibit interleukin-2 production
Nucleotide inhibitors	• Mycophenolate mofetil (CellCept, Myfortic): Disrupts inosine monophosphate dehydrogenase involved in de novo synthesis of purines in lymphocytes • Azathioprine (Imuran): Purine analog that interferes with DNA and RNA synthesis
Mechanistic target of rapamycin (mTOR) inhibitors	• Sirolimus, everolimus; inhibit lymphocyte response to interleukin-2
Rituximab	• Anti CD20 inhibitor on B cells

Table 4.5 Rejection types

Type	Cause	Time	Management
Hyperacute	Preformed antibodies (ABO incompatibility)	Minutes	Removal of organ
Acute cellular	Activated T-cells	Weeks to months	Steroids, increased immunosuppression, antibody therapy
Acute humoral/ antibody-mediated	Reactivation of low-level preformed antibodies or *de novo* formation of antibodies	Weeks to years	Plasmapheresis, intravenous immunoglobulin, steroids, increased immunosuppression, antibody therapy
Chronic	Antibodies, cell-mediated, toxicity from immunosuppression	Months to years	Poor response to medication changes; reduced risk by avoiding acute rejection episodes

○ Recent advances in liver transplantation include using human immunodeficiency virus (HIV)–positive donor organs in HIV-positive recipients, use of hepatitis C organs in both hepatitis C–positive and –negative recipients and postoperatively using new antiviral regimens to treat the hepatitis C.

4.7.2 Renal Transplantation

• Indications[17]:
  ○ End-stage renal disease: Transplantation improves long-term patient survival and also decreases health care costs when compared with long-term dialysis.
  ○ Absolute contraindications: Active, untreated malignancy except nonmelanocytic skin cancer and incidental renal cell cancer, active infection, cardiopulmonary disease, acute viral hepatitis.

- ○ Relative contraindications: Substance abuse, poor social support, untreated HIV infection, renal diseases with high recurrence rate.
- ○ Renal transplantation improves long-term survival depending on comorbidities of recipient.
- Evaluation:
  - ○ ABO blood type and human leukocyte antigen matching required.
  - ○ Glomerular filtration rate (GFR) ≤ 30 mL/min (chronic kidney disease stage 4) evaluated for transplantation, GFR < 20 mL/min referred for transplantation.
  - ○ Pretransplantation nephrectomy recommended if: Chronic renal infection, infected stones or reflux, significant proteinuria, intractable hypertension, significant polycystic kidney disease, adenocarcinoma.
  - ○ Kidney Donor Profile Index (KDPI):
    - – Scoring system predicting graft failure after transplantation, with higher score associated with shorter estimated function.
    - – Factors: Patient age, weight, height, race, diabetes, hypertension, hepatitis C, creatinine; cause of donor death, DCD status.
- Organ type:
  - ○ Living donor:
    - – 96% 1-year and 58% 10-year graft survival.
    - – Donor nephrectomy mortality rate 0.03%, reoperation rate < 1%, readmission rate < 1%, postoperative complications 3%.
    - – Exclusion criteria: Psychiatric disease, substance abuse, renal disease, abnormal renal anatomy, recurrent or bilateral nephrolithiasis, other organ system disease, active infection or malignancy, hereditary hypercoagulability disorders, donating due to suspected financial incentives provided by recipient.
  - ○ SCD:
    - – 92% 1-year and 44% 10-year graft survival.
  - ○ Extended-criteria donor (ECD):
    - – 85% 1-year and 26% 1-year graft survival.
    - – Age ≥ 60 years or age 50–59 years with two of following: hypertension, death from stroke, Cr ≥ 1.5 mg/dL.
    - – 70% risk of renal failure within 2 years.
  - ○ DCD: Longer warm ischemic time and therefore higher incidence of delayed graft function after transplantation.
- Surgical technique:
  - ○ Left kidney preferred because of longer vein; laparoscopic with or without hand-assisted nephrectomy preferred technique.
  - ○ Renal artery and vein divided with stapler.
  - ○ Ureter ligated distally and kidney delivered through hand port or Pfannenstiel incision.
  - ○ Transplantation into right iliac fossa offers easier surgical access because of more superficial iliac vessels; can be transplanted on either side if necessary because of anatomic considerations or prior transplantation.
  - ○ Extraperitoneal approach classically used; double J stent employed across ureterocystostomy.
- Postoperative care and complications:
  - ○ Hourly monitoring of urine output; electrolyte replacement, volume replacement ensured; central venous pressure monitoring can guide volume status; Foley catheter left for 2–5 days; urinalysis can monitor for infection and acute renal injury; serial vascular ultrasounds can be performed to evaluate vascular inflow, outflow, and graft perfusion.
  - ○ Decreased urine output can be from hypovolemia, urinary obstruction, ureteral compromise, vascular compromise, acute tubular necrosis, or rejections.
  - ○ Creatinine decrease indicates graft functioning.
  - ○ Ultrasound used after decrease in urine output or laboratory abnormalities; can evaluate for vessel function, fluid collection, and hydronephrosis.
  - ○ Wound infection (1–10%).

- Delayed graft functioning (5% living donors, 20% deceased donors): dialysis within first week after transplantation.
- Bleeding can result in graft compression and decreased urine output.
- Graft thrombosis (< 1%): Results in graft loss; occurs within first week.
- Lymphocele (1–10%): Mostly asymptomatic; treated with intraperitoneal window.
- Renal artery stenosis (1–10%): Occurs 3–48 months after transplantation; presents with refractory hypertension or increase in creatinine.
- Ureteral stricture (2–15%): Early onset due to hematoma or kinking, late onset due to fibrosis from ischemia or BK virus.
- Urine leak (3–10%): Occurs within 1 month; results from ureteral ischemia and anastomosis failure; treated with percutaneous nephrostomy, stenting, or operative revision.
- Malignancy: Post-transplant lymphoproliferative disorder or Kaposi sarcoma caused by immunosuppression.
- Distinct immunosuppression protocols used by institution to manage organ rejection (▶ Table 4.3 and ▶ Table 4.4).

4.7.3 Pancreas Transplantation

- Indications[18,19]:
  - Treatment of insulin-dependent/type 1 diabetics with C-peptide deficiency, some insulin-independent/type 2 diabetics, brittle diabetics (insulin dependence with glucose fluctuation, hypoglycemic unawareness), end-stage renal disease secondary to diabetes.
- Evaluation:
  - ABO blood-type compatibility and donor organs from age 5–50 years evaluated.
  - Absolute contraindications: Patients with malignancy, generalized complications from diabetes, nonrenal organ failure, impaired and irreversible cardiac function, substance abuse or psychiatric factors, morbid obesity.
  - Organs evaluated for history of diabetes, chronic pancreatitis, pancreatic trauma, and alcohol abuse.
- Organ type:
  - Simultaneous pancreas and kidney (SPK) transplant:
    - 80% 5-year transplant survival.
    - 80% of pancreas transplants.
    - Improves insulin control, renal graft survival, diabetic neuropathy, and diabetic nephropathy.
    - Lowest rate of pancreas graft thrombosis (5%) and organ rejection (2%).
  - Pancreas after kidney (PAK) transplant:
    - 62% 5-year transplant survival.
    - 15% of pancreas transplants.
    - Patients of prior renal transplantation and poor diabetes control.
  - Pancreas transplant alone (PTA):
    - 59% 5-year transplant survival.
    - 5% of pancreas transplants.
    - Patients with brittle diabetes with hypoglycemic unawareness without renal dysfunction.
  - Islet cell transplantation:
    - Alternative to PTA in brittle diabetics without hypoglycemic unawareness.
    - Rare procedure but lower risk.
    - Involves enzymatic digestion of pancreatic tissue from pancreatectomy or cadaver, purification of islet cells, microencapsulation and injection into liver via portal vein.
    - 70% 1-year and 35% 3-year insulin independence.
- Surgical technique:
  - Transplanted to right iliac fossa, systemic or portal venous drainage; arterial anastomosis using donor external iliac to superior mesenteric artery, donor internal iliac to splenic artery, or donor common iliac to recipient common iliac.
  - Exocrine secretions placed in donor duodenum harvested with pancreas and anastomosed to small bowel or to bladder.

- Postoperative care and complications:
  - Patients anticoagulated with aspirin, systemic heparinization, or low-molecular-weight heparin to reduce vascular thrombosis.
  - Graft function monitored by amylase levels and glucose levels.
  - Insulin supplementation limited immediately postoperatively to evaluate organ function.
  - Duplex ultrasound or radionucleotide scans used to evaluate transplant viability and blood supply.
  - Creatinine levels monitored for rejection; 32% loss in first year.
  - Graft pancreatitis (up to 30%): Due to transplant ischemia/reperfusion or injury, peripancreatic collection, or infection; pain located over graft; amylase level increases.
  - Graft thrombosis (5–15%): Sudden graft lost with alterations in amylase, glucose, and insulin requirement; venous thrombosis more common than arterial injury.
  - Anastomotic leak (2–10%): Diagnosed with CT and oral contrast.
  - Bleeding (6–8%): GI bleeding from vessel anastomosis; associated with systemic anticoagulation.
  - Transplant rejection (30%): Highest risk in first year.
  - Distinct immunosuppression protocols used by institution to manage organ rejection (▸ Table 4.3 and ▸ Table 4.5).

References

[1] Shah AP, Mourad MM, Bramhall SR. Acute pancreatitis: current perspectives on diagnosis and management. J Inflamm Res. 2018; 11: 77–85

[2] Forsmark CE, Vege SS, Wilcox CM. Acute pancreatitis. N Engl J Med. 2016; 375(20):1972–1981

[3] Foster BR, Jensen KK, Bakis G, Shaaban AM, Coakley FV. Revised Atlanta classification for acute pancreatitis: a pictorial essay. Radiographics. 2016; 36(3):675–687

[4] Sanders G, Kingsnorth AN. Gallstones. BMJ. 2007; 335(7614):295–299

[5] Wiegand J, Berg T. The etiology, diagnosis and prevention of liver cirrhosis: part 1 of a series on liver cirrhosis. Dtsch Arztebl Int. 2013; 110(6):85–91

[6] Tsochatzis EA, Bosch J, Burroughs AK. Liver cirrhosis. Lancet. 2014; 383(9930):1749–1761

[7] MacConmara M, Brunt LM. Spleen: The Washington Manual of Surgery. 6th ed. Philadelphia, PA: Lippincott Williams & Wilkins; 2015;16:387–395

[8] Beauchamp RD, Evers BM, Mattox K. Spleen. Sabiston Textbook of Surgery. 2017; 56:1560–1566

[9] Trunkey A. Splenic injuries. Therapy of Trauma and Surgical Critical Care. Amsterdam, Netherlands: Elsevier Health Sciences; 2016:373–379

[10] Coccolini F, Montori G, Catena F, et al. Splenic trauma: WSES classification and guidelines for adult and pediatric patients. World J Emerg Surg. 2017; 12:40

[11] Crooker KG, Howard JM, Alvarado AR, et al. Splenic embolization after trauma: an opportunity to improve best immunization practices. J Surg Res. 2018; 232:293–297

[12] Feliciano DV. Abdominal trauma revisited. Am Surg. 2017; 83(11):1193–1202

[13] Shamim AA, Zafar SN, Nizam W, et al. Laparoscopic splenectomy for trauma. JSLS. 2018; 22:e2018.00050

[14] Neuberger J. An update on liver transplantation: a critical review. J Autoimmun. 2016; 66:51–59

[15] Zarrinpar A, Busuttil RW. Liver transplantation: past, present and future. Nat Rev Gastroenterol Hepatol. 2013; 10(7):434–440

[16] Loupy A, Lefaucheur C. Antibody-mediated rejection of solid-organ allografts. N Engl J Med. 2018; 379(12):1150–1160

[17] Nieto T, Inston N, Cockwell P. Renal transplantation in adults. BMJ. 2016; 355:i6158

[18] Meirelles Júnior RF, Salvalaggio P, Pacheco-Silva A. Pancreas transplantation: review. Einstein (Sao Paulo). 2015; 13(2):305–309

[19] Gruessner RW, Gruessner AC. The current state of pancreas transplantation. Nat Rev Endocrinol. 2013; 9(9):555–562

5 Vascular Surgery

Edited by Anthony Ocon

5.1 Atherosclerotic Disease and Ischemia

Michael Karsy

5.1.1 Anatomy

- Some key palpable pulses and locations (▶ Fig. 5.1):
  - Radial: Lateral wrist.
  - Ulnar: Medial wrist.
  - Brachial: Antecubital fossa or medial brachial surface.
  - Carotid: Midneck region, anterior to sternocleidomastoid.
  - Femoral: Midpoint of inguinal ligament from anterosuperior iliac spine to pubis.
  - Popliteal: Lateral popliteal fossa between two heads of gastrocnemius.
  - Dorsal pedis: Dorsal foot between first and second metatarsal bones.
  - Posterior tibial: Medial malleolus.
- Head, neck, and upper-extremity vessels:
  - Ascending aorta:
    – Coronary vessels.
  - Brachiocephalic/innominate:
    – Common carotid (left common carotid off subclavian) → internal/external carotid.
  - Right subclavian → right axillary → right brachial → right ulnar/radial → same branches as left:
    – Vertebral.
- Aortic arch:
  - Common carotid (bovine arch defines left common carotid sharing origin with brachiocephalic/innominate common trunk):
    – Internal carotid: Ophthalmic, superior hypophyseal, posterior communicating, anterior choroidal, anterior cerebral, middle cerebral.
    – External carotid: Superior thyroid, ascending pharyngeal, facial, lingual, occipital, posterior auricular, maxillary.
  - Left subclavian artery:
    – Vertebral: Posterior inferior cerebellar, basilar.
    – Internal thoracic/left internal mammillary artery (LIMA).
    – Thyrocervical trunk: Inferior thyroid, transverse cervical, ascending cervical, suprascapular.
    – Dorsal scapular.
    – Costocervical trunk: Deep cervical, superior intercostal.
  - Left axillary artery:
    – Superior thoracic.
    – Thoracoacromial.
    – Subscapular.
    – Anterior humeral circumflex.
    – Posterior humeral circumflex.
  - Left brachial:
    – Profunda brachii.
    – Ulnar.
    – Radial.
    – Deep palmar arch, superficial palmar arch, common palmar digital, radial artery index finger, proper palmar digital, princeps pollicis.
- Abdominal vessels:
  - Descending aorta (intercostal and lumbar radicular branches).
  - Inferior phrenic:

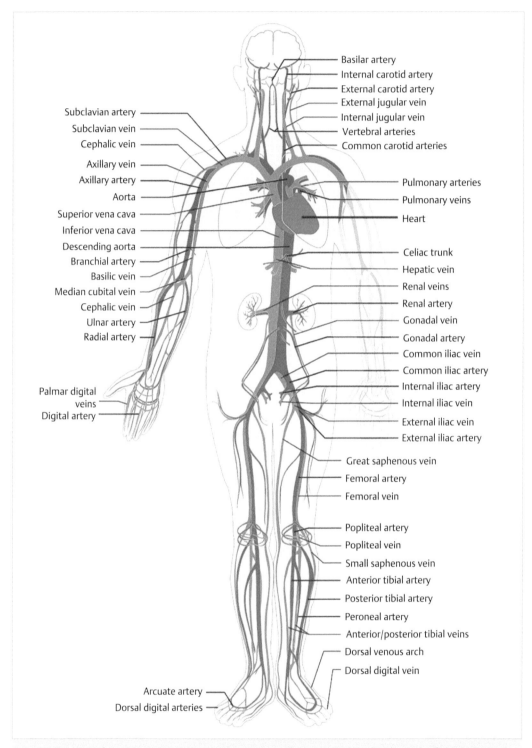

Fig. 5.1 Overview of circulatory system. Source: Mariana Ruiz Villarreal (LadyofHats [Public Domain]).

- Recurrent branch of esophagus.
- Suprarenal.
- Celiac trunk:
  - Left and right gastric.
  - Splenic: Short gastric, left gastric.
  - Common hepatic: Left and right hepatic, right gastroepiploic and gastroduodenal, cystic.
- Superior mesenteric:
  - Inferior pancreaticoduodenal.
  - Middle colic.
  - Right colic.
  - Ileocolic.
  - Intestinal arteries: Jejunal and ileal arteries.
- Left and right renal.
- Inferior mesenteric:
  - Left colic (ascending and descending branches; ascending joins marginal artery of Drummond).
  - Sigmoid arteries.
  - Superior rectal.
- Lower extremity vessels:
  - Descending aorta (median sacral branch).
  - Common iliac:
    - Internal iliac: Iliolumbar, inferior and superior gluteal, inferior vesical, obturator, middle rectal, lateral sacral, umbilical, uterine, artery to ductus deferens, internal pudendal, external iliac (inferior epigastric and deep circumflex; continues as common femoral).
    - Common femoral: Superficial femoral and profunda femoris/deep femoral (lateral and medial circumflex; perforating arteries), superficial epigastric, superficial circumflex iliac, superficial external pudendal, deep external pudendal, descending genicular.
    - Popliteal: Middle genicular, sural, tibial-peroneal trunk.
    - Tibial Peroneal trunk: posterior tibial, peroneal, circumflex fibular, medial malleolar, medial and lateral plantar, anterior tibial (dorsal pedis, anterior and posterior tibial recurrent, anterior medial and lateral malleolar).

5.1.2 Vascular Imaging

- Ultrasound:
  - Doppler:
    - Velocity < 50 cm/s signifies slowed flow from proximal stenosis or occlusion.
    - Velocity > 300 cm/s signifies elevated velocity within or adjacent to stenosis.
    - B-mode: Image soft tissue.
    - Pulse Doppler: Samples velocity at visualized location.
  - Ankle-brachial index: ratio of systolic occlusion pressure in dorsal pedalis or posterior tibial artery (toe-brachial index can be used in diabetic patients, patients > 80 years, or those with critical ischemia; use higher value of dorsal pedalis or posterior tibial) vs. brachial pulses:
    - 0.9–1.3: normal.
    - 0.7 to < 0.9: mild.
    - 0.4 to < 0.7: moderate.
    - < 0.4: critical.
  - Specific cutoffs for different diseases and areas exist with varying sensitivity and specificity (▶ Table 5.1).
- Computed tomography (CT) angiography: Used for vascular imaging; risk of contrast-induced nephrotoxicity in patients with renal dysfunction.
- Magnetic resonance (MR) angiography: Uses noncontrast forms (e.g., time of flight, arterial spin labeling) and contrast-enhanced forms; risk of nephrogenic systemic fibrosis in patients with diabetes and renal dysfunction receiving gadolinium.

Table 5.1 General duplex findings of occlusive disease

Stenosis (%)	Peak systolic velocity (cm/s)	Velocity ratio across stenosis	Waveform
0–30	<150	<1.5	Triphasic
30–49	150–200	1.5–2.0	Tri/biphasic
50–75	200–300	2.0–3.9	Bi/monophasic
>75	>300	>4.0	Flattened

Wave patterns: triphasic (normal, anterograde–retrograde–anterograde blood flow), biphasic (mild stenotic disease), monophasic (severe disease).

- Invasive imaging:
  - Digital subtraction angiography shows best resolution of vessels but invasive, risk of contrast nephropathy.
  - Catheters sized by French (Fr) sizing; 1 French = 0.33 mm; Fr/3 = approximate catheter size in mm.
  - Sheaths sized by inner diameter.
  - Catheters sized by outer diameter (e.g., 5 Fr catheter passes through a 5 Fr sheath), passive catheters used as shaped and multipurpose, active catheters that must be shaped intravascularly.
  - Wires sized in inches (0.014" wire commonly used in renal, mesenteric, carotid, and tibial interventions); coated with hydrophilic coating and vary in stiffness and tip softness.
  - ≥ 8 Fr femoral sheath and ≥ 6 Fr brachial sheath increases complication rate.

5.1.3 Vascular Occlusion and Ischemia

- Atherosclerosis:
  - Systemic disease involving narrowing of vessels due to buildup of cholesterol plaque.
  - Multifactorial; involves coronary, carotid, large vessels, and peripheral arteries.
  - Initial lesion undergoes accumulation of lipids forming a fatty streak; formation of an atheroma results from intracellular lipid accumulation; later multilayered fibroatheroma forms from fibrous and calcified tissues; final complicated lesion involves ulcerated plaques with potential for thrombosis formation, hemorrhage, vessel injury, and embolism.
  - Modifiable risk factors: Smoking, diabetes, dyslipidemia, hypertension, transfats.
  - Nonmodifiable risk factors: advanced age, male sex, family history, genetic abnormalities, infectious agents, inflammatory cytokines.
  - Antiplatelet drugs are used for patients with coronary artery, carotid artery, and peripheral artery disease (PAD); there is no clear evidence for one agent over another.
  - Identification of vulnerable plaques and patients is key for recommendation of surgical treatments; risks of surgical treatment are balanced against risk of continued disease progression.[1,2]
- Acute limb ischemia:
  - Symptoms can occur within 2 weeks of onset of symptoms but usually presents acutely, include any combination of 6 Ps (pain, paralysis, paresthesias, pulselessness, poikilothermia, pallor); 90% embolism commonly from cardiac source.
  - Require emergent attention; first treated by balloon embolectomy using Fogarty catheter; all patients are started on heparin drip, and direct or systemic thrombolytic therapy is considered if unable to receive surgical treatment; various revascularization approaches can be used; fasciotomy of limbs is considered to reduce later risk of limb ischemia in patients with compartment syndrome.
  - 30% risk of limb loss within 30 days.
  - 80% of embolic events are from atrial fibrillation or a recent myocardial infarction; also likely in individuals with previous interventions or hypercoagulable stages.
  - Locations: Common femoral (30–35%, classic water-hammer femoral pulse), aortoiliac (20–25%, bilateral ischemia, saddle embolism), popliteal (15%), brachial (10%, mostly left upper extremity).
  - Surgical treatment:
    - Open surgical and endovascular treatment options are complementary.[3]

- Access for open surgical treatment: brachial (S-type incision in antecubital fossa), femoral (vertical or transverse groin incision), tibial (below knee popliteal incision 2 fingerbreadths below inferior tibial tuberosity).
  - Fogarty size dilates to double size (e.g., #3 dilates to 6 mm): iliac (5/white), femoropopliteal/brachial (4/red), tibial/radial (3/green).
- Blue toe syndrome/atheroembolic disease: microscopic cholesterol containing debris usually from aneurysm, cardiac embolism, or aortic atherosclerosis; can be spontaneous or iatrogenic from endovascular procedures; patients are treated with antiplatelet agents and statins; warfarin is generally contraindicated due to cholesterol emboli release except for patients with symptomatic aortic plaques ≥ 4 mm.
- Carotid disease:
  - Stroke is the fifth leading cause of death and disability in the United States.
  - 90% ischemic (thrombotic, embolic, systemic hypoperfusion, venous thrombosis), 10% hemorrhagic (intracerebral vs. subarachnoid).
  - In general, carotid endarterectomy (CEA) superior to medical treatment for symptomatic patients with carotid stenosis > 50% or asymptomatic patients with stenosis > 70%; carotid artery stenting (CAS) can be used in patients with high risk for surgical treatment.
  - Stenosis measured by North American Symptomatic Carotid Endarterectomy Trial (NASCET) compares diseased vessel to normal vessel diameter, correlates with European Carotid Surgery Trial (ECST) measurement.
  - Symptoms: transient ischemic attacks (TIAs) (neurological deficits lasting < 24 hours), cerebral infarction (with permanent or resolved deficits), or amaurosis fugax (transient monocular blindness).
  - Diastolic bruit suggests a > 70% stenosis.
  - NASCET evaluated 659 patients with stroke or TIA with internal carotid artery (ICA) stenosis > 70%; randomized to CEA vs. medical management; patients with CEA had a lower 2-year stroke rate (9% vs. 26%), patients with 50–69% stenosis had moderate benefit in 5-year stroke rates.[4]
  - ECST evaluated 3,024 patients with stroke in the last 6 months; patients with stenosis > 80% showed benefit from CEA in 3-year stroke rate (2.8% vs. 16.8%).[5]
  - Asymptomatic Carotid Atherosclerosis Study (ACAS)[6] and Asymptomatic Carotid Surgery Trial (ACST)[7] evaluated patients with > 60% ICA stenosis; showed reduction in 5-year stroke risk.
  - Stenting and Angioplasty with Protection in Patients at High Risk for Endarterectomy Investigators (SAPPHIRE) trial[8] evaluated 334 patients with symptomatic 50% ICA stenosis or asymptomatic 80% stenosis to receive CEA vs. CAS; composite end point of death, stroke, or myocardial infarction up to 1 year; noninferior at 1 year.
  - Carotid Revascularization Endarterectomy versus Stenting Trial (CREST)[9] evaluated 2,502 patients to receive CEA vs. CAS; no difference in composite end point of death, stroke, or myocardial infarction at 4 years, higher risk of stroke during CAS and higher risk of myocardial infarction with CEA helped to define subgroups where one treatment may be preferred.
  - Treatment:
    - CEA: Linear incision is made parallel to sternocleidomastoid; requires identification of common, internal, and external carotid; vessel occluded while patient is monitored with or without a temporary shunt; heparin is administered to reduce clots resulting in stroke; plaque is removed; patch is sewn in.
    - Endovascular CAS: Femoral access with navigation to common carotid artery; embolization prevention parachute is deployed distal to plaque; carotid stent is measured and deployed with angioplasty balloon; patients are then treated with dual antiplatelet agents.
    - Treatment cutoff values for stenosis vary by trial (▶ Table 5.2).
    - CEA shows higher risk of myocardial infarction compared with CAS; CAS shows a higher risk of stroke compared with CEA; institutional complication rate for CEA recommended < 3% to provide patient benefit.
    - CAS is used for high-riding carotid stenosis (above C2) or low-riding stenosis (below clavicle); CAS is used for patients with recurrent disease, contralateral occlusion preventing occlusion of disease vessel during treatment, recurrent laryngeal nerve injury, prior neck radiation, or tracheostomy.

Table 5.2 Cutoff values for occlusive carotid disease

Study	Stenosis	Sample size	End point	End point with medical therapy	End point with surgical therapy	Absolute risk reduction	Relative risk reduction
NASCET symptomatic	50–69%	858	5-y ipsilateral stroke	22.2%	15.7%	6.5%	29%
ECST symptomatic	80–99%	576	3-y ipsilateral stroke	20.6%	6.8%	13.8%	67%
NASCET asymptomatic	70–99%	659	2-y ipsilateral stroke	26%	9%	17%	65%
ACAS asymptomatic	60–99%	1662	5-y ipsilateral stroke	11%	5.1%	6.1%	53%
ACST asymptomatic	60–99%	3120	5-y any stroke	11.8%	6.4%	5.4%	46%

Abbreviations: ACAS, Asymptomatic Carotid Atherosclerosis Study; ACST, Asymptomatic Carotid Surgery Trial; ECST, European Carotid Surgery Trial; NASCET, North American Symptomatic Carotid Endarterectomy Trial.

- Controversial order of treatment for patients with need for coronary artery bypass graft and carotid stenosis.
- Controversial whether to reduce heparin treatment with protamine and increasing risk of stroke.
- Brachiocephalic:
  - Less likely to require intervention than carotid vessels.
  - Stenosis most likely due to atherosclerosis (80%) but also due to vasculitis, aneurysms, and radiation.
  - Associated syndromes:
    - Vertebrobasilar insufficiency: Transient vertigo, dizziness, focal neurological symptoms localized to brainstem, visual symptoms, drop attacks.
    - Subclavian steal: Vertebrobasilar insufficiency secondary to upper-extremity activity, due to occlusion proximal to vertebral artery causing retrograde blood flow to the arms with activity.
    - Coronary-subclavian steal: Coronary symptoms in patients with coronary artery bypass grafting using LIMA.
    - Upper-extremity claudication: Reduced pulses and limb fatigue with use.
    - Arterial thoracic outlet syndrome: Arterial obstruction and remodeling via occlusion in the scalene triangle (first rib, anterior and middle scalene).
  - Treatment by stenting (> 70% patency at 5 years), direct reconstruction (innominate endarterectomy, aortocarotid bypass with > 80% patency at 10 years), or indirect reconstruction (carotid–carotid, carotid–subclavian, > 80% patency at 5 years).
- Occlusive PAD:
  - Occurs in 15% of the population > 70 years; 5% risk of amputation at 5 years for patients with intermittent claudication.
  - Claudication: Pain in hips, thighs, or calves worse with ambulation; resolves within 5 minutes; occurs at reproducible distance; not always associated with burning, tingling, or numbness; can be associated with tissue loss.
  - Nonatherosclerotic arterial disease[10]:
    - Considered in patients without history of vascular disease, nonexertional leg symptoms or symptoms with extreme exertion, younger patients, waxing/waning pattern, associated symptoms (e.g., fever, malaise, weight loss), known systemic diseases, atypical atherosclerosis imaging.
    - Popliteal artery entrapment syndrome: Exertion on popliteal artery from muscles or ligaments; five anatomic types; results in pain and paresthesias after exercise; treated by resection of compression site.
    - Cystic adventitial disease: collection of mucinous material within the adventitial layer of the artery; seen in middle-aged men mainly in the popliteal artery.

- Endofibrosis of iliac artery: Arterial stenosis in highly functional cyclists and runners from repetitive trauma.
- Fibromuscular dysplasia: Noninflammatory, nonatherosclerotic disease in women age 20–60 years.
- Vasculitis: inflammation of vessels, associated systemic features and systemic vascular distribution (e.g., Takayasu arteritis, giant-cell arteritis, Behçet disease).
- Midaortic syndrome: Form of aortic coarctation; results in hypertension of children and young adults with pressure differences in the upper and lower extremities.
- Buerger disease: Inflammatory segmental disease in adults associated with tobacco use; involves > 2 extremities and can be subclinical.
- Lumbar stenosis/neurogenic claudication: Similar claudication to PAD but imaging shows lower lumbar stenosis neurogenic claudication relieved with bending forward.
○ Diabetic PAD classically seen in aortoiliac artery in young females and superficial femoral in males; both show infrapopliteal and microvascular disease.
○ Distribution segments:
  - Aortoiliac: 5–10%.
  - Abdomen and external iliacs: 25%.
  - Widespread above inguinal ligament: 65%.
○ Important vascular collaterals:
  - Internal mammary to inferior epigastric.
  - Intercostal to circumflex iliac.
  - Lumbar and hypogastric to common femoral and deep femoral.
  - Superior mesenteric artery (SMA) to inferior mesenteric artery (IMA) and superior hemorrhoidal via marginal artery of Drummond and arc of Riolan.
  - Celiac to SMA via gastroduodenal and pancreaticoduodenal.
  - Angiosomes: Vascular territories with associated muscle, soft tissue, and neurological dermatomal territory; greater variance in lower extremities potentially explaining variability in clinical impacts of ischemia.
○ Rutherford classification of acute and chronic limb ischemia can be useful to track severity and recommend treatment (▶ Table 5.3 and ▶ Table 5.4); multiple other grading systems[11]; tissue loss is the best predictor for needing both arterial and venous procedures.
○ Medical management: Antiplatelet medications (aspirin), antihypertensive medications, statins, cilostazol (treatment for 3–6 months improves walking distances in 50% of patients, contraindicated in congestive heart failure).
○ Endovascular and open treatment can both be options depending on disease severity.
○ Interventions graded by Trans-Atlantic Inter-Society Consensus Document II (TASC II) determining treatment efficacy for patterns of disease; helps classify the multiple variations in vascular disease.[12]
  - A: endovascular results excellent.
  - B: endovascular results good and used unless open indication in same area.

Table 5.3 Rutherford classification of acute limb ischemia

Category	Description	Sensory loss	Muscle weakness	Arterial Doppler	Venous Doppler
I: Viable	Not immediately threatened	None	None	Audible	Audible
IIa: Marginally threatened	Salvageable if treated	Minimal/none	None	Inaudible	Audible
IIb: Immediately	Salvageable with immediate revascularization	More in toes, rest pain	Mild, moderate	Inaudible	Audible
III: Irreversible	Major tissue loss, permanent nerve damage inevitable	Numb	Severe, paralysis	Inaudible	Inaudible

Table 5.4 Rutherford classification of chronic limb ischemia

Grade	Category	Description	Diagnosis
0	0	Asymptomatic	Normal stress test
I	1	Mild	Can complete stress test, ankle pressure > 50 mm Hg after exercise and < 25 mm Hg more than brachial
I	2	Moderate	Between 1 and 3
I	3	Severe	Cannot complete stress test, ankle pressure < 50 mm Hg
II	4	Ischemic rest pain	Resting ankle pressure < 40 mm Hg, toe pressure < 30 mm Hg, minimal distal pulsatility
III	5	Minor tissue loss	Resting ankle pressure < 60 mm Hg, toe pressure < 40 mm Hg, minimal distal pulsatility
III	6	Major tissue loss	Same as 5

Note: Classic stress test includes walking at 1.5 mph at 12% for 5 min until symptoms cause patient to stop.

Table 5.5 TASC II classification of aortoiliac disease

Type	Finding	Treatment
A	• Uni/bilateral common iliac stenosis • Uni/bilateral < 3-cm external iliac stenosis	Endovascular favored
B	• < 3-cm stenosis infrarenal aorta • Unilateral common iliac occlusion • Unilateral stenosis > 3 cm or occlusion of external iliac artery not involving internal iliac or common femoral	Endovascular unless other indication for open
C	• Bilateral common iliac occlusion • Calcified external iliac occlusion • Bilateral external iliac stenosis or unilateral external iliac occlusion extending into common femoral or internal iliac	Open preferred, endovascular used for high-risk patients
D	• Infrarenal aortic occlusion • Unilateral common iliac and external iliac occlusion • Bilateral external iliac occlusion • Iliac stenosis in patients needing abdominal aortic aneurysm repair • Diffuse occlusive disease	Open favored

Abbreviation: TASC II, Trans-Atlantic Inter-Society Consensus Document II.

- – C: open result better than endovascular, endovascular used for high-risk patients.
    - – D: endovascular worse than open.
    - ○ Early graft failure (< 3 months) due to technical issues vs. late graft failure (3 months–2 years) due to intimal hyperplasia.
- Aortoiliac disease:
    - ○ 50% of aortic occlusions progress to the level of the renal arteries and 50% occlude below the IMA or lumbar arteries.
    - ○ Leriche syndrome triad: Buttock claudication, decreased femoral pulses, impotence.
    - ○ Endovascular stenting shows 80% patency at 5 years; less effective in chronic occlusions and external iliac arteries.
    - ○ Endovascular management reasonable for all lesions except proximal aortic occlusion above the IMA.
    - ○ Treated according to TASC II classifications (► Table 5.5).
    - ○ Surgical treatment:
        - – Aortobifemoral bypass: 80% patency at 5 years; uses a midline incision and retroperitoneal approach.
        - – Axillobifemoral bypass: 50–80% patency at 5 years; used for high-risk patients or patients with infected aortic grafts before explantation; uses a subclavicular incision and midline incision.
        - – Femoral–femoral bypass: 60% primary patency at 5 years; used for unilateral iliac disease and minimal disease in ipsilateral iliac.

Table 5.6 TASC II classification of infrainguinal disease

Type	Finding	Treatment
A	• Single stenosis < 10 cm or occlusion < 5 cm	Endovascular favored
B	• Multiple < 5-cm stenosis/occlusions • Single < 15-cm stenosis/occlusion not involving the infrageniculate popliteal artery • Calcified < 5-cm occlusion • Single popliteal stenosis	Endovascular unless other indication for open
C	• Multiple stenosis/occlusion 0.15 cm • Recurrent stenosis/occlusion after two endovascular interventions	Open preferred, endovascular used for high-risk patients
D	• Chronic total occlusion of common femoral or superficial femoral > 20 cm involving popliteal • Chronic total occlusion of popliteal and proximal trifurcation	Open favored

Abbreviation: TASC II, Trans-Atlantic Inter-Society Consensus Document II.

  – Ileo-femoral bypass: Retroperitoneal approach using a groin incision.
  ○ Infrainguinal disease:
  – Treated according to TASC II classifications (▶ Table 5.6).
  – Common femoral/profunda: Open treatment used except in high-risk cases.
  – Saphenous vein bypass grafting shows 75% patency at 5 years and is the gold standard compared with conduit bypasses.
- Mesenteric ischemia:
  ○ Found in 5–10% of the population over 65 years; 45% embolic and 25% thrombotic, 10% venous occlusion, 20% nonocclusive.
  ○ Presents with sudden abdominal pain, gut emptying, elevated white blood cell count, lactate and serum amylase.
  ○ Imaging shows portal venous air, pneumatosis intestinalis, and/or SMA filling defect.
  ○ Disease of at least two vessels classically required for symptoms; poor collateralization can cause symptoms.
  ○ Presents with postprandial abdominal pain occurring reproducibly after eating; requires high index of suspicion.
  ○ Can be subdivided into acute, chronic, nonocclusive, and venous etiologies.
  ○ Endovascular treatments involve embolectomy with stenting or open surgical bypass treatment (aorta to celiac/SMA, aorta or iliac to stenosed mesenteric vessel); exploratory laparotomy is used to assess bowel viability.
  ○ Acute ischemia from embolism, thrombosis, venous thrombosis, or nonocclusive mesenteric ischemia; treated with anticoagulation, imaging, resection of dead bowel, and bypass grafting; classically embolism stops at middle colic artery whereas thrombus stops proximal to duodenum.
- Renal artery occlusive disease:
  ○ Types: Atherosclerotic (90%, involves ostium or proximal segment, symptomatic later in life, mediated by hypertension and ischemic neuropathy) vs. fibromuscular (10%, involves mid or distal segment of artery, symptomatic in late teens to early 30 s, not associated with ischemic neuropathy).
  ○ Unilateral stenosis results in euvolemic hypertension; bilateral stenosis results in hypervolemic hypertension.
  ○ Seen in 40% of end-stage renal disease.
  ○ Favors surgical treatment: Hemodynamically significant stenosis with recurrent pulmonary edema; resistant hypertension not controlled with three antihypertensive medications; hypertension with unilateral small kidney; hypertension with medication intolerance; bilateral stenosis and chronic kidney disease; stenosis with a solitary functioning kidney; stenosis with unstable angina.
  ○ Treated with stenting or renal artery bypass using autologous saphenous, autologous hypogastric, or synthetic graft.

5.2 Venous Insufficiency and Occlusion

Michael Karsy

5.2.1 Venous Anatomy

- Divided into deep and superficial veins depending on position above or below deep fascia; multiple anastomotic channels and patient variation; multiple communicating veins connecting deep to deep or superficial to superficial (▸ Fig. 5.1).
- Named perforators:
  - Dodd's perforator: Inferior 1/3 of thigh.
  - Boyd's perforator: Level of knee.
  - Cockett's perforator: Inferior 2/3 of leg; superior, middle, and inferior; newly termed paratibial perforator.
  - Hunterian perforator: Mid-thigh perforator.
  - May's perforator: Posterior tibial perforator.
  - Medial gastrocnemius.
  - Fibular perforators.
- Upper extremity:
  - Superior vena cava (SVC)←Subclavian:
    - Internal jugular←sigmoid sinus←transverse sinus←superior and inferior sagittal sinus.
    - External jugular.
    - Axillary.
    - Cephalic.
    - Basilic (subscapular, lateral thoracic, brachial ← radial, ulnar, palmar venous branches, and median cubital; median cubital ← cephalic, median antebrachial, palmar venous arches, and digital).
- Lower extremity:
  - Inferior vena cava (IVC) ← common iliac ← external iliac ← common femoral:
    - Femoral vein: meets at saphenofemoral junction.
    - Profunda vein/deep femoral.
    - External pudendal.
    - Circumflex (medial and lateral).
    - Accessory saphenous (anterior and posterior).
    - Great saphenous: Meets at saphenofemoral junction.
    - Popliteal: small saphenous, tibial (anterior and posterior), peroneal, gastrocnemius (medial and lateral), soleal, paratibial perforators, lateral leg perforators, posterior tibial perforators, and plantar (median and lateral); plantar ← posterior arch/Leonardo's vein, posterior tibial, medial malleolar, dorsal venous arch.

5.2.2 Venous Disease

- Varicose veins:
  - 2% of health care expenses; 20% of males and 60% of females show varicose veins.
  - CEAP (clinical, etiology, anatomic, pathophysiologic) classification is used to grade and describe.
  - Symptomatic lesions result in pain, swelling of the leg/foot without skin changes, dermatitis, lipodermatosclerosis, ulceration, bleeding, and cosmesis.
  - Treatment with compression stockings, microphlebectomy, ligation and stripping, and endovascular venous ablation.
  - Vein ablations result in deep vein thrombosis (DVT) risk of < 3% with extension to saphenofemoral junction, 20% risk of paresthesias, 5% risk of recurrence.
- Chronic venous insufficiency:
  - Buildup of blood in lower extremities due to poor vessel compliance, venous obstruction, valvular insufficiency, and calf muscle atrophy or fibrosis; results in tissue edema.
  - Associated with skin changes (e.g., edema, hyperpigmentation, stasis dermatitis, eczema, telangiectasias, venous ulcers) and venous claudication.

○ Diagnosed with venous duplex scanning.

○ Treated with compression devices, percutaneous laser ablation, venous sclerotherapy, varicose vein phlebectomy, saphenous vein stripping/ablation, iliac vein stenting or bypass, venous valvuloplasty.

5.2.3 Venous Thromboembolism

- One million annual cases in the United States; 200,000 deaths/year in the United States; long-term complication of venous hypertension (post-thrombotic syndrome).
- Venous thromboembolism (VTE) describes DVT and pulmonary embolism (PE); risk of 1–2:1,000 patients annually.
- CHEST Guideline and Expert Panel Report provides frequently updated recommendations for DVT diagnosis and treatment.[13]
- Virchow triad: Venous stasis, hypercoagulability, venous wall/endothelial injury.
- Risk factors: Prior DVT, malignancy, surgery/trauma, critical care, pregnancy, hypercoagulability (see ▸ Table 2.17).
- Presentation: Calf pain with dorsiflexion (Homan sign), leg swelling with or without cyanosis, venous gangrene (full-thickness skin necrosis), palpable if superficial thrombophlebitis, asymptomatic PE; only 1/3 show physical examination findings.
- Diagnosis: Complete blood count (CBC) with platelet count is evaluated prior to anticoagulation; basic metabolic panel (BMP) with blood urea nitrogen (BUN)/Cr is evaluated to dose with low-molecular-weight heparin, arterial blood gas to evaluate hypoxemia with PE; D-dimer shows negative predictive value.
- Wells criteria for DVT (▸ Table 5.7) with multiple iterations have been developed to aid in decision making; PE rule-out criteria (▸ Table 5.8) are also used to identify patients requiring further testing; Wells PE criteria also used.
- Hypercoagulopathy work-up in select cases can include: Factor V Leiden, factor II mutation, protein C and S, lupus anticoagulant, antithrombin III, JAK2 mutation anticardiolipin (IgM, IgG, IgA), prothrombin gene mutation (G2021A), beta-2-glycoprotein (IgM, IgG, IgA), homocystine; hematology consultation; screening for malignancy.
- Duplex findings:
  ○ Acute: Dilated, noncompressible, low echogenicity, absence of phasicity, augmentation (increased flow at level of insonation due to squeezing of leg above level, suggests no obstruction of flow transmitted).
  ○ Chronic: Nondilated, echogenic, partially compressible, present collaterals.
- Other imaging studies: CT and MR venogram (more sensitive for proximal thrombosis), digital subtraction venogram.

Table 5.7 Wells criteria for DVT

Clinical characteristic	Points
Active cancer (treatment or palliation within 6 mo)	+ 1
Bedridden recently > 3 d or major surgery within 12 wk	+ 1
Calf swelling > 3 cm compared with contralateral leg (measured 10 cm below tibial tuberosity)	+ 1
Collateral (superficial) veins present	+ 1
Entire leg swollen	+ 1
Localized tenderness along deep vein system	+ 1
Pitting edema confined to symptomatic leg	+ 1
Paralysis, paresis, or recent plaster immobilization of lower extremity	+ 1
Previously documented deep vein thrombosis (DVT)	+ 1
Alternative diagnosis to DVT as likely or more likely	−2
Score of 0: low risk, DVT prevalence of 5%, proceed to D-dimer testing	
Score 1–2: moderate risk, DVT prevalence of 17%, proceed to high-sensitivity d-dimer testing	
Score 3: high risk, DVT prevalence of 17–53%, D-dimer testing, consider ultrasound testing	

Table 5.8 Pulmonary embolism exclusion criteria

Clinical characteristic	Points
Age ≥ 50 y	+1
Heart rate ≥ 100 beats/min	+1
SaO$_2$ on room air < 95%	+1
Unilateral leg swelling	+1
Hemoptysis	+1
Recent surgery or trauma ≤ 4 wk requiring general anesthesia	+1
Prior pulmonary embolism (PE) or deep vein thrombosis (DVT)	+1
Hormone use (e.g., oral contraceptives, hormone replacement)	+1
Any positive criteria do not allow exclusion of PE.	

- Paget-Schroetter syndrome: axillary-subclavian vein thrombosis due to strenuous or repetitive upper extremity activity; requires aggressive treatment with catheter-directed thrombolysis and surgical decompression as well as anticoagulation.
- May Thurner syndrome: Left iliac vein compressed by right iliac artery, treated with catheter thrombolysis with stenting.
- PE:
  - Presents with tachypnea, pleuritic chest pain, hemoptysis, tachycardia, hypotension, hypoxemia, hypocarbia.
  - Electrocardiogram: Tachycardia is the most commonly seen pattern (44% of patients), right bundle branch blocks predict increased mortality, T-wave inversion or ST changes are possible and nonspecific, right axis deviation or dominant R-wave in V1 suggest ventricular strain, peaked P-wave indicates enlarged R atrium and other atrial tachyarrhythmias are possible, S1Q3T3 pattern (deep S-wave in lead 1, Q-wave in III, and inverted T-wave in 3 are classic findings).
  - Chest X-ray: Westermark sign (segmental or lobar perfusion loss).
  - Ventilation/perfusion scan, CT angiogram, pulmonary angiography.
  - Treated with systemic anticoagulation or thrombolysis with cardiopulmonary failure.
- Treatment locations:
  - Iliofemoral: Catheter-directed thrombolysis through saphenous or popliteal vein.
  - Femoropopliteal, axillary, subclavian, jugular: Intravenous or subcutaneous anticoagulation.
  - Infrapopliteal or superficial veins: Controversial; can repeat duplex in 5–7 days to assess for propagation in high-risk patients.
  - Subsegmental PE without DVT: Clinical surveillance anticoagulation generally recommended.
  - Subsegmental PE without DVT but high risk of recurrence: anticoagulation recommended.
- Medical treatment:
  - Treatment balanced against risk of bleeding.
  - Options:
    - Unfractionated heparin (80 IU/kg bolus followed by up to 18 IU/kg with partial thromboplastin time goal of 1.5–2.5 × control).
    - Low-molecular-weight heparin (enoxaparin; 1 mg/kg twice/day or 1.5 mg/kg once/day).
    - Warfarin (5 mg starting, titrated to international normalized ratio [INR] 2–3).
    - Direct oral anticoagulant (DOAC)/Novel oral anticoagulants (NOAC) (apixaban, rivaroxaban, dabigatran, argatroban, bivalrudin).
  - General adult population: First line is apixaban, or rivaroxaban, second line is warfarin with LMWH and less commonly dabigatran.
  - Pregnant women: First line is LMWH; second line is unfractionated subcutaneous heparin.
  - Adults with cancer: First line is enoxaparin or NOAC.
  - Provoked PE:
    - Adults treated for 3 months.
    - Pregnant women treated for 3 months and 6 weeks postdelivery.

Table 5.9 Pulmonary embolism severity index

Clinical characteristic	Points
Age	+1/y
Male sex	+10
Heart failure	+10
Chronic lung disease	+10
Arterial oxygen saturation < 90%	+20
Pulse ≥ 110 beats/min	+20
Respiratory rate ≥ breaths/min	+20
Temperature < 36 °C	+20
Cancer	+30
Systemic blood pressure < 100 mm Hg	+30
Altered mental status	+60

Risk	PESI score	30-d mortality	Recommendations
Class I (very low risk)	<65	0.1–1.6%	Outpatient treatment can be offered
Class II (low risk)	66–85	1.7–3.5%	
Class III (intermediate risk)	86–105	3.2–7.1%	Inpatient treatment
Class IV (high risk)	106–125	4.0–11.4%	
Class V (very high risk)	>125	10–24.5%	

- ○ Unprovoked PE:
  - – Adults treated indefinitely unless high risk of bleeding.
  - – Adults with cancer treated indefinitely regardless of bleed risk.
  - – Pregnant women treated for 3 months and 6 weeks postdelivery.
  - ○ Outpatient treatment can be used in clinically stable patients (class I or II) with good cardiopulmonary reserve; risk classification with PE severity index can be performed (▶ Table 5.9).
- IVC filter: Used after failure of anticoagulation, contraindication of anticoagulation, recurrent DVT, prophylactic in patients with high risk of PE (e.g., bariatric surgery, organ injury, brain injury), after pulmonary embolectomy, free-floating ileofemoral thrombus.
- PREPIC trial[14]: 400 patients randomized to anticoagulation vs. anticoagulation with filter, PE decreased with filter (6 vs. 15%), DVT increased with filter (35% vs. 27%), similar long-term survival, 8-year follow-up.
- Open surgical thrombectomy used in patients with contraindication to thrombolysis, mechanical thrombectomy, or poor response to thrombolytics.
- Mechanical thrombectomy with rotational or hydrodynamic thrombotic devices can be used for acute ileofemoral DVT.

5.3 Vascular Aneurysms and Dissections

Michael Karsy

5.3.1 Aneurysms

- Definition:
  - ○ Aneurysm: > 1.5 × diameter of normal adjacent vessel; most commonly due to degenerative pathology with risk factors from genetics, smoking, atherosclerotic or other vascular disease, and infectious causes.
  - ○ Ectasia: < 1.5 × diameter of normal adjacent vessel.
  - ○ Aneurysmosis: Patient with multiple discrete aneurysms.
  - ○ True aneurysm: All layers of vessel involved.

Table 5.10 Abdominal and thoracic aortic aneurysm size and risk of rupture

AAA size (cm)	Risk of rupture (%)	TAA size (cm)	Risk of rupture (%)
4–4.9	1–5	<5	2
5–5.9	5–10	5–5.9	3
6–6.9	10–20	>6	7
7–7.9	20–40	–	–
>8	30–50	–	–

Abbreviation: AAA, Abdominal aortic aneurysm; TAA, thoracic aortic aneurysm.

- ○ Pseudoaneurysm: Contained rupture.
- Abdominal aortic aneurysm (AAA)[15]:
  - ○ Found in 3% of men > 65 years; 5% of patients with coronary artery disease, 10% of patients with PAD, 50% patients with popliteal aneurysms.
  - ○ More common in men and associated with genetics, smoking, and hypertension.
  - ○ Average growth 10%/y, with 50% requiring repair within 3 years.
  - ○ 95% are below the renal artery.
  - ○ Can be identified via pulsatile abdominal mass; evaluation of other aneurysms is required.
  - ○ United States Preventive Services Task Force recommends men of 65–75 years of age who have ever smoked be screened at least once by ultrasound.
  - ○ Imaging:
    - – X-rays: 70% of aneurysms have calcium that can be seen.
    - – Ultrasound: Most common primary modality for screening and diagnosis.
    - – Computed tomography angiogram (CTA): Used for surgical planning; used to evaluate location of renal vein, size, position, and thrombus of aneurysm neck, distance of aneurysm from renal arteries, aortic bifurcation, and iliac arteries, patency of arteries, diameter of aortic bifurcation and iliac arteries, and the number of lumbar vessels.
    - – Magnetic resonance angiogram (MRA): Uncommon for diagnosis; often incidentally discovered when other findings are evaluated.
  - ○ Rupture risk depends on size (▶ Table 5.10).
  - ○ Treatment performed for symptomatic aneurysms of any size or asymptomatic sizes of 5.5 cm in men and 5.0 cm in women; treatment thresholds have some variation.
  - ○ Open repair vs. endovascular aneurysm repair (EVAR):
    - – Open repair uses a transperitoneal or retroperitoneal approach.
    - – Open repair has a < 3% risk of perioperative mortality, 5% death rate, 15% myocardial infarction rate, risk of hypotension, 2% risk of ischemic colitis, risk of renal failure, limb ischemia, abdominal compartment syndrome, < 0.5% risk of paraplegia.
    - – EVAR is sized according to configuration of aorta and branches.
    - – EVAR has lower perioperative mortality compared with open AAA repair (1.2 vs. 4.8%) but higher rates of late rupture (5.4 vs. 1.4%).
    - – Fenestrated endovascular aneurysm repair (FEVAR) can use patient-customized thoracoabdominal grafts.
  - ○ EVAR has 15% risk of endoleak; endoleak types:
    - – Ia: Proximal aortic leak; requires repair.
    - – Ib: Distal iliac leak; requires repair.
    - – II: Back bleeding from lumbar, accessory renal, or inferior mesenteric arteries; can be observed if stable and grows < 5 mm; most common type.
    - – III: Device failure/separation; requires repair.
    - – IV: Fabric porosity; often resolves spontaneously; seen in older-generation grafts.
    - – V: Endotension causing bowing of vessel at stent site.
  - ○ Ruptured AAA:
    - – 50% patients make it to the hospital alive and 50% survive surgery; overall 75% mortality rate.
    - – Triad of abdominal pain, pulsatile abdominal mass, and hypotension.

- Work-up requires CBC, BMP, blood type and cross-match, urinalysis for hematuria, ultrasound most commonly used to diagnose, CT used in hemodynamically stable patients; Foley catheter, arterial line, and vascular sheath in jugular can be placed before surgery.
    - Mortality predictors: Coagulopathy from bleeding, renal failure, ischemic colitis, respiratory failure.
    - Open repair used for unstable, nonendovascular candidates; otherwise, endovascular treatments are possible.
  - Aortoenteric fistulas: Present with gastrointestinal hemorrhage; require emergent laparotomy for repair.
  - Graft infections: Early infections due to *Staphylococcus aureus*, late due to *S. epidermidis*; first-line therapy antibiotics, lastly axillary-bifemoral or other bypass with graft excision.
- Iliac artery aneurysm:
  - Associated with 30% of AAA, rarely isolated (1–2% cases).
  - 75% involve common iliac artery, 10–20% involve internal iliac artery, external iliac artery involvement is rare, 1–2 mm growth/year.
  - Commonly presents with lower abdominal and flank pain due to compression; rarely palpable.
  - Repaired when > 3 cm diameter, symptomatic with pain, or > 2 cm at time of open AAA repair.
  - Open and endovascular repair are both options depending on patient anatomy.
- Thoracic aortic aneurysm:
  - 10% operative mortality, 15–20% secondary to dissections.
  - 60% involve ascending aorta and 40% involve descending aorta.
  - 1 cm/y growth rate, greater growth rate in descending aneurysm, dissecting aneurysms, or Marfan disease.
  - Rupture risk depends on size (▶ Table 5.10).
  - Crawford classification:
    - Type 1: Subclavian to renal.
    - Type 2: Subclavian to aortic bifurcation.
    - Type 3: Midthoracic aorta to aortic bifurcation.
    - Type 4: Thoracic aorta at diaphragm to aortic bifurcation.
  - Repaired if symptomatic or > 6 cm in diameter.
  - Open vs. thoracic endovascular aortic repair (TEVAR) is used; ascending aneurysm requires open surgery with cardiac bypass; descending aneurysms distal to the subclavian can undergo TEVAR.
  - Lumbar drains have been used to improve spinal cord perfusion after TEVARs; mean spinal perfusion pressure (goal 60 mm Hg) = mean arterial pressure – spinal compartment pressure; used for 24–48 hours if no neurological deficits.
- Peripheral artery aneurysm:
  - Associated with 5% of AAA, associated with nonpopliteal aneurysm in > 50% of cases, 50% bilateral.
  - Most commonly asymptomatic but 50% become symptomatic over time.
  - Peripheral aneurysms more often have thromboembolic complications due to slowed flow and propensity for clot formation.
  - Presents with claudication, thromboembolic occlusion (25%), venous compression, widened pulse on exam, associated with other aneurysms, risk of rupture is rare (5%).
  - Work-up initially includes ultrasound to determine size of aneurysm and presence of thrombus; other imaging includes CT, MR imaging, or angiography.
  - Aneurysms are treated if > 2 cm, asymptomatic but with thrombus, or symptomatic.
  - Symptomatic aneurysms are treated by combinations of thrombolysis, stenting, or open repair; controversial for treatment strategy.
- Femoral artery aneurysm:
  - True aneurysms are uncommon but 50% are associated with contralateral femoral aneurysm or AAA; anastomotic aneurysm can be due to graft failure or infection.
  - Iatrogenic pseudoaneurysm from angiography is most common.
  - Commonly involve common femoral; < 1% involve superficial femoral or deep femoral.
  - Presents with thromboembolic symptoms, compressive symptoms, or leg pain; deep femoral aneurysm classically present with rupture.
  - Diagnosed with ultrasound; CT imaging can be used for operative repair.

- ○ Treatment includes ultrasound-guided thrombin injection for small pseudoaneurysms; symptomatic aneurysms at any size or asymptomatic aneurysm > pseudoanerysms 3 cm require surgical repair; pseudoaneurysms < 3 cm can be monitored at 1- to 2-week intervals because 90% resolve within 6 weeks.
- Popliteal artery aneurysms:
  - ○ AAA present in 1/3 of patients with popliteal aneurysms; 50–60% are bilateral requiring surveillance of contralateral popliteal artery and abdominal aorta.
  - ○ Distal thromboembolism is the most common complication.
  - ○ Repaired if asymptomatic and > 2 cm or all symptomatic patients.
- Visceral artery aneurysm:
  - ○ Rare, found in 0.01–0.2% of autopsies, 22% present as emergencies.
  - ○ Treated if > 2 cm, growing rapidly, or causing symptoms; generally treated for all women of child-bearing age, and pregnant women due to rupture risk with pregnancy, and liver transplant recipients.
  - ○ Endovascular and open treatment options are used; thrombin injection can be used for small, accessible pseudoaneurysms or patients for whom endovascular treatment fails.
  - ○ Visceral aneurysms associated with vasculitis and infection (fungal or bacterial, rarely viral or mycobacterial).
  - ○ Splenic artery aneurysms:
    - – 60–80% of visceral aneurysm cases; most are small (2–4 cm), saccular, and asymptomatic; 2% rupture rate with 36% mortality rate.
    - – Present with left upper quadrant pain in subscapular region with hypotension.
    - – More likely true aneurysms.
    - – Repaired in pregnant women of child-bearing age, symptomatic patients at any size, or asymptomatic patients if > 2 cm.
  - ○ Hepatic artery aneurysms:
    - – 20% of visceral aneurysms.
    - – Usually solitary, extrahepatic; rare.
    - – Present with epigastric pain, hemobilia, and obstructive jaundice (Quincke triad); rupture occurs into visceral compartment with 21–25% mortality.
  - ○ Gastroduodenal, pancreaticoduodenal, and pancreatic artery aneurysms:
    - – 6% of visceral aneurysms, 90% rupture.
    - – Presents with epigastric pain; ruptures can result in gastrointestinal hemorrhage.
  - ○ Celiac artery aneurysms:
    - – 4% of visceral aneurysms, 13% rupture.
    - – Associated with AAA in 20% of cases; rupture presents as intraperitoneal hemorrhage and gastrointestinal hemorrhage.
    - – All types repaired.
  - ○ SMA aneurysms:
    - – 5.5% of visceral artery aneurysms, 38–50% present with rupture.
    - – Associated with bacterial endocarditis.
    - – Present with upper abdominal pain, frequently contain thrombus, and palpable mass is felt in 50% of patients.
  - ○ IMA aneurysms:
    - – 1% of visceral artery aneurysms.
    - – Commonly asymptomatic.
    - – Usually arise as a result of increased blood flow from stenosis of the celiac and SMA.

5.3.2 Dissections

- Disruption of one or more layers of the artery usually the intima, resulting in a false lumen running parallel to a blood vessel.
- Can occur from rupture of the vasa vasorum with bleeding in the media; bleeding can result in pseudoaneurysm or vessel occlusion.

- Associated with trauma, vascular collagen diseases (e.g., hypertension, Marfan syndrome, Ehlers-Danlos syndrome, radiation therapy, vasculitis, infection, iatrogenic from endovascular procedures).
- Cervical/vertebrobasilar dissection:
  - Found in 20% of young adults with stroke, 2% strokes overall.
  - Often symptomatic but can present with ipsilateral headache or neck pain, partial Horner syndrome (ipsilateral miosis, pitosis, and without hidrosis) symptoms, stroke-like symptoms depending on vascular territory (cerebral in cervical dissection and brainstem in vertebrobasilar dissection), cranial nerve palsies.
  - Diagnosed with CTA predominantly, also by ultrasound, MRA, and angiography.
  - Treatment depends on Biffl grading (see ▶ Table 14.8).
- Aortic dissection[16]:
  - 20% preadmission mortality, 30% in-hospital mortality.
  - Risk factors include age > 40 years with hypertension, age < 40 years with Marfan syndrome, other connective tissue disorder, or bicuspid aortic valve.
  - Present with stabbing neck, interscapular, or chest pain and loss of consciousness or ischemic limb from poor perfusion.
  - Diagnosed with CT aortography (sensitivity 100%, specificity 98%) or an esophageal echocardiography, MRA used for surveillance.
  - Differential diagnosis: Myocardial infarction, PE, spontaneous pneumothorax, ureteric colic, perforated viscus, mesenteric ischemia, embolism, stroke, cauda equina.
  - Stanford type:
    - A: All dissections affecting ascending aorta; surgically treated.
    - B: All dissections not involving ascending aorta; classically managed with medications but generally treated endovascularly.
  - DeBakey classification:
    - I: Originates in ascending aorta, propagates to aortic arch or beyond; equivalent to Stanford A; surgically treated.
    - II: Confined to ascending aorta; equivalent to Stanford A; surgically treated.
    - III: Originates in descending aorta and extends distally; equivalent to Stanford B; medically, surgically, or endovascularly treated.
  - Managed with CBC, BMP, two large-bore intravenous (IV) lines, blood type and cross-match, close hemodynamic monitoring, beta-blockers, nitroprusside, and/or calcium channel blockers to reduce heart rate to 60–80 beats, systolic blood pressure ≤ 100–120 mm Hg, electrocardiogram to rule out myocardial infarction, arterial line for blood pressure monitoring.
  - Stanford type A/DeBakey type I or II dissections have 1-week mortality of 50–91% due to aortic rupture, stroke, visceral ischemia, cardiac tamponade, and circulatory failure; urgent surgical treatment is indicated.
  - Stanford type B dissections show 78% 3-year survival with medical management, goal systolic blood pressures 100–120 mm Hg with beta-blockers as first-line agents.
  - Open or endovascular treatments possible depending on clinical features but both with substantial risk.
  - Regular surveillance using MRA performed annually for nonoperatively treated patients.

5.4 Other Vascular Topics

Michael Karsy

5.4.1 Lymphatic Disease

- Cause:
  - Lymphedema[17]:
    - Accumulation of extracellular, interstitial fluid due to excessive production or obstructed drainage into the venous system; can result in progressive fibrosis and disruption of limb function in the setting of elephantiasis.

- Initially liquid phase/pitting edema followed by solid phase/nonpitting edema as transitions from acute to chronic phase and fibrosis sets in.
    - Increased risk of cellulitis and infection from static fluid.
    - Rare risk of lymphangiosarcoma, Kaposi sarcoma, and lymphoma.
  ○ Primary lymphedema: rare, congenital disruption of lymphatic circulation.
  ○ Secondary lymphedema: more common; associated with tumor resection and occurs mostly in breast (49%), gynecological (20%), melanoma (16%), genitourinary (10%), and head/neck cancer (6%) patients; can occur after sentinel lymph node dissection; commonly occurs due to filariasis in developing countries.
  ○ Incidence from 0–3% after lumpectomy to 65–70% after radical mastectomy, underreported in oncology generally.
- Diagnosis:
  ○ Limb circumference discrepancy of 2 cm.
  ○ Volume increases of 200 mL or > 10–20% compared with baseline or contralateral arm.
  ○ Bioimpedance measurement.
- Treatments:
  ○ Treatments used in combination are more effective; surgery is rarely done.
  ○ Complete decongestive therapy: Involves certified lymphedema therapist performing manual drainage, massage, compression, therapeutic exercises, and skin care.
  ○ Compressive garments have been used.
  ○ Diuretics have been tried without consistent benefit.
  ○ Charles procedure: Surgical debulking of limb; used as last resort for fibrotic elephantiasis and limb dysfunction.
  ○ Vascularized lymph node transfer: Microsurgical transfer of lymphatic-containing soft tissue flap with arteriovenous supply to recipient site; typical donor sites include lateral groin, chest wall, or neck; typical recipient sites include affected limb, groin, or axilla; can be used in principle with vascularized free flaps (e.g., deep inferior epigastric perforator, omentum).
  ○ Lymphaticovenous anastomosis: Connection of lymphatic vessels with adjacent venules; dyes used to identify venules; most common surgical treatment method.
  ○ Lymphaticolymphatic bypass: Transfer of healthy lymphatic vessels from healthy donor site to recipient site.
  ○ Suction-assisted protein lipectomy: Proteinaceous fatty tissue aspirated using liposuction cannula, followed by compression therapy.

5.4.2 Endovascular Procedures and Complications

- Access:
  ○ Retrograde femoral (95% cases), brachial, radial, or other access; less commonly anterograde access.
- Catheters/Sheaths:
  ○ French = 0.33 mm; French size/3 = approximate catheter diameter in mm.
  ○ Sheath diameter defined by inner diameter.
  ○ Femoral sheaths ≥ 8 Fr and brachial sheaths ≥ 6 Fr increase risk.
  ○ Catheters defined by outer diameter as they pass through sheaths.
  ○ Catheter types: flush, selective (passive, intermediate, active), guide, microcatheter.
- Balloons:
  ○ Rated burst pressure: pressure where 99.9% of balloons do not rupture with 95% confidence.
  ○ Nominal pressure: pressure where balloon reaches designed diameter.
  ○ Compliance defines change of volume with pressure, different levels used for different purposes.
  ○ Placed "over-the-wire" or via a monorail system with different advantages and disadvantages.
- Stents:
  ○ Balloon expandable if low radial force vs. self-expandable.
  ○ Bare-metal stents vs. drug-eluting stents; drug elution reduces risk of thrombosis.
  ○ Open- or closed-cell design: Open cells are more flexible whereas closed cells lower risk of plaque rupture and distal embolization.

- ○ Covered stents: Covered with expanded polytetrafluoroethylene (ePTFE) used for venous stenosis in arteriovenous fistulas.
  - ○ Dual antiplatelet therapy used for reduction of thromboembolism; more critical in sensitive vascular distributions (e.g., carotid arteries) at risk for patient deficits.
- Thrombolysis:
  - ○ Mechanical (e.g., Fogarty catheter) vs. chemical (recombinant tissue plasminogen activator or urokinase).
  - ○ Used for patients with clots < 14 days old in Paget-Schroetter syndrome, ileofemoral DVT, acute limb ischemia, thrombosed popliteal artery aneurysms, acute PE.
  - ○ Absolute contraindications: Cerebrovascular event < 2 months, active bleeding, gastrointestinal bleeding < 10 days, neurosurgery < 3 months, intracranial trauma < 3 months.
  - ○ Relative contraindications: Cardiopulmonary resuscitation < 10 days, major surgery or trauma < 10 days, systolic > 180 mm Hg or diastolic > 110 mm Hg, puncture of noncompressible vessel, intracranial tumor, recent eye surgery.
  - ○ Complications: Intracranial hemorrhage (2%), major bleeding (10%), compartment syndrome (4%), embolization (5%).
  - ○ STILE trial[18]: 393 patients randomized for catheter-based (e.g., recombinant tissue plasminogen activator or urokinase) vs. surgical thrombolysis after nonembolic arterial and graft occlusion for lower limb ischemia; study terminated at interim analysis because equal effect shown between interventions; secondary analysis showed patients treated ≤ 14 days after symptoms had better limb salvage and amputation-free survival at 6 months.
  - ○ TOPAS trial[19]: 514 patients randomized to catheter-based vs. surgical thrombolysis; amputation-free survival at 6 months similar for catheter and surgical groups (71.8% vs. 74.8%); four episodes of intracranial hemorrhage in catheter group and none in surgical group.
- Intravascular ultrasound:
  - ○ 8 Fr system used for aortic cases; 5–6 Fr system used for other areas.
  - ○ Used in cases where limited contrast necessary, treatment of dissection, and evaluation of IVC filter placement.
- Complications:
  - ○ Range for low-risk (< 1%) to high-risk (> 3%) procedures; depends on patient features and technique features (► Table 5.11).
  - ○ Closure devices: Compression devices (e.g., Femostop, Safeguard), topical hemostatic agents (e.g., D-Stat, Syvek), invasive devices (Perclose, Angio-seal, Starclose), invasive without foreign plug (Cardiva catalyst).
  - ○ Surface hemorrhage treated with manual pressure or compression device.

5.4.3 Hemodialysis Vascular Access and Management

- Dialysis access:
  - ○ Intermittent renal dialysis access types:
    - Nontunneled and tunneled catheters for short-term use.
    - Arteriovenous fistula (AVF) or grafts for long-term use.
  - ○ Peritoneal dialysis: uses peritoneal catheter; break-in wait time 2 weeks after catheter placement before use to allow wound healing; most common dialysis in children; can be placed at time of AVF.
- Arteriovenous (AV) access:
  - ○ AVF: Direct arteriovenous anastomosis; best long-term patency rates but longest time to maturation; accessible within 6–8 weeks.
  - ○ AV graft: Synthetic material (e.g., polytetrafluoroethylene) used to connect artery and vein; shorter time to maturation but higher risk of infection and thrombosis; accessible within 2–3 weeks; Hemodialysis Reliable Outflow (HeRO) catheter is an accessible synthetic catheter connecting a peripheral artery to central venous circulation.
  - ○ AVF and AV graft used for patients with need for long-term access (glomerular filtration rate < 25 mL/min and expected dialysis within 1 year).
  - ○ Autogenous fistulas show 70% 6-month patency and 50% 18-month patency.
  - ○ Nondominant arm used first.

Table 5.11 Complication frequency and management after angiography

Complication	Frequency (%)	Notes
Groin hematoma	1–3	Caused by puncture above femoral head and inguinal ligament, noncompressible
		Results initially in extensive hemorrhage that is difficult to compress, then expansion of the thigh can be seen
		Last run of case should include access site to reverify localization of puncture in common femoral artery
		Sheath should not be pulled with systolic > 170 mm Hg or activated clotting time > 180 s
		Surgery used if progressively enlarging hematoma, skin compromise, femoral nerve compression, severe pain, life-threatening hemorrhage
		20% risk of infection
Pseudoaneurysm	≤ 1	< 3 cm undergoes repeat duplex in 1–2 wk as 90% resolve
		≥ 3 cm undergo thrombin injection or surgical treatment if unsuccessful
Retroperitoneal hematoma	0.5	Usually from high puncture above inguinal ligament into external iliac arteries
		Presents with back pain, decreasing hematocrit, and decreasing blood pressure
Arteriovenous fistula	< 1%	Puncture through profunda femoris artery and vein
		80% resolve in 1 mo
Dissection	< 1%	Due to rupture of plaque; identified when unable to aspirate blood or poor waveform
Wire perforation	< 1%	Mostly in inferior epigastric or deep circumflex arteries
		Can result in retroperitoneal bleeding
		Treated with selective embolization
Vessel rupture	< 1%	Seen from oversizing balloon-expandable stents, balloons, or calcified vessels
		Treated with covered stent
Atheroembolism	< 1%	Shows as neurological compromise, livedo reticularis, blue toe syndrome, renal failure, limb compromise, or acute gastric pain depending on distribution

- Order of AVF placement sites to maintain vessels for as long as possible (starts distal and moves proximally): radiocephalic, brachiocephalic, transposition brachiobasilic, forearm loop, upper arm brachioaxillary.
- Evaluation for prior access procedures, central vein catheters, arm or neck surgery, pressure differences of > 20 mm Hg between arms, or poor pulses throughout arm.
- Arterial requirement: Unobstructed inflow, patent palmar arch, luminal diameter 2 mm.
- Venous requirements: Unobstructed outflow, diameter > 2.5 mm, depth < 1 cm.
- Complications:
  - Thrombosis: Technical complication; 90% due to poor venous outflow; AVF or AV grafts should have a thrill or bruit; pulsatility suggests stenotic outflow; requires 12–16 weeks for maturation and quicker maturation suggests high central vein pressure, evaluated for rule of 6's (i.e., flow of 600 mL/min, diameter > 6 mm, depth < 6 mm, cannula length of 6 inches).
  - Infection: 5% rate; requires partial or total graft removal.
  - Edema: Poor venous outflow; requires repair of stenosis or access ligation if persistent.
  - Maturation failure: Occurs in 30% of wrist fistulas, 15% of basilic transpositions; due to poor inflow or excessive outflow.

– Steal syndrome: 2–8% patients; higher frequency in diabetics and those with more proximal access.
– Access pseudoaneurysm: due to repeated punctures; treated with covered stents or interposition repair.
– High-output congestive heart failure: 1% of fistulas; seen with high-flow fistulas.
– Venous hypertension: Due to central venous stenosis; can result in edema, nonhealing skin ulcers.

5.4.4 Diabetes in Vascular Medicine

- Epidemiology:
  - Diabetic foot ulcers occur in 15% of diabetic patients; located on bottom of feet; results in hospitalization in 6% of diabetic patients; 14–24% with a diabetic foot ulcer require amputation.
  - Foot ulcers occur from poor circulation, foot deformities, poor sensation with irritation, and trauma.
- Recommendation guideline by the Society for Vascular Surgery[20]:
  - Diabetic foot ulcers:
    - Annual foot inspections; testing for peripheral neuropathy using Semmes-Weinstein filament testing; education of patients/families regarding foot care.
    - Against specialized footware for average-risk diabetics but custom footware for those with significant neuropathy, foot deformities, or previous amputation.
    - Glycemic control with A1C < 7% to reduce risk of foot ulcers, infections, and amputations.
    - Against prophylactic revascularization to prevent foot ulcers.
  - Offloading diabetic foot ulcers:
    - Total contact cast or irremovable fixed-ankle walking boot for plantar ulcers; removable cast for those requiring frequent dressing changes.
    - Any modality to relieve pressure at ulcer sites for nonplantar wounds or those with healed ulcers.
  - Diabetic foot osteomyelitis:
    - Bone probing test to confirm osteomyelitis with diabetic foot infections.
    - Serial radiography to evaluate deformity, soft tissue gas, and radiopaque foreign bodies.
    - Magnetic resonance imaging (MRI) for those with suspected soft tissue abscess or inconclusive radiographs; leukocyte or antigranulocyte scan if MRI is contraindicated.
    - Confirmed diagnoses based on bone culture and histology.
  - Wound care:
    - 1–4 week evaluations for infection, moist dressings with control of exudation, and avoidance of intact skin maceration.
    - Debridement of infected diabetic ulcers with urgent surgical intervention for those with abscess, gas, or necrotizing fasciitis.
    - Wounds without improvement (> 50% area reduction) after 4 weeks to undergo adjunctive wound therapies (e.g., negative pressure therapy, biologics, living cell therapy, extracellular matrix products, amniotic membrane products, hyperbaric oxygen).
  - PAD:
    - Risk factors: Diabetic patients age > 50 years, prior foot ulcers, abnormal vascular examinations, prior interventions for vascular disease, atherosclerotic cardiovascular (e.g., coronary, cerebral, renal) disease to undergo ankle-brachial index measurements with toe pressure and transcutaneous oxygen pressure measurement annually.
    - Patients with diabetic foot ulcers and PAD recommended for surgical bypass or endovascular therapy.

References

[1] Stone NJ, Robinson JG, Lichtenstein AH, et al. American College of Cardiology/American Heart Association Task Force on Practice Guidelines. 2013 ACC/AHA guideline on the treatment of blood cholesterol to reduce atherosclerotic cardiovascular risk in adults: a report of the American College of Cardiology/American Heart Association Task Force on Practice Guidelines. J Am Coll Cardiol. 2014; 63 25 Pt B:2889–2934

[2] Liapis CD, Avgerinos ED, Kadoglou NP, Kakisis JD. What a vascular surgeon should know and do about atherosclerotic risk factors. J Vasc Surg. 2009; 49(5):1348–1354

[3] Wang JC, Kim AH, Kashyap VS. Open surgical or endovascular revascularization for acute limb ischemia. J Vasc Surg. 2016; 63(1):270–278

[4] Barnett HJM, Taylor DW, Haynes RB, et al. North American Symptomatic Carotid Endarterectomy Trial Collaborators. Beneficial effect of carotid endarterectomy in symptomatic patients with high-grade carotid stenosis. N Engl J Med. 1991; 325(7):445–453

[5] Randomised trial of endarterectomy for recently symptomatic carotid stenosis: final results of the MRC European Carotid Surgery Trial (ECST). Lancet. 1998; 351(9113):1379–1387

[6] Executive Committee for the Asymptomatic Carotid Atherosclerosis Study. Endarterectomy for asymptomatic carotid artery stenosis. JAMA. 1995; 273(18):1421–1428

[7] Halliday A, Mansfield A, Marro J, et al. MRC Asymptomatic Carotid Surgery Trial (ACST) Collaborative Group. Prevention of disabling and fatal strokes by successful carotid endarterectomy in patients without recent neurological symptoms: randomised controlled trial. Lancet. 2004; 363(9420):1491–1502

[8] Yadav JS, Wholey MH, Kuntz RE, et al. Stenting and Angioplasty with Protection in Patients at High Risk for Endarterectomy Investigators. Protected carotid-artery stenting versus endarterectomy in high-risk patients. N Engl J Med. 2004; 351(15):1493–1501

[9] Brott TG, Hobson RW, II, Howard G, et al. CREST Investigators. Stenting versus endarterectomy for treatment of carotid-artery stenosis. N Engl J Med. 2010; 363(1):11–23

[10] Weinberg I, Jaff MR. Nonatherosclerotic arterial disorders of the lower extremities. Circulation. 2012; 126(2):213–222

[11] Hardman RL, Jazaeri O, Yi J, Smith M, Gupta R. Overview of classification systems in peripheral artery disease. Semin Intervent Radiol. 2014; 31(4):378–388

[12] Norgren L, Hiatt WR, Dormandy JA, et al. TASC II Working Group. Inter-society consensus for the management of peripheral arterial disease (TASC II). Eur J Vasc Endovasc Surg. 2007; 33 Suppl 1:S1–S75

[13] Kearon C, Akl EA, Ornelas J, et al. Antithrombotic therapy for VTE. Chest. 2016; 149(2):315–352

[14] Decousus H, Leizorovicz A, Parent F, et al. A clinical trial of vena caval filters in the prevention of pulmonary embolism in patients with proximal deep-vein thrombosis. Prévention du Risque d'Embolie Pulmonaire par Interruption Cave Study Group. N Engl J Med. 1998; 338(7):409–415

[15] Aggarwal S, Qamar A, Sharma V, Sharma A. Abdominal aortic aneurysm: a comprehensive review. Exp Clin Cardiol. 2011; 16(1):11–15

[16] Thrumurthy SG, Karthikesalingam A, Patterson BO, Holt PJ, Thompson MM. The diagnosis and management of aortic dissection. BMJ. 2011; 344 d8290:d8290

[17] Granzow JW, Soderberg JM, Kaji AH, Dauphine C. Review of current surgical treatments for lymphedema. Ann Surg Oncol. 2014; 21(4):1195–1201

[18] Results of a prospective randomized trial evaluating surgery versus thrombolysis for ischemia of the lower extremity. The STILE trial. Ann Surg. 1994; 220(3):251–266, discussion 266–268

[19] Ouriel K, Veith FJ, Sasahara AA, Thrombolysis or Peripheral Arterial Surgery (TOPAS) Investigators. A comparison of recombinant urokinase with vascular surgery as initial treatment for acute arterial occlusion of the legs. N Engl J Med. 1998; 338(16):1105–1111

[20] Hingorani A, LaMuraglia GM, Henke P, et al. The management of diabetic foot: a clinical practice guideline by the Society for Vascular Surgery in collaboration with the American Podiatric Medical Association and the Society for Vascular Medicine. J Vasc Surg. 2016; 63(2) Suppl:3S–21S

6 Cardiothoracic Surgery

Edited by Line Kemeyou and Milos Buhavac

6.1 Assistive Ventricular Devices and Cardiac Transplantation

Michael Karsy and Milos Buhavac

6.1.1 Durable Left Ventricular Assist Devices (LVADs)

- Introduction[1,2,3,4]:
  - Longer term mechanical circulatory support (MCS) with LVADs can be used to improve survival and quality of life compared to medical management alone.
  - Heart failure occurs in 1–2% of the population in western countries; estimated to affect 8 million patients in the United States annually by 2030.
  - 81% 1-year survival and 70% 2-year survival with variation depending on functional class.
  - See Chapter 6.3 Heart Failure.
- Indications for LVADs:
  - New York Heart Association (NYHA) Class III or IV advanced heart failure (see Chapter 6.3 Heart Failure); further categorized into seven Interagency Registry for Mechanically Assisted Circulatory Support (INTERMACS) categories.
  - Ejection fraction < 25%.
  - Reduced functional capacity (VO$_2$ < 14 mg/kg/min).
  - Clinical trial protocol inclusion criteria.
- Contraindications for LVADs:
  - Limited life expectancy, age > 80 years.
  - Active malignancy with poor prognosis.
  - Severe comorbidities not explained by heart failure; end-stage renal, liver, or lung disease; neuromuscular disorder.
  - Hematological abnormalities (e.g., coagulopathy).
  - Anatomic limitations (e.g., congenital heart disease, hypertrophic cardiomyopathy, large ventricular septal defect [VSD]), obesity.
  - Independent right heart failure, uncorrectable aortic insufficiency, severe vascular disease.
  - Poor psychosocial support, active smoking, alcohol or drug abuse.
- Four strategies for usage:
  - Bridge to transplant: Patient listed for transplantation; 21% of LVADs in 2012.
  - Bridge to candidacy: Patient not listed for transplantation; no absolute contraindications to transplantation; unclear recovery; 33% of LVADs in 2012.
  - Destination therapy: Patient ineligible/absolute contraindication for transplantation; nonsurvivable treatment; 44% of LVADs in 2012.
  - Bridge to recovery: Temporary support with expected recovery and no need for transplantation; 1.0% of LVADs in 2012.
- LVAD versions:
  - First generation: Pulsatile pumps (i.e., HeartMate I, Thoratec PVAD; Novacor N100); implantation required sternotomy and cannula insertion; pump chamber in abdomen or preperitoneal space; required long-term anticoagulation.
  - Second generation: Decreased pump size and continuous flow (i.e., HeartMate II, Jarvik 2000, Micromed DeBakey); implantation required sternotomy with cannula implantation.
  - Third generation: Pump with magnetic levitation to reduce device wear (i.e., DuraHeart, HeartWare HVAD, Incor, Levacor, HeartMate III); continuous flow; use of centrifugal flow.
  - HeartMate III BTT trial resulted in replacement of pulsatile pumps with continuous flow LVADs.
  - Randomized Evaluation of Mechanical Assistance for the Treatment of Congestive Heart Failure (REMATCH) trial first to show superior outcome of VADs compared to medical management alone.[4]
  - INTERMACS registry aims to follow patients with LVAD placement.

- Complications:
  - 31% readmission within 30 days; 60% readmission within 6 months; 65–80% readmission within 1 year.
  - Thrombotic events: 1–12%; diagnosed by hemolysis, echocardiography, and intraoperatively; treated with thrombolytics and device exchange.
  - Right heart failure: 15–25%; diagnosed by echocardiography; treated with inotropy and right VAD.
  - Gastrointestinal bleeding: 15–30%; diagnosed by endoscopy; treated with proton pump inhibitors and cauterization by gastroenterology.
  - Driveline infection: 15–24%; diagnosed clinically; treated with antibiotics and possible device exchange.
  - Stroke: 13–30%; diagnosed by brain imaging; treated by variety of methods.
  - Aortic insufficiency: 30% at 2 years; diagnosed with echocardiography; treated surgically or by transcatheter valve repair.

6.1.2 Temporary Mechanical Circulatory Support

- Introduction:
  - Short-term MCS device used for circulatory support in cardiogenic shock, acute decompensated heart failure, myocarditis with cardiogenic shock, or cardiopulmonary arrest.
  - Provide temporary bridge to recovery or more definitive surgical therapy.
  - Can be used for left, right, or bilateral heart failure.
  - Can improve end-organ perfusion, coronary perfusion, reduction of pulmonary congestion, and reduction in infarct size.
  - Contraindicated with aortic valve regurgitation, metallic aortic valves, aortic aneurysm/dissections, vascular disease, left heart thrombi, bleeding diathesis, or sepsis.
- Four types:
  - Intra-Aortic Balloon Pumps (IABPs):
    - Least expensive, placed by interventional cardiologists, moderate hemodynamic support.
    - Blood displaced to proximal aorta and coronary arteries by inflation during diastole; balloon reduced during systole.
  - Non-IABP percutaneous mechanical circulatory arrest devices:
    - Greater cardiac support, more expensive.
    - Left-ventricle–to-aorta assist device: Axial flow pump using Archimedes screw (e.g., Impella System); smaller device version placed percutaneously while larger device version placed surgically; reduced rate of adverse cardiovascular events in patients with three-vessel or unprotected left main coronary disease and severely depressed left ejection fraction.
    - Left-atrium-to-aorta assist device: Centrifugal pump with spinning impeller; blood pumped from left atrium to iliofemoral artery; right-atrium-to-iliofemoral artery system can be used with oxygenator to mimic extracorporeal membrane oxygenation.
    - Right ventricular assist device (RVAD): Pumps from vena cava to pulmonary arteries (e.g., Impella RP catheter); provides temporary right ventricular (RV) support; contraindicated in biventricular failure.
  - Extracorporeal membrane oxygenator pumps:
    - Venoarterial or venovenous bypass methods for improving blood oxygenation; see Chapter 2.3 Ventilator Management.
  - Nonpercutaneous centrifugal pumps:
    - Small centrifugal pumps used for short-term flow assistance; used for cardiopulmonary bypass during open heart cases.
  - Total artificial heart:
    - Biventricular mechanical system replacing the function of the heart completely; can be used as a bridge to transplantation.

6.1.3 Cardiac Transplantation

- Epidemiology[5]:
  - > 5,000 cases annually worldwide.
  - Greater demand than supply of hearts.

- Increased number of patients who are complex, older, and on MCS.
- Currently 1-year survival of 85% with median survival of 12 years or more in adults and 18 years in kids.
- Indications for cardiac transplantation:
  - Advancing heart failure with limiting symptoms on exertion despite optimal medical therapy:
    - Patients with frequent hospital admission (≥2 admissions in 12 months) despite medical therapy.
    - Need to decrease medications due to side effects (e.g., renal dysfunction or hypotension).
    - Worsened RV function or rising pulmonary artery pressures.
    - Rising natriuretic peptide levels.
    - Increased refractory frequency of ventricular arrhythmias.
    - Worsening anemia, weight loss, hyponatremia, liver or renal dysfunction, secondary to heart failure.
  - Persistent cardiogenic shock with inotropy dependence and/or need for MCS.
- Indications for urgent inpatient referral:
  - Inability to wean intravenous inotropic treatment.
  - Need for percutaneous MCS.
  - Ventilator support with positive airway pressure for worsening pulmonary edema.
  - Refractory ventricular arrhythmia.
- Contraindications for cardiac transplantation:
  - Active infectious disease.
  - Symptomatic central or peripheral vascular disease.
  - Diabetes mellitus with end-organ injury or uncontrolled diabetes.
  - Recent neoplasm with risk of recurrence.
  - Severe lung, renal, or liver dysfunction.
  - Recent pulmonary thromboembolism; elevated pulmonary artery systolic pressures.
  - Poor psychosocial factors, active smoking/alcohol/drug abuse.
  - Obesity.
  - Comorbidities, organ failure, or other issues portending poor survival.
- Evaluation:
  - Comprehensive laboratory, infectious, psychosocial, as well as cancer screening.
  - Echocardiogram evaluates ventricular function, pulmonary artery systolic pressure, and valvular function.
  - Right heart catheterization performed to evaluate hemodynamics including presence of pulmonary hypertension that may preclude transplant candidacy.
  - Seattle Heart Failure Model uses 20 variables including clinical, medication, laboratory, and assistive device data to predict 1-, 2-, and 5-year survival; used for risk stratification.
  - Heart Failure Survival Scores uses seven parameters including peak VO2 to predict risk stratification for cardiac transplantation.
- Complications:
  - Primary graft dysfunction: Occurs within 24 hours; occurs in 31% of cases; 1-year survival of 44%.
  - Graft rejection:
    - Can be acute or chronic; different categories (e.g., antibody, cellular, etc.).
    - Immunosuppression commonly performed with calcineurin inhibitor, antimetabolite agent, and corticosteroids; corticosteroids may be weaned after 6–12 months with 50–80% weaned off completely; see Chapter 4.7 Transplantation.
    - Depending on its severity, rejection is generally managed with optimization of maintenance immunosuppression therapy, pulse dose steroid followed by steroid taper, or in moderate to severe cases, IVIG, plasmapheresis, immunemodulator agents, with consideration of hemodynamic support (temporary mechanical devices) in those with cardiogenic shock.
    - Rejection ranges from mild to severe; rates of rejection have decreased over time.
    - Acute cell-mediated rejection: Severe types occur in 5–21% of patients; rare after 12 months, milder forms diagnosed by biopsy; treated with high-dose steroids.
    - Antibody-mediated rejection: Occurs early or late; late occurrence correlated with poor survival; treated with plasma exchange, intravenous immunoglobulins, and monoclonal antibodies.
  - Infection: Highest risk within first year, prophylaxis used against *Pneumocystis jirovecci*, cytomegalovirus, *Candida* spp., and sometimes *Herpes* virus.

- Cardiac allograft vasculopathy: Progressive narrowing of coronary arteries effecting 29% of transplants at 5 years.
- Renal dysfunction can occur in 9% of transplants within the first year.
- Increased rate of hypertension, hyperlipidemia, and diabetes due to immunosuppressant use.

6.2 Coronary Artery Bypass Grafting and Percutaneous Coronary Intervention

Michael Karsy and Milos Buhavac

6.2.1 Coronary Artery Bypass Grafting (CABG)

- Introduction:
  - CABG is generally used for patients with survival benefit and high risk for future cardiovascular event.
  - 90% of patients show improvement in angina symptoms after CABG; long-term benefit limited by atherosclerosis in nonvascularized vessels and graft stenosis.
  - SYNTAX score can be used to determine risk of coronary artery disease.
  - Greater evidence in improving survival compared to PCI but depends on patient subgroup; type 1 diabetic patients may benefit from CABG; patients with low/intermediate SYNTAX scores and an unprotected left main may benefit from cardiac stenting.
  - Most common cardiac procedure (> 200,000 cases in the United States annually).
- Indications for CABG[6,7]:
  - ≥ 1 significant coronary artery stenosis treatable with revascularization and disabling medical therapy.
  - Left main coronary disease with ≥ 50% stenosis.
  - Three-vessel disease (≥ 70% stenosis) with proximal left anterior descending (LAD) disease.
  - Two-vessel disease with > 75% stenosis in LAD artery proximal to first major septal artery.
  - Patients undergoing noncoronary cardiac surgery with > 50% narrowing of LAD or 70% narrowing of other major coronary arteries.
  - Emergent CABG:
    - Acute myocardial infarction where primary percutaneous coronary intervention (PCI) has failed or cannot be performed, coronary artery anatomy is suitable for CABG, and ischemia or hemodynamic instability exists at rest.
    - Repair of postinfarction mechanical complication such as myocardial infarction, ventricular septal rupture, mitral valve insufficiency.
    - Cardiogenic shock.
    - Life-threatening arrhythmia due to ischemia and left main stenosis or ≥ 50% three-vessel coronary artery disease.
  - Weak recommendations:
    - Two-vessel disease without significant proximal LAD disease but extensive ischemia.
    - Mild-to-moderate left ventricular (LV) systolic dysfunction (ejection fraction 35–50%) and multivessel coronary artery disease or proximal LAD stenosis with potential viable myocardium.
- Complications:
  - Perioperative myocardial infarction:
    - Defined by elevated biomarkers > 5 × 99% percentile of upper reference limit, new pathological Q waves, new left bundle branch block, graft occlusion, native coronary artery occlusion, or evidence of myocardium loss.
    - 3–6% of patients develop symptomatic postoperative ischemia.
    - PCI performed within 30 days after CABG if feasible with potentially salvageable myocardium.
  - Low cardiac output: Incidence of 6–12% postoperatively; can occur for ischemic injury, reduced preload, reduced afterload from hypertension, arrhythmia, perioperative myocardial infarction, or mechanical complications; can be treated with IABP or ventricular assist device (VAD).
  - Distributive shock: Occurs from low vascular tone, treated with norepinephrine.

- Arrhythmia: Atrial fibrillation occurs in 15–40% of patients undergoing CABG; nonsustained ventricular tachycardia (VT) occurs in 17–97% of patients; sustained VT or ventricular fibrillation (VF) occurs in 1–3% of patients; bradyarrhythmia occurs in 0.8–4% of patients.
- Postpericardiotomy syndrome: Pericarditis after CABG occurs in up to 85% of patients; usually small effusion but can result in tamponade and hemodynamic instability.
- Sternal wound infection and mediastinitis: Occurs in 0.3–1.3% of patients; detected within 2 weeks.
- Leg wound complications: 0.65–4% risk.
- Bacteremia: Seen in 3% of patients within 90 days.
- Acute kidney injury (AKI): Mild elevations in creatinine are common; 0.9–1.7% develop AKI severe enough to need dialysis.
- Venous thromboembolism: Underdiagnosed but can be seen in as high as 20% of patients.
- Aortic dissection: Rare complication of CABG from use of pump which can be acute or delayed.
- Gastrointestinal bleeding: Can be seen in 4% of patients.

6.2.2 Percutaneous Coronary Intervention (PCI)

- Introduction:
  - Revascularization considered after maximal medical treatment including aspirin, statins, and risk reduction.
  - Risk stratification with stress testing or significant dysfunction can be helpful.
  - Drug-eluting stents (DES) show improvement in outcomes compared to bare metal stents (BMS); improved outcomes for stenting compared to angioplasty alone.
  - Biodegradable polymer stents are currently in development and trial.
  - Door-to-balloon time for revascularization is critical for improving outcome and reducing mortality.
  - Dual antiplatelet therapy is important to maintain after stenting with different trials aiming to evaluate the shortest potential duration.
- Indications:
  - Patients with stable angina where maximal medical therapy has not improved treatments or is not tolerated.
  - High-risk patients and some intermediate-risk patients for cardiovascular events.
  - Patients who cannot tolerate CABG and have multivessel disease.
  - Some patients with ischemic cardiomyopathy and reduced LV systolic function.
  - Patients with large area of ischemia (> 10% of left ventricle) and proximal LAD stenosis (> 50%).
- Complications:
  - Stent thrombosis: Uncommon but usually uniformly fatal; 1.5–2% risk over 2 years which is similar for BMS and first-generation DES; occurs at any time point within the first year but most cases for DES occur within the first 30 days for drug and 2 days for BMS; longer dual antiplatelet therapy used for DES than BMS.
  - Contrast-induced nephropathy.

6.3 Heart Failure

Line Kemeyou and Josef Stehlik

6.3.1 Epidemiology and Pathophysiology

- Heart failure (HF): Progressive condition resulting from an injury to the heart muscle and gradual loss of its ability to pump adequate blood to meet the body's needs.[8,9,10,11]
- HF types:
  - HF with reduced ejection fraction (HFrEF): Also known as systolic HF; defined by a reduced LV ejection fraction (LVEF) ≤ 50%.
  - HF with preserved ejection fraction (HFpEF): Also known as diastolic HF; LVEF is preserved but abnormality results from abnormal filling due to stiff myocardium.
  - Right HF: Resulting from pathologies predominantly affecting the right ventricle, or as a result of long-standing left heart disease that eventually affects the right ventricle through development of pulmonary hypertension.

- Pathophysiology of HF is complex and involves adaptive and compensatory mechanisms from the subcellular level all the way through organ-to-organ interactions.
- HF ensues when network of compensatory mechanisms becomes overwhelmed, and patient develops symptoms related to fluid retention and/or low cardiac output.
- Adaptive mechanisms:
  - Activation of neurohormonal system: The release of norepinephrine by the adrenergic system augments myocardial contractility and leads to activation of the renin–angiotensin–aldosterone system (RAAS), the sympathetic nervous system (SNS), and other neurohormonal pathways that act to maintain arterial pressure and perfusion of vital organs. While useful during acute myocardial injury, this activation becomes maladaptive in the long term.
- HF remains an epidemic:
  - Nearly 6.5 million Americans over the age of 20 years have HF.
  - One million new cases of HF are diagnosed annually in the United States.
  - Prevalence in the United States is estimated to be 8 million by 2030.
- HF is a disease with high mortality:
  - Accounts for about 8.5% of all heart disease deaths in the United States.
  - Mortality of 50% at 5 years from diagnosis; over 300,000 deaths per year.
  - Mortality is highest for patients with New York Heart Association (NYHA) class IV, stage D HF.
- Incidence and prevalence:
  - Higher in Blacks, Hispanics, Native Americans.
  - Can occur at any age, but prevalence increases with age.
  - Similar cumulative incidence in men and women.
  - Women tend to develop HF later in life than men, are more likely to have HFpEF, and have better survival, but their symptoms are more severe.
- HF hospitalization is a burden on health care system:
  - Nearly one in four patients hospitalized with HF is readmitted within 30 days of discharge.
  - Direct costs > $30 billion/y.

6.3.2 Common Etiologies of HF

- Ischemic heart disease: HF secondary to coronary artery disease (CAD).[12]
  - Remains the most common identifiable cause of HF in the United States.
  - Approach to diagnosis and management should focus on identifying patients in whom coronary revascularization—either percutaneous (PCI) or surgical (CABG)—may alleviate symptoms, relieve ischemia, improve cardiac function, and extend survival.
- Nonischemic HF[12]:
  - Dilated cardiomyopathy: Abnormality in myocardial contraction in the absence of CAD resulting in four-chamber enlargement with relatively thin cardiac walls. Specific examples include:
    - Result of inflammatory diseases/myocarditis, including viral, protozoal (Chagas disease), fungal, giant cell myocarditis.
    - Familial cardiomyopathy: Genetic abnormality of the myocardium that may result in dilated cardiomyopathy (e.g., titin mutation, mitochondrial myopathies).
    - Toxic injury to the myocardium: Alcohol-induced cardiomyopathy, anthracycline-induced cardiomyopathy.
    - Peripartum cardiomyopathy.
    - Cardiomyopathy associated with muscular dystrophies.
    - Arrhythmogenic RV dysplasia: Genetic disease, affects predominantly the right ventricle.
  - Restrictive cardiomyopathy: Abnormality of diastolic relaxation of the myocardium resulting in restricted ventricular filling, high filling pressures, and a reduced stroke volume. Examples include amyloidosis, sarcoidosis, hemochromatosis, myocardial storage diseases, endomyocardial fibrosis, radiation-induced myocardial injury.
  - Hypertrophic cardiomyopathy: Autosomal-dominant genetic disease resulting in impaired ventricular compliance and dynamic obstruction of the LV outflow as a consequence of inappropriate myocardial hypertrophy.

○ Valvular cardiomyopathy: HF resulting from severe valvular diseases such as aortic stenosis, aortic regurgitation (AR), mitral regurgitation (MR), and mitral stenosis (MS).
○ HF due to congenital heart disease.
• Right HF: May result from dysfunctional RV myocardium, excessive load on the right ventricle, or obstruction to RV outflow.
○ The clinical expression of right HF is similar regardless of cause and is mediated via a combination of elevated systemic venous pressure and depressed cardiac output.
○ Etiologies include RV myocardial infarction, RV dysplasia, left HF, cor pulmonale, tricuspid and pulmonary valvular disease.
• Constrictive pericarditis: Results from thickening of the pericardium and shares many features of right HF of other etiologies.

6.3.3 Precipitating Causes of HF

• HF is a chronic condition characterized by acute decompensations with worsening symptoms. Common causes of decompensation include[13]:
○ Dietary indiscretion: Nonadherence to sodium and fluid restriction.
○ Suboptimal medical therapy with drug nonadherence or other reasons for drug regimen reduction.
○ Uncontrolled hypertension.
○ Cardiac arrhythmias (atrial fibrillation, ventricular arrhythmias).
○ Worsening of underlying heart disease, such as acute coronary syndrome, progression of valvular pathologies, progression of myocardial dysfunction.
○ Systemic infection or other unrelated illness with increase of total metabolism demand and hemodynamic burden on the heart.

6.3.4 Clinical Assessment

• Careful evaluation of the patient's history[14]:
○ Symptoms: Shortness of breath, fatigue, extremity swelling, abdominal bloating, dyspnea with exertion, paroxysmal nocturnal dyspnea, weight gain, orthopnea, bendopnea, poor concentration, altered mental status.
• Physical examination: Presence of pulmonary rales, tachycardia, S3 gallop, jugular venous distention, abdominal distension, positive hepatojugular reflux, hepatomegaly, extremity edema, poor capillary refill, cool extremities, central or peripheral cyanosis.
• Classifications:
○ Framingham criteria: Can help with the diagnosis of HF; requires that either two major criteria or one major and two minor criteria be present concurrently (▶ Table 6.1).

Table 6.1 Framingham diagnostic criteria for heart failure

Major criteria	Minor criteria
Paroxysmal nocturnal dyspnea	Nocturnal cough
Weight loss of 4.5 kg in 5 days in response to treatment	Dyspnea on ordinary exertion
Neck vein distention	A decrease in vital capacity by one-third the maximal value recorded
Rales	Pleural effusion
Acute pulmonary edema	Tachycardia (rate of 120 bpm)
Hepatojugular reflux	Hepatomegaly
S3 gallop	Bilateral ankle edema
Central venous pressure > 16 cm water	
Circulation time of ≥ 25 s	
Radiographic cardiomegaly	
Pulmonary edema, visceral congestion, or cardiomegaly at autopsy	

○ NYHA functional classification of HF: Reflection of the patient's symptom severity and the amount of exertion that is needed to provoke symptoms (▶ Table 6.2).
○ American College of Cardiology/American Heart Association (ACC/AHA) staging of HF:
  – Describes the development and progression of HF.
  – Acknowledges established risk factors and structural prerequisites for the development of HF.
  – Emphasizes implementation of therapeutic interventions even before the development of LV dysfunction or symptoms as a way to reduce the population HF morbidity and mortality (▶ Table 6.3).

6.3.5 Diagnosis/Testing

- Imaging[15,16,17]:
  ○ Echocardiogram: Recommended in the initial evaluation of patients with known or suspected HF.
    – Allows evaluation of ventricular function, primary and secondary valvular abnormalities, and diastolic function.
    – Can also be used to determine pulmonary and ventricular filling pressures.
  ○ EKG: May help detect arrhythmia as the cause of HF, detect acute myocardial ischemia or infarction, prior myocardial infarction, or the presence of CAD.
  ○ Chest radiograph:
    – Posterior–anterior and lateral views are recommended.
    – Assesses heart size and shape, pulmonary congestion, pulmonary or thoracic causes of dyspnea, and proper positioning of any implanted cardiac devices.
    – Up to 50% of patients with HF and documented elevation of PCWP do not manifest typical radiographic findings of pulmonary congestion.
  ○ Cardiac computed tomography (CT) and magnetic resonance imaging (MRI).
  ○ More advanced imaging techniques that provide detailed functional and morphological information.

Table 6.2 NYHA functional classification of heart failure

Class	Functional capacity
I	Patients without limitation of physical activity
II	Patients with slight limitation of physical activity, in which ordinary physical activity leads to fatigue, palpitation, dyspnea, or anginal pain; they are comfortable at rest
III	Patients with marked limitation of physical activity, in which less than ordinary activity results in fatigue, palpitation, dyspnea, or anginal pain; they are comfortable at rest
IV	Patients who are not only unable to carry on any physical activity without discomfort but who also have symptoms of HF or the anginal syndrome even at rest; the patient's discomfort increases if any physical activity is undertaken

Abbreviations: HF, heart failure; NYHA, New York Heart Association.

Table 6.3 ACC/AHA stages of heart failure development

Level	Description	Examples
A	At high risk for heart failure but without structural heart disease or symptoms of HF	Patients with coronary artery disease, hypertension, or diabetes mellitus without impaired LV function, LVH, or geometric chamber distortion
B	Structural heart disease but without signs/symptoms of HF	Patients who are asymptomatic but who have LVH and/or impaired LV function
C	Structural heart disease with current or past symptoms of HF	Patients with known structural heart disease and shortness of breath and fatigue, reduced exercise tolerance
D	Refractory HF requiring specialized interventions	Patients who have marked symptoms at rest despite maximal medical therapy

Abbreviations: ACC, American College of Cardiology; AHA, American Heart Association; HF, heart failure; LV, left ventricular; LVH, left ventricular hypertrophy.

- May be useful in delineating congenital and valvular abnormalities, and presence of pericardial disease.
- Can be used to assess ischemic versus nonischemic cause, infiltrative disease, and hypertrophic disease or to determine viability.
- Laboratory testing: The following tests may be useful during the initial evaluation of a patient with suspected HF.
  - Natriuretic peptides:
    - Rapid measurement of B-type natriuretic peptide (BNP) or N-terminal proBNP (NT-proBNP) levels can aid in differentiating between cardiac and noncardiac causes of dyspnea.
    - BNP and NT-proBNP levels are higher in older patients, women, and patients with renal dysfunction or sepsis. Atrial fibrillation has been associated with increased BNP levels in the absence of acute HF.
    - BNP levels may be disproportionately lower in patients who are obese or who have hypothyroidism.
    - Sacubitril/valsartan elevates serum BNP; NT-proBNP should be tested in patients on this drug.
  - Other tests: Complete blood count (CBC), serum electrolyte levels, fasting blood glucose levels, renal and liver function testing, thyroid stimulating hormone (TSH) level, lipid profile, iron studies, urinalysis, pulse oximetry or arterial blood gas; genetic testing: considered in selected group of patients when indicated.
- Endomyocardial biopsy: Indicated when a specific diagnosis is suspected that cannot be ruled out without biopsy and would influence management in patients presenting with HF.
- Heart catheterization:
  - Coronary angiogram: Done when atherosclerosis is suspected as the cause of HF.
  - Right heart catheterization: Indicated to better define a patient hemodynamics and guide treatment, measures filling pressures and pulmonary arterial pressures, and provides calculated cardiac output.

6.3.6 Management

- Nonpharmacological therapies[17,18,19,20]:
  - Dietary measures with fluid intake (1.5–2 L/d) and sodium (2 g/d) restriction.
  - Physical activity: Cardiac rehabilitation, lifestyle changes to include routine physical activity.
  - Nutritional management: Weight loss in obesity and proper nutrition in cachexia.
- Pharmacological therapies:
  - Neurohormonal antagonists:
    - Activation of the RAAS and the adrenergic system has a pivotal role in the progression of HF. These systems are activated by increased myocardial stretch and peripheral hypoperfusion and cause vasoconstriction, fluid retention, myocardial hypertrophy and fibrosis, fetal gene expression, and accelerated cell death.
    - The administration of neurohormonal antagonists is the basis of the current medical treatment of chronic HF and has been shown to reduce HF morbidity and mortality. The medications are typically started at a low dose and titrated up to target doses as tolerated.
    - Angiotensin-converting enzyme inhibitors (ACEIs): Main mechanisms of action include inhibition of LV remodeling and myocardial dysfunction as well as reducing ischemic events in patients with CAD. Key side effects include hyperkalemia, renal dysfunction, hypotension, cough, angioedema.
    - Angiotensin receptor blockers (ARBs): Block the effects of angiotensin II on type I angiotensin II receptors. Unlike the ACEIs, ARBs do not increase kinin level, and therefore do not produce cough. Other key side effects are similar to ACEIs.
    - Aldosterone antagonists: Spironolactone and eplerenone block the aldosterone receptor. Key side effects include hyperkalemia and renal failure. Spironolactone may cause gynecomastia.
    - β-Blockers: β-blockers shown to benefit patients with HF include metoprolol succinate, carvedilol, and bisoprolol. Key side effects include bradycardia, hypotension worsening symptoms in acute decompensated HF, or cardiogenic shock.
    - Hydralazine and nitrates used in combination is an alternative for patients intolerant to ACEIs and ARBs. Addition of hydralazine and nitrate combination to ACEIs and β-blockers has also been shown to decrease mortality and hospitalizations in a population self-described as African Americans. Key side effect is hypotension.

– Angiotensin receptor/neprilysin inhibitor: Currently available as one formulation (Sacubitril/valsartan); shown in a randomized clinical trial to reduce mortality and hospitalization when compared with ACEI. Key side effects are similar to ARBs.
○ Additional pharmacotherapy without proven mortality benefit:
  – Diuretics: Recommended in patients who have evidence of fluid retention for relief of symptoms.
  – Digitalis: Oldest recognized therapy for HF increases contractility, but clinical studies did not show reduction of mortality. It can be beneficial in patients with HFrEF unless contraindicated to reduce hospitalizations for HF. Therapeutic range is narrow and key side effects include gastrointestinal symptoms, visual disturbances, and rhythm abnormalities.
  – Ivabradine: Inhibits hyperpolarization-activated cyclic nucleotide-gated channel present in the SA node, leading to slowing of heart rate. Has been shown to reduce hospitalization in patients with HF and is approved for HFrEF patients who have a resting heart rate > 70 bpm despite taking the highest tolerable dose of a β-blocker.
- Device therapies: Include interventions such as pacemakers, implantable cardioverter-defibrillators, cardiac resynchronization therapy (CRT). A newer device therapy used for diagnosis of decompensating HF is a pulmonary artery pressure monitor (Cardiomems).
- Surgical options:
  ○ Heart transplantation is used when progressive end-stage HF occurs despite maximal medical therapy, and when the prognosis is poor with continuation of medical therapy alone
  ○ MCS devices such as durable VADs and total artificial heart can bridge the patient to transplantation.
  ○ VADs are increasingly being used as permanent therapy.
- Role of palliative care: Treatment of refractory symptoms and compromised quality of life in advanced HF should be addressed with palliative care resources. These resources should be integrated into comprehensive HF care and strategies to facilitate communication about prognosis with HF patients.

6.4 Open Heart Surgery

Michael Karsy and Milos Buhavac

6.4.1 Cardiopulmonary Bypass

- First utilized in 1952 for treatment of atrial septal defect (ASD).[21]
- Limited access coronary artery surgery:
  ○ Port-access coronary artery bypass (PACAB) and minimally invasive coronary artery bypass (MIDCAB) graft are alternatives to CABG surgery via the use of endoscopic techniques.
  ○ PACAB involves a bypass machine while MIDCAB does not use the bypass machine.
- Utilizes cardiopulmonary bypass pump run by a perfusionist in close collaboration with the cardiac anesthesiologist and cardiothoracic surgeon.
- Components (▶ Fig. 6.1):
  ○ Pumps, cannulas, tubing, venous reservoir, oxygenator, heat exchanger, line filters, temperature and blood gas monitors, and alarms.
  ○ Roller and centrifugal pumps can be used.
  ○ Venous cannulas are usually inserted into the superior and inferior vena cava or the right atrium; can also be threaded from the femoral vein into the right atrium.
  ○ Arterial cannulas are placed in the ascending aorta, femoral, innominate, or axillary artery; cannulas are right angled or straight and can have beveled or diffusive tips.
  ○ Oxygenators use polypropylene fibers (100–200 μm in diameter) separating blood and gas flow.
  ○ Tubing and cannula are composed of polyvinylchloride and wire reinforced when able.
  ○ Open venous reservoirs are more common and require a safe level of blood to avoid air entry; closed reservoirs reduce blood contact with containers.
  ○ Cardioplegia involves placement of crystalloid or blood-containing fluid given continuously or intermittently containing potassium-based solutions to stop the heart.

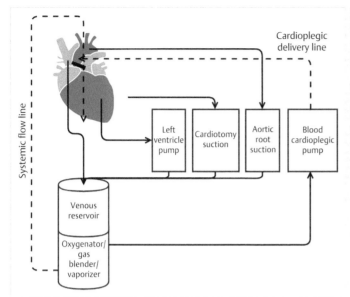

Cardioplegic delivery line

Left ventricle pump

Cardiotomy suction

Aortic root suction

Blood cardioplegic pump

Systemic flow line

Venous reservoir

Oxygenator/ gas blender/ vaporizer

Fig. 6.1 Schematic of cardiopulmonary bypass system. A simplified schematic of a cardiopulmonary bypass circuit is shown. Blood is suctioned from the left ventricle, surgical field (i.e., cardiotomy suction) and aortic root to a venous reservoir. Blood is oxygenated and gas is blended before it is returned to systemic circulation and the cardioplegic delivery line. Not shown are various filters, gas and pressure analyzer, one-way valves, heat exchangers, exit points for blood gas sampling, and entry point for plegic solution mixing.

- Usage:
  - Pump priming involves heparin to improve fluid flow during hypothermia; activated clotting time is used to offer real-time evaluation of anticoagulation.
  - Each 1 °C decrease in temperature reduces cardiac output by 7%.
  - Patient cooling (0.5–1.5 °C/min) can be faster than patient warming (0.3–0.5 °C/min) due to physical properties of fluids and goal to not create microbubbles or denature proteins with heating.
  - Mean arterial pressure of 50–70 mm Hg is maintained with higher pressures needed for patients with hypertension at base line or risk of stroke.
  - Cerebral monitoring (e.g., evoked potentials, transcranial Doppler) can be used to monitor perfusion.
  - Line and patient vasculature constantly monitored for pressure, acid/base status, electrolytes, and temperature during pump usage.
  - Pump weaning involves gradual temperature warming, normalization of metabolism, monitoring for air embolism, treatment of arrhythmia (e.g., amiodarone, lidocaine, magnesium), use of defibrillation with internal paddles (5–20 J), heparin reversal.
  - Deairing involves removal of air from surgical, anesthetic, pump, and dead space components; transesophageal echocardiography is used to ensure no residual air
  - Circuit is dismantled when condition requiring pump is completed, no residual air is present, pacing and ventilation are adequate, and physiological normalization has occurred.
  - When circuit is dismantled, return to pump may be necessary; thus, pump is reprimed and readied.
- Complications:
  - Cannula malposition or dissection, bleeding, air embolism, and mechanical pump failure are possible.
  - Coagulopathy can occur during blood loss and perfusion; monitored with thromboelastography (see Chapter 2.8 Hematology and Coagulation), fibrinolysis treated with tranexamic acid or aminocaproic acid.
  - AKI or cerebral injury can occur depending on bypass time, comorbidities, and perfusion pressure.
  - Systemic inflammatory response can occur from blood contact with artificial surfaces, ischemia-reperfusion injury, or operative trauma; requires clinical support and metabolic normalization.
  - Acute respiratory distress can occur from bypass; lung protective ventilation is utilized when possible.
  - Vasoplegia is treated with resuscitation, vasopressors, and/or methylene blue to compete with nitric oxide.

6.4.2 Aortic Valve Surgery

- Introduction[22,23]:
  - ~180,000 valve surgeries performed annually in the United States with most being aortic valve replacement (AVR) or mitral valve replacement (MVR).
  - Most common congenital heart defect in adults is the bicuspid aortic valve, which increases risk of insufficiency.
  - Increased prevalence of aortic valve repair with newer endovascular approaches.
- Aortic valve repair[24]:
  - Indications:
    - Dilated aortic annulus.
    - Conjoint cusp prolapses in bicuspid aortic valves.
    - Single cusp prolapses in tricuspid aortic valves.
    - Perforation from endocarditis.
    - Younger patients with AR and no stenosis, aims to avoid postoperative anticoagulation.
  - Reduces area of aortic valve to improve leaflet coaptation.
  - Annular dilation repair: Surgical repair performed on pump, transverse aortotomy performed to allow suture closure of subcommisural triangles, plication above the commissure and downsizing of the sinotubular junction with a Dacron graft can be performed.
  - Bicuspid aortic valve repair: Usually involves conjoint cusp of right and left coronary cusps, repair performed on pump, cut edges of cusp are reapproximated by suture and tethered tissue to the aortic wall is released.
  - Cusp prolapse in tricuspid valve: Usually caused by prolapse of one or more cusps due to rupture of a small fenestration, repaired by various methods to plicate the defect.
- AVR[7,25]:
  - Surgical aortic valve replacement (SAVR) and transcatheter aortic valve replacement (TAVR) methods exist.
  - Aortic valve sclerosis affects 25% of adults > 65 years and stenosis impacts 2.9% of adults > 65 years.
  - Patients present with heart failure, exertional syncope or angina; low volume and slow carotid pulse seen; loud mid-late systolic murmur in right second intercostal space or single second heart sound can be heard due to delay of A2 sound.
  - Aortic stenosis (AS) grading:
    - Stage A: Asymptomatic patients, maximum transvalvular aortic velocity (V_{max}) < 2 m/s, includes bicuspid aortic valve or aortic sclerosis, patients at risk for further aortic valve disease.
    - Stage B: Mild-to-moderate leaflet calcification, V_{max} 2–2.9 m/s, mean transvalvular pressure < 20 mm Hg.
    - Stage C: Severe obstruction, C1 and C2 subclasses, severe calcification, $V_{max} \geq 4$ m/s, aortic valve area ≤ 1.0 cm^2; ejection fracture can be normal or reduced.
    - Stage D: Severe symptomatic stenosis; D1, D2, and D3 subclasses; mean transvalvular gradient ≥ 40 mmHg or peak velocity ≥ 4 m/s; aortic valve area ≤ 0.6 cm^2/m^2; ejection fracture usually reduced.
  - AR grading:
    - Stage A: Bicuspid aortic valve or sclerosis, rheumatic heart disease, no hemodynamic changes.
    - Stage B: Progressive AR, mild-to-moderate calcification, regurgitation fraction < 30% (mild) or 30–49% (moderate).
    - Stage C: Asymptomatic severe AR, divided into C1 and C2 subclasses depending on ejection fracture, regurgitation fraction ≥ 50%, exercise testing can be performed.
    - Stage D: Symptomatic severe AR, regurgitation fracture ≥ 50%, LV dilatation, ejection fraction may or may not be decreased, exertional dyspnea is noted.
  - Evaluation may include electrocardiogram, ultrasound, chest radiography, serial clinical evaluation, stress testing, angiography, CT imaging; MRI and PET imaging are not commonly used.
  - Important to distinguish subvalvular (e.g., thick fibromuscular ridge, diffuse obstruction, abnormal mitral valve attachments, accessory endocardial cushion) and supravalvular disease (e.g., thickened ascending aorta at sinuses of valsalva, congenital syndromes) when treating aortic stenosis.

○ AVR indications[22,23]:
  – Symptomatic patients with severe AS (stage D) and asymptomatic patients with severe AS (stage C) who meet indication for AVR with low or intermediate surgical risk.
  – Symptomatic patients with severe (AS) and high risk for SAVR are considered for TAVR.
  – TAVR is recommended for symptomatic patients with severe AS (stage D), prohibitive risk for SAVR, and predicted survival > 12 months.
  – TAVR alternative to SAVR for symptomatic patients with severe AS (stage D) and intermediate surgical risk.
  – Percutaneous aortic balloon dilation can be bridged to SAVR or TAVR for symptomatic patients with severe AS.
  – Symptomatic patients with severe AR (class D) regardless of LVEF.
  – Asymptomatic patients with chronic severe AR (stage C2) and LVEF < 50% at rest.
  – Severe AR (stage C or D) while undergoing other cardiac surgery.
  – Asymptomatic patients with severe AR, normal LVEF, but severe or worsening left ventricle dilation.
  – Asymptomatic patients with moderate AR undergoing surgery on ascending aorta, CABG or mitral valve.
○ Valve types:
  – Mechanical bileaflet (e.g., St Jude, Carbomedic, On-X valve); mechanical low thrombogenicity tilt disc (e.g., Medtronic hall); bioprosthetic valve (e.g., porcine, bovine, equine, cadaveric aortic valve); Ross procedure (pulmonary autograft with replacement of pulmonary valve with pulmonary homograft).
  – Mechanical valves: preferred for patients < 50 years, no contraindications to anticoagulation, high risk of morbidity/mortality with reintervention (e.g., porcelain aorta).
  – Bioprosthetic valve: preferred for patients > 70 years, preferred in patients with shorter life expectancy, reoperation for mechanical valve thrombosis, anticoagulation is contraindicated.
  – Uncertainty in type of valve for patients age 50–70.
○ TAVR introduction[25]:
  – Endovascular aortic valve replacement; Similar indications to traditional SAVR; used for patients with > 1 year of life expectancy with symptomatic severe calcific aortic stenosis with high surgical risk.
  – Placement of Aortic Transcatheter Valves (PARTNER) multicenter trial showed reduced mortality and improved outcomes compared to medical treatment alone;[7] mortality reduced compared to SAVR in meta-analysis depending on surgical risk; TAVR offers lower rates of major bleeding and atrial fibrillation but higher rates of aortic valve retreatment, pacemaker placement, and AR compared to SAVR.
  – Society of Thoracic Surgeons Predicted Risk of Mortality (STS-PROM) used to calculate surgical risk.
  – Increasing trend of TAVR use in older patients who otherwise would not have been candidates for SAVR.
○ TAVR indications:
  – Symptomatic aortic stenosis but not suitable candidate for SAVR.
  – Patients with ≥ 50% probability of death or disability or absolute contraindication recommended for transfemoral TAVR when able.
  – Patients with high surgical risk (STS-PROM > 8 and < 50% probability of death) evaluated individually.
  – Patients with intermediate (STS-PROM 4–8) or low (STS-PROM < 4) surgical risk and anatomy precluding SAVR are considered for TAVR.
  – Asymptomatic patients with severe aortic stenosis and indications for valve replacement are considered individually for TAVR.
○ SAVR complications:
  – Paravalvular AR: 0.9% over 30 days and 0.5% risk over 1 year, 0.1–1.3% risk long term.
  – Aortic dissection: 0.6% risk.
  – Coronary artery occlusion: 0.3–5% risk.
  – Stroke: 7–17% risk.
  – Mediastinitis: 0.9–20%.
  – Infective endocarditis: 1–6%.
  – Sternal osteomyelitis: 1–3%.
  – Hemolysis: 5–15% risk.

○ TAVR complications:
  – Registry data: In-hospital mortality of 5–7%, in-hospital stroke rate of 1.1–4.1%, 1-year mortality of 21–23%.
  – Shock: Acute postoperative change; can arise from hemorrhage due to access complication, annular rupture or aortic dissection; can result from cardiac tamponade or intracardiac flow dysfunction (e.g., VSD, papillary muscle rupture, AR, outflow obstruction); arrhythmia.
  – Bleeding and access complications: Major early bleeding 7–24% but has improved with improvement of technique; early bleed risks include larger sheaths, vessel calcification or tortuosity, and closure device failure; late bleeding occurs in 6% of cases mostly from gastrointestinal, neurological, and traumatic causes.
  – Transapical tear/rupture: 0.4–0.8% risk.
  – Aortic dissection: 0.12% risk.
  – Ventricular perforation: 1% risk.
  – Aortic valve rupture: 0.17% risk, life-threatening requiring emergent sternotomy with aortic root and valve replacement.
  – Valve malpositioning or migration: 0.3% risk.
  – Stroke: 2–5% 30-day stroke risk; larger rate of subclinical stroke; embolic protection devices have not been completely effective.
  – Myocardial infarction: 0.7% risk of acute coronary occlusion; 0.22% risk of delayed coronary occlusion; 1% of subclinical injury.
  – Arrhythmia: 2–8% risk of arrhythmia; may require a permanent pacemaker.
  – Paravalvular AR: 7–70% risk of mild regurgitation, 0–24% risk of moderate/severe regurgitation.
  – Valvular stenosis: Subclinical thrombosis occurs in 4% of patients and treated with anticoagulants; 3–4% risk of causing hemodynamic instability.
  – Endocarditis: 0.3–3% risk but most patients do not need surgical retreatment.

6.4.3 Mitral Valve Surgery

• Second most common form of valvular defect in adults, prevalence of 2–3% population in the United States and 13% in patients > 75 years.[22,23,26]
• Treatment of MS and MR can be more challenging and controversial; evidence for increased benefit for treatment in asymptomatic and earlier disease.
• MR is divided into chronic primary and secondary reasons.
• Mitral valve repair/valvulplasty[27]:
  ○ Operative mortality of 2–4% for valvuloplasty vs. 5–9% for replacement; greater survival after valvuloplasty compared to replacement; similar rates of reoperation; morbidity and mortality depend on causes of mitral valve deficiency and other patient factors (e.g., atrial fibrillation).
  ○ Goals to repair leaflet coaptation and correct annular dilatation.
  ○ Carpentier's technique: Resection of abnormal tissue with reconstruction of normal anatomy.
  ○ Multiple techniques for repair with or without prosthetic reinforcement have been described.
  ○ Minimally invasive techniques have been developed for repair.
  ○ MR repair preference:
    – Chronic severe primary MR limited to posterior leaflet.
    – Chronic severe primary MR involving anterior or both leaflets and likely durable repair.
    – Symptomatic patients with chronic severe primary MR but prohibitive surgical risk.
    – Asymptomatic patients with chronic severe MR (stage C1), preserved left ventricle ejection fraction, likely durable repair, and < 1% mortality risk.
    – Asymptomatic patients with chronic nonrheumatic primary MR (stage C1), preserved left ventricle ejection fraction, likely durable repair, and new-onset atrial fibrillation or pulmonary hypertension.
    – Chronic moderate primary MR (stage B) undergoing cardiac surgery for other indications.
    – Rheumatic heart disease where reliability of long-term anticoagulation management is questionable.
• MS staging:
  ○ Stage A: Mild valve doming without hemodynamic compromise.

- Stage B: Progressive MS, rheumatic changes with increased transmitral flow and mild-to-moderate left atrial enlargement, normal pulmonary pressure at rest.
- Stage C: Asymptomatic severe MS, rheumatic changes, decreased mitral valve area with severe left atrial enlargement, elevated pulmonary artery pressure.
- Stage D: Symptomatic severe MS, rheumatic valve changes, valve doming, decreased mitral valve area and increased pressure, severe left atrial enlargement, elevated pulmonary pressure, exertional dyspnea.
- Primary MR staging:
  - Stage A: Mild valve prolapse or thickening, small central jet < 20% of left atria.
  - Stage B: Progressive MR, severe prolapse with rheumatic changes, central jet 20–40%, mild left atrial enlargement, normal pulmonary pressure.
  - Stage C: Asymptomatic severe MR, divided into C1 and C2, severe valve prolapse with rheumatic changes or thickening, central jet > 40%, moderate-to-severe left atrial enlargement, pulmonary hypertension, preserved or reduced ejection fraction.
  - Stage D: Symptomatic severe MR: severe valve prolapse with loss of coaptation, rheumatic changes with loss of coaptation, central jet > 40%, large regurgitant fraction, moderate-to-severe left atrial enlargement, pulmonary hypertension, exertional dyspnea.
- Mitral valve repair or MVR indications:
  - Percutaneous mitral balloon commissurotomy considered for symptomatic patients with severe MS (stage C or D), favorable morphology, absence of left atrial thrombus, and absence of moderate-to-severe MR; can be considered for patients who are high risk for surgery or with suboptimal valve anatomy.
  - Mitral valve surgery is recommended for severely symptomatic patients with severe MS (mitral valve area ≤ 1.5 cm^2, stage D), not high risk for surgery, and not candidates for percutaneous balloon commissurotomy.
  - Severe MS (stage C or D) undergoing other cardiac surgery including excision of left atrial appendage for recurrent embolic events; chronic severe MR (stage C or D) undergoing other cardiac surgery.
  - Symptomatic patients with chronic severe primary MR (stage D) and decreased or maintained LVEF.
  - Asymptomatic patients with chronic severe primary MR (stage C2) and LV dysfunction.
  - Chronic severe secondary MR (stage C or D) undergoing CABG or AVR.
  - Severely symptomatic patients with chronic severe secondary MR (stage D).
  - Chronic moderate secondary MR (stage B) undergoing other cardiac surgery.
- Similar decision point when considering mechanical or bioprosthetic valves as in AVR.

6.4.4 Tricuspid Valve

- Much less frequent and less commonly treated than MVR or AVR.
- Grading of tricuspid stenosis (TS):
  - Stage C or D: Severe TS, thickened or distorted leaflets, decreased valve area, right atrial or inferior vena cava enlargement, variable symptoms depending on obstruction.
- Grading of tricuspid regurgitation (TR):
  - Stage A: Mild prolapse or rheumatic changes without hemodynamic compromise.
  - Stage B: Mild-to-moderate TR or prolapse, no right atrial enlargement, central jet < 5 cm^2 (mild) or 5–10 cm^2 (moderate).
  - Stage C: Asymptomatic severe TR, elevated right atrial pressure, dilated right atrium or ventricle.
  - Stage D: Symptomatic severe TR, distorted or tethered leaflets, annular dilation, central jet area > 10 cm^2, dilated right atrium or right ventricle, clinical symptoms (e.g., fatigue, palpitations, dyspnea, edema).
- Tricuspid valve surgery indications:
  - Severe TS (stage D) at time of other left-sided valve disease, severe symptomatic TS (stage D), or severe symptomatic TR (stage D) unresponsive to medical treatment.
  - Percutaneous balloon tricuspid commissurotomy considered for patients with severe symptomatic TS without TR.
  - Severe TR (stage C and D) undergoing left-sided valve surgery.

○ TR (stage B) at time of left-sided valve surgery with tricuspid annular dilatation or right heart failure.
○ Moderate TR (stage B) and pulmonary artery hypertension at time of left-sided valve surgery.
○ Asymptomatic severe primary TR (stage C) and progressive right ventricle dilatation.
○ Persistent symptoms from severe TR (stage D) in patients with prior left-side valve surgery without severe pulmonary hypertension or right ventricle systolic dysfunction.

6.4.5 Infective Endocarditis

- Introduction[22,23,28]:
  ○ Impacts 15:100,000 people in the United States annually; hospital mortality is 20% and 6-month mortality 30%.
  ○ Increased incidence due to older age of population, increased rates of interventional cardiac procedures, and increased rates of intravenous drug abuse (IVDA) in younger patients.
  ○ Most commonly from *S. aureus*; less commonly from fastidious gram-negative bacteria or fungal sources.
  ○ Antibiotic prophylaxis is recommended during dental procedures for patients at risk (e.g., prosthetic cardiac valves repair or replacement, prior infective endocarditis, congenital heart disease, cardiac transplantation).
- Diagnosis:
  ○ Presents with high fever, rigor, and sepsis; murmur can be identified.
  ○ Subclinical symptoms can include fatigue, dyspnea, and weight loss.
  ○ Fever may not always be present.
  ○ Duke criteria can be helpful but are not definitive in diagnosis.
  ○ Janeway lesion or Osler nodes are present in < 5% of cases.
  ○ Risk factors: Age > 60 years, male, structural heart disease, prosthetic valve, prior infective endocarditis, IVDA, hemodialysis, indwelling cardiovascular devices, skin infection, or poor oral hygiene.
  ○ Multiple blood cultures from separate sites are recommended.
  ○ Transthoracic echocardiography (sensitivity 70%) and transesophageal echocardiography (sensitivity 95%, specificity 90%) are critical to diagnosis.
  ○ Imaging of other infected sites (e.g., joints, soft tissue, spine, brain) is important to obtain disease control and prevent tissue injury.
  ○ Other imaging modalities include PET.
- Treatment:
  ○ Broad-spectrum, appropriate antibiotics are utilized; commonly include vancomycin, cefazolin, nafcillin, daptomycin, and linezolid.
  ○ Surgical treatment is performed in approximately 50% of first-time left-side infections.
  ○ Controversial with surgical treatment in IVDA due to risk of repeat drug use.
  ○ Surgical treatment performed early except in situations with extensive neurological damage or hemorrhage from stroke which delays it for at least 4 weeks.
  ○ Surgical treatment:
    – Patients with valvular dysfunction resulting in heart failure.
    – Treatment of highly resistant organisms.
    – Patients with heart block, annular or aortic abscess, destructive penetrating lesions.
    – Persistent infection with bacteremia lasting > 5–7 days.
    – Prosthetic valves with relapsing infection.
    – After removal of pacemaker or defibrillator systems with valvular infective endocarditis.
    – Recurrent emboli or persistent vegetations despite antibiotic therapy.
    – Mobile vegetations > 1 cm in length.

6.4.6 Septal Defects

- ASD:
  ○ Second most common congenital lesion in adults.
  ○ ASD increase risk of arrhythmia, paradoxical emboli, cerebral abscess, and right heart failure.

- Indications for repair of ASDs:
  - ASD with decreased functional capacity, increased left-to-right shunt and elevated pulmonary artery pressure.
  - Asymptomatic patients without symptoms but significant left-to-right shunt, right atrial enlargement, RV enlargement or elevated pulmonary artery pressure.
  - Documented platypnea-orthodeoxia: Dyspnea and arterial desaturation in upright position.
  - Paradoxical emboli in younger patients (e.g., age < 60 years) without other sources of stroke.
  - Repair performed endovascularly, or using full sternotomy, partial sternotomy, right anterior thoracotomy, or right axillary approaches.
- VSD:
  - Most small VSDs close spontaneously, larger defects decrease in size, smaller rate of spontaneous closure in adults.
  - Five types: Infundibular, membranous, inlet, muscular or atrioventricular/Gerbode defect.
  - Increased risk of AR, sinus of Valsalva aneurysm, pulmonary hypertension and Eisenmerger syndrome, endocarditis, arrhythmia, and heart failure.
  - Indications for repair of VSDs:
    - Small defects without pulmonary hypertension can be observed which increases risk of endocarditis, right heart failure, or AR over time.
    - Medium-to-large VSDs with increased pulmonary hypertension, cyanosis, heart failure, and arrhythmia are indicated for treatment.
    - VSD with worsening AR.
    - History of infective endocarditis if patient remains at risk.
    - During repair of concomitant cardiac issues.
  - Contraindicated closure in patients with irreversible pulmonary artery hypertension.
  - Repair performed by endovascular or surgical methods.
  - Women of reproductive age have small risk with small shunts; higher risk of arrhythmias, ventricular dysfunction, and heart failure with larger shunt showing pulmonary hypertension.

6.4.7 Arrhythmia Surgery

- See Chapter 2.5 Cardiac Arrhythmia in Surgical Patients
- Catheter ablation:
  - Used for atrioventricular reentrant tachycardia with Wolff-Parkinson-White syndrome or accessory pathway, atrioventricular nodal reentrant tachycardia, atrial tachycardia, atrial fibrillation/flutter, frequent ventricular ectopy, VT, arrhythmia-induced cardiomyopathy, and rarely premature ventricular contractions with polymorphic VT or VF.
  - Contraindicated for unstable angina, bacteremia, congestive heart failure not due to arrhythmia, bleeding disorders, lower extremity venous thrombosis, intracardiac mass.
- Cox maze IV procedure:
  - Commonly used for atrial fibrillation.
  - Surgical generation of linear scars by incision or ablation to prevent errant cardiac rhythms from passing effectively through myocardium; performed at time of other cardiac surgery.
  - Multiple iterations of the procedure (e.g., Maze I, Maze II, Maze III) have aimed to improve treatment safety.
  - Procedure aimed to create conduction blocks, reestablish atrioventricular synchrony, and restoration of atrial mechanical function.

6.4.8 Hypertrophic Cardiomyopathy

- Present in 0.2% of the population.
- Genetically caused disease resulting in cardiac myocyte hypertrophy and left ventricular outflow tract (LVOT) obstruction, diastolic dysfunction, myocardial ischemia, and MR.
- LVOT obstruction due to systolic anterior motion (SAM) of the mitral valve resulting in anterior leaflet pulled into the ventricular septum causing MR and obstruction.

- Presents with heart failure, chest pain, or arrhythmia.
- Increased risk of sudden cardiac death (SCD).
- Treatment:
  - Pharmacology: β-blockers attempted initially followed by nondihydropyridine calcium channel blockers; disopryramide used as second-line agent due to arrhythmic side effects; diuretics used for volume management; ACE inhibitors, aldosterone antagonists, diuretics, and cardiac resynchronization considered for patients with < 50% ejection fraction.
  - Septal myectomy: Improved relief of LVOT obstruction compared to alcohol septal ablation, immediate improvement of LVOT instead of improvement after 3 months with alcohol, lower incidence of complete heart block and improved treatment durability.
  - Ethanol septal ablation: Avoids risk of sternotomy and cardiopulmonary bypass.
  - Dual chamber pacing: Rarely used for patients with refractory symptoms who are not candidates for surgical treatment.
  - MVR: Less often performed due to improvement with medications and ablative treatments.
  - Cardiac transplantation in select patients with progressive symptoms/HF despite medical treatment.
- Complications of myectomy:
  - VSD (2%).
  - Complete heart block (5%).
  - AR.
  - Perioperative mortality (1–2%).

6.5 Cardiopulmonary Neoplasms

Michael Karsy and Milos Buhavac

6.5.1 Pulmonary Neoplasms

- Introduction:
  - Very common pathology; affects 230,000 patients annually in the United States and causes 140,000 deaths annually in the United States.
  - Decreased rates after reduction in smoking.
  - 95% of lung cancers are small cell lung cancer (SCLC) or non-small cell lung cancer (NSCLC); NSCLC accounts for 80% of lung cancers and 50% are adenocarcinomas.
  - Risk factors: Smoking, radiation, environmental heavy metal exposure, pulmonary fibrosis, HIV, alcohol.
  - Low-dose CT scan has moderate benefit in screening, covered by Medicare for patients age 55–77 without symptoms of lung cancer if they had a prior 30-pack year smoking history and quit 15 years prior.
  - NSCLC survival: 5-year total survival is 23%; 5-year survival ranges from 92% in stage IA to 1–10% in stage 4.
  - SCLC survival: Limited disease (median survival 15–20 months, 5-year survival 10–13%), extensive disease (median survival 8–13 months, 5-year survival 1–2%).
  - Common sites of metastasis: Liver, adrenal glands, bone, and brain.
  - Treatments and survival highly dependent on target therapy of ALK and epidermal growth factor receptor (EGFR) mutations.
- Present with:
  - Cough (50–75% patients), hemoptysis (20–50%), chest pain (20–40%), dyspnea (25–40%).
  - Hoarseness, pleural effusion.
  - Superior vena cava syndrome: Dilated neck veins, facial edema, widening of mediastinum or right hilar mass.
  - Pancoast syndrome: Pain in shoulders or forearms, Horner syndrome, bone destruction, and atrophy of hand muscle.
- Work-up:
  - NSCLC staging performed clinically and by imaging (▶ Table 6.4).
  - SCLC staging more commonly divided into limited stage (ipsilateral lung disease, 30% of patients) or extensive stage (bilateral lung disease or spread to distant organs) than TNM staging (▶ Table 6.4).

Table 6.4 Lung carcinoma TNM staging

TNM classification	Description
Tx	Tumor in sputum/bronchial washings
To	No evidence of tumor
Tis	Carcinoma in situ
T1 (T1a–T1c)	≤ 3 cm
T2 (T2a–T2b)	3–5 cm or involvement of main bronchus without carina
T3	5–7 cm or invasion of chest wall, pericardium, phrenic nerve or ipsilateral satellite nodules
T4	> 4 cm or invasion of mediastinum, diaphragm, heart, great vessels, recurrent laryngeal nerve, carina, trachea, esophagus, spine or separate ipsilateral tumor
N1	Ipsilateral peribronchial or hilar nodes and intrapulmonary nodes
N2	Ipsilateral mediastinal or subcarinal nodes
N3	Contralateral mediastinal or hilar nodes, scalene or supraclavicular nodes
M1	Distant metastasis
Stage	
Ia	T1a, T1b
Ib	T2a
IIa	T2b, N0; T1a–T2a, N1
IIIa	T1a, N2; T1b–T2a, N2; T2b, N2; T3–T4, N1; T4, N0
IIIb	T1a–T1b, N3
IV	Any T, any N, M1

- ○ PET-CT imaging can be used to evaluate tumor burden and location.
- Paraneoplastic effects of lung cancer:
  - ○ Hypercalcemia.
  - ○ Syndrome of inappropriate antidiuretic hormone secretion resulting in hyponatremia.
  - ○ Immune-mediated neurological dysfunction resulting in central or peripheral nervous system dysfunction.
  - ○ Hematological deficits including anemia and leukocytosis.
  - ○ Hypertrophic pulmonary osteoarthropathy.
  - ○ Dermatomyositis/Polymyositis.
  - ○ Cushing syndrome.
- NSCLC treatment:
  - ○ Surgical resection strongly considered for stage I or II NSCLC; postoperative adjuvant therapy used for stage IB, II, or III disease; immunotherapy can be useful depending on tumor mutations and stage (e.g., epidermal growth factor receptor, EML4-ALK fusion oncogene, PD-L1).
  - ○ Patients not candidates for resection can be treated with radiofrequency ablation, cryoablation, or radiation.
  - ○ Stage IV disease treated with systemic therapy or palliative approaches (e.g., resection of brain lesions, stabilization of spine lesions, bronchoscopy-directed catheter brachytherapy).
- SCLC treatment:
  - ○ Disease is usually disseminated at time of treatment and is responsive to chemotherapy.
  - ○ Limited disease is treated with chemoradiotherapy; initial treatment for extensive disease is also radiochemotherapy.
  - ○ Surgery is rarely used for solitary pulmonary nodule without metastasis or lymph node involvement.
  - ○ Prophylactic cranial radiotherapy decreases risk of brain lesions.
  - ○ Immunotherapy is also utilized in some patients but is less common than NSCLC treatment.

6.5.2 Pleural Neoplasms

- Mesothelima:
  - ○ Rare cancer of the pleural and pericardial cavities, less commonly in the abdomen or testes.

Table 6.5 TNM staging of mesothelioma

TNM classification	Description
T1	Ipsilateral parietal or visceral pleura
T2	Ipsilateral pleura with invasion of diaphragmatic muscle or pulmonary parenchyma
T3	Ipsilateral pleural with invasion of endothoracic fascia, mediastinal fat, chest wall/rib or pericardium
T4	Ipsilateral pleura with invasion of chest wall, peritoneum, contralateral pleura, mediastinal organs, vertebrae, or pericardium
N0	No regional lymph node metastasis
N1	Ipsilateral lymph node metastasis
N2	Contralateral lymph node metastasis
M1	Distant metastasis
Stage	
IA	T1
IB	T2, T3
II	T1, T2, N1
IIIA	T3, N1
IIIB	T1–T3, N2; T4, N0–N2
IV	Any T, any N, M1

- o Affects ~3,000 people annually in the United States, increased incidence overall with higher rates internationally than the United States.
- o Presents with shortness of breath, pleural effusions, and pain.
- o 80% of cases due to asbestos exposure with 40-year period between exposure and cancer onset.
- o 5-year survival of 8%, average survival of 12–21 months.
- o Staging by TNM classification (▶ Table 6.5) performed.
- o Treatment: Surgical resection, radiochemotherapy, pleurodesis to reduce pleural effusion.

6.5.3 Cardiac Neoplasms

- Introduction:
  - o Extremely rare primary cancers with incidence 0.1% of U.S. population.
  - o More commonly metastatic cancers.
  - o Identified incidentally on imaging.
  - o Symptoms can include embolization to systemic or pulmonic vessels, obstruction with heart failure, valvular regurgitation, LV arrhythmia, or adjacent pulmonary symptoms.
  - o Evaluated by echocardiography primarily; cardiac MRI and CT are adjunct imaging methods.
  - o Transvenous biopsy for some tumors but increases risk of embolization.
  - o Surgical treatment is commonly performed due to risk of embolism, thrombus and valvular obstruction with SCD.
- Benign tumors:
  - o Myxomas:
    - – Most common primary tumors, scattered cells within mucopolysaccharide stroma.
    - – 80% arise in left atrium and 20% within right atrium.
    - – Present with constitutional symptoms (e.g., weight loss, fevers) due to cytokine secretion.
    - – Commonly obstruct mitral valve.
    - – Carney complex: Autosomal-dominant syndrome with atrial and extracardiac myxomas, schwannomas, and endocrine tumors; pigmented lentigines and blue nevi seen on skin.
    - – Treated with surgical resection.
  - o Papillary fibroelastoma:
    - – Second most common primary cardiac tumor.
    - – Present in older adults.

- Presents with symptoms from embolism (e.g., stroke, transient ischemic attack, angina, myocardial infarction); 30% asymptomatic.
    - Treated with surgical resection.
  ○ Rhabdomyoma:
    - Present in children within ventricular walls or atrioventricular valves.
    - Most regress spontaneously and do not require treatment.
  ○ Fibroma:
    - Second most common pediatric tumor, rare.
    - More common in left ventricle.
    - Treated with surgical resection.
  ○ Teratoma:
    - Embryonic tumors from two or three germinal layers, rare, < 1% cardiac tumors.
    - Fetal types are benign but grow quickly.
    - Cystic portions treated by aspiration may not completely relieve symptoms.
    - Treated with surgical resection.
  ○ Purkinje cell hamartomas:
    - Small tumors requiring electrophysiologic localization occurring in young children with VT.
    - Surgical resection depends on size and location of lesion.
  ○ Lipomas:
    - Benign fatty tumors in subendocardial region, can occur on valves, usually small but can grow very large.
    - Lipomatous hypertrophy of interatrial septum must be distinguished as growth of normal fat, developmental disorder of fat trapped in septum during embryogenesis.
    - Surgical resection depends on size and location of lesion.
- Intermediate risk tumors:
  ○ Paragangliomas:
    - Neuroendocrine tumors that can be hormonally active, more frequently hormonally inactive in pericardium but hormonally active in thorax.
    - Challenging to surgically resect due to vascularity.
  ○ Mesothelioma:
    - Most commonly in pleura but can rarely occur in pericardium or atrioventricular node.
    - Treated with surgical resection and chemoradiotherapy.
- Malignant tumors:
  ○ 15% of primary cardiac tumors.
  ○ Sarcoma:
    - Rare.
    - Types: Angiosarcoma, rhabdomyosarcoma, fibrosarcoma, undifferentiated sarcoma, leiomyosarcoma.
    - Treated by complete resection but poor survival (median 6–12 months); other strategies include cardiac transplantation and cardiac autotransplantation with ex vivo tumor resection.
    - Treated with surgical resection and chemoradiotherapy.
  ○ Lymphoma:
    - Very rare, handful of cases with poor outcome.

6.6 Implantable Cardiovert Defibrillators and Pacemakers

Michael Karsy and Milos Buhavac

6.6.1 Implantable Cardiovert Defibrillators (ICDs)

- Also see Chapter 1.1 Perioperative Risk.
- First created in 1980 and approved in 1985 for secondary prevention in survivors after cardiac arrest.
- Indications:
  ○ Secondary prevention of SCD after VT, VF, or hemodynamically unstable/resuscitated SCD thought to be due to ventricular tachyarrhythmia.

- Primary prevention for patients at increased risk of VT/VF including prior myocardial infarction and reduced LVEF ($\leq 30\%$).
- VT/VF from congenital long QT syndrome, presence of valvular disease with arrhythmia, channelopathies (e.g., Brugada syndrome, catecholaminergic polymorphic VT), high-risk hypertrophic cardiomyopathy.
- Cardiomyopathy with New York Heart Association (NYHA) class II or III symptoms and LVEF $\leq 35\%$.
- Contraindications:
  - Reversible ventricular tachyarrhythmias.
  - Poor patient survival.
  - VT/VF with possibility of catheter ablation or other therapies.
  - Patient not psychologically sound for surgical treatment.
  - NYHA class IV heart failure not a candidate for transplantation or CRT.
  - Syncope of unknown or noncardiac origins.
  - Active infections or other acute illnesses.
- Components:
  - Pacing and sensing electrodes; distal lead at the tip of an electrode and proximal lead several mm more proximal.
  - Defibrillation electrode consists of a coil along the lead; multiple electrodes are present in the system; ICD housing can serve as a defibrillation site also.
  - Single chamber systems use right ventricle lead; dual chamber systems use right atrial and ventricle leads.
  - Pulse generator placed subclavicularly; subcutaneous ICD also possible.
  - ICDs can store and monitor rhythms allowing telemetry of shocks.
  - Synchronized and desynchronized defibrillation possible.
  - ICD can be combined with biventricular pacemakers, termed cardiac resynchronization therapy-defibrillator (CRT-D).
  - Wearable ICDs are potential modalities for patients at high risk for device placement or early young age otherwise requiring multiple ICDs.

6.6.2 Implantable Cardiac Pacemakers

- Introduction:
  - > 3 million devices placed globally; increased trend of dual-chamber pacemakers in the United States in older patients with increased medical comorbidities.
  - Detection of myocardial infarction in the setting of a pacemaker can be challenging, findings approximate a left bundle branch block (Sgarbossa criteria can be used to define infarction), may require high degree of suspicion and expert consultation.
- Permanent pacemaker indications:
  - Symptomatic bradyarrhythmia; symptoms include lightheadedness, syncope, fatigue, poor exercise tolerance; heart rate < 40 beats/min or inability to achieve 85% of age-predicted maximal heart rate during exercise; includes bradycardia-induced ventricular arrhythmia.
  - Conduction blocks of His-Purkinje system due to greater likelihood of progression.
  - Sinus node dysfunction.
  - Acquired atrioventricular block (second most common indication; includes Mobitz type I, Mobitz type II, and complete blocks depending on symptoms).
  - Postmyocardial infarction.
  - Neurocardiogenic syncope (controversial).
  - Complete congenital heart block.
  - Neuromuscular diseases with atrioventricular heart block.
  - Long QT syndrome in high-risk patients.
  - Hypertrophic cardiomyopathy.
  - Cardiac resynchronization.
- Temporary pacemaker indications:
  - Medication-related atrioventricular block or bradycardia.

- Toxic or metabolic disturbances.
- Acute myocardial infarction.
- Cardiac trauma.
- Infectious disease.
- Bacterial endocarditis with damage to His-Purkinje system.
- Components:
  - Internal pulse generator placed subclavicularly, transvenous leads most commonly used, epicardial systems less often used.
  - Nomenclature:
    - 5 letter code: First position indicates chamber paced (A: atrium, V: ventricle, D: dual); second position indicates chamber sensed (A, V, D, O: absence of sensing); third position indicates pacemaker response to sensing (I: inhibits, T: triggered, D: dual with event in atrium triggering ventricle; O: no response); fourth position indicates rate modulation (R: rate modulation and adjusts to patient activity; O: unavailable or disabled); fifth position indicates multisite pacing (A, V, D, O).
    - Mode switching allows biventricular pacers to switch from responsive mode (e.g., DDD) to an automatic mode (e.g., VVI, DDI, DVI) in the setting of atrial tachyarrhythmia to prevent VT.
    - Physiologic pacing: Aim to approximate normal cardiac activity which can reduce rates of atrial fibrillation, thromboembolic events, and cardiac dyssynchrony (e.g., pacemaker syndrome) while improving some hemodynamics.
- Pacer modes:
  - Single-chamber pacing: Sensing and pacing of single chamber.
  - VVI: Most commonly used mode; utilized for bradycardia; capable in most devices.
  - AAI: Utilized for sinus node dysfunction with intact atrioventricular node; do not protect against atrioventricular conduction block.
  - DDD: Pacemaker inhibit with sinus rhythm and adequate atrioventricular conduction; sinus bradycardia with adequate atrioventricular conduction results in atrial pacing; sinus bradycardia with inadequate atrioventricular conduction results in synchronous atrial and ventricular pacing; utilized for patients with atrioventricular block or combined sinus/atrioventricular nodal dysfunction.
  - DDI: During atrioventricular block, ventricular pacing occurs at a programmed rate; less often used with current pacemakers since mode switching is available.
  - Less common modes: VDD, DVI.
  - Asynchronous pacing (e.g., AOO, VOO, DOO) is used during surgical procedures so electrocautery is not misinterpreted as cardiac activity resulting in pacemaker triggering.

6.6.3 Perioperative Management of Pacemakers and ICDs

- Electromagnetic interference (EMI): can cause misinterpretation of rhythm, causing bradycardia, asystole, tachycardia, or inappropriate shocks; device failure; resetting to device VVI pacing mode (ventricular pace of 60–72.5 beats/min) which can result in acute heart failure.
- Electrosurgical units:
  - Monopolar causes more EMI than bipolar electrosurgery.
  - Coagulation mode causes more EMI than cutting mode.
  - Highest risk of EMI when near an internal pulse generator (e.g., above the umbilicus).
- Elective surgery steps:
  - Device interrogation recommended 3–12 months prior to surgical treatment.
  - Pacemaker dependence determined (e.g., symptomatic bradycardia); pacer-dependent modes should be reprogrammed to asynchronous pacing modes.
  - ICD antitachycardia therapy must be suspended.
  - Transcutaneous pacing/defibrillator pads are placed for ICDs with defibrillation turned off.
  - Magnet reprogramming should be performed only when device specifications are known.
- Emergency situations:
  - Placement of magnet for a pacemaker usually initiates asynchronous pacing with a fixed rate and atrioventricular delay.
  - Placement of magnet for ICD usually suspends anti-tachyarrhythmia therapy.

References

[1] Rodriguez LE, Suarez EE, Loebe M, Bruckner BA. Ventricular assist devices (VAD) therapy: new technology, new hope? Methodist DeBakey Cardiovasc J. 2013; 9(1):32–37

[2] Han JJ, Acker MA, Atluri P. Left ventricular assist devices. Circulation. 2018; 138(24):2841–2851

[3] Birati E, Jessup M, E YB. Left ventricular assist devices in the management of heart failure. Card Fail Rev. 2015; 1(1):25–30

[4] Rose EA, Gelijns AC, Moskowitz AJ, et al. Randomized Evaluation of Mechanical Assistance for the Treatment of Congestive Heart Failure (REMATCH) Study Group. Long-term use of a left ventricular assist device for end-stage heart failure. N Engl J Med. 2001; 345 (20):1435–1443

[5] Bhagra SK, Pettit S, Parameshwar J. Cardiac transplantation: indications, eligibility and current outcomes. Heart. 2019; 105(3): 252–260

[6] Hillis LD, Smith PK, Anderson JL, et al. American College of Cardiology Foundation/American Heart Association Task Force on Practice Guidelines. 2011 ACCF/AHA guideline for coronary artery bypass graft surgery: executive summary: a Report of the American College of Cardiology Foundation/American Heart Association Task Force on Practice Guidelines. J Thorac Cardiovasc Surg. 2012; 143(1):4–34

[7] Leon MB, Smith CR, Mack M, et al. PARTNER Trial Investigators. Transcatheter aortic valve implantation for aortic stenosis in patients who cannot undergo surgery. N Engl J Med. 2010; 363(17):1597–1607

[8] Harrison TR. Tinsley Randolph Harrison 1900-1978. "The pathogenesis of congestive heart failure": then and now. 1935. Medicine (Baltimore). 1991; 70(1):67–80, discussion 80–81

[9] Dharmarajan K, Rich MW. Epidemiology, pathophysiology, and prognosis of heart failure in older adults. Heart Fail Clin. 2017; 13(3): 417–426

[10] Levy D, Kenchaiah S, Larson MG, et al. Long-term trends in the incidence of and survival with heart failure. N Engl J Med. 2002; 347 (18):1397–1402

[11] Benjamin EJ, Blaha MJ, Chiuve SE, et al. American Heart Association Statistics Committee and Stroke Statistics Subcommittee. Heart Disease and Stroke Statistics—2017 update: a report from the American Heart Association. Circulation. 2017; 135(10):e146–e603

[12] Hosenpud JD, Greenberg BH. Congestive Heart Failure. 3rd ed. Springfield, IL: Charles C. Thomas; 2007

[13] Kapoor JR, Kapoor R, Ju C, et al. Precipitating clinical factors, heart failure characterization, and outcomes in patients hospitalized with heart failure with reduced, borderline, and preserved ejection fraction. JACC Heart Fail. 2016; 4(6):464–472

[14] Hauptman PJ, Rich MW, Heindenreich PA, et al. The heart failure clinic: a consensus statement of the heart failure society of America. J Cardiac Fail. 2008; 14:801–e815

[15] Gupta VA, Nanda NC, Sorrell VL. Role of echocardiography in the diagnostic assessment and cause of heart failure in older adults: opacify, quantify, and rectify. Heart Fail Clin. 2017; 13(3):445–466

[16] Ritchie JL, Bateman TM, Bonow RO, et al. Guidelines for clinical use of cardiac radionuclide imaging. Report of the American College of Cardiology/American Heart Association Task Force on Assessment of Diagnostic and Therapeutic Cardiovascular Procedures (Committee on Radionuclide Imaging), developed in collaboration with the American Society of Nuclear Cardiology. J Am Coll Cardiol. 1995; 25(2):521–547

[17] Ponikowski P, Voors AA, Anker SD, et al. ESC Scientific Document Group. 2016 ESC Guidelines for the diagnosis and treatment of acute and chronic heart failure: the task force for the diagnosis and treatment of acute and chronic heart failure of the European Society of Cardiology (ESC) developed with the special contribution of the Heart Failure Association (HFA) of the ESC. Eur Heart J. 2016; 37(27): 2129–2200

[18] Yancy CW, Jessup M, Bozkurt B, et al. 2017 ACC/AHA/HFSA Focused Update of the 2013 ACCF/AHA Guideline for the Management of Heart Failure: a report of the American College of Cardiology/American Heart Association Task Force on Clinical Practice Guidelines and the Heart Failure Society of America. Circulation. 2017; 136(6):e137–e161

[19] Starling RC, Naka Y, Boyle AJ, et al. Results of the post-U.S. Food and Drug Administration-approval study with a continuous flow left ventricular assist device as a bridge to heart transplantation: a prospective study using the INTERMACS (Interagency Registry for Mechanically Assisted Circulatory Support). J Am Coll Cardiol. 2011; 57(19):1890–1898

[20] Park SJ, Tector A, Piccioni W, et al. Left ventricular assist devices as destination therapy: a new look at survival. J Thorac Cardiovasc Surg. 2005; 129(1):9–17

[21] Sarkar M, Prabhu V. Basics of cardiopulmonary bypass. Indian J Anaesth. 2017; 61(9):760–767

[22] Nishimura RA, Otto CM, Bonow RO, et al. American College of Cardiology/American Heart Association Task Force on Practice Guidelines. 2014 AHA/ACC guideline for the management of patients with valvular heart disease: executive summary: a report of the American College of Cardiology/American Heart Association Task Force on Practice Guidelines. J Am Coll Cardiol. 2014; 63(22):2438–2488

[23] Nishimura RA, Otto CM, Bonow RO, et al. 2017 AHA/ACC focused update of the 2014 AHA/ACC guideline for the management of patients with valvular heart disease: a report of the American College of Cardiology/American Heart Association Task Force on clinical practice guidelines. J Am Coll Cardiol. 2017; 70(2):252–289

[24] McKellar S, Zehr K. Aortic valve repair for aortic insufficiency. CTSNet 2010. Accessed July 27, 2019

[25] Thonghong T, De Backer O, Søndergaard L. Comprehensive update on the new indications for transcatheter aortic valve replacement in the latest 2017 European guidelines for the management of valvular heart disease. Open Heart. 2018; 5(1):e000753

[26] Yanagawa B, Latter D, Verma S. Year in review: mitral valve surgery. Curr Opin Cardiol. 2016; 31(2):148–153

[27] Madesis A, Tsakiridis K, Zarogoulidis P, et al. Review of mitral valve insufficiency: repair or replacement. J Thorac Dis. 2014; 6 Suppl 1: S39–S51

[28] Wang A, Gaca JG, Chu VH. Management considerations in infective endocarditis: a review. JAMA. 2018; 320(1):72–83

7 Otolaryngology

Edited by Hilary McCrary

7.1 Airway Management/Tracheostomy

Eric Babajanian, Hilary McCrary, and Richard Cannon

7.1.1 Summary

- Definitive airway management is essential in the patient who exhibits a failure to adequately oxygenate, ventilate, or maintain their airway.
- There are various classification systems that aid in identification of patients that are anticipated to be difficult to intubate.
- Difficult airways are characterized by either difficult tracheal intubation, difficult laryngoscopy, or difficult mask ventilation.
- In patients that are unable to be either intubated or mask ventilated, establishing a surgical airway is indicated, via either cricothyroidotomy or tracheotomy.

7.1.2 Definitions

- Difficult airway: Involves at least one of the following three distinct scenarios[1]:
  - Difficult tracheal intubation: One that requires multiple attempts by multiple operators or is performed with excessive effort/manipulation or without adequate glottic exposure.
  - Difficult laryngoscopy: Grade 3 or 4 laryngoscopies as defined by the Cormack–Lehane classification system.[2]
  - Difficult mask ventilation: Inability to provide adequate facemask ventilation, due to either inadequate mask seal or inadequate patency of airway.
- Cricothyroidotomy: Incision made through skin and cricothyroid membrane to obtain airway typically in an airway emergency.
- Tracheotomy: The tracheal incision.
- Tracheostomy: The opening that provides a connection to the trachea from the external neck through which a tracheostomy tube is often placed.

7.1.3 Epidemiology

- Data obtained from Nation Emergency Airway Registry examining 17,500 emergency department intubations[3]:
  - Orotracheal rapid sequence intubation: 85% first-pass success rate (initial method in 85% of all encounters).
  - Direct laryngoscope: Most common initial device (84% of cases).
  - Surgical airway: Needle, surgical, or rescue cricothyroidotomy (0.45% of cases).
    - Rescue cricothyroidotomy more likely in trauma-indicated intubations compared with medical- or other-indicated intubations.
- Difficult laryngoscopy: Data obtained from selected cases in the operating room; incidence in the emergency department is likely higher.[4]
  - Grade 3 laryngoscopy: ~5%.
  - Grade 4 laryngoscopy: ~1%.
- Tracheostomy (data obtained from Healthcare Cost and Utilization Project): Over 100,000 tracheostomy procedures performed per year for any indication.[5]

7.1.4 Diagnosis

- Deciding when to establish a definitive airway may sometimes not be immediately clear. If any of the following scenarios are true, then a definitive airway needs to be established[6]:
  - Failure of airway maintenance/protection.

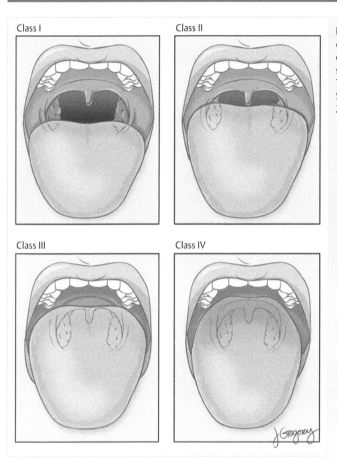

Fig. 7.1 Modified Mallampati classification system for determining ease of orotracheal intubation. (Source: Dyleski R, Linstrom C, Pitman M, et al, eds. Total Otolaryngology: Head and Neck Surgery. 1st ed. New York, NY: Thieme; 2014.)

- ○ Failure of oxygenation/ventilation.
- ○ Anticipated need for intubation as a result of the patient's most likely clinical course.
- Patients in whom intubation is expected to be difficult can be identified using different grading systems based on physical examination findings.
- Modified Mallampati classification:
  - ○ Classified according to pharyngeal structures seen while examining patient at eye level using only pen light[7] (▶ Fig. 7.1).
  - ○ Common classification system among anesthesiologists:
    - – Class I: Soft palate, fossas, uvula, pillars.
    - – Class II: Soft palate, fossas, uvula.
    - – Class III: Soft palate, base of uvula.
    - – Class IV: Soft palate not visible.
- Cormack–Lehane classification:
  - ○ Classified according to the view obtained at laryngoscopy[2] (▶ Fig. 7.2):
    - – Grade 1: Most of glottis visible.
    - – Grade 2: Posterior extremity of glottis visible.
    - – Grade 3: Only epiglottis is visible.
    - – Grade 4: Epiglottis is not visible.
- Thyromental distance:
  - ○ Determined as the distance between the anterior portion of the mandibular mental prominence and the thyroid prominence while the head is fully extended.
  - ○ Thyromental distance ≤ 6.5 cm predictive of difficult laryngoscopy.

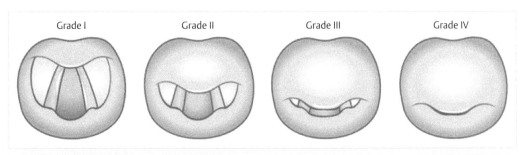

Fig. 7.2 Cormack–Lehane classification system for determining ease of endotracheal intubation. (Source: Goldenberg D, Goldstein B, eds. Handbook of Otolaryngology: Head and Neck Surgery. 2nd ed. New York, NY: Thieme; 2017.)

7.1.5 Imaging

- Imaging is not indicated and not particularly useful in the acute setting of airway management.
- Obtaining a computed tomography (CT) scan with intravenous contrast of the neck can be useful in determining the cause of respiratory compromise in the patient in whom an anatomical obstruction is suspected; however, it is imperative to ensure patient stability before obtaining imaging.

7.1.6 Medical Management

- Oxygen delivery methods.[8]
- Low-flow systems: Depends on inspiration of room air to satisfy peak inspiratory and minute ventilator demands.
  - Can be used to deliver both low and high values of FiO_2, but is less predictable compared with high-flow systems.
  - Examples: Nasal cannula, partial rebreathing mask, nonrebreathing mask, simple face mask, tracheostomy collar.
- High-flow systems: Do not depend on inspiration of room air and provide the entire inspiratory atmosphere required to satisfy peak inspiratory and minute ventilator demands.
  - Can be used to consistently and predictably deliver both low and high values of FiO_2.
  - Examples: High-flow nasal cannula, Venturi mask, aerosol masks with nebulizers or air-oxygen blenders.
- Manual resuscitation bags: Used primarily for resuscitation of ventilator-dependent patients.
  - Can deliver high levels of FiO_2 with use of oxygen reservoir and connection to an oxygen source.
- Noninvasive ventilation[9]: Can be used prophylactically to prevent respiratory distress or therapeutically to reduce symptoms associated with hypoxemia or hypoventilation and resulting respiratory distress.
  - Requires patients to be able to protect their airway and spontaneously ventilate.
  - Examples: Continuous positive airway pressure (CPAP) and bilevel positive airway pressure (BiPAP).
- Conventional (invasive) mechanical ventilation: Can either fully or partially replace spontaneous breathing in the setting of acute or chronic respiratory failure.
  - Requires a definitive airway, either via endotracheal intubation or tracheostomy placement.
  - Discussion regarding the types, settings, and management of mechanical ventilation is outside the scope of this chapter; see Chapter 2.3 Ventilator Management.

7.1.7 Types of Airways

- Extraglottic devices[10,11]:
  - Laryngeal mask airway (LMA): Inflatable mask that occupies the hypopharyngeal space and forms a seal in the supraglottis.
  - Cuffed pharyngeal sealers with esophageal cuff: Allow for blind insertion.
    - Examples: Esophageal tracheal Combitube (Combitube; Medtronic, Minneapolis, MN, USA), EasyTube (Well Lead, Guangzhou, China), Laryngeal Tube (VBM, Medizintechik, Sulz, Germany).

- ○ Cuffed pharyngeal sealers without esophageal cuff: Similar to LMA, should not be used in patients at risk for regurgitation/aspiration.
  - – Example: Cobra perilaryngeal airway (Cobra PLA, Engineered Medical Systems, Indianapolis, IN).
- ○ Anatomically preshaped noninflatable supraglottic airway device: easily inserted but require appropriate sizing for adequate seal.
  - – Examples: I-gel (Intersurgical, Wokingham, United Kingdom), streamlined liner of pharynx airway (Hangzhou Fushan Medical Appliances Co., Ltd., China).
- Endotracheal intubation: Airway assessment should be completed before intubation is attempted to identify features associated with difficult airways.
  - ○ There are a multitude of approaches and devices available to guide successful endotracheal intubation in difficult airways.[12]
    - – Stylets: Endotracheal tube introducers, optical stylets, flexible endoscope.
    - – Extraglottic devices: Ideally should use a device that can be used as a conduit to pass an endotracheal tube for a definitive airway.
    - – Video or optical laryngoscopes: Allow indirect laryngoscopy and visualization of glottic anatomy for guidance of endotracheal tube placement.
    - – Rigid direct laryngoscopes: The authors of this chapter prefer the Dedo laryngoscope to guide difficult airway intubation.
    - – Nasal intubation: Can be performed blindly or under flexible endoscopic guidance; useful in patients with limited jaw opening; contraindications: coagulation status, nasal pathology.
  - ○ Absolute contraindications: Blunt laryngeal trauma resulting in laryngeal fracture or disruption of the laryngotracheal junction, penetrating trauma of the upper airway.[13,14]
- Tracheostomy tube: Allows for a definitive airway with or without mechanical ventilation or pressure support (▶ Fig. 7.3).
  - ○ Various types of tubes available, with selection of tracheostomy tube varying by scenario and patient anatomy.

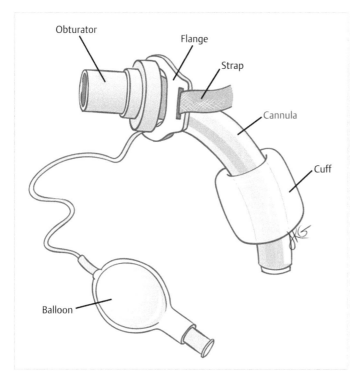

Fig. 7.3 Cuffed, nonfenestrated tracheostomy tube with labeled components. (Source: Dyleski R, Linstrom C, Pitman M, et al, eds. Total Otolaryngology: Head and Neck Surgery. 1st ed. New York, NY: Thieme; 2014.)

- Tubes are defined by inner and outer diameter, length, curvature, material of construction, and the presence of fenestration and a cuff.
- Indications, placement technique, and care will be discussed in detail later in the chapter.

7.1.8 Surgical Management

- Surgical anatomy:
  - It is important for any clinician that is routinely exposed to patient's requiring airway management interventions to have a comprehensive understanding of laryngotracheal anatomy and the corresponding palpable anatomical landmarks (▶ Fig. 7.4).
- Cricothyroidotomy[1]:
  - Indications: Failure to orally or nasally intubate or mask ventilate a patient of immediate need for a definitive airway.
  - Technique:
    - Identify landmarks: Sternal notch, thyroid notch, cricoid cartilage, cricothyroid membrane.
    - Midline vertical incision over cricoid cartilage while stabilizing upper airway with nondominant hand.
    - Horizontal incision through the cricothyroid membrane just superior to the cricoid cartilage.
    - Dilate incision with a tracheal dilator or hemostat.
    - Tracheal cartilage may be elevated using a cricoid hook (if available) to facilitate opening the airway.
    - Insert small endotracheal tube into incision.
    - If necessary, can convert to formal tracheostomy in the operating room (OR) after stabilization of patient.
  - Complications:
    - Pneumothorax/pneumomediastinum: relatively uncommon and often does not require intervention; thus, routine postprocedure imaging is not warranted.
    - Vocal cord injury: Can be avoided by making incision as inferiorly as possible in the cricothyroid membrane.

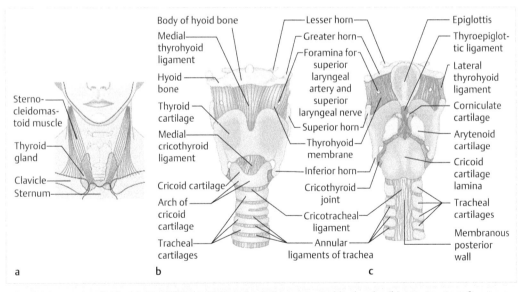

Fig. 7.4 Laryngotracheal anatomy. (a) External view of palpable anatomical landmarks. **(b)** Anterior view of laryngotracheal anatomy. **(c)** Posterior view of laryngotracheal anatomy. (Source: Probst R, Grevers G, Iro H, eds. Basic Otorhinolaryngology: A Step-by-Step Learning Guide. 2nd ed. New York, NY: Thieme; 2017.)

- Tracheotomy[15]:
  - Advantages compared with endotracheal intubation:
    - Decreased risk of laryngeal damage.
    - Decreased need for sedation.
    - Earlier return to oral nutrition.
    - Decreased incidence of ventilator-associated pneumonia given more efficient pulmonary toilet.
    - Shortened ICU stay.
  - Indications: Upper airway obstruction, prolonged mechanical ventilation, pulmonary toilet, surgical access.
  - Technique:
    - Identify landmarks: Sternal notch, hyoid bone, thyroid cartilage, cricoid cartilage.
    - Inject planned incision with 1% lidocaine with 1:100,000 epinephrine.
    - Horizontal incision 2–3 cm in length roughly 1 cm inferior to the cricoid cartilage.
    - Vertically divide superficial layer of the deep cervical fascia, avoid anterior jugular veins if possible.
    - Divide midline raphe and reflect strap muscles laterally.
    - Thyroid isthmus can be mobilized or divided to expose the anterior trachea.
    - The authors prefer to mobilize the isthmus if possible to avoid bleeding; if divided, bleeding should be addressed prior to entering the airway.
    - Clear pretracheal fascia using a Kittner sponge for identification of tracheal rings.
    - Insert cricoid hook superior to the second tracheal ring in order to elevate and expose the trachea.
    - Enter the airway: This can be accomplished with a number of approaches; the authors prefer a roughly 1.5-cm horizontal incision between the second and third tracheal rings, followed by dilation using a tracheal dilator.
    - Pull back endotracheal tube so tip is just superior to opening and insert tracheostomy tube.
    - Connect tube to ventilator circuit and confirm return of end-tidal CO_2.
    - Remove cricoid hook.
    - Secure tracheostomy tube in four quadrants with suture in addition to tracheostomy collar.
  - Complications:
    - Airway fire: Can be prevented by ideally maintaining $FiO_2 < 40\%$ while electrocautery is in use and discontinuing use of electrocautery after entry into airway.
    - Pneumothorax/pneumomediastinum: Relatively uncommon and often does not require intervention; thus, routine postoperative imaging is not warranted.
    - Postoperative pulmonary edema: Secondary to release of pressure after tracheostomy placement; can be prevented/treated with positive pressure ventilation.
- Percutaneous dilational tracheotomy[15]:
  - Can be performed at bedside using guidewire placement followed by sequential dilation and tracheostomy tube introduction with or without videobronchoscopic assistance.
  - Advantages compared with open procedure:
    - Decreased cost.
    - Decreased physiologic stress on critically ill patients by avoiding need for transport from intensive care setting.
    - Decreased amount of procedural time and related stressors.
  - Contraindications:
    - Pediatric patients: Difficult to stabilize trachea; difficult to simultaneously ventilate patient while managing bronchoscope through endotracheal tube.
    - Coagulation abnormalities.
    - Obscured anatomical landmarks secondary to midline pathology or body habitus.
    - High level of respiratory support ($FiO_2 > 70\%$, positive end-expiratory pressure > 10).
    - Cervical spine injuries.
  - Complications:
    - Injury to surrounding neurovascular and cartilage structures.
    - Loss or kinking of the guidewire.
    - Lateralization of the stoma.
    - Posterior tracheal wall injury, including injury to the esophagus.

7.1.9 Additional Topics

- Tracheostomy care:
  - Cuff pressure: Important to ensure that cuff pressure is less than capillary pressure (<25 cm H_2O) to prevent pressure necrotic injury.
  - Note: Feeding may be difficult while cuff is inflated.
  - Suctioning: Can be accomplished by regularly passing an appropriately sized suction through the tracheostomy tube and slowly retracting suction; the authors prefer to use a 14 g or 10 g red rubber catheter (depending on the size of the tracheostomy tube) attached to a suction circuit to prevent mucosal irritation and damage.
  - Skin care: It is important to routinely clean secretions and crusting around the tracheostomy tube to prevent skin breakdown and infection.
  - Various dressings can be used if pressure injury or skin breakdown is of concern based on positioning of tracheostomy tube.
  - Cuff deflation: Cuff can be deflated on postoperative day 1 at the earliest and once patient is no longer ventilated.
  - Suction patient just before and after deflation to assist with clearing of secretions.
  - Capping: Prevents air flow through tube and requires breathing around tube; useful as tool to evaluate readiness for decannulation; imperative to never cap with an inflated cuff as this causes complete airway obstruction.
  - Speaking valve: If the patient is able to tolerate, a one-way (inspiratory) speaking valve may be placed to facilitate speech; should never be placed while cuff is inflated.
  - Decannulation: In preparation for decannulation, the tracheostomy tube should be downsized on postoperative day 3 at the earliest to allow for tract maturation and the patient should be able to maintain a stable respiratory status with tracheostomy capping for 24 hours.
    - Once the patient has been decannulated, the authors prefer to place a nonocclusive dressing with an electrocardiogram lead for ease in providing finger pressure while coughing or speaking to promote stoma healing.
    - It is important to decannulate a patient as early and as safely possible to prevent tracheal injury and subglottic stenosis.
- Tracheostomy emergencies:
  - Tube dislodgement:
    - Important for supplies to be easily accessible for urgent replacement.
    - If necessary, can replace with a smaller size tube or endotracheal tube.
    - Supplies necessary at bedside: obturator, suction, spare tube.
    - Can be prevented by suturing tube to skin in four quadrants during placement.
  - Acute tube occlusion:
    - Remove inner cannula and attempt suctioning.
    - Often secondary to a mucus plug.
    - Other possibilities include a false passage (will be unable to easily pass suction) or obstructing granuloma.
    - Can be prevented with use of humidified air to prevent crusting/mucus plugs in addition to regular cleaning of inner cannula.

7.2 Head and Neck Infections

Alana Aylward, Bridger Battaglia, and Eric W. Cerrati

7.2.1 Sialadenitis

- Epidemiology:
  - Sialadenitis is inflammation of any salivary gland, most commonly the parotid (also known as parotitis). This can be acute or chronic, bacterial or viral.[16] This section primarily addresses acute bacterial sialadenitis.

- While most common in the elderly, this condition can affect people of all ages including children.[17]
- Sialolithiasis (formation of calculi in the duct) can contribute to inflammation or infection, most commonly in the submandibular gland.[16]
- Diagnosis:
  - Risk factors: Recent surgical intervention, use of medications such as antihistamines, antidepressants, or anticholinergic agents which lead to decreased salivary production, dehydration, or systemic volume depletion secondary to disease.[16,17]
  - Symptoms:
    - Painful, edematous, erythematous salivary glands that may be unilateral or bilateral.[16,17]
    - Purulent drainage from the duct with gland massage is observed in about 75% of cases.[16]
    - Compromise of the airway, while uncommon, should be acutely assessed—see Chapter 7.1 Airway Management/Tracheostomy.
- Imaging (▶ Fig. 7.5)[16,18]:
  - Consider CT or ultrasound to rule out abscess if the patient does not improve with 2–3 days of medical management.
  - 90% of sialoliths over 2 mm are detected with ultrasound; thin-slice CT without contrast is even more accurate.
  - 90% of submandibular sialoliths are radiopaque while 90% of parotid sialoliths are radiolucent (▶ Fig. 7.5).
  - CT with contrast or magnetic resonance imaging (MRI) is recommended if underlying neoplasm is suspected.
- Medical management:
  - Warm compresses, sialagogues, hydration, and antibiotics are the mainstays of treatment.[16,18]
  - Antibiotics should cover gram-positive and anaerobic bacteria. Anti-staphylococcal penicillin with β-lactamase is most commonly used.[16]

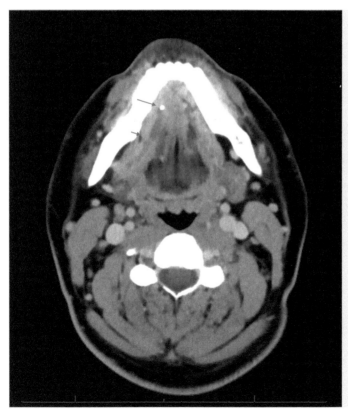

Fig. 7.5 Computed tomography (CT) demonstrating sialolith in submandibular gland. Radiopaque sialolith marked by *long arrow*. Proximal duct distention marked with *short arrow*.

- ○ Continue antibiotics for 7 days after symptom improvement.[16]
- ○ Consider culture of drainage from ducts if present, but contamination with oral flora is likely.[16]
- ○ Follow white blood count as well as inflammatory markers (c-reactive protein, erythrocyte sedimentation rate) to monitor response to treatment.
- ○ If recurrent episodes occur, investigate for underlying causes such as sialolithiasis or ductal stricture.
- Surgical intervention:
  - ○ Acute surgical intervention is indicated in cases where an abscess is present or in cases of an obstructing stone of the floor of mouth[16]—see Chapter 7.2.4. Neck Space Infections/Abscesses.
  - ○ Recurrent acute sialadenitis may require minimally invasive sialendoscopy for diagnostic and therapeutic purposes.

7.2.2 Pharyngitis (aka Tonsillitis)

- Epidemiology:
  - ○ Majority of pharyngitis has viral cause, including rhinovirus, adenovirus, coxsackievirus, Epstein–Barr virus (EBV), and many others.[19]
  - ○ Most common bacterial source of pharyngitis is Group A β-hemolytic *Streptococcus*, causing 15–30% of pharyngitis in children. Peak incidence is at 5–6 years of age.[20]
- Diagnosis[19,20]:
  - ○ Rhinorrhea, cough, sneezing, conjunctivitis, and oral ulcers strongly suggest viral cause and no further diagnostic testing is needed.
  - ○ Sudden onset, high fever, odynophagia, dysphagia, headache, enlarged tonsils with exudate, tonsillar/palatal petechiae, tender adenopathy are consistent with bacterial cause.
  - ○ If bacterial cause is suspected, streptococcal rapid antigen test and culture should be performed. Rapid antigen test is highly specific but less sensitive, culture is more sensitive but takes days.
  - ○ Also consider monospot testing for Epstein–Barr virus, as it may present very similarly to bacterial tonsillitis.
- Imaging:
  - ○ Does not play a role in diagnosis unless secondary abscess is suspected—see Chapter 7.2.4 Neck Space Infections/Abscesses.
- Medical management[20,21]:
  - ○ Viral pharyngitis, including mononucleosis, is treated with supportive care.
  - ○ Bacterial pharyngitis should be treated with antibiotics to prevent complications such as abscess formation, as well as complications of Streptococcal infection including rheumatic fever, acute poststreptococcal glomerulonephritis, scarlet fever, and pediatric autoimmune neuropsychiatric disorders associated with streptococcal infections (PANDAS).
  - ○ First-line treatment is a penicillin with/without β-lactamase inhibitor. In penicillin allergic patients, use first-generation cephalosporin or clindamycin.
- Surgical intervention:
  - ○ Only indicated acutely for secondary abscess—see Section 7.2.4 Neck Space Infections/Abscesses.
  - ○ Per current guidelines tonsillectomy is recommended for patients with recurrent pharyngitis, defined as sore throat accompanied by positive Streptococcal testing, fever over 38.5 °C, cervical lymphadenopathy, or tonsillar exudates, which occurs seven or more times in 1 year, five or more times per year for 2 years, or three or more times per year for 3 years.[22]
- Additional topics:
  - ○ Diphtheria[20,21]:
    - – Rare in the United States since immunization, but endemic in many developing countries.
    - – Symptoms are sore throat, thick grey-green plaques with friable exudate on tonsils.
    - – Treatment involves airway management, antibiotics (erythromycin and penicillin), diphtheria antitoxin.
  - ○ Periodic fever, aphthous stomatitis, pharyngitis, cervical adenitis (PFAPA)[20,21]:
    - – Most common cause of pediatric recurrent fever. Fevers last 3–5 days accompanied by aphthous stomatitis, cervical adenitis, or pharyngitis. May also have malaise, headache, abdominal pain, diarrhea.

– Symptoms recur every 3–8 weeks with asymptomatic period in between.
– Thought to have autoimmune cause, although has not been definitively established.
– Treat with nonsteroidal anti-inflammatory drugs.

7.2.3 Lymphadenitis

- Epidemiology[19]:
  - Most cases caused by viruses including EBV, cytomegalovirus (CMV), herpes simplex virus (HSV), adenovirus.
  - Group A *Streptococcus* and *Staphylococcus aureus* are most frequently implicated bacteria.
  - Atypical mycobacteria: *Mycobacterium avium* complex, *M. scrofulaceum, M. kansasii.*
  - Less frequently encountered organisms include *Bartonella henselae* (aka cat scratch disease), tuberculosis, syphilis, toxoplasmosis.
- Diagnosis[19,23]:
  - Low-grade fevers, preceding upper respiratory infection, conjunctivitis, pharyngitis, and time course around 2 weeks along with small, bilateral, and diffuse lymphadenopathy suggest viral cause.
  - Acute, unilateral, erythematous, solitary, larger (2–3 cm) tender lymphadenopathy is consistent with bacterial cause. Symptoms include fever, irritability, and malaise.
  - Sudden appearance of mass followed by slow enlargement over 2–3 weeks with overlying violaceous skin changes indicates likely atypical mycobacteria.
- Imaging[23]:
  - Ultrasound or CT is indicated for evaluation of suspected lymph node abscess.
- Medical management[19,23]:
  - Viral lymphadenitis is managed with supportive care and symptomatic treatment.
  - First-line treatment for bacterial lymphadenitis is ampicillin-sulbactam or amoxicillin-clavulanate, which give broad coverage of gram-positive, gram-negative, and anaerobic organisms. Clindamycin is used in penicillin allergic patients. However, incidence of *methicillin-resistant S. aureus* infection has increased in recent years, for which clindamycin or trimethoprim-sulfamethoxazole is appropriate.
  - Atypical mycobacterial lymphadenitis is treated with macrolide antibiotics.
- Surgical intervention[19,23]:
  - Bacterial lymphadenitis may devolve into suppurative node and abscess requiring incision and drainage.
  - Atypical mycobacterial frequently necessitates surgical excision especially with bulky disease; avoid incision and drainage which may lead to draining fistula.
- Additional topics:
  - Kawasaki disease[21,23]:
    - Acute vasculitis of unclear etiology occurring in children.
    - Diagnostic criteria include fever lasting 5 or more days plus four or more of the following: erythematous rash, conjunctival injection, oropharyngeal changes ("strawberry tongue," oropharyngeal erythema, erythema or cracking of lips), peripheral extremity changes (edema of hands and feet, erythema of soles and palms) and cervical lymphadenopathy.
    - Requires echocardiogram because of coronary involvement.
    - Treat with intravenous immunoglobulin (IVIG) and aspirin.

7.2.4 Neck Space Infections/Abscesses

- Epidemiology[24]:
  - Most common cause in adults: Dental infection; in children: oropharyngeal infection (i.e., "strep throat").
  - Other causes include sialadenitis, penetrating trauma, IV drug use, and underlying congenital or malignant lesion.[24]
  - Approximately 5% of deep neck infections in adults over age 40 years are associated with malignant lymph nodes.
  - Majority of odontogenic infections contain mixed flora including gram-negative anaerobes; most common pathogens include *Streptococci, Staphylococci, Bacteroides.*[24]

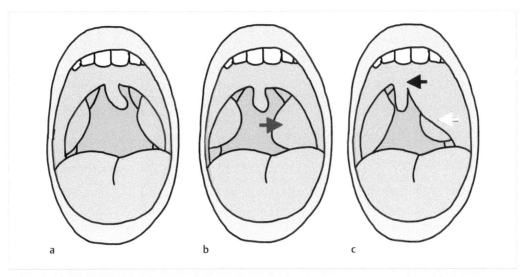

Fig. 7.6 Normal and abnormal pharyngeal exams. (a) Normal exam with tonsils visible between anterior and posterior pillars. Note uvula may lean slightly to one side or the other without being "deviated." **(b)** Bilateral tonsillar enlargement, left greater than right (*gray arrow*) which short term is consistent with acute pharyngitis/tonsillitis. **(c)** Deviation of uvula base toward the right (*black arrow*) and fullness of the left soft palate (*white arrow*) consistent with left-sided peritonsillar abscess.

- Diagnosis:
  - Peritonsillar space:
    - Boundaries: Palatine tonsil medially, superior pharyngeal constrictor laterally.
    - Symptoms: Odynophagia, trismus, deviation of uvular base away from affected side, unilateral soft palate fullness, drooling, hot-potato voice.[19]
    - This is a clinical diagnosis and does not usually require imaging (▶ Fig. 7.6).
  - Submandibular/Sublingual spaces:
    - Sublingual boundaries: Floor of mouth superiorly to mylohyoid inferiorly, mandible laterally and anteriorly, open to submandibular space posteriorly.
    - Submandibular boundaries: Mylohyoid superiorly to digastric inferiorly, open to sublingual and parapharyngeal space posteriorly.
    - Symptoms: Odynophagia, tenderness.[19]
  - Masticator space:
    - Boundaries: Superficial fascia of masseter laterally, deep fascia of pterygoids medially, contains ramus and posterior body of mandible.
    - Symptoms: Trismus.[19]
  - Parapharyngeal space:
    - Boundaries: Inverted pyramid bounded by pharynx medially, parotid laterally, prevertebral fascia posteriorly, and skull base superiorly with inferior tip at hyoid.
    - Symptoms: Trismus, muffled voice, intraoral bulge, dysphagia, drooling.[19]
  - Retropharyngeal space (▶ Fig. 7.7):
    - Boundaries: Pharyngeal constrictors anteriorly, alar fascia posteriorly, skull base superiorly, mediastinum inferiorly—this space has a midline raphe dividing it, and abscesses will be found on right or left.
    - Symptoms: Stiff neck, odynophagia, drooling, hot potato voice, spiking fevers, stridor.[19]
  - Danger space:
    - Boundaries: Alar fascia anteriorly, prevertebral fascia posteriorly, skull base superiorly, diaphragm inferiorly. No midline dividing raphe and abscess will be midline.
    - Symptoms: same as retropharyngeal space.[19]

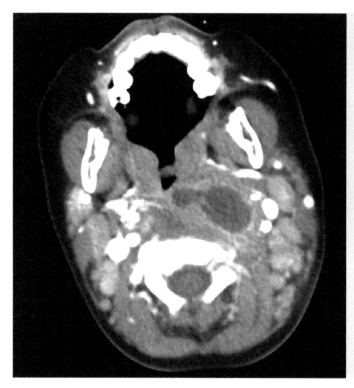

Fig. 7.7 Computed tomography (CT) demonstrating retropharyngeal abscess. Note fluid collection is lateralized to the left side.

- Prevertebral space:
  - Boundaries: Prevertebral fascia anteriorly, vertebral bodies posteriorly, skull base superiorly, coccyx inferiorly. No midline dividing raphe and abscess will be midline.
  - Symptoms: Same as retropharyngeal and danger spaces.[19]
- Imaging:
  - CT neck with IV contrast.
  - Ultrasound—less widely used because of difficulty differentiating spaces and identifying deeper fluid collections such as retropharyngeal.[24]
- Medical management:
  - For patient in respiratory distress, airway should be addressed immediately; see Chapter 7.1 Airway Management/Tracheostomy.
  - Empiric broad-spectrum antibiotic treatment.[24]
  - First-line treatment: Ampicillin-sulbactam 1.5–3.0 g IV every 6 hours OR clindamycin 600–900 mg IV every 8 hours (if penicillin is allergic).
  - Up to 60% of cases respond to antibiotic therapy alone.[24]
  - 48- to 72-hour trial of medical management is appropriate in stable patient with abscess less than 2.5 cm in single neck space;[24] children tend to be more responsive than adults.
  - Follow white blood count and inflammatory markers to monitor response to treatment.
- Surgical management[24]:
  - Tooth extraction if dental cause.
  - Needle aspiration, particularly in areas of high risk for nerve injury such as in the parotid.
  - In other areas, either transoral or external incision and drainage is appropriate.
- Additional topics:
  - Ludwig angina[19,24]:
    - Bilateral cellulitis of submental, sublingual, and submandibular spaces with infection spreading throughout all inframandibular areas.
    - Generally caused by mixed flora including streptococci.

- Symptoms include trismus, drooling, dysphagia, dyspnea, and tachypnea; examination shows firm edema and induration of floor of mouth and submandibular tissue.
- Leads to rapidly worsening airway compromise.
- Treat with early flexible fiberoptic intubation, possible tracheotomy, parenteral antibiotics, possible external incision.
  ○ Necrotizing fasciitis[24]:
- Mainly in immunocompromised patients, especially those with poorly controlled diabetes.
- Usually due to mixed aerobic and anaerobic bacteria including group A β-hemolytic streptococci, staphylococci, gram-negative rods including gram-negative anaerobes.
- Symptoms: Rapidly progressing pain, edema, erythema. Orange peel skin appearance and crepitus.
- Characteristic CT findings include tissue gas, widespread hypodense areas consistent with liquefaction necrosis.
- Requires prompt surgical management with aggressive serial debridement followed by prolonged parenteral antibiotics (first line is clindamycin 600–900 mg IV every 8 hours plus vancomycin 1 g IV every 12 hours).

7.2.5 Sinusitis

- See Chapter 7.4, Endoscopic Sinus Surgery.

7.2.6 Laryngotracheitis (aka "Croup")

- Epidemiology:
  ○ Most frequently caused by parainfluenza virus, but may be caused by a variety of other viruses.
  ○ Common in children ages 6 months to 3 years. Atypical under age 6 months, consider other diagnosis.[20]
- Diagnosis:
  ○ Symptoms: Usually begin with nasal discharge, congestion, and inflammation and progress over 12–48 hours to include low-grade fever, hoarseness, barking cough, and stridor.[20,21]
  ○ Severe upper airway obstruction is suggested by presence of biphasic stridor, retractions, decreased lower airway breath sounds, tachypnea, oxygen desaturations, or altered consciousness[20]—see Chapter 7.1, Airway Management/Tracheostomy.
  ○ Toxic appearance, high fever, duration of symptoms over 7 days, or lack of response to croup treatment should raise suspicion for other diagnosis particularly supraglottitis or bacterial tracheitis.[20,21]
- Imaging/laboratory studies[20]:
  ○ Diagnosis is generally clinical, not necessitating labs or radiographs; however, if patient is stable and diagnosis is in question, can consider plain films of the neck.[20]
  ○ Subglottic narrowing on anterior–posterior X-ray, called the "steeple sign," is consistent with croup (▶ Fig. 7.8).
  ○ Presence of indistinct opacities within the airway on lateral view suggests bacterial (exudative) tracheitis.
- Medical management:
  ○ Viral croup is generally self-limited and resolves in 3–7 days.[20,21]
  ○ IV dexamethasone 0.6 mg/kg, racemic epinephrine or L-epinephrine alone, humidified oxygen, consider heliox if airway narrowing.[20,21]
- Surgical management:
  ○ Intubation is rarely required for viral croup; however, patients with bacterial tracheitis often require bronchoscopy and intubation.[20]
- Additional topics:
  ○ Consider other more acutely dangerous airway diagnoses, particularly epiglottitis, airway foreign body, and thermal/caustic airway injury.[20]

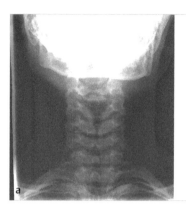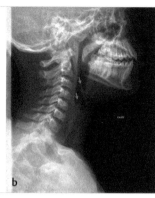

Fig. 7.8 Anteroposterior (AP) and lateral neck X-rays demonstrating croup. (a) AP view demonstrating characteristic narrowing in the subglottis or "steeple sign" (*long arrow*). (b) Lateral view again with narrowing. Note the epiglottis and arytenoids (*short arrows*) are crisp, ruling out supraglottitis/epiglottitis.

7.2.7 Epiglottitis/Supraglottitis

- Epidemiology:
  - Incidence among children declined dramatically after the addition of routine *Haemophilus influenzae type b* (Hib) vaccine in the United States.[25]
  - Epiglottitis is now diagnosed more frequently in adults than children.[25]
  - Alternate pathogens are commonly seen, most frequently *S. pneumoniae, S. pyogenes,* and *S. aureus.*[20]
- Diagnosis:
  - Airway management is the first priority for patients with signs of respiratory distress. Airway obstruction can advance very rapidly in this condition; therefore, it needs to be recognized and treatment initiated as soon as possible before emergent respiratory distress ensues—see Chapter 7.1, Airway Management/Tracheostomy.
  - Epiglottitis refers specifically to inflammation and edema of the epiglottis, however other supraglottic structures are often also involved including the aryepiglottic folds, vallecula, and arytenoids; therefore, the term supraglottitis is more accurate.[20]
- Risk factors:
  - In children: Lack of immunization for Hib and/or immunodeficiency syndromes.
  - In adults: Hypertension, diabetes mellitus, substance abuse, and immune deficiency.[25]
- Symptoms:
  - Children: Abrupt onset and rapid progression (within hours) of classic symptoms dysphagia, drooling, and respiratory distress; may have preceding upper respiratory infection. Generally have severe throat pain and muffled voice, less frequently cough and hoarseness.[20]
  - Adults: Sore throat or odynophagia, dysphagia, fever, muffled voice, inability to handle secretions (drooling, spitting out or suctioning secretions), less commonly stridor and respiratory distress; may have preceding upper respiratory infection.[25]
- Imaging/laboratory studies:
  - Plain lateral neck films can be helpful in diagnosis of the stable patient, enlarged epiglottis, known as "thumbprint sign," accompanied by thickening of the aryepiglottic folds is diagnostic.[20]
- Medical management:
  - Patients with epiglottitis should be started on empiric therapy with a third-generation cephalosporin.[20]
  - Blood cultures should be taken as soon as possible, and if airway intervention is needed, cultures should be taken of infected tissue. Cultures should then be used to direct therapy.
  - Patients usually require less than 72 hours of intubation, as edema resolves rapidly with treatment.[20] Consider the possibility of antibiotic resistance if patient is not improving appropriately with antibiotics.
  - Can transition to oral antibiotics after extubation, treat for 7–10 days total.[20]
  - Patients should be monitored in intensive care unit setting for assessment of response to therapy.

- Surgical management:
  - Patients with suspected supraglottitis requiring airway management with intubation should be taken to the operating room, where otolaryngologist can visualize the airway to make diagnosis then intubate with minimal attempts.[20]
  - Surgical airway may rarely be necessary if intubation fails, see Chapter 7.1 Airway Management/ Tracheostomy.

7.2.8 Otologic Infections

- Epidemiology:
  - Otitis externa affects 1 in 123 people in the United States annually; just less than half are children ages 5–14 years.[26]
  - Children average four episodes a year of otitis media with effusion, and 90% of children will have an effusion before school age.[27]
- Otitis externa:
  - Infection of ear canal skin, usually bacterial.[26,28]
  - Risk factors: Immune compromise, recent water exposure or trauma (including from cleaning).
  - Symptoms: Otalgia, tenderness with palpation of pinna or tragus, pruritis, purulent otorrhea, edema and erythema of canal, normal mobility of tympanic membrane on pneumatic otoscopy if it can be visualized.
- Acute otitis media:
  - Inflamed middle ear.
  - Risk factors: Age < 2 years.[28]
  - Symptoms: Otalgia, otorrhea, aural fullness, hearing loss, tinnitus, fever, tympanic membrane erythematous, bulging, opaque yellowish hue, reduced mobility on pneumatic otoscopy.[28,29]
- Serous otitis media/otitis media with effusion:
  - Persistent middle ear fluid without infection.[27,28]
  - Risk factors: Prolonged intubation or nasogastric tube, nasopharyngeal mass, recent upper respiratory infection.
  - Symptoms: Aural fullness, hearing loss, tinnitus, retracted/nonmobile tympanic membrane, translucent serous fluid, reduced mobility on pneumatic otoscopy.
- Imaging:
  - CT scan of temporal bone with contrast only if suspect complication/abscess—mastoid effusion means there is fluid in the middle ear, DOES NOT necessarily indicate acute mastoiditis.
- Medical management:
  - Otitis externa[26]:
    - Treat with topical antimicrobials.
    - If there is a possibility of tympanic membrane perforation, nonototoxic drops should be chosen.
    - Prior to administration, debris should be removed and wick placed if there is significant edema.
    - Systemic antibiotics are indicated only if there is spread of inflammation outside the ear canal or cartilage is involved.
  - Acute otitis media[29]:
    - Prescribe antibiotics for children over 6 months with severe symptoms (severe pain or fever over 102.2 °F), or patients 6–24 months with bilateral otitis media.
    - For patients over age 6 months with unilateral without severe symptoms or over 24 months with bilateral nonsevere symptoms, consider a 48- to 72-hour period of observation before antibiotics.
    - Amoxicillin is first line unless patient has received amoxicillin in the past 30 days, has purulent conjunctivitis, or has a history of recurrent otitis media resistant to amoxicillin, in which case amoxicillin with β-lactamase should be given.
    - Alternatives with penicillin allergy include cefdinir, cefuroxime, cefpodoxime, and ceftriaxone.
    - Consider change of antibiotic if no improvement in 72 hours.
  - Serous otitis media[27]:
    - Majority will resolve within 3 months without intervention.
    - Recommendation against decongestants, steroid, or antibiotic treatment.

- Hearing test if patient is at high risk for hearing loss, has known preexisting loss, or effusion lasts more than 3 months.
- Surgical management:
  - Not indicated in otitis externa.
  - Tympanostomy tubes may be indicated for recurrent acute otitis media or persistent serous otitis media.[27,29]
- Additional topics:
  - Temporal bone osteomyelitis (aka "malignant otitis externa")[28,30]:
    - Risk factors: Immune compromise (especially poorly controlled diabetes), radiation.
    - *Pseudomonas aeruginosa* causes the vast majority of cases.
    - Symptoms: Severe otalgia, otorrhea, granulation tissue in external auditory canal, cranial nerve deficits (VII, X, XI, facial nerve is most common).
    - Initial diagnosis with CT of the temporal bone showing bony erosion. For high clinical suspicion and negative CT, consider technetium-99 bone scan which is very sensitive for osteoblastic activity but stays positive even after treatment. Gallium-67 citrate and indium-111–labeled leukocyte scans are used to follow progression of disease.
    - Aggressive antibiotic treatment with pseudomonal coverage and treatment of any reversible immunocompromise, particularly blood glucose control in diabetics, are mainstays of treatment. Early disease may be treated with oral fluoroquinolone; more advanced disease requires initial IV antibiotics then transition to long-term oral fluoroquinolone, generally for a total of 6 weeks.
  - Acute mastoiditis[19]:
    - Symptoms: Edema causing proptosis of the pinna, tenderness over mastoid tip, fever, associated acute otitis media.
    - CT demonstrates opacification of mastoid, may also note breakdown of bony septae termed "coalescence," and/or ring enhancement of mastoid fluid collection.
    - Treatment includes parenteral antibiotics, possible tympanostomy tube placement.

7.3 Facial Trauma

Brent Geffen, Christopher Ian Newberry, and Eric W. Cerrati

7.3.1 Summary

- Facial trauma is a common component of emergency evaluation for injuries to the head, neck, and spine.
- The highest incidence of facial trauma is in young men, and is often due to aggravated assault, fall, and motor vehicle accidents (MVAs).
- There are a number of telltale signs on physical exam and imaging that may indicate need for specialist consult and/or operative intervention.

7.3.2 Epidemiology

- There are over 200,000 incidences of facial trauma in the United States each year.[31]
- Facial trauma is more frequent in males (M:F of 2:1); highest incidence in the 20- to 40-year-old range.
- Significantly associated with tobacco, alcohol, and drug use.
- Most common etiology: Aggravated assault (37%), fall (24.6%), MVA (12.1%).[32]
- Most common fracture sites: Nasal bones (58.6%), mandible (16.9%).[33]
- Up to 76% of facial fractures are associated with other injuries, including open wounds, orthopaedic fractures (spine, extremities, pelvic), organ lacerations, and intracranial injuries.[34]

7.3.3 Diagnosis

- History:
  - Establish time since injury, location, and mechanism of injury.
    - MVA: Details should include speed, seatbelt use, and airbag deployment.
    - Gunshot wound (GSW): Details should include caliber, distance from barrel, and rounds fired.

- High-yield head-and-neck review of systems:
  - Eyes: Diplopia, decreased acuity.
  - Ears: Otorrhea (possible cerebrospinal fluid [CSF] leak), vertigo, tinnitus, hearing loss.
  - Nose: Anosmia, rhinorrhea, epistaxis, nasal obstruction.
  - Mouth: Odynophagia, malocclusion, trismus, dysarthria.
  - Throat: Hoarseness, globus sensation, dyspnea.
- Examination:
  - Evaluation begins with the primary trauma survey in airway assessment:
    - Remove obstructive foreign bodies (e.g., teeth) and suction any blood clots or secretions visualized.
    - Bilateral maxillary or mandibular fractures may produce pharyngeal collapse; reduce fractures as necessary, and augment the airway with tongue pull or jaw thrust.
    - Due to the frequent coincidence of cervical spine injury, nasotracheal intubation can be considered to minimize neck extension, if there are no significant skull base fractures.
  - Facial trauma assessment continues in the secondary and tertiary trauma assessments.
    - Visually examine the face and palpate for any depressions, step-offs, or mobile segments as well as pain, which can signify underlying fractures.
    - For lacerations, the area should be thoroughly cleaned and the wounds examined.
    - All injured structures must be identified and repaired. All lacerations are closed in a multilayered fashion. For GSW, the entry and exit points are identified.
    - CNs: Pupillary response (afferent: CN II and efferent: CNIII) including the "swinging light test" (▶ Fig. 7.9). is used to detect a relative afferent pupil defect; extraocular muscle function (CN III, IV, VI); sensation of forehead (V1), maxilla (V2), and lower lip/chin as well as masseter and temporalis

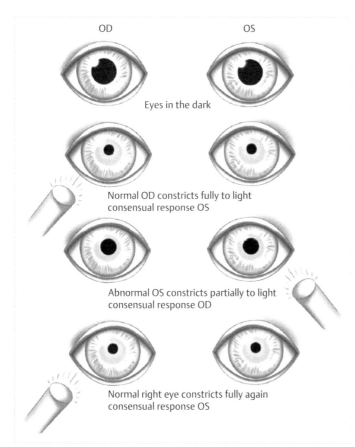

OD   OS

Eyes in the dark

Normal OD constricts fully to light
consensual response OS

Abnormal OS constricts partially to light
consensual response OD

Normal right eye constricts fully again
consensual response OS

Fig. 7.9 Swinging flashlight test for relative afferent pupillary defect. Light shone in one eye should lead to constriction, with equal constriction (consensual) in the contralateral eye. When swinging to the contralateral eye, lack of constriction or frank dilation of both eyes indicates decreased sensitivity to light. (Source: Pupils. In: Di Ieva A, Lee J, Cusimano M, eds. Handbook of Skull Base Surgery. 1st ed. Thieme; 2016.)

function with jaw clenching (V3); facial symmetry at rest and motion (VII). Symmetric palate elevation (X); midline tongue extension (XII).

- Otologic: Foreign body, tympanic membrane (TM) perforation, otorrhea, hemotympanum, "Battle's sign" (mastoid ecchymosis indicating skull base fracture), auricular hematoma. Tuning fork tests (Weber and Rinne) for sensorineural vs. conductive hearing loss.
- Ophthalmic: Ptosis, laceration, subconjunctival hemorrhage, chemosis, hyphema, or raccoon eyes (periorbital ecchymosis, indicating possible cribriform fracture). Globe position: hypoglobus (globe inferior), proptosis, enophthalmos (globe posterior), medial canthal ligament integrity via the bowstring test and its associated telecanthus (increased palpebral aperture width, or > 1/2 interpupillary distance). If the patient cannot follow commands, forced duction testing on anesthetized conjunctiva should be undertaken to rule out extraocular muscle entrapment.
- Rhinologic: Step-offs, crepitus, epistaxis, foreign body, septal hematoma, rhinorrhea.
- Oral: Hematomas, tongue position and swelling, loosened or missing teeth, trismus (interincisal opening < 4–5 mm), malocclusion, cross bite, anteriorly open bite (subcondylar fracture) or posteriorly open bite (symphyseal fracture), and lacerations.

7.3.4 Imaging

- Nasal bone fracture: Primarily a clinical diagnosis. No need for radiographs if solely to evaluate for nasal fracture; however, fractures can be visualized on plain X-rays.
- All other suspected facial fractures should be evaluated with CT maxillofacial without contrast usually with thin-slice (< 2 mm cuts) and possible 3D reconstruction to evaluate the horizontal and vertical buttresses of the midface.[35]

7.3.5 Upper Face Trauma

- Anatomy:
  ○ Above the eyebrows, the frontal bone forms the forehead and orbital roof. Within the forehead are pneumatized frontal sinuses that separate the frontal bone into an anterior and posterior wall (i.e., anterior table and posterior table of the cranium).
- Pathology:
  ○ The frontal sinuses absorb mechanical forces to protect the brain. Fractures here are often the result of high velocity trauma, such as with MVA, falls, and assaults.
  ○ Anterior table fractures are most common. Fractures involving the posterior table are significantly associated with intracranial injuries and CSF leak risk.[36,37]
  ○ Complications of frontal sinus fractures: cosmetic defect, meningitis, CSF leaks, and nasofrontal outflow tract (NFOT) obstruction leading to mucocele or sinusitis.
- Management of frontal sinus fractures:
  ○ Anterior table fractures: Observation for minimally displaced (< 2 mm) fractures or in more significant factures if no NFOT and minimal concern for cosmesis. If concern for cosmesis, endoscopic reduction and/or fixation or open reduction with internal fixation (ORIF) using metallic or bioabsorbable plates and/or meshes or solely endoscopically camouflage.
  ○ Posterior table fractures (▸ Fig. 7.10): Require neurosurgery consultation. Treatment depends on severity and complications, especially CSF leak. If only mild posterior wall facture (minimal displacement and comminution) and no CSF leak: observation. If CSF leak is present without catastrophic posterior table fracture, 1 week of observation is indicated, as 50–90% will resolve spontaneously.[38] If severe comminution, significant displacement, or persistent CSF leak, cranialization or obliteration is indicated.
  ○ NFOT injury: If gross obstruction on CT scan or suspected due to severe frontal fracture involves the ethmoids, medial sinus, or sinus floor, then sinus obliteration or endoscopic frontal sinus reconstruction.

7.3.6 Nasal Trauma

- Anatomy:
  ○ Upper bony pyramid comprised of paired nasal bones which articulate with the frontal bone superiorly, maxilla laterally, and upper lateral cartilages and septum caudally.[39] The nose is perfused

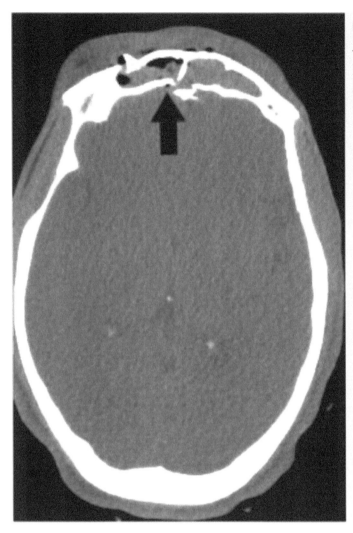

Fig. 7.10 Frontal sinus fracture involving the anterior and posterior table, with pneumocephalus (*arrow*). (Source: Frontal sinus osteoplastic flap. In: Kennedy D, Hwang P, eds. Rhinology: Diseases of the Nose, Sinuses, and Skull Base. 1st ed. Thieme; 2012.)

by a rich arterial plexus with contributions from the internal carotid (anterior and posterior ethmoid vessels) and external carotid (sphenopalatine, infraorbital, superior labial and angular arteries).

- Pathology:
  - Nasal bones are the most commonly fractured bones of the face.
  - Numerous fracture patterns exist; fractures can be characterized as unilateral (often depressed), bilateral, open-book (splayed), comminuted, or impacted.[40]
  - Close examination of the septum should be undertaken in order to rule out septal hematomas. Failure to recognize and treat a hematoma separating the vascular supply between the mucosa and underlying cartilage risks septal necrosis and collapse, and may lead to "saddle nose" deformity (▶ Fig. 7.11). Furthermore, patients with severely deviated noses almost always have a major septal deformity.[40]
  - Clinical examination within the first 1–2 hours is best to access for cosmetic deformity. The ensuing edema limits aesthetic examination, which should be repeated in 3–5 days.
- Management of acute nasal fractures:
  - Timing: Best repaired within the first 2 hours before edema develops, otherwise fractures should be repaired on days 7–10, once the edema has resolved.[40]

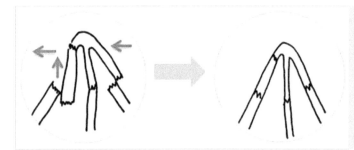

Fig. 7.11 Nasal fracture before and after closed reduction. Reduction required disimpaction with anterior elevation. (Source: Loyo M, Wang T. Management of the deviated nasal dorsum. Facial Plastic Surg 2015; 31(03): 216–227.)

- ○ Methods:
  - – Closed reduction techniques using the Boies elevator and external digital manipulation are sufficient in most cases to achieve favorable outcomes. Asch forceps may also be employed to realign an impacted or depressed segment of septum.[41]
  - – Open repairs using intranasal or external/open approaches are indicated for cases with significant comminution, severe septal deformity, involvement of the nasal orbital ethmoid (NOE) complex, or after failed closed reduction.

7.3.7 Midface Trauma

- Anatomy:
  - ○ The middle face includes the orbits, maxilla, and zygomatic bones.
  - ○ The maxilla contributes to the orbital floor, supports the maxillary teeth, and forms the medial cheek in articulation with the zygoma.
  - ○ The zygoma comprises the "cheek bone" and contributes the inferior and lateral orbital walls. Zygoma is anchored to the face via articulations with the frontal bone, maxillary bone, temporal bone, and lesser wing of the sphenoid.
- Pathology:
  - ○ Le Fort classification (▶ Fig. 7.12): identifies common fracture patterns, but must involve the nasal septum and pterygoid plates[42]:
    - – Le Fort I: Transverse maxillary fracture extending through the inferior nasal septum and including the pterygoid plates posteriorly disrupting the nasomaxillary and zygomaticomaxillary buttresses. Typically caused by an anterior force to lower midface. This separates the upper alveolus from the rest of the midface, and is seen on exam with upper alveolus mobility relative to the face when rocked back and forth.
    - – Le Fort II: Pyramidal fracture creating a nasomaxillary segment separates from the other upper craniofacial skeleton, and disrupts the nasomaxillary and zygomaticomaxillary buttresses more superiorly along with orbital floor and nasofrontal suture. Typically caused by anterior force at the level of the nose or a midline inferior impact with force directed superiorly into midface.
    - – Le Fort III: Craniofacial separation with complete midface disarticulation from skull base/upper face. Fracture crosses the zygomaticofrontal and nasofrontal sutures, zygoma, lateral and medial orbits, nasal bones and septum, and pterygoid plates. Typically requires a high-velocity impact.
  - ○ Zygomaticomaxillary complex (ZMC): There are no major forces acting on the zygomatic bone, but injuries dislocating the zygoma or separating it at multiple points may produce significant cosmetic deformities or globe malposition. ZMC fractures are also known as tripod (misnomer) or tetrapod fractures, as all four connections must be fractured to create displacement.
  - ○ NOE fractures (▶ Fig. 7.13 and ▶ Fig. 7.14): Fracture involving the area of confluence of the nose, orbit, ethmoids, frontal sinus, and anterior cranial fossa.[43] The area includes the insertion of the medial canthal tendon (MCT). Therefore, telecanthus as well as decreased nasal projection can be seen on physical exam.
    - – Type I: Single noncomminuted central fragment without MCT disruption.
    - – Type II: Comminution of the central fragment, but the MCT remains firmly attached to a definable segment of bone.
    - – Type III: Severe central fragment comminution with disruption of the MCT attachment.

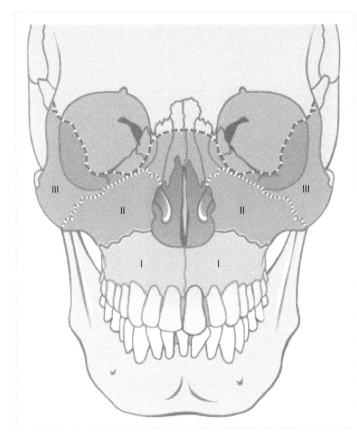

Fig. 7.12 Le Fort fracture patterns. Type I (*blue solid line*), Type II (*green dashed line*), and Type III (*red dashed line*). (Source: Classification of nasal and paranasal sinus trauma. In: Georgalas C, Fokkens W, eds. Rhinology and Skull Base Surgery: From the Lab to the Operating Room—An Evidence-Based Approach. 1st ed. Thieme; 2013.)

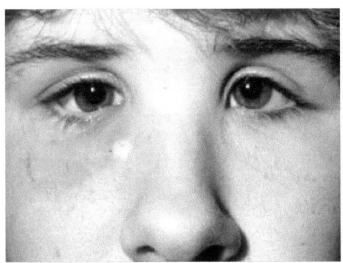

Fig. 7.13 Naso-orbito-ethmoid (NOE) fracture with posttraumatic telecanthus and dacrocystitis. (Source: Late repair of orbital fractures. In: Codner M, McCord C, eds. Eyelid & Periorbital Surgery. 2nd ed. Thieme; 2016.)

- Management of midface fractures:
  ○ Generally involve disimpaction, open reduction, and internal fixation. Approaches vary depending on site of injury, and often include sublabial, subciliary or transconjunctival, lateral brow, and coronal incisions.

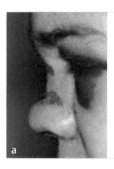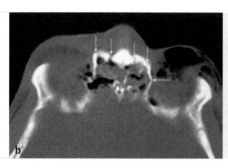

Fig. 7.14 (a, b) Depressed fracture of the naso-orbito-ethmoid (NOE) complex with "raccoon eye" indicating fracture involvement of the skull base. (Source: Diagnosing injuries of the midface. In: Ernst A, Herzog M, Seidl R, eds. Head and Neck Trauma: An Interdisciplinary Approach. 1st ed. Thieme; 2006.)

- Orbital wall fractures become a time-sensitive concern if displacement or intraorbital hematoma elevates intraorbital pressure or there is extraocular muscle entrapment. A surgical emergency is only present if the oculocardiac reflex is activated.
- NOE: Type I and II can often be repaired with rigid fixation of the central fragment(s) whereas Type III additionally requires tendon repair.
- Antibiotics: Not routinely administered without evidence of a dirty or contaminated wound, but perioperatively cefazolin or clindamycin are indicated before skin incision.

7.3.8 Mandibular Trauma

- Anatomy:
  - U-shaped bicortical bone that articulates with the glenoid fossa of the skull base at the temporomandibular joint (TMJ).
  - Contains 16 permanent teeth (six molars, four premolars, two canines, four incisors).
  - The anterior midline from canine to canine contains the symphysis and adjacent parasymphysis transitioning into the mandibular body until the third molar where it becomes the angle in its transition from the horizontal body to the vertical ramus. The vertical ramus divides giving a "Y" shape with an anterior coronoid process (temporalis muscle attachment) and a posterior condyle with its thin inferior neck and superior head that contributes to the TMJ.
  - Mandibular nerve (V3): The inferior alveolar nerve and blood vessels enter mandible at the ramus through the mandibular foramen then extends anteriorly curving superiorly before exiting the mental foramen below the second premolar as the mental nerve supplying the chin, lower lip, mucosa, and gingiva.
- Pathology:
  - Classified according to location (e.g., parasymphyseal) and type (▶ Fig. 7.15). Simple (closed) has intact covering whereas compound (open) communicates externally through mucosa, skin, or periodontal ligaments. Comminuted has multiple fragments while a greenstick is a monocortical fracture.
  - An anterior impact typically causes a symphyseal fracture with or without condylar involvement, whereas lateral impacts often result in body/angle fractures. The vast majority of fractures include two lacerations on opposite sides.
- Management of mandible fractures[44] (▶ Fig. 7.16):
  - Observation: appropriate for greenstick, nondisplaced condylar fractures, coronoid fractures, and seldomly for single nondisplaced, noncomminuted noncondylar fractures. Management includes soft, non-chew diet, and follow-up in 4–6 weeks to assess healing or persistent defect (nonunion).
  - Surgical intervention if displaced condylar fractures, malocclusion, minimally (and most nondisplaced) single noncondylar mandibular fractures, comminuted fractures, or multiple (unilateral or bilateral) mandibular fractures.
  - There are few definitive treatment paradigms for mandible fractures. Treatment choice involves patient factors (i.e., dentition, atrophy, aspiration risk, compliance), as well as clinician skill set and experience with various treatment modalities.
    - *Maxillomandibular fixation (MMF/IMF):* "Wiring" mandible to intact maxilla. Closed method of stabilizing nondisplaced fractures, minimally displaced reducible fractures, and most condylar

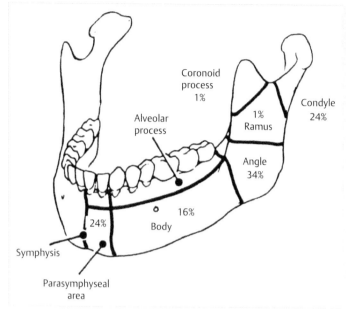

Fig. 7.15 Mandible anatomy and pattern of common fractures with relative frequency of incidence. (Source: Craniomaxillofacial trauma. In: Goldenberg D, Goldstein B, eds. Handbook of Otolaryngology: Head and Neck Surgery. 2nd ed. Thieme; 2017.)

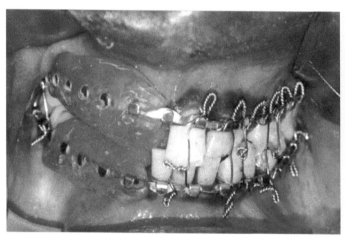

Fig. 7.16 Maxillomandibular fixation with arch bars and stainless-steel wiring. Acrylic resin is used to secure edentulous segments. (Source: Shanti R, Braidy H, Ziccardi V. Application of maxillomandibular fixation for management of traumatic macroglossia: a case report. Craniomaxillofac Trauma Reconstr 2015; 08(04): 352–355.)

fractures. Patients typically remain in MMF for 4–6 weeks on a liquid diet. They should always be in possession of wire cutters in case of choking emergencies. MMF may be contraindicated in patients with psychiatric disorders, seizure disorders, and alcoholics.

- Open reduction internal fixation (ORIF): Open method of reducing fractures using load-sharing or load-bearing plates across the fracture line. Indication for most multiple fractures, most edentulous atrophic fractures, severely comminuted or with missing segments, and certain condylar fractures such as condylar displacement into the middle fossa, inability to obtain reduction with closed treatments, significant displacement with need to reestablish vertical mandibular height, lateral extracapsular displacement, and foreign body within TMJ.

○ Antibiotics: Preoperative antibiotics are indicated as prophylaxis for open mandibular fractures. Perioperative antibiotics (cefazolin, ampicillin/sulbactam, clindamycin) are recommended for all fractures before surgery. Postoperative antibiotics are not routinely indicated, except in cases of anticipated poor wound healing (current tobacco use, diabetes, advanced age).

7.4 Endoscopic Sinus Surgery

Michael Yim and Jeremiah Alt

7.4.1 Epidemiology of Rhinosinusitis

- Number of adults with diagnosed sinusitis: 26.9 million.
- Percent of adults with diagnosed sinusitis: 11%.[45]
- Has been associated with air pollution, cigarette smoking, allergies, gastroesophageal reflux, aspirin sensitivity, immune system disorders.[46]
- Significant economic burden: Direct and indirect health-care costs exceeds US$22 billion annually. These include office visits, antibiotic prescriptions, lost work/school days, decreased productivity.
- More than one in five antibiotics prescribed in adults is for sinusitis.
- Severity of disease has been shown to have a significant impact on pain, depression, sleep, fatigue, and health-related quality of life.
- Patients with chronic rhinosinusitis (CRS) have worse health utility scores than congestive heart failure, coronary artery disease, and chronic obstructive pulmonary disease.[47]

7.4.2 Diagnosis

- Important to clarify acute vs. chronic sinusitis, viral vs. bacterial vs. fungal.
- Viral and bacterial sinusitis:
  - Acute viral rhinosinusitis:
    - Symptoms typically last less than 10 days and gradually improve over time.
  - Acute bacterial rhinosinusitis:
    - Symptoms for 10 to 30 days.
    - Symptoms are typically either persistent, or worsen after initial improvement (double worsening).
    - Must have nasal obstruction or nasal discharge and facial pain/pressure or loss of smell.
  - Recurrent acute rhinosinusitis (RARS):
    - Episodes as above, four or more per year, with symptom-free intervals between.
  - CRS:
    - Symptoms > 12 weeks duration.
    - Pathophysiology: Still many unknowns, but better thought of as a chronic *inflammatory* condition rather than a chronic *infectious* condition, although infection certainly plays a significant role.
    - Must have *subjective* symptoms, at least two of the following: nasal obstruction, nasal discharge, facial pain/pressure, or loss of smell.
    - Also must have *objective* findings, at least one of the following: sinus opacification on CT imaging, or purulence draining from the sinuses on nasal endoscopy.
    - Typically divided into two broad phenotypes:
    - CRS with nasal polyposis (CRSwNP): Th2-mediated, eosinophilic, aspirin exacerbated respiratory disease (AERD) falls into this category.
    - CRS without nasal polyposis (CRSsNP): Th1-mediated, neutrophilic.
- Fungal sinusitis:
  - Allergic fungal sinusitis (AFS):
    - Allergic response to fungal antigens, *NOT* a fungal infection.
    - Typically caused by aerosolized dematiaceous fungi: *Alternaria, Bipolaris, Culvularia.*
    - Characterized by thick allergic fungal mucin (peanut butter-like appearance and consistency) filling the paranasal sinuses.
  - Invasive fungal sinusitis:
    - Found in severely immunocompromised patients, uncontrolled diabetics, or hematologic malignancies.
    - Typically caused by *Aspergillus* or *Mucormycosis.*
    - Diagnosis is based on fungal hyphae present within vasculature on tissue biopsy.

– Once diagnosed, prompt surgical intervention is paramount.
– Survival is highly dependent on recovery of patient's immune system.
- Nasal endoscopy is typically utilized in conjunction with a thorough history and physical examination.
  ○ Lund-Kennedy score: edema, polyps, discharge, crusting, scarring.
    – 0–2 score given for each criterion: absent (0), mild-to-moderate (1), severe (2).
    – Total score ranges from 0 to 10.

7.4.3 Imaging

- CT face/orbit/sinus without contrast is most sensitive study in the work-up of sinusitis:
  ○ Best reviewed on coronal slices, bone window.
  ○ Lund-Mackay score: frontal, ethmoid, maxillary, sphenoid, ostiomeatal complex.
    – 0–2 score given for each sinus: normal (0), partial opacification (1), total opacification (2).
    – Ostiomeatal complex is graded only 0 or 2.
    – Total score ranges from 0 to 24.
  ○ Use the CLOSE method when reviewing scans.
  ○ C: cribriform plate:
    – Assess the depth of the cribriform plate into the sinonasal cavity and its relationship to the skull base.
    – Keros subtypes (measure the lateral lamella).
    – Shallow (1–3 mm), intermediate (4–7 mm), and deep (≥ 8 mm).
    – Most common location of iatrogenic CSF leaks is penetration of the lateral lamella.
  ○ L: lamina papyracea:
    – Assess for any dehiscence in the bilateral lamina papyracea.
    – Evaluate the relationship of the orbit to the ipsilateral maxillary sinus.
  ○ O: other cells:
    – Agger nasi cell: Anteriormost ethmoid cell and anterior boundary of the frontal recess.
    – Haller cell: Infraorbital ethmoid cell. If present can lead to ostiomeatal complex obstruction (and subsequently maxillary sinus obstruction).
    – Onodi cell: Posterior ethmoid cell that pneumatizes superolateral to the sphenoid sinus. If present can complicate approach and visualization of the opticocarotid recess.
  ○ S: skull base:
    – Best viewed on sagittal and coronal images.
    – Evaluate for dehiscence in the skull base as well as overall slope (up-sloping, down-sloping, flat).
  ○ E: ethmoid arteries:
    – Anterior ethmoid artery is best seen on coronal images; pointy protrusion visible along the medial bony orbit around the level of the beginning of the optic nerve; key to note location below skull base (bony mesentery).
    – Posterior ethmoid artery is typically located just anterior to the anterior face of the sphenoid sinus.
- Important to thoroughly review imaging prior to sinus surgery to avoid pitfalls and unwarranted complications.
- Magnetic resonance imaging (MRI) face/orbit/sinus is typically obtained when there is concern for sinonasal malignancy or skull base dehiscence. Not recommended for routine sinus surgery procedures.
  ○ T1-weighted precontrast bright: Fat, proteinaceous material, blood, metabolic depositions.
  ○ T1-weighted precontrast dark: Nasal mucosa, turbinates, fluid.
  ○ T2-weighted precontrast bright: Nasal mucosa, turbinates, fluid.
  ○ T1- and T2-weighted postcontrast: Everything is bright ("the nose knows," look at the nose to see if there is contrast or not).

7.4.4 Medical Management

- Acute viral rhinosinusitis:
  ○ Nasal saline rinses.
  ○ Topical nasal steroid sprays.
  ○ Supportive management (guaifenesin, nasal decongestants, etc.).

- Acute bacterial rhinosinusitis:
  - Nasal saline rinses.
  - Oral antibiotic therapy:
    - Amoxicillin or amoxicillin-clavulanate.
    - Third-generation cephalosporins (cefixime, cefpodoxime, etc.).
    - Doxycycline.
    - Clindamycin.
    - Fluoroquinolones should be reserved for patients who cannot tolerate any of the above.
    - Trimethoprim-sulfamethoxazole and macrolides (azithromycin and clarithromycin) are typically not recommended for empiric therapy due to high rates of *S. pneumoniae* resistance.[47]
- CRS without nasal polyposis (CRSsNP):
  - Nasal saline rinses.
  - Topical nasal steroid sprays.
  - Oral antibiotics:
    - Long-term low-dose macrolides have been shown to have anti-inflammatory benefit.
  - Oral steroids are an option.
- CRS with nasal polyposis (CRSwNP):
  - Nasal saline rinses.
  - Topical nasal steroid sprays.
  - Oral antibiotics are an option.
  - Oral steroids.
  - Antileukotrienes are an option.
- AFS:
  - Nasal saline rinses.
  - Oral steroids.
  - Antifungals are not indicated.
- Invasive fungal sinusitis:
  - Antifungals.

7.4.5 Surgical Management

- Surgery is indicated when medical therapy has failed for RARS or CRS.[48]
  - CRSwNP: Trial of nasal steroid sprays, nasal saline rinses, oral steroids. Antibiotics are optional.
  - CRSsNP: Trial of nasal steroid sprays, nasal saline rinses, and antibiotics. Oral steroids are optional.
- No strong evidence to dictate extent of surgery, but general tenets are to open sinuses with evidence of disease, and minimize manipulation of healthy sinuses to avoid unnecessary scarring and iatrogenic obstruction.
- Subcomponents of functional endoscopic sinus surgery (FESS):
  - Maxillary antrostomy:
    - Involves taking down the uncinate process, identifying the natural ostia, and widening it posteriorly as nasolacrimal duct can be injured inadvertently anteriorly. Important to identify natural ostia, otherwise can develop recirculation syndrome with mucous retention within the sinus.
  - Anterior ethmoidectomy:
    - Involves removing the ethmoid bulla and cells anterior to the basal lamella of the middle turbinate.
    - Anterior ethmoid artery is usually located in close proximity to the suprabullar ethmoid cell, posterior to the frontal recess.
  - Posterior ethmoidectomy:
    - Removal of all ethmoid cells between the basal lamella of the middle turbinate and the anterior face of the sphenoid sinus.
  - Sphenoidotomy:
    - Posterior septal artery arises from the sphenopalatine artery that courses across the inferior aspect of the anterior sphenoid face and can be injured when widening the natural sphenoid ostia inferolaterally. The nasoseptal flap is based off this artery.

- The optic nerve and carotid artery are adjacent to the superolateral sphenoid sinus and care must be taken to avoid inadvertent injury to these structures.
  - Frontal sinusotomy—Frontal recess boundaries:
    - Anterior: Agger nasi cell.
    - Medial: Middle turbinate attachment to the skull base.
    - Lateral: Lamina papyracea.
    - Posterior: Ethmoid bulla/bulla lamella.
  - Frontal sinusotomy—Draf classification:
    - Draf I: Anterior ethmoidectomy, no instrumentation of the frontal drainage tract.
    - Draf IIa: Removal of the agger nasi ("uncapping the egg"), opening between middle turbinate and lamina papyracea.
    - Draf IIb: Middle turbinate resection, opening between the nasal septum and the lamina papyracea.
    - Draf IIc: Extension of Draf IIb across midline without including the contralateral frontal recess.
    - Draf III: Otherwise known as a modified Lothrop procedure, removal of the entire frontal sinus floor including the superior nasal septum from orbit to orbit.
- Risks of surgery:
  - Overall rate of significant complications is ~1%.[49]
  - Postoperative hemorrhage:
    - Highest rate of all complications.[49]
    - Start with oxymetazoline and firm pressure for 20 minutes.
    - Nasal endoscopy, attempt to identify source.
    - Local control with cauterization.
    - Absorbable packing.
    - Consider cauterization in operating room for severe bleeding.
    - Close follow-up to ensure no scarring/synechiae.
  - Orbital injury:
    - Diplopia, blurry vision, vision loss.
    - Medial rectus is most commonly injured orbital muscle.
    - Nasolacrimal duct/epiphora: Majority do not become symptomatic.
    - Orbital penetration: Avoid injured area, avoid postoperative nasal packing.
    - Orbital hemorrhage: Ophthalmology consultation, elevate head of bed, steroids, topical vasoconstrictor eye drops, mannitol, acetazolamide, lateral canthotomy/cantholysis.
  - Injury to the skull base:
    - CSF rhinorrhea, pneumocephalus.
    - If identified intraoperatively then repair immediately.
    - If there is concern postoperatively, conduct nasal endoscopy, collect fluid for β-2 transferrin, diagnostic imaging studies. Lumbar drain is typically not indicated.
  - Loss of smell:
    - Preserve olfactory mucosa (olfactory cleft, superior turbinate, superior septum) as much as possible to avoid this.
- General postoperative management:
  - Start nasal saline rinses on postoperative day #1.
  - Sinus precautions for 2 weeks to minimize risk of postoperative hemorrhage: no nose blowing, no heavy lifting or strenuous activity, sneezing with mouth open, etc.
  - Antibiotics can be considered if evidence of active infection is discovered, otherwise typically not indicated.

7.5 Head and Neck Neoplasms

Hilary C. McCrary, Marcus M. Monroe, and Richard Cannon

7.5.1 Epidemiology

- Head and neck neoplasms covers a broad differential; determining malignant from benign masses is an important distinguishing factor.

- Head-and-neck cancers (HNCs) can arise from several anatomical subsites in the head and neck, with nearly 50,000 estimated new cases arising each year in the United States.[50]
- Collectively, HNC is the seventh most common type of cancer worldwide and the ninth most common cancer in the United States.[51]
- Major risk factors for HNC include the following: tobacco and alcohol use, exposure to human papilloma virus (HPV), male sex, elderly age, and betel quid use (a leaf chewed in various parts of the developing world).[51]
- There is an unequal sex distribution associated with HNC, with men accounting for 71.9% of all new HNCs.[50] This increased risk of HNC in men is likely related to increased tobacco and alcohol abuse.
- The median age for diagnosis of HPV-negative HNC is on average between the sixth and seventh decades of life. HPV-positive HNC affects younger individuals with a median age of diagnosis between 50 and 56 years.[51]
- Historically, there has been an increased incidence of HNC among African Americans; however, there has been a steady shift over the years where there is now a lower incidence of HNC among African Americans compared with Caucasian patients. The age-adjusted incidence of HNCs from 2011 to 2015 among African Americans is 8.98 per 100,000, compared with Caucasian patients with an age-adjusted incidence of 11.87 per 100,000.[52] This change is attributed to an increased incidence of HPV-positive HNCs.[53]
- Over the years there has been a steady increase in the incidence of oropharyngeal cancers, which has largely been attributed to the HPV. From 1998 to 2004 there was an estimated 225% increase in HPV-positive oropharyngeal cancers.[54]

7.5.2 Diagnosis

Surgical Head and Neck Anatomy

- Neck:
  - Divided into anterior and posterior neck, divided by the sternocleidomastoid muscle (SCM).
  - Anterior neck anatomy includes prevertebral musculature, the great vessels, anterior cervical musculature.
  - Posterior neck anatomy comprises the cervical vertebrae, cervical segment of the spinal cord, and the postvertebral musculature.
  - The carotid sheath which surrounds the internal jugular vein, common carotid artery, and the vagus nerve is formed by all three layers of the deep cervical fascia.
  - The left common carotid artery arises from the aortic arch, while the right arises from brachiocephalic trunk. The common carotid bifurcates into the external and internal carotid at the upper border of the thyroid cartilage.
  - The internal jugular vein originates from the jugular foramen, where it ultimately joins the subclavian vein to form the brachiocephalic vein. It lies lateral to the internal carotid artery, then common carotid artery.
  - The thyroid is comprised of the isthmus, lateral lobes, and inconsistently the pyramidal lobe, which overlies the trachea at the second to sixth tracheal rings. It has a rich blood supply including two arteries and three veins.
  - There are four parathyroid glands (a superior and inferior gland on both sides), with a close relationship with the thyroid.
  - Lymphatic drainage of the neck is composed of six levels, which spans the central, anterior, and posterior portions of the neck.
- Parotid gland:
  - Anterior to the ear, divided into a deep and superficial lobe with the facial nerve spanning between the two lobes.
- Nose and paranasal sinuses:
  - Nose is composed of boney and cartilaginous structures. Arterial supply via a branch of the angular artery.

- Lateral walls of the nose formed by nasal turbinates with drainage via the meatus, inferior to the corresponding turbinate. Arterial supply via the anterior and posterior ethmoid arteries and the sphenopalatine artery.
  - Paranasal sinuses include paired frontal, ethmoid, maxillary, and sphenoid sinuses.
- Maxilla and palate:
  - The maxilla is the bony portion of the upper jaw. Branches of V2 provide sensation over the maxilla.
  - Hard palate is composed of maxilla, horizontal process of the palatine bone, and ptyergoid plates.
  - Soft palate is a boundary between the nasopharynx and oropharynx, with the uvula appreciated at the posterior edge of the soft palate.
- Tongue and floor of mouth:
  - The tongue is formed by extrinsic and intrinsic muscles.
  - Blood supply is via the lingual artery.
  - Nerve supply includes the following: anterior two-third has sensation via the lingual branch of the cranial nerve (CN) V and taste via the chorda tympani (CN VII), posterior one-third has sensation and taste derived from CNs IX and X. The tongue muscles are largely supplied by CN XII.
  - The floor of mouth is formed by the mylohyoid muscles, which separate the oral cavity from the neck. The sublingual salivary gland and the deep aspect of the submandibular gland lie below the floor of mouth mucosa, with the Warthin duct on either side.
- Mandible:
  - Consists of the following subsites: Symphyseal/parasymphyseal, body, angle, ramus, coronoid process, condyle, and alveolar process.
  - Muscles associated with jaw movement include the masseter, temporalis, and two pterygoid muscles; innervated by V3.
- Pharynx:
  - From superior to inferior, the pharynx has three portions including the nasopharynx (above soft palate), oropharynx (behind the mouth and tongue), and laryngopharynx (from tip of epiglottis to distal end of pharynx).
  - The blood supply to the pharynx includes branches from the superior thyroid artery and ascending pharyngeal branches of the external carotid. CNs IX and X apply sensory and motor function.
- Larynx:
  - The structures that make up the larynx include the epiglottis, thyroid cartilage, cricoid, and the arytenoids.
  - The epiglottis lies behind the tongue base, connected laterally to the arytenoid by the aryepiglottic folds.
  - The thyroid cartilage forms a shield over the larynx, which joins with the cricoid via the cricothyroid joint.
  - Overlying these structural components of the larynx are the infrahyoid muscles.
  - The recurrent laryngeal nerve lies in the tracheoesophageal groove, which supplies all the intrinsic muscles of the larynx, except the cricothyroid muscles (innervated by superior laryngeal nerve).

7.5.3 Clinical History and Exam

- History[55]:
  - Important aspects of history for neoplasms of the head and neck include the following: location, size (including fluctuation), and duration.
  - Determine if patient has any hoarseness, voice changes, or dysphagia.
  - Rule out infectious symptoms, including fever, chills, sore throat, or cough.
  - Social history is of utmost importance; determine if patient has history of using alcohol, smoking, or chewing tobacco.
  - History of childhood radiation or family history of head and neck neoplasms should be determined.
- Oral cavity: Begin with evaluation of the lips and teeth, including mucosal surfaces. Examine tongue for mobility and symmetry. Examine the hard palate, soft palate, and uvula (▶ Fig. 7.17). Then assess the oropharynx, including the palatine tonsils. Using tongue depressors to lift the tongue, assess the floor

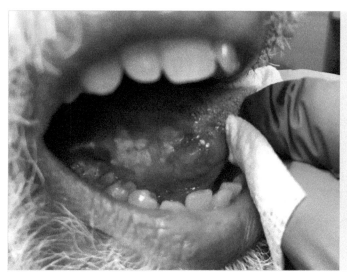

Fig. 7.17 Lesion of the lateral tongue concerning for malignancy; appropriate biopsy should be obtained.

of mouth, assess for ulcerations, mass, and growths. Complete bimanual palpation of the floor of mouth, tongue, and buccal mucosa.

- Face and nose: Examine for asymmetry and for facial nerve function through the following actions: wrinkling forehead, closing eyes, wrinkling nose, smiling, pursing lips, and tightening of the neck. Palpate the bony and cartilaginous structures of the nose. Assess the nasal ala and columella, composed of lower lateral cartilage. Use a speculum and otoscope to evaluate the turbinates, mucosa, and septum.
- Neck: Preferably performed behind the patient. Examine the posterior and anterior triangles on the neck, including the submental and submandibular spaces. Ensure palpation along the length of the SCM. Palpate along the mandible and behind the angle of the mandible to assess the tail of the parotid. Then palpate the remainder of the parotid gland anterior to the ear, along the cheek.
- Thyroid: In the midline neck, palpate superiorly to inferiorly the hyoid cartilage, thyroid cartilage (commonly larger in men than women), cricoid cartilage, and thyroid gland. The thyroid gland sits along the lateral aspects of the trachea, with the isthmus of the thyroid just inferior to the thyroid cartilage. Neck extension may bring the outline of the thyroid into view. Swallowing allows for improved palpation of the thyroid gland, because the gland moves with the airway as it elevates. Palpable thyroid nodules are typically at least 1.5 cm.
- Ear: Has three components (external, middle, and internal); examine the external ear: the concha, including the helix, antihelix, tragus, antitragus, concha bowl, and lobule. Assess for lesions or ulcerations. Then gently pull the helix posteriorly; using an otoscope examine the tympanic membrane, appreciate the handle of the malleus and light reflex. Pneumatic otoscopy can evaluate for movement of the tympanic membrane to determine if there is a possible effusion. Unilateral effusion can be suspicious for a possible neoplasm.
- Nasopharynx and larynx: Requires flexible or direct laryngoscopy for evaluation (▶ Fig. 7.18).

7.5.4 Imaging

- Several factors to consider when selecting an imaging modality, including the histology of the mass, stage of disease, and anticipated treatment.[56,57,58]
- Ultrasound (US), CT, MRI, and positron emission tomography (PET)/CT are the primary imaging modalities used for head and neck neoplasms (▶ Table 7.1).
- Swallowing can cause artifact on head and neck imaging, limiting full evaluation of soft tissue.
- Combinations of imaging are frequently obtained when evaluating head and neck neoplasms.
- Obtain appropriate studies to evaluate renal function before obtaining contrast-enhanced imaging.

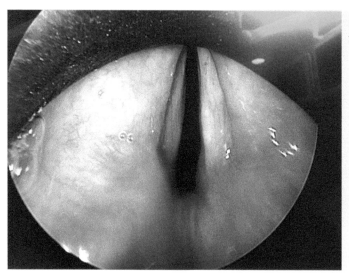

Fig. 7.18 View of the false and true vocal folds under direct laryngoscopy.

Table 7.1 Imaging of head and neck neoplasms

Imaging	Advantages and uses	Disadvantages
Ultrasound	• Effective for evaluating lymph nodes, salivary gland disease, and thyroid nodules • Able to assess vascularity of lesions and lymph nodes • Commonly used for image-guided biopsy, via fine-needle aspiration • Often the first imaging modality of choice for children	• Limited use in anatomically complex areas
CT	• Mainstay imaging to evaluate most head and neck cancers • Increased patient tolerance • Preferable for evaluated necrotic lymph nodes (when > 3 cm in size) and bony architecture • CT-guided biopsy utilized for lesions with poor accessibility • Mainstay imaging to evaluate the larynx and hypopharynx • Chest CT is typically obtained to evaluate for distant metastasis	• Radiation exposure and exposure to iodinated contrast agents
MRI	• Improved soft tissue contrast resolution, ability to evaluate extent of tumor, particularly perineural spread, via T1- and T2- weighted imaging • Preferable for nasopharyngeal and skull base tumors	• Timely • Poor patient tolerance • Exposure to gadolinium contrast • Metallic implant noncompliance
PET/CT	• Improved evaluation of cervical, supraclavicular, and mediastinal lymph node involvement • Allows for accurate evaluation of treatment response • Includes metabolic activity, which can allow distinct between benign and malignant pathologies	• Radiation exposure and exposure to iodinated contrast agents • Need to wait up to 3 mo after treatment to assess for response to treatment, due to possible inflammatory changes that will lead to false-positive results

Abbreviations: CT, computed tomography; MRI, magnetic resonance imaging; PET, positron emission tomography.

7.5.5 Differential Diagnosis

- Squamous cell carcinoma (SCC) is the most common malignancy of the head and neck (▶ Fig. 7.19).[59]
- Infectious masses can occur virtually anywhere in the head and neck, should be correlated clinically.
- Differential diagnosis is commonly broken up into benign and malignant disease processes (▶ Table 7.2).
- Mesenchymal, neuroectodermal sarcomas, vascular tumors, and secondary tumors can be found essentially anywhere in the head and neck.

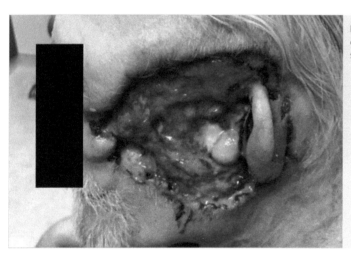

Fig. 7.19 Invasive squamous cell carcinoma invading through the skin and soft tissues.

Table 7.2 Differential diagnosis for benign and malignant tumors

	Non-neoplastic	Benign neoplastic	Malignant
Oral cavity	Nonodontogenic cysts	Chondromyxoid tumor	Leukoplakia
	Odontogenic cysts	Peripheral nerve sheath tumors	Erythroplakia
	Hamartomas	Odontogenic tumors (i.e., ameloblastoma, keratocyst)	Actinic cheilitis
	Ranulas		SCC
	Necrotizing sialometaplasia	Ductal papillomas	Minor salivary gland tumor
	Salivary duct cyst		Adenocarcinoma of salivary gland
	Mucous retention cyst		Mucosal melanoma
	Mucous extravasation phenomenon		Neuroendocrine carcinoma
			Lymphoma
			Malignant odontogenic tumors
Pharynx	Nasopharyngeal cysts	Squamous papilloma	SCC
	Hamartomas	Angiofibroma	HPV or EBV related SCC
	Dermoid	Craniopharyngioma	Neuroendocrine carcinoma
	Lymphangiomatous polyp	Paraganglioma	Minor salivary gland tumor
	Salivary gland anlage tumor		Nasopharyngeal papillary adenocarcinoma
			Lymphoma
			Mucosal melanoma
			Cordoma
			Malignant peripheral nerve sheath tumor
Face/Neck	Brachial cleft anomalies	Fibromatosis	Lymphoma
	Thyroglossal duct cyst	Nodular fasciitis	Metastatic cervical carcinoma from

Table 7.2 (*Continued*) Differential diagnosis for benign and malignant tumors

	Non-neoplastic	Benign neoplastic	Malignant
	Thymic cyst	Paraganglioma	head and neck, including SCC and adenocarcinoma
	Bronchogenic cyst	Pleomorphic adenoma	
	Dermoid cyst	Warthin tumor	Thyroid cancer
	Mesenchymal lesion	Myoepithelioma	Malignant paraganglioma
	Parathyroid cyst	Oncocytoma	Mucoepidermoid carcinoma
	Lingual thyroid	Sclerosing polycystic adenosis	Acinic cell adenocarcinoma
		Cystadenoma	Adenoid cystic carcinoma
		Sebaceous adenoma/lymphadenoma	Polymorphous low-grade adenocarcinoma
		Nodular goiter	Carcinoma ex pleomorphic adenoma
		Amyloid goiter	Epithelial-myoepithelial carcinoma
		Teratoma	Cystadenocarcinoma
		Parathyroid hyperplasia	Myoepithelial carcinoma
		Parathyroid cyst	Salivary duct carcinoma
		Parathyroid adenoma	Intraductal carcinoma
			Lymphoepithelial carcinoma
			Neuroendocrine carcinomas
			Oncocytic carcinoma
			Cribriform adenocarcinoma of the minor salivary glands
			Sebaceous carcinoma
			Sialoblastoma
			Parathyroid carcinoma
Larynx	Vocal cord nodules/polyp	Papilloma	Premalignant epithelial lesions
	Laryngocele	Granular cell tumor	SCC (several variants exist)
	Laryngeal cysts	Nodular fasciitis	Verrucous carcinoma
	Contact ulcer	Myofibroblastic tumors	Adenosquamous carcinoma
	Subglottic stenosis	Fibrous histiocytoma	Lymphoepithelial-like carcinoma
		Paraganglioma	Giant cell carcinoma
			Minor salivary gland tumors
			Neuroendocrine carcinomas
			Hematolymphoid
Ear	Keloid	Keratoacanthoma	Basal cell carcinoma
	Epidermal and sebaceous cysts	Ceruminal gland neoplasms	SCC (several variants)
	Chondromalacia	Seborrheic keratosis	Verrucous carcinoma
	Chondrodermatitis nodularis helicis chonicus	Squamous papilloma	Ceruminal gland adenocarcinomas
	Exostosis	Melanocytic nevi	Malignant melanoma
	Synovial chrondromatosis	Dermal adnexal neoplasm	Merkel cell carcinoma
	Autoimmune conditions	Pilomatrixoma	Atypical fibroxanthoma
	Otic or aural polyp	Neurilemmoma/Neurofibroma	Middle ear adenocarcinoma
	Cholesteatoma	Osteoma/Chondroma	Endolymphatic sac papillary tumor
	Langerhans cell histiocystosis	Middle ear adenoma or papilloma	Kaposi sarcoma
	Heterotopias	Acoustic neuroma	Lymphoproliferative
		Meningioma	
		Paraganglioma	

Abbreviations: EBV, Epstein–Barr virus; HPV, human papilloma virus; SCC, squamous cell carcinoma.

7.5.6 Surgical Management

- Surgical excision remains the mainstay of treatment in HNC, with selective or therapeutic neck dissection commonly being performed simultaneously for lymph node groups at highest risk of metastasis.[60,61,62,63,64]
- Due to defects formed by HNC surgery, microvascular free tissue transfer is commonly used for reconstruction. Free flaps can be considered fasciocutaneous, musculocutaneous, or osteocutaneous, used depending on the reconstructive needs. Free flap donor sites include the radial forearm, lateral arm, anterolateral thigh, fibula, scapula, latissimus dorsi, rectus abdominis, or even visceral donor sites like the jejunum (▶ Fig. 7.20 and ▶ Fig. 7.21).
- Each free flap consists of a neurovascular pedicle, with the vein and artery undergoing end-to-end anastomosis with vessels at the reconstructive site.
- Transoral endoscopic head and neck surgery is an evolving field that is used primarily in oropharyngeal cancers, consists of transoral laser microsurgery (TLM) or transoral robotic surgery (TORS).
- TORS frequently used in HPV-positive oropharyngeal cancer, which is associated with decreased treatment morbidity without sacrificing survival outcomes.
- Larynx preservation is increasingly used for laryngeal cancer, which offers chemoradiation as an alternative to open surgery or total laryngectomy to maintain optimal voice outcomes.
- Thyroid cancer is moving toward less invasive approaches with more patients being offered thyroid lobectomy, particularly when there is no evidence of lymph node metastasis, or when the size is < 4 cm. Lobectomy typically avoid thyroid hormone replacement therapy.

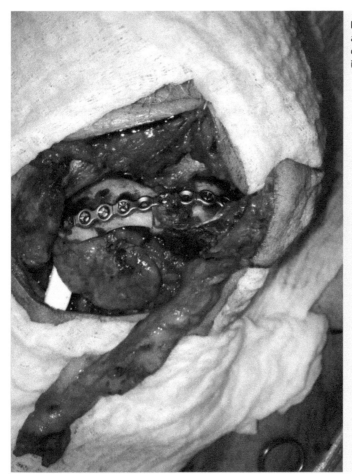

Fig. 7.20 Radial forearm with bone and soft tissues placed into the mandible for squamous cell carcinoma invading the mandible.

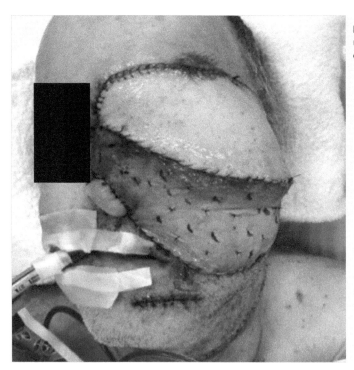

Fig. 7.21 A two-paddle scapula flap used to reconstruct a large facial defect.

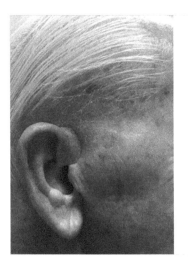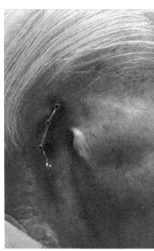

Fig. 7.22 Patient with a history of invasive squamous cell carcinoma of the ear, now with a prosthetic ear.

- Thyroid lesions < 1 cm are typically not biopsied and do not need treatment.
- Adjuvant radiation is commonly used in HNC, particularly for advanced stage disease, positive lymph nodes at multiple levels of the neck, or if there is extracapsular extension of disease, perineural or lymphatic invasion.
- Common complications after HNC surgery include the following: infection, bleeding, fistulas, chyle leak, edema, apnea, jugular vein thrombosis.
- Emergent complications can include hematoma with airway compression, carotid or jugular blowout, which warrants urgent surgical exploration.
- Prosthetic devices are evolving and are frequently used when cancer resection drastically alters normal facial structures (▶ Fig. 7.22).

7.5.7 Medical Management

- For HNC, chemotherapy used in the following capacities: Induction chemotherapy, concomitant with radiation therapy, or as adjuvant therapy following surgery.[65,66,67]
- Chemotherapy is commonly used in patients found to have lymph nodes with extracapsular spread of disease or positive surgical margins.
- High-dose cisplatin is the most common chemotherapy agent used, and benefit does not vary by tumor site.
- Use of immunotherapy agents has been increasing in HNC, with nivolumab and pembrolizumab (both anti-PD-1 antibody drugs) being used in recurrent and metastatic HNC; there are ongoing trial evaluating the effectiveness in combination with surgery and radiation as upfront therapy.

References

[1] Bhatti NI. Surgical management of the difficult airway. In: Flint PW, Haughey BH, Lund V, eds. Cumming's Otolaryngology. Philadelphia, PA: Elsevier/Saunders; 2015:86–94

[2] Cormack RS, Lehane J. Difficult tracheal intubation in obstetrics. Anaesthesia. 1984; 39(11):1105–1111

[3] Brown CA, III, Bair AE, Pallin DJ, Walls RM, NEAR III Investigators. Techniques, success, and adverse events of emergency department adult intubations. Ann Emerg Med. 2015; 65(4):363–370.e1

[4] Burkle CM, Walsh MT, Harrison BA, Curry TB, Rose SH. Airway management after failure to intubate by direct laryngoscopy: outcomes in a large teaching hospital. Can J Anaesth. 2005; 52(6):634–640

[5] HCUP Databases. Healthcare Cost and Utilization Project (HCUP). 2006–2014. Rockville, MD: Agency for Healthcare Research and Quality

[6] Brown CA III, Walls RM. The decision to intubate. The Walls Manual of Emergency Airway Management. Philadelphia, PA: Lippincott Williams & Wilkins; 2018: 3

[7] Samsoon GL, Young JR. Difficult tracheal intubation: a retrospective study. Anaesthesia. 1987; 42(5):487–490

[8] Tokarczyk AJ, Katz J, Vender JS. Oxygen delivery systems, inhalation, and respiratory therapy. In: Hagberg CA, Artime CA, Aziz MF, eds. Hagberg and Benumof's Airway Management. Philadelphia, PA: Elsevier; 2018:288–308

[9] Jaber S, Chanques G, Jung B. Postoperative noninvasive ventilation. Anesthesiology. 2010; 112(2):453–461

[10] Lindsay HA, Cook TM, Russo SG, et al. Supraglottic airway techniques: laryngeal mask airways. In: Hagberg CA, Artime CA, Aziz MF, eds. Hagberg and Benumof's Airway Management. Philadelphia, PA: Elsevier; 2018:328–348

[11] Vaida S, Gaitini L, Frass M. Supraglottic airway techniques: nonlaryngeal mask airways. In: Hagberg CA, Artime CA, Aziz MF, eds. Hagberg and Benumof's Airway Management. Philadelphia, PA: Elsevier; 2018:349–370

[12] Mark LK, Hillel AT, Herzer KR, et al. General considerations of anesthesia and management of the difficult airway. In: Flint PW, Haughey BH, Lund V, eds. Cumming's Otolaryngology. Philadelphia, PA: Elsevier/Saunders; 2015:64–85

[13] Ford HR, Gardner MJ, Lynch JM. Laryngotracheal disruption from blunt pediatric neck injuries: impact of early recognition and intervention on outcome. J Pediatr Surg. 1995; 30(2):331–334, discussion 334–335

[14] Kendall JL, Anglin D, Demetriades D. Penetrating neck trauma. Emerg Med Clin North Am. 1998; 16(1):85–105

[15] Kraft SM, Schindler JS. Tracheotomy. In: Flint PW, Haughey BH, Lund V, eds. Cumming's Otolaryngology. Philadelphia, PA: Elsevier/Saunders; 2015:95–103

[16] Jackson NM, Mitchell JL, Walvekar RR. Inflammatory disorders of the salivary glands. In: Cummings CW, Flint PW, Haughey BH, et al., eds. Cummings Otolaryngology: Head & Neck Surgery, 6th ed. Philadelphia: Elsevier; 2014:1223–1237

[17] Laskawi R, Schaffranietz F, Arglebe C, Ellies M. Inflammatory diseases of the salivary glands in infants and adolescents. Int J Pediatr Otorhinolaryngol. 2006; 70(1):129–136

[18] Cornetta AJ, Sataloff RT, Pasha R. Salivary glands. In: Pasha R, Golub JS, eds. Otolaryngology Head and Neck Surgery. 5th ed. San Diego, CA: Plural Publishing; 2014

[19] Stachler RJ, Shibuya TY, Golub JS, Pasha R. General otolaryngology. In: Pasha R, Golub JS, eds. Otolaryngology Head and Neck Surgery. 5th ed. San Diego, CA: Plural Publishing; 2014

[20] Meyer A. Pediatric infectious disease. In: Cummings CW, Flint PW, Haughey BH, et al., eds. Cummings Otolaryngology: Head & Neck Surgery. 6th ed. Philadelphia: Elsevier; 2014:3045–3054

[21] Cote V, Dimachkieh A, Prager JD, et al. Pediatric otolaryngology. In: Pasha R, Golub JS, eds. Otolaryngology Head and Neck Surgery. 5th ed. San Diego, CA: Plural Publishing; 2014

[22] Baugh RF, Archer SM, Mitchell RB, et al. American Academy of Otolaryngology-Head and Neck Surgery Foundation. Clinical practice guideline: tonsillectomy in children. Otolaryngol Head Neck Surg. 2011; 144(1) Suppl:S1–S30

[23] Alper CM, Robison JG. Head and neck masses in children. In: Johnson J, ed. Bailey's Head and Neck Surgery: Otolaryngology. 5th ed., Vol. 1. Philadelphia: Lippincott Williams & Wilkins; 2013:1591–1604

[24] Christian JM, Goddard AC, Gillespie MB. Deep neck and odontogenic infections. In: Cummings CW, Flint PW, Haughey BH, et al., eds. Cummings Otolaryngology: Head & Neck Surgery. 6th ed. Philadelphia: Elsevier; 2014:164–175

[25] Guardiani E, Bliss M, Harley E. Supraglottitis in the era following widespread immunization against Haemophilus influenzae type B: evolving principles in diagnosis and management. Laryngoscope. 2010; 120(11):2183–2188

[26] Rosenfeld RM, Schwartz SR, Cannon CR, et al. Clinical practice guideline: acute otitis externa. Otolaryngol Head Neck Surg. 2014; 150 (1) Suppl:S1–S24

[27] Rosenfeld RM, Shin JJ, Schwartz SR, et al. Clinical practice guideline: otitis media with effusion executive summary (update). Otolaryngol Head Neck Surg. 2016; 154(2):201–214

[28] McRackan TR, Hatch JL, Carlson ML, et al. Otology and neurotology. In: Pasha R, Golub JS, eds. Otolaryngology Head and Neck Surgery. 5th ed. San Diego, CA: Plural Publishing; 2014

[29] Lieberthal AS, Carroll AE, Chonmaitree T, et al. The diagnosis and management of acute otitis media. Pediatrics. 2013; 131(3): e964–e999

[30] Brant JA, Ruckenstein MJ. Infections of the external ear. In: Cummings CW, Flint PW, Haughey BH, et al., eds. Cummings Otolaryngology: Head & Neck Surgery. 6th ed. Philadelphia: Elsevier; 2014:2115–2122

[31] Stewart RM, Chang MC. 2016

[32] VandeGriend ZP, Hashemi A, Shkoukani M. Changing trends in adult facial trauma epidemiology. J Craniofac Surg. 2015; 26(1): 108–112

[33] Allareddy V, Allareddy V, Nalliah RP. Epidemiology of facial fracture injuries. J Oral Maxillofac Surg. 2011; 69(10):2613–2618

[34] Alvi A, Doherty T, Lewen G. Facial fractures and concomitant injuries in trauma patients. Laryngoscope. 2003; 113(1):102–106

[35] Wikner J, Riecke B, Gröbe A, Heiland M, Hanken H. Imaging of the midfacial and orbital trauma. Facial Plast Surg. 2014; 30(5): 528–536

[36] Chouake RJ, Miles BA. Current opinion in otolaryngology and head and neck surgery: frontal sinus fractures. Curr Opin Otolaryngol Head Neck Surg. 2017; 25(4):326–331

[37] Joshi UM, Ramdurg S, Saikar S, Patil S, Shah K. Brain injuries and facial fractures: a prospective study of incidence of head injury associated with maxillofacial trauma. J Maxillofac Oral Surg. 2018; 17(4):531–537

[38] Echo A, Troy JS, Hollier LH, Jr. Frontal sinus fractures. Semin Plast Surg. 2010; 24(4):375–382

[39] Chegar BE, Tatum SA. Nasal fractures. In: Cummings Otolaryngology, Vol. 1. 6th ed. Saunders; 2015:493–505

[40] Newberry CI, Mobley S. Correction of the crooked nose. Facial Plast Surg. 2018; 34(5):488–496

[41] Basheeth N, Donnelly M, David S, Munish S. Acute nasal fracture management: a prospective study and literature review. Laryngoscope. 2015; 125(12):2677–2684

[42] Hopper RA, Salemy S, Sze RW. Diagnosis of midface fractures with CT: what the surgeon needs to know. Radiographics. 2006; 26(3): 783–793

[43] Nguyen M, Koshy JC, Hollier LH, Jr. Pearls of nasoorbitoethmoid trauma management. Semin Plast Surg. 2010; 24(4):383–388

[44] Koshy JC, Feldman EM, Chike-Obi CJ, Bullocks JM. Pearls of mandibular trauma management. Semin Plast Surg. 2010; 24(4):357–374

[45] National Center for Health Statistics. Chronic sinusitis. Available at: https://www.cdc.gov/nchs/fastats/sinuses.htm. Accessed November 11, 2018

[46] Hamilos DL. Chronic rhinosinusitis: epidemiology and medical management. J Allergy Clin Immunol. 2011; 128(4):693–707, quiz 708–709

[47] Rosenfeld RM, Piccirillo JF, Chandrasekhar SS, et al. Clinical practice guideline (update): adult sinusitis. Otolaryngol Head Neck Surg. 2015; 152(2) Suppl:S1–S39

[48] Orlandi RR, Kingdom TT, Hwang PH, et al. International consensus statement on allergy and rhinology: rhinosinusitis. Int Forum Allergy Rhinol. 2016; 6 Suppl 1:S22–S209

[49] Ramakrishnan VR, Kingdom TT, Nayak JV, Hwang PH, Orlandi RR. Nationwide incidence of major complications in endoscopic sinus surgery. Int Forum Allergy Rhinol. 2012; 2(1):34–39

[50] Siegel RL, Miller KD, Jemal A. Cancer Statistics, 2017. CA Cancer J Clin. 2017; 67(1):7–30

[51] Rettig EM, D'Souza G. Epidemiology of head and neck cancer. Surg Oncol Clin N Am. 2015; 24(3):379–396

[52] National Cancer Institute. Surveillance E, and End Results Program. SEER Cancer Statistics Review 1975–2015. Available at: https://seer.cancer.gov/csr/1975_2015/browse_csr.php?sectionSEL=20&pageSEL=sect_20_table.22. Accessed November 13, 2018

[53] Settle K, Posner MR, Schumaker LM, et al. Racial survival disparity in head and neck cancer results from low prevalence of human papillomavirus infection in black oropharyngeal cancer patients. Cancer Prev Res (Phila). 2009; 2(9):776–781

[54] Chaturvedi AK, Engels EA, Pfeiffer RM, et al. Human papillomavirus and rising oropharyngeal cancer incidence in the United States. J Clin Oncol. 2011; 29(32):4294–4301

[55] Surgery AAoO-HaN. ENT Exam Video Series. Available at: https://www.entnet.org/content/ent-exam. Accessed November 18, 2018

[56] Abraham J. Imaging for head and neck cancer. Surg Oncol Clin N Am. 2015; 24(3):455–471

[57] Alberico RA, Husain SH, Sirotkin I. Imaging in head and neck oncology. Surg Oncol Clin N Am. 2004; 13(1):13–35

[58] Stern JS, Ginat DT, Nicholas JL, Ryan ME. Imaging of pediatric head and neck masses. Otolaryngol Clin North Am. 2015; 48(1):225–246

[59] Wenig B. Atlas of Head and Neck Pathology. Philadelphia, PA: Elsevier; 2016

[60] Holsinger FC, Ferris RL. Transoral endoscopic head and neck surgery and its role within the multidisciplinary treatment paradigm of oropharynx cancer: robotics, lasers, and clinical trials. J Clin Oncol. 2015; 33(29):3285–3292

[61] Mydlarz WK, Chan JY, Richmon JD. The role of surgery for HPV-associated head and neck cancer. Oral Oncol. 2015; 51(4):305–313

[62] Gooi Z, Fakhry C, Goldenberg D, Richmon J, Kiess AP, Education Committee of the American Head and Neck Society (AHNS). AHNS series: do you know your guidelines? Principles of radiation therapy for head and neck cancer: a review of the National Comprehensive Cancer Network guidelines. Head Neck. 2016; 38(7):987–992

[63] Grover S, Swisher-McClure S, Mitra N, et al. Total laryngectomy versus larynx preservation for T4a larynx cancer: patterns of care and survival outcomes. Int J Radiat Oncol Biol Phys. 2015; 92(3):594–601

[64] Haugen BR, Alexander EK, Bible KC, et al. 2015 American Thyroid Association management guidelines for adult patients with thyroid nodules and differentiated thyroid cancer: The American Thyroid Association Guidelines Task Force on thyroid nodules and differentiated thyroid cancer. Thyroid. 2016; 26:1–133

[65] Pfister DG, Spencer S, Brizel DM, et al. National Comprehensive Cancer Network. Head and neck cancers, Version 2.2014. Clinical practice guidelines in oncology. J Natl Compr Canc Netw. 2014; 12(10):1454–1487

[66] Blanchard P, Baujat B, Holostenco V, et al. MACH-CH Collaborative group. Meta-analysis of chemotherapy in head and neck cancer (MACH-NC): a comprehensive analysis by tumour site. Radiother Oncol. 2011; 100(1):33–40

[67] Adelstein D, Gillison ML, Pfister DG, et al. NCCN guidelines insights: head and neck cancers, Version 2.2017. J Natl Compr Canc Netw. 2017; 15(6):761–770

8 Ophthalmology

Edited by Michael Burrow

8.1 Ophthalmological Trauma and Other Emergencies

Michael Karsy

8.1.1 Orbital Trauma

- Anatomy[1,2]:
  - Orbital bones: Zygoma, sphenoid (lesser and greater wing), maxillary, frontal, palatine, lacrimal, and ethmoid bones.
  - Superior orbital fissure: Lacrimal and frontal branches of V1, superior and inferior divisions of cranial nerve (CN) III, CN IV, CN VI, ophthalmic vein, sympathetic fibers.
  - Inferior orbital fissure: Zygomatic branch of V2, pterygopalatine branches, ophthalmic vein.
  - Optic canal: Contains optic nerve (CNII) and ophthalmic artery.
  - Contains eye, orbital and retrobulbar fascia, extraocular muscles, CN, lacrimal gland (lateral) and nasolacrimal duct (medial), medial and lateral canthal/palpebral ligaments.
  - Pupil response: Retinal ganglion cells → optic nerve → optic chiasm → pretectal nuclei → Edinger-Westphal nuclei → preganglionic parasympathetic travel along CN3 → ciliary ganglion → postganglionic parasympathetic fibers innervate sphincter muscle.
  - CN injuries:
    - CN3: Eye down and out, pupils dilated on affected side.
    - CN4: Difficulty to look down (e.g., going down flight of stairs), patient may tilt head toward affected side.
    - CN6: Inability looking directly lateral toward affected side.
- Epidemiology:
  - Most common trauma in young adult males, less common in children where head and face show injury.
  - Orbital fractures highly associated with intracranial and intraocular injury.
  - Open globe injuries occur in 3.5:100,000 people per year globally.
- Diagnosis:
  - Fracture types:
    - Orbital zygomatic: Most common; from lateral blow to orbit; commonly associated with orbital floor fracture.
    - Nasoethmoid: Medial fracture that can injure the medial canthal ligament and lacrimal duct system or entrap the medial rectus.
    - Orbital floor/blowout: Direct trauma or indirectly from elevated intraocular pressure; can entrap inferior muscles, cause enophthalmos (affect eye receded), or orbital dystopia (affect eye lower horizontally); can injure infraorbital nerve.
    - Orbital roof: More common in children; highly associated with cranial injuries.
  - Evaluation of other polytrauma injuries takes precedence; evaluation of extraocular muscles, sinus injury, medial canthal ligament, lacrimal duct, and globe performed; evaluation of visual acuity and pupillary constriction routinely performed; intraocular pressure, dilated funduscopic examination, and fluorescein examination performed by ophthalmologist when able.
  - Initial imaging with 1-mm cut computed tomography (CT) images to evaluate orbital fracture pattern; orbital magnetic resonance less commonly used in emergency situation.
  - Vagal symptoms (nausea, vomiting, and bradycardia) seen with extraocular muscle entrapment.
  - Features of significant injury: Proptosis/orbital hematoma, extraction of intraocular contents, widened intercanthal distance, limited extraocular movement, orbital dystopia, enophthalmos.
  - Orbital compartment syndrome: Elevated intraorbital pressure with decreased visual acuity and/or marked proptosis, emergent intervention required as 60–100 minutes of elevated pressure can result in permanent vision loss.

- Treatment:
  - Ophthalmologist consulted early during evaluation of orbital trauma with planned follow-up within 1 week.
  - Oculoplastic surgeons consulted within 24 hours for entrapment, enophthalmos, orbital dystopia, injury to medial canthal ligament, or injury to lacrimal gland.
  - Mild globe injuries treated with elevation of head, intravenous fluids, pain control, and ice to reduce swelling; corticosteroids can be used to reduce swelling after injury and potentially reduce diplopia sooner.
  - Antibiotic prophylaxis (vancomycin and ceftazidime) used for open globe injury to reduce risk of endophthalmitis despite limited evidence; tetanus prophylaxis used in cases with intraorbital foreign bodies (IOFB) or contaminated wounds.
  - Eye shield used for lacerations or perforations to prevent accidental eye pressure.
  - Emergent lateral canthotomy to decompress orbit if needed for significant injury or worsening globe edema.
  - Surgical treatment is complex, controversial, and variable depending on types of injury; early treatment for ocular entrapment or persistent diplopia may have improved ocular motility outcomes.
  - Close follow-up of vision is required even with mild injury due to retinal detachment or reduced perfusion.
- Specific conditions:
  - Open globe injury:
    - Globe rupture is disruption of the globe commonly at the insertion of rectus muscles; decreased globe or anterior chamber size can be seen compared to normal eye.
    - Orbital laceration involves penetrating injury to the globe.
    - Divided by thickness of injury: Corneal, corneal-scleral, and scleral laceration.
    - Divided by zone of injury: Cornea and limbus (zone 1); < 5 mm of anterior sclera but not retina (zone 2); full thickness or > 5 mm posterior from limbus (zone 3).
    - Deeper injury and/or higher zone injuries have worsened risk of visual acuity and scarring.
    - 2–7% risk of endophthalmitis, 13% risk with IOFB, most common infection from *Staphylococcus* species, *Streptococcus* species, and gram-negative organisms.
    - Early ophthalmology consultation and early primary closure performed if possible.
    - Ocular trauma score (▶ Table 8.1 and ▶ Table 8.2) can be predictive of 6-month visual acuity.[3]
    - Traumatic cataract formation can occur days to years after injury.
  - Orbital hematoma:
    - Orbital septum arises from the periosteum and fuses with the tarsus; estimated by imaginary line connecting palpebral fissures to anterior globe.

Table 8.1 Ocular trauma score

Visual factor	Points
Visual acuity	
• Nil perception of light	60
• Light perception to hand movement	70
• 1/200 to 19/200	80
• 20/200 to 20/50	90
• ≥ 20/40	100
Ocular injuries	
• Globe rupture	−23
• Endophthalmitis	−17
• Perforating injury	−14
• Retinal detachment	−11
• Afferent pupillary defect	−10

Table 8.2 Estimated probability of follow-up visual acuity at 6 mo based on ocular trauma score

Raw score	Ocular trauma score	Nil perception of light	Light perception to hand movement	1/200–19/200	20/200–20/50	≥20/40
0–44	1	73%	17%	7%	2%	1%
45–65	2	28%	26%	18%	13%	15%
66–80	3	2%	11%	15%	28%	44%
81–91	4	1%	2%	2%	21%	74%
92–100	5	0%	1%	2%	5%	92%

- Preseptal hematoma may have lower risk of visual loss than postseptal hematoma which can cause a compartment syndrome.
- Preseptal imaging can be observed or drained.
- Postseptal hematoma in the setting of worsening visual function treated emergently with a lateral canthotomy or surgical evacuation.
- Retrobulbar hematoma: Hemorrhage behind the globe; more commonly postoperative or in patients on anticoagulation but can be seen after trauma; high risk of compartment syndrome.
○ Retinal and choroidal hemorrhages:
    - Retinal hemorrhages occur between retinal pigment epithelium and sensory retinal layers; has a V-shaped appearance on CT imaging.
    - Choroidal hemorrhages have a biconvex shape sparing the optic disk and posterior one-third of the globe.
    - Intraocular hemorrhage 95% specific for nonaccidental trauma and should prompt additional workup.
    - Optic nerve sheath hematoma.
○ Lens dislocation:
    - Partial or complete disruption of the lens due to trauma.
    - Surgical emergency as can result in acute angle-closure glaucoma.
○ Hyphema:
    - Layered hemorrhage or hyperattenuation of anterior chamber on CT imaging.
    - Detection on exam should prompt additional workup of intraocular injuries.
○ Traumatic optic neuropathy:
    - 5% of patients with close head trauma.
    - Loss of vision after trauma without findings on funduscopic examination.
    - Direct type involves disruption of nerve; indirect type involves blunt force transmission to intracanalicular optic nerve.
    - Treatment is controversial.
○ Carotid cavernous fistula:
    - Abnormal communication between carotid artery and cavernous sinus that can be due to trauma or other vasculopathy.
    - Direct type (type A) involves high flow between intracavernous carotid artery and cavernous sinus.
    - Indirect types involve low flow between internal (type B), external (type C), or both internal and external (type D) carotid arteries and cavernous sinus.
    - Results in ipsilateral proptosis with enlargement of the superior ophthalmic vein, extraocular muscles, and cavernous sinus enhancement.
    - Treated emergently in patients with progressive vision loss, ophthalmoplegia, elevated intraocular pressure, or high risk for hemorrhage.
○ Corneal injury:
    - 3% of all emergency department visits; 80% due to corneal abrasions or foreign bodies; ocular burns involve 7–18% of injuries in the emergency department with most due to chemicals; seen in 0.013–0.17% of nonocular surgeries.
    - Range of minor injury from abrasions to vision-threatening perforation; includes burns from chemical, radiation, and thermal injury.

– Presents with pain, conjunctival erythema, lid swelling, chemosis, and/or blepharospasm.
– Seidel test: Leaking of aqueous humor on fluorescein exam suggests corneal perforation.
– Most abrasions heal spontaneously; abrasions >2 mm treated with cycloplegic agent to help with blepharospasm; artificial tears used to maintain hydration; topical nonsteroidal anti-inflammatory agent can help with pain; antibiotics (erythromycin ointment; ciprofloxacin or ofloxacin for contact wearers; foreign bodies removed if safe; chemical burns treated with irrigation until pH normalization).
– Urgent referral required for corneal infiltrate or opacity, suggesting ulceration, foreign body that cannot be removed, hypopyon, purulent discharge, drop in vision of one to two lines on Snellen chart, infant or child unwilling to keep eye open, or corneal abrasion that has not healed after 3–4 days.

- Lateral canthotomy:
  - Can be used emergently to preserve visual function.
  - Should not wait for ophthalmology in the setting of acute severe injury with worsening visual function.
  - Procedure:
    – Consent, cleaning of skin, and arrangement of sedation performed when able but should not delay procedure.
    – Betadine prep can be used to clean the skin lateral to the orbit, no risk of chemical injury to the eye or cornea.
    – Lateral cantus infiltrated with lidocaine if able.
    – Scissors used to incise lateral eye lid skin and canthal tendon; tendon is slightly posteroinferior to the lateral canthal fold.
    – Mosquito hemostat placed across tissue can be used for hemostasis.

8.1.2 Other Ophthalmological Emergencies

- Central retinal artery occlusion[4]:
  - Sudden painless unilateral loss of vision; can present with amaurosis fugax (transient, painless unilateral vision loss).
  - Bilateral vision loss suggests migraines, heart failure, or hypertensive emergencies.
  - Evaluated by funduscopic examination; higher risk in older patients with hyperlipidemia, diabetes, atherosclerosis, hypercoagulability.
  - Emergent referral to ophthalmologist performed; ocular digital massage, lowering of intraocular pressure with intravenous mannitol (0.25–2 g/kg once), intravenous acetazolamide (500 mg once), high-flow oxygenation, oral nitrates, or lying flat can be used.
  - Further evaluation of carotid disease and referral to stroke neurology performed to reduce stroke risk.
- Acute angle-closure glaucoma[4]:
  - Presents with blurred vision, conjunctivitis, headaches, eye pain, nausea, vomiting, and decrease in visual function; elevated intraocular pressure (> 30 mm Hg), and shallow anterior chamber seen on examination.
  - Attacks precipitated by medications (e.g., dilating drops, anticholinergics, antidepressants), sulfa drugs, topiramate, or dim light.
  - Treated with 1 drop each of 0.5% timolol maleate, 1% apraclonidine, and 2% pilocarpine repeated every 3–5 minutes; acetazolamide (500 mg once) can be emergently given; urgent referral to ophthalmologist performed; laser or surgical iridotomy can provide more definitive treatment.
- Retinal tear/detachment[4]:
  - Detachment of the retina from the choroid and retinal pigment epithelium; results in ischemia and photoreceptor degeneration resulting in permanent vision loss; rare (1:10,000 people per year in the United States).
  - Presents with unilateral photopsia (flashing lights), floaters, decrease acuity, metamorphopsia (wavy distortion), cloudy/curtain-like vision loss; diagnosed with ophthalmoscopic exam or ultrasound imaging.
  - Risk factors: Myopia, cataract surgery, diabetic retinopathy, family history of retinal detachment, older age, trauma.

○ Treated by laser surgery (photocoagulation) or freezing (cryopexy) for retinal tears; treated with injection of air or gas in the eye (pneumatic retinopexy), indenting eye surface (scleral buckling), or replacement of fluid of the eye (vitrectomy) for retinal detachment.

8.2 Ophthalmology Neoplasms

Michael Burrow

8.2.1 Epidemiology

- A wide range of tumors involve the orbit. The most frequently used classification is by anatomic location including tumors of the eyelids, tumors of the conjunctiva, tumors of the orbit, and intraocular tumors.[5]
- Literature-reported frequencies of different types of orbital lesions vary greatly.[6,7] These discrepancies are thought to be due to reporting bias of various study populations.
- In one large review article that examined 2,480 patients over a 35-year period, the following demographics of patients with orbital lesions were identified: 53.6% male, 46.4% female; mean age of female patients: 43.4, mean age of male patients: 41.7; 68% lesions were benign, 32% were malignant. The following types of lesions and their percentage of total were identified in this series: vasculogenic (24%), cystic (21%), lymphoproliferative (13%), neurogenic (12%), lacrimal gland (10%), secondary tumors (9%), mesenchymal (7%), metastatic tumors (3%).[8]

8.2.2 Diagnosis

- Presentation: Variable depending on the location and etiology, but can include periorbital or eyelid abnormalities, ptosis, proptosis, globe displacement, erythema, ecchymosis, pain, diplopia, extraocular motility deficits, anisocoria, relative afferent pupillary defect, leukocoria, optic nerve pallor, optic nerve edema, poor visual acuity, visual field deficits, dyschromatopsia.
- Tumor location (▶ Table 8.3), symptoms, and patient age can help with initial differential diagnosis.
- Ophthalmological signs and symptoms can help localize tumor (▶ Table 8.4).

Table 8.3 Most common neoplasms by orbital location

Orbital location	Most common neoplasms (more common to less common)
All orbital locations	Dermoid cyst > orbital lymphoma > cavernous hemangioma > mucocele > lymphangioma > meningioma
Upper-inner quadrant	Mucocele > dermoid cyst > orbital lymphoma >> cavernous hemangioma
Upper-outer quadrant	Dermoid cyst >> lacrimal gland adenoma > orbital lymphoma > cavernous hemangioma
Lower-inner quadrant	Basal cell epithelioma > orbital lymphoma > cavernous hemangioma
Lower-outer quadrant	Cavernous hemangioma >> orbital varix > orbital lymphoma > basal cell epithelioma

Table 8.4 Ocular signs and symptoms based on tumor location

Tumor location	Possible signs and symptoms
Periorbital	Eyelid/periorbital skin abnormalities, mechanical ptosis, globe displacement, erythema, ecchymosis, diplopia, blurred vision, extraocular motility deficits
Intraocular	Anisocoria, leukocoria, decreased vision, photopsia, floaters, pain
Orbital extraconal	Globe displacement, proptosis, extraocular motility deficits, diplopia
Orbital intraconal	Proptosis, extraocular motility deficits, anisocoria, relative afferent pupillary defect, optic nerve pallor, optic nerve edema, diplopia, decreased vision, visual field deficits, dyschromatopsia
Intracanalicular (optic canal) or intracranial	Extraocular motility deficits, anisocoria, relative afferent pupillary defect, optic nerve pallor, optic nerve edema, diplopia, decreased vision, visual field deficits, dyschromatopsia, neurologic deficits

- Capillary hemangioma:
  - Primary benign tumor of the orbit present at birth or within the first weeks of life.
  - Most common in the superonasal orbital quadrant or medial upper eyelid; usually enlarge in the first 6–12 months, then begin to spontaneously involute, with 75% of lesions resolving in the first 3–7 years of life.
  - Associations include female sex, prematurity/low birth weight, maternal chorionic villus sampling.
  - Magnetic resonance imaging (MRI) can be helpful in distinguishing from other vascular abnormalities.
  - Usually benign and self-limiting, but physicians must be aware of possible complication of amblyopia in children.
  - Treatment is generally observational, but if affecting vision then medical therapy with topical or oral β-blocker therapy is the first line.
- Cavernous hemangioma:
  - Most common benign orbital neoplasm in adults; women > men.
  - Large encapsulated (with smooth muscle) cavernous spaces containing red blood cells.
  - Classic presentation is slowly progressive proptosis with or without decreased vision, diplopia, pain.
  - Limited communication with systemic circulation, thus arteriography and venography are of limited use.
  - If lesion compromises vision, then treatment is primarily surgical.
- Lymphatic malformation (aka lymphangioma).
  - Usually appear in the second to fourth decades of life and can appear in the orbit, but less commonly in the conjunctiva, eyelids, or sinuses.
  - Often consist of dysgenic lymphatic channels and venous components; histologically, they are nonencapsulated lesions.
  - Presentation can be slowly progressive or rapid-onset proptosis, especially if the lesion acutely hemorrhages.
  - Pathognomonic MRI findings are grapelike cystic lesions with fluid–fluid layering of serum and erythrocytes.
  - Treatment generally consists of either surgical excision or more recently intralesional sclerosing agents.
- Orbital varix (venous malformation):
  - Low-flow dysgenic vascular lesion that exhibits proptosis accentuated during Valsalva maneuver or when the head is in a dependent location.
  - Contrast-enhanced CT during Valsalva maneuver can highlight the lesion.
  - Conservative treatment or observation.
- Arteriovenous malformation:
  - Similar presentation to orbital varix, but are often treated surgically or with coiling of selective occlusion of feeding vessels.[9,10]
- Optic pathway glioma (optic nerve glioma):
  - Typically benign lesions considered to be pilocytic astrocytomas.
  - Almost exclusively diagnosed in childhood (3–5% of all pediatric brain tumors; 70% are found within the first decade of life and 90% within the second decade).
  - Majority of patients with optic nerve glioma have neurofibromatosis type 1 (NF-1), but only 15–20% of patients with NF-1 have optic nerve gliomas.
  - Typical presentation is gradual, painless proptosis with or without vision loss, afferent pupillary defect, or dyschromatopsia.
  - Classically show fusiform enlargement of the optic nerve on CT or MRI.
  - Treatment varies widely depending on visual compromise and can range from observation to surgery with or without radiation/chemotherapy.[8]
- Plexiform neurofibroma:
  - Schwann cell proliferation within nerve sheath endings that can appear in the periorbital region, eyelid, or orbit as well as extraorbital sites.
  - Occur in NF-1, although likely occur in only ~10% of patients with NF-1.

- Classic presentation of an "**S**-shaped" configuration to the upper eyelid with ptosis, usually identified within the first year of life.
- Treatment is observational unless visual compromise exists, then surgical.[11]
- Optic nerve meningioma:
  - Arise from arachnoid cells of the optic nerve sheath.
  - Most common in women in their third to fourth decades of life.
  - Present with gradual, painless, unilateral decrease in vision often accompanied by relative afferent pupillary defect, proptosis, extraocular motility deficits.
  - Imaging with CT or MRI shows diffuse, contrast-enhancing, tubular enlargement of the optic nerve; classic CT finding is "tram-tracking," caused by calcification.
  - Management is variable and may include observation with repeat MRI scans, radiation therapy, and rarely surgical excision from the posterior globe to the chiasm.[12]
- Rhabdomyosarcoma:
  - Malignant proliferation of undifferentiated pluripotent mesenchymal cells histologically categorized into four categories, in order of decreasing frequency: embryonal (60%), alveolar (20%), pleomorphic (10%), and botryoid (< 10%).
  - Most common primary orbital malignancy of childhood, but still rare.
  - Average age of onset is 6 years; slight male predominance (1.3:1).
  - Classic presentation is sudden onset and rapid progression of unilateral proptosis often associated with edema, erythema, or discoloration of the eyelid.
  - Urgent workup is warranted for suspicion of rhabdomyosarcoma and should include CT or MRI as well as biopsy (often by anterior orbitotomy).
  - Metastasis is frequent; thus, further evaluation for metastatic disease should occur and may include lymph node examination, chest radiography, bone marrow biopsy, lumbar puncture.
  - Radiation therapy and chemotherapy are the mainstays of treatment, with orbital exenteration reserved for recurrent or locally invasive cases.[13]
- Orbital lymphoma (ocular adnexal lymphoma):
  - Lymphocyte proliferation, most often B-cell non-Hodgkin type, can involve the eyelids, conjunctiva, periorbital tissues, and lacrimal gland.
  - Account for more than 20% of all orbital tumors, with incidence increasing more than 50% over the last 20 years (thought to be due to increasing population age).
  - Recent classification includes the Revised European-American Lymphoma (REAL) classification, with the most common types being mucosa-associated lymphoid tissue lymphomas; chronic lymphocytic lymphoma; follicular center lymphoma; and high-grade lymphoma.
  - Typical presentation is gradually progressive, painless mass often located in the anterior orbit or beneath the conjunctiva; diplopia, vision loss, and extraocular motility deficits are less common because lesions usually mold around adjacent structures rather than invade; imaging can be helpful in this respect.
  - Open biopsy is important and subsequent morphologic, cytogenetic, and immunologic studies should be undertaken for diagnostic, management, and prognostic purposes; fine-needle aspiration can also be performed.
  - Workup by oncology may include physical examination, blood and serum testing, bone marrow biopsy, chest and abdominal imaging, and other imaging as clinically indicated.
  - Management typically includes radiotherapy for localized ocular lymphoma; if systemic disease is found, treatment is individualized to symptoms.[14,15]
- Neuroblastoma:
  - Typically pediatric, embryonal tumor involving the sympathetic nervous system.
  - Orbital involvement is due to metastasis from distant site (in children metastasis from distant site is most common to the orbit, whereas in adults metastasis is most common to the choroid/globe).
  - Accounts for 15% of deaths in pediatric cancer; 1–2% of individuals with neuroblastoma exhibit a family history of neuroblastoma.
  - Classic presentation includes abrupt onset of proptosis with ecchymosis (raccoon eyes) that can be bilateral; Horner syndrome can be present with involvement of the cervical ganglia.
  - Primary tumor may be detected on physical examination in the abdomen or neck and with imaging in those locations as well as the mediastinum.

- Better prognosis linked with earlier age of diagnosis and early treatment (diagnosis before 1 year of age portends a 90% survival).
- Mainstay of treatment is chemotherapy with radiotherapy in select cases of vision loss from compressive lesions.[16]
- Retinoblastoma:
  - Most common intraocular malignancy in childhood with an estimated incidence of 1 in 16,000–18,000 live births and 8,000 new cases annually.
  - Average age of diagnosis varies geographically but is approximately 27 months for unilateral cases and 15 months for bilateral cases.
  - Nonheritable retinoblastoma is always unilateral, whereas heritable retinoblastoma is bilateral in 80% of cases and unilateral in 15% of cases with 5% trilateral retinoblastoma referring to involvement of both eyes in addition to a pineal/midline neuroectodermal tumor.
  - A parent with a history of heritable retinoblastoma confers a 45% chance of retinoblastoma to offspring (90% penetrance), but most cases of retinoblastoma are first cases; genetic testing and counseling are very important.
  - In delayed diagnosis, metastasis is frequent and occurs through invasion into the central nervous system or by way of the vasculature to bone marrow or visceral organs.
  - Most commonly presentation is with leukocoria, but delayed presentation may include ocular misalignment/strabismus.
  - Diagnosis is made by history, clinical examination, and imaging, in particular ultrasonography; CT is avoided because of radiation risk; fine-needle aspiration confers considerable risk of tumor dissemination.
  - Tumor, node, metastasis, heritable trait staging has become the gold standard for defining retinoblastoma and deciding treatment strategy.
  - Primary goal of treatment is life-saving, while secondary goal is sight saving and may include a combination of chemotherapy, focal therapy, radiotherapy, or surgical therapy.[16,17]
- Uveal melanoma:
  - Uncommon, accounting for < 5% of all melanomas, but is the most common primary intraocular tumor in adults; incidence is 5 cases per 1 million per year.
  - Average age of presentation is the fifth to sixth decades of life.
  - Arise from melanocytes of the choroid, ciliary body, or iris, which make up the uvea; identified as pigmented, dome-shaped, and often subretinal lesions.
  - Presenting symptoms can be vague and mild (blurry vision, floaters, visual field defect, etc.), and lesions can sometimes be difficult to assess on examination depending on location in the eye.
  - In addition to fundus examination, imaging with ultrasound is especially helpful for showing medium internal echogenicity and also can measure dimensions that help stratify risk.
  - Primary goal of treatment is life-saving (prevent metastasis) with secondary goal of preserving vision.
  - Brachytherapy is often used with the option of external beam radiation or enucleation; less commonly, localized ophthalmic treatments are used, such as transpupillary thermotherapy, photodynamic therapy, or photocoagulation.
  - Recurrence rates vary from 4 to 20% depending on the mode of treatment.
  - Despite treatment, ~50% of patients end up with metastatic disease; new directions of therapy are aimed at molecular profiling tumors and developing genetically targeted therapy.[18]
- Lacrimal gland tumors:
  - Incidence of 1 per 1 million people per year; 10% of all orbital tumors; can present at any age, but most common in middle-aged adults.
  - Divided into nonepithelial tumors (lymphoid tumors, dacryoadenitis, other mesenchymal tumors), which comprise 55–80%, and epithelial tumors, which comprise 20–45%.
  - Half of epithelial tumors are benign mixed tumors (pleomorphic adenoma) and half are carcinomas (adenoid cystic carcinoma, pleomorphic adenocarcinoma, malignant mixed, etc.).
  - Imaging is helpful, especially CT scan; lymphoid tumors tend to mold around the globe, but epithelial neoplasms will displace or indent the globe; there can be bony remodeling in response to epithelial tumors, whereas this is rare in lymphoid tumors.

- Pleomorphic adenoma:
  - Progressive, painless proptosis sometimes associated with downward and inward displacement of the globe; may have a firm mass near the upper-outer quadrant of the orbit.
  - Histologically, benign epithelial cells are present with occasional metaplasia surrounded by a pseudocapsule.
  - Treatment is complete excision with pseudocapsule and surrounding margin of normal orbital tissue with long-term follow-up; if excision is incomplete, recurrence is extremely high (up to 32%) and there is a 10% risk of malignant transformation per decade.
- Adenoid cystic carcinoma:
  - More rapid progression than pleomorphic adenoma, progressive, and often painful proptosis with associated downward and inward displacement of the globe; may have a firm mass near the upper-outer quadrant of the orbit.
  - Histologically, benign-appearing cells that grow in nests or tubules, sometimes described as a Swiss-cheese pattern.
  - Perineural extension, often into the cavernous sinus and ultimately to the central nervous system, is common even after treatment.
  - Treatment consists of a combination of high-dose radiation therapy, surgical debulking, intracarotid chemotherapy, or radical exenteration; mortality rates remain high.[19]
- Mucocele:
  - Cystic structure most often arising from the ethmoid or frontal sinus that can invade the orbit by bony remodeling/erosion.
  - Present with progressive proptosis and displacement of the globe that can lead to diplopia or extraocular motility restriction.
  - Imaging is helpful and often shows the cystic space filled with fluid (often mucoid secretions or pus in the case of pyoceles).
  - Treatment is surgical, with evacuation of the mucocele and reconstruction of the sinus drainage or obliteration of the sinus by mucous stripping and sinus packing.[12,20]
- Dermoid:
  - Choristoma consisting of an epithelial-line cyst encasing dermal structures (hair follicles, smooth muscle, sebaceous glands, sweat glands, etc.).
  - Can occur anywhere, but > 80% are found in the head/orbit region and comprise ~10% of all orbital masses (up to 46% in children).
  - Occur at suture lines, most frequently at the frontozygomatic suture line in the upper-outer quadrant of the orbit, but also at the frontoethmoidal or frontomaxillary suture in the upper-inner quadrant of the orbit.
  - Present as a slowly enlarging, nontender, cyst-like mass often identified in the first year of life.
  - Imaging by CT can be done to rule out encephalocele, mucocele, or a dumbbell configuration for surgical planning purposes.
  - Treatment can consist of observation, but most often surgical removal is planned to avoid the risk of traumatic rupture and subsequent inflammatory reaction; complete, intact excision without rupture should be the goal of surgical removal.[21]
- Orbital metastasis:
  - Intraocular metastases are uncommon in children; adults can have metastases found in the orbit or intraocular compartments (choroid, ciliary body, or iris).
  - 75% of patients have a known primary tumor, but in 25% the orbital metastasis is the presenting sign.
  - In men, the most common primary tumor is lung/bronchogenic carcinoma; in women, the most common primary tumor is breast cancer.
  - Presentation is often rapidly progressive, painful proptosis, and inflammation with bone destruction on physical examination or imaging often associated with decreased vision or diplopia.
  - Diagnosis can be done with imaging (CT/MRI), ultrasound, fine-needle aspiration, or a combination of the above.
  - Treatment is largely palliative and usually consists of local radiation therapy, but in extreme circumstances may require surgical excision.[22]

8.2.3 Imaging

- Imaging techniques used to evaluate orbital neoplasms include MRI, CT, angiography, variations on ultrasound including B-scan, A-scan, ultrasound biomicroscopy, color Doppler ultrasound, and ophthalmology-specific imaging techniques including optical coherence tomography and fluorescein or indocyanine green angiography.
- CT imaging is especially helpful when examining bone or soft tissue–bone interactions; it can be helpful in detecting calcification in certain tumors (e.g., meningiomas).
- Disadvantages to CT imaging include poor soft-tissue differentiation (especially in spaces such as the orbital apex), exposure to ionizing radiation, and iodine sensitivities.
- MRI provides better soft-tissue detail as well as optic nerve and orbital apex resolution while avoiding ionizing radiation; MRI is preferred if there is suspicion for coexistent neurologic, cerebral, or intraparenchymal brain pathology.
- Disadvantages to MRI scans include cost, longer acquisition time, and artifact susceptibility from metal and even eye make-up, which often contains metal.
- In both CT and MRI, contrast-enhanced imaging is helpful in cases of vascular abnormality, for tumor identification, and for enhancing soft-tissue details.
- Often, a CT or MRI of the orbits is preferred over brain imaging because they provide thinner slices with higher details and more windows that are helpful in examining orbital and periorbital tissues.
- Ultrasound can be useful as a quick, inexpensive, noninvasive method with nearly no contraindications to evaluate the periorbita, globe, and adjacent structures (e.g., periorbital skin, eyelids, lacrimal gland, globe and intraocular contents, extraocular muscles).
- Ultrasound is limited with deeper structures, e.g., optic nerve or orbital apex lesions.
- Color Doppler ultrasound can be especially useful in evaluating vascular lesions, but many suspected vascular abnormalities require evaluation with other vascular imaging such as CT or MRI angiography or venography.[23]

8.2.4 Medical Management

- In many orbital tumors, observation with close follow-up can be a useful strategy if there is no visual compromise and the tumor is aesthetically acceptable.
- Treatment plans are often multidisciplinary, especially when dealing with oncologic neoplasia; additional disciplines may include neurology, hematology-oncology, neuro-oncology, radiation oncology, otolaryngology, neurosurgery, dermatology, or plastic surgery because of the close association of the orbits with maxillofacial anatomy, sinus system, intracranial compartments, and systemic disease ramifications.

8.2.5 Surgical Management

- When surgical management is indicated, preoperative imaging is often of great importance to successful postsurgical outcomes.
- Goals of surgical intervention include maximal safe resection or debulking with preservation of neurovascular structures including the optic nerve.
- Multidisciplinary surgical intervention may be required involving neurosurgery, otolaryngology, plastic surgery, or dermatology.
- Commonly, subsequent extraocular muscle surgery and/or oculoplastic surgery will be required to treat diplopia from strabismus/ocular misalignment, exposure keratopathy from lagophthalmos, vision-obstructing ptosis, epiphora, or cosmetically unacceptable postoperative states.

8.3 Ophthalmological Infections

Michael Karsy

8.3.1 Orbital Infection

- Epidemiology[2,24]:
  - Infections involve half of orbital abnormalities with two-thirds due to sinusitis and one-fourth due to intraocular foreign bodies.
  - More common in pediatric population than in adults.
  - Preseptal commonly spreads from adjacent structures, trauma, or insect bites.
- Diagnosis:
  - Anterior periorbital/preseptal vs. posterior deep/orbital cellulitis performed emergently as deep infections require more aggressive treatment to prevent vision loss and intracranial spread of infection.
  - Orbital septum is barrier to infection spread.
  - Most commonly spreads from ethmoid sinusitis.
  - Orbital cellulitis results in proptosis/exophthalmos, ophthalmoplegia, and vision loss.
  - Orbital abscess is a complication of cellulitis.
  - Fungal infections most commonly from *Mucormycoses* and *Aspergillus* species; more common in immunocompromised patients and diabetics.
  - Treatment:
    - Fungal infections treated with aggressive debridement, antifungal treatment, and correction of immunodeficiency.

8.3.2 Other Conditions

- Infection location:
  - Conjunctivitis: Eye surface.
  - Blepharitis: Eyelid.
  - Keratitis: Cornea.
  - Uveitis: Uvea, inner layer of eye.
  - Vitritis: Intraocular fluid.
  - Neuroretinitis: Optic nerve and retina.
- Conjunctivitis:
  - Most commonly viral cause with 65–90% due to adenovirus; can also be due to herpes simplex or zoster virus.
  - Bacterial conjunctivitis more common in children; due to *Haemophilus influenza*, *Streptococcus pneumonia*, and *Staphylococcus aureus*.
  - Viral conjunctivitis treated with artificial tears, topical antihistamines, and acyclovir if due to herpes; severe cases or recurrence warrants ophthalmology referral to exclude immune post-viral keratitis; bacterial conjunctivitis treated with antibiotics.
  - Gonococcal and chlamydial conjunctivitis are other considerations.
- Keratitis:
  - Most commonly due to bacteria (*S. aureus*, coagulase-negative *Staphylococci*, *S. pneumonia*, and *P. aeruginosa*); can be due to herpes simplex; high risk of corneal blindness or visual impairment; can be due to fungal causes.
  - Presents with pain, photophobia, hypopyon (pus inside eye).
  - Patients with contact lenses referred to ophthalmology for corneal scraping and examination, empiric treatment started (ciprofloxacin, ofloxacin, cefalotin/gentamicin, and chloramphenicol).
- Superior ophthalmic vein thrombosis:
  - Occlusion of the superior ophthalmic vein commonly from infection of the paranasal sinus; can also be due to inflammation, hypercoagulability, or orbital masses.

- Patients present with orbital pain, swelling, decreased visual function, CN palsy, chemosis, and/or proptosis.
- Identified with MR imaging earlier than CT imaging.
- Treatment of underlying condition is performed.

- Endophthalmitis:
  - Bacterial or fungal infection of globe involving the vitreous or aqueous humor.
  - Can spread from corneal infection in aqueous humor to vitreous humor.
  - Risk factors: Cataract surgery, intravitreal injections, trauma, filtering bleb, keratitis, bacteremia, fungemia; most commonly due to trauma or ocular surgery (e.g., cataract surgery).
  - Imaging shows periocular inflammation and enhancement.
  - Treated with aggressive antibiotics including intravitreal antibiotics and/or vitrectomy; urgent referral to ophthalmology required.

References

[1] Joseph JM, Glavas IP. Orbital fractures: a review. Clin Ophthalmol. 2011; 5:95–100

[2] Nguyen VD, Singh AK, Altmeyer WB, Tantiwongkosi B. Demystifying orbital emergencies: a pictorial review. Radiographics. 2017; 37 (3):947–962

[3] Kuhn F, Maisiak R, Mann L, Mester V, Morris R, Witherspoon CD. The Ocular Trauma Score (OTS). Ophthalmol Clin North Am. 2002; 15 (2):163–165, vi

[4] Pokhrel PK, Loftus SA. Ocular emergencies. Am Fam Physician. 2007; 76(6):829–836

[5] Shields JA, Shields CL. Eyelid, Conjunctival, and Orbital Tumors: An Atlas and Textbook. 3rd ed. Philadelphia, PA: Wolters Kluwer Health; 2016

[6] Bonavolontà G, Strianese D, Grassi P, et al. An analysis of 2,480 space-occupying lesions of the orbit from 1976 to 2011. Ophthal Plast Reconstr Surg. 2013; 29(2):79–86

[7] Shields JA, Shields CL, Scartozzi R. Survey of 1264 patients with orbital tumors and simulating lesions: the 2002 Montgomery Lecture, part 1. Ophthalmology. 2004; 111(5):997–1008

[8] Rasool N, Odel JG, Kazim M. Optic pathway glioma of childhood. Curr Opin Ophthalmol. 2017; 28(3):289–295

[9] Sullivan TJ. Vascular anomalies of the orbit—a reappraisal. Asia Pac J Ophthalmol (Phila). 2018; 7(5):356–363

[10] Lally SE. Update on orbital lymphatic malformations. Curr Opin Ophthalmol. 2016; 27(5):413–415

[11] Avery RA, Katowitz JA, Fisher MJ, et al. Orbital/Peri-orbital plexiform neurofibromas in children with neurofibromatosis Type 1. Ophthalmology. 2017; 124(1):123–132

[12] Jørgensen M, Heegaard S. A review of nasal, paranasal, and skull base tumors invading the orbit. Surv Ophthalmol. 2018; 63(3):389–405

[13] Panda SP, Chinnaswamy G, Vora T, et al. Diagnosis and management of rhabdomyosarcoma in children and adolescents: ICMR consensus document. Indian J Pediatr. 2017; 84(5):393–402

[14] Demirci H, Shields CL, Shields JA, Honavar SG, Mercado GJ, Tovilla JC. Orbital tumors in the older adult population. Ophthalmology. 2002; 109(2):243–248

[15] Olsen TG, Heegaard S. Orbital lymphoma. Surv Ophthalmol. 2019; 64(1):45–66

[16] Kamihara J, Bourdeaut F, Foulkes WD, et al. Retinoblastoma and neuroblastoma predisposition and surveillance. Clin Cancer Res. 2017; 23(13):e98–e106

[17] AlAli A, Kletke S, Gallie B, Lam WC. Retinoblastoma for pediatric ophthalmologists. Asia Pac J Ophthalmol (Phila). 2018; 7(3):160–168

[18] Álvarez-Rodríguez B, Latorre A, Posch C, Somoza Á. Recent advances in uveal melanoma treatment. Med Res Rev. 2017; 37(6):1350–1372

[19] Gündüz AK, Yeşiltaş YS, Shields CL. Overview of benign and malignant lacrimal gland tumors. Curr Opin Ophthalmol. 2018; 29(5):458–468

[20] Hicks KL, Moe KS, Humphreys IM. Bilateral transorbital and transnasal endoscopic resection of a frontal sinus osteoblastoma and orbital mucocele: a case report and review of the literature. Ann Otol Rhinol Laryngol. 2018; 127(11):864–869

[21] Eldesouky MA, Elbakary MA. Orbital dermoid cyst: classification and its impact on surgical management. Semin Ophthalmol. 2018; 33(2):170–174

[22] Shields CL, Shields JA, Gross NE, Schwartz GP, Lally SE. Survey of 520 eyes with uveal metastases. Ophthalmology. 1997; 104(8):1265–1276

[23] Héran F, Bergès O, Blustajn J, et al. Tumor pathology of the orbit. Diagn Interv Imaging. 2014; 95(10):933–944

[24] Watson S, Cabrera-Aguas M, Khoo P. Common eye infections. Aust Prescr. 2018; 41(3):67–72

9 Plastic Surgery

Jacob Veith, Fatma Tuncer, and Faizi Siddiqi

9.1 Overview

- Combination of reconstructive and cosmetic surgery.
- The goal of plastic surgery is to restore function and appearance.
- Encompasses many subspecialties (craniofacial surgery, hand surgery, microsurgery, general reconstructive surgery, breast and oncologic reconstructive surgery, and aesthetic surgery).

9.2 General Principles and Techniques

9.2.1 Skin Closure and Favorable Scar Techniques

- Skin type: Pigmented, oily skin produces more unsightly scars. Pale and dry skin produces less conspicuous scars.
- Location: Shoulder and sternal incisions produce wide, hypertrophic scars. Periorbital and preauricular incisions heal with a fine-line scar. Incisions hidden in anatomic boundaries (nasofacial groove, nasolabial fold, upper eyelid fold) are less noticeable.
- Wound direction: Lacerations or excisions in the direction of relaxed skin tension lines (Langer's lines) leave favorable scars.
- Systemic or local factors: Smoking, vascular disease, crush injury, etc.
- The four most important factors in attempting to gain a favorable scar are:
  ◦ Debridement of necrotic tissue, removal of foreign material.
  ◦ Sutures that are not excessively tight (tension-free).
  ◦ Minimizing damage to the skin edges with atraumatic technique.
  ◦ Wound-edge eversion.
  ◦ Removing sutures promptly enough to avoid railroad scars.
    – Face: 5–7 days.
    – Body: 7–10 days.
    – Hands/feet: 10–14 days.

9.2.2 Excision

- Unsightly and contracted scars can be avoided with proper excision technique of skin lesions.
- Elliptical excision:
  ◦ Most common technique.
  ◦ Avoid dog ears with adequate length.
- Wedge excision (▶ Fig. 9.1):
  ◦ Lesions near or on free margins (i.e., lips, eyelids).
- Serial excision:
  ◦ Used for large lesions such as congenital nevi, where single-stage excision is not possible or desired because of longer scar. Skin stretches over time.

9.2.3 Reconstructive Ladder

- Applicable to simple and complex wounds.
- Options should be evaluated from simplest to most complex (▶ Fig. 9.2).
- Should be tailored to the situation as sometimes a more complex option will provide better aesthetic and functional results when technically a simpler reconstructive option would suffice.
- New methods in wound healing (i.e., dermal matrices, negative pressure wound therapy, tissue expansion) have led to an updated version.

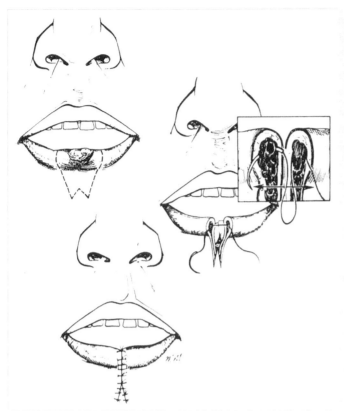

Fig. 9.1 Wedge excision of the lip and primary closure. (Reproduced with permission from Papel I, Frodel J, Holt R, et al, eds. Facial Plastic and Reconstructive Surgery. 4th ed. Thieme; 2016.)

Free flap
Tissue expansion
Distant flaps
Local flaps
Dermal matrices
Skin graft
Negative pressure wound therapy
Closure by secondary intention
Primary closure

Fig. 9.2 Modern reconstructive ladder (in ascending complexity). *Source*: Janis JE, Kwon RK, Attinger CE. The new reconstructive ladder: modifications to the traditional model. Plast Reconstr Surg 2011;127(Suppl 1):205S–212S

9.3 Grafts

- Standard tool for closing defects that cannot be closed primarily and when local tissue is unavailable.
- Definitions:
  - Graft: A part of tissue that is transferred from one part of body to another part without its vascular blood supply.
  - Skin graft: Consists of epidermis and some or all of the dermis.
  - Split-thickness skin grafts contain various amounts of dermis.
  - Full-thickness skin grafts contain all of the dermis.
- Contraction:
  - Primary: Graft becomes smaller immediately after harvest due to elastin.
  - Secondary: Due to myofibroblasts in healing skin graft (greater in thinner grafts).
- Full-thickness skin grafts:
  - Some degree of hair regrowth (vs. none in split thickness).
  - Greater reinnervation than split thickness due to greater presence of neurilemmal sheaths.
- Meshing:
  - Increases the surface area of the graft.
  - Allows for drainage of serum and blood through the holes.
  - Leads to "pebbled" or "meshed" scar.
- Application:
  - Staple graft to wound edges.
  - Suture for small defects/full-thickness grafts.
- Care of the recipient site:
  - Common causes of failure include seroma, hematoma, shearing or movement of the graft, and infection.
  - Negative pressure wound therapy.
  - Bolster dressing.
  - Leave initial dressing for 5 days.
- Contraindications:
  - Infection in recipient bed.
  - Poor vascularization of wound bed (i.e., radiation, microvascular disease).
    - Debridement to bleeding tissue is always necessary.
  - Exposed bone/tendon/nerve/cartilage:
    - If necessary, it can be placed over periosteum, paratenon, or perichondrium.
    - Exceptions: Inside of orbit, temporal bone.
  - Area expected to experience sheering trauma from motion or trauma.
  - Staged reconstruction of structures in wound bed (i.e., nerves, tendons).
- Phases of healing in skin grafts:
  - Plasma imbibition lasts for 24–48 hours.
  - Inosculation (alignment) of donor and recipient capillary ends.
  - Revascularization of the graft through these new capillary connections.
- Donor site:
  - Location:
    - Based on patient preference of scar.
    - Most common—anterolateral thigh.
    - Other sites: Back, abdomen, upper inner arm, scalp.
  - Skin is best with similar skin (i.e., color, hair presence).
  - Dressing:
    - Moistness.
    - Semiocclusive now most common (i.e., Tegaderm).
  - Healing:
    - Split thickness: Regenerates from wound edges and epidermal cells in hair follicle shafts.
    - Full thickness: Will need primary closure because no epithelial structures remain.

9.4 Flaps

- Also see Chapter 13.2.7 Flap Techniques.
- A part of tissue that is transferred with its own blood supply (unlike grafts, which are revascularized from recipient bed).
- Good choice for covering recipient sites with poor vascularity, covering vital structures, reconstructing facial structures, covering bony prominences, or for providing functional units.
- Local flaps:
  - Rotational flaps:
    - Local tissue rotated around a pivot point to cover a defect.
    - Secondary defect created—direct closure or skin graft.
  - Transpositional flaps:
    - Bilobed flap, Limberg (rhomboid) flap (▶ Fig. 9.3).
  - Advancement flaps:
    - Rectangular flaps with Burow triangle.
    - V–Y advancement (▶ Fig. 9.4).
  - Z-plasty (▶ Fig. 9.5):
    - Scar revision: Changes direction of scars.
    - Contracture release: Lengthens the scar in expense of the width.
- Free flaps: Donor-site tissue detached from blood supply and anastomosed at another location by microsurgical techniques.
- Flaps based on tissue composition:
  - Cutaneous flap.
  - Fascia or fasciocutaneous flaps.
  - Muscle or musculocutaneous flap.
  - Osseous, osteocutaneous, or osteomyocutaneous flaps.
- Tissue expansion:
  - Expander in subcutaneous plane is gradually inflated until desired skin expansion is achieved.
  - Mechanical stress leads to increased surface area.
  - Used for both local reconstruction and eventual transfer.

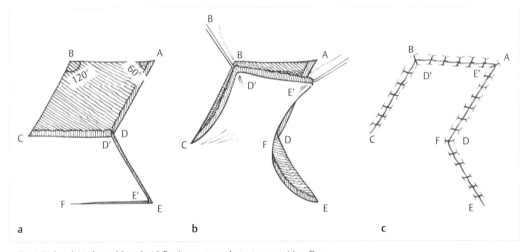

Fig. 9.3 (a–c) Limberg (rhomboid flap), an example to transposition flap.

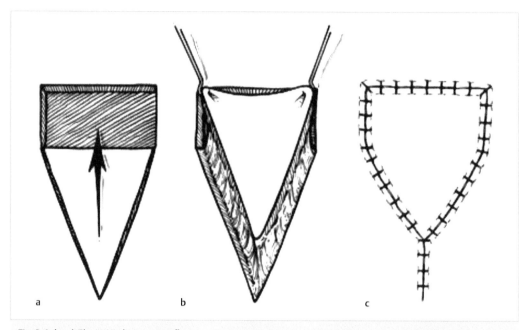

Fig. 9.4 (a–c) The V–Y advancement flap.

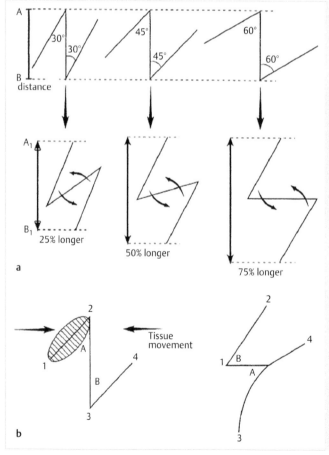

a

b

Fig. 9.5 Z-plasty. (a) The standard Z-plasty advances tissue from the lateral margins and expands the tissue along the 2–3 axis. A defect may be placed in any one of the three limbs of the Z-plasty. The A and B flaps must transpose across one another. The transposition of the A and B flaps occurs with all transposition flaps, although it may not be as obvious as in the Z-plasty flap. **(b)** A Z-plasty design used to close a defect placed along one of its three limbs. (Source: Murakami CS, Nishioka GJ. Essential concepts in the design of local skin flaps. Facial Plast Surg Clin North Am 1996;4:455–468.)

Suggested Readings

Hallock GG, Morris SF. Skin grafts and local flaps. Plast Reconstr Surg. 2011; 127(1):5e–22e

Harii K. Microvascular surgery in plastic surgery: free-tissue transfer. J Microsurg. 1979; 1(3):223–230

Hove CR, William EF, 3rd, Rodgers BJ. Z-plasty: a concise review. Facial Plast Surg. 2001; 17(4):289–94

Jaibaji M, Morton JD, Green AR. Dog ear: an overview of causes and treatment. Ann R Coll Surg Engl. 2001; 83(2):136–138

Janis JE, Kwon RK, Attinger CE. The new reconstructive ladder: modifications to the traditional model. Plast Reconstr Surg. 2011; 127 Suppl 1:205S–212S

Khouri RK. Free flap surgery. The second decade. Clin Plast Surg. 1992; 19(4):757–761

McCraw JB, Vasconez LO. Musculocutaneous flaps: principles. Clin Plast Surg. 1980; 7(1):9–13

Simman R. Wound closure and the reconstructive ladder in plastic surgery. J Am Col Certif Wound Spec. 2009; 1(1):6–11

Takei T, Mills I, Arai K, Sumpio BE. Molecular basis for tissue expansion: clinical implications for the surgeon. Plast Reconstr Surg. 1998; 102 (1):247–258

Taylor GI. The current status of free vascularized bone grafts. Clin Plast Surg. 1983; 10(1):185–209

10 Pediatrics

Edited by Katie W. Russell

10.1 Pediatric Physiology and Surgical Preparation

Michael Karsy

10.1.1 Physiology Basics

- Age:
  - Premature: Birth < 37 weeks of gestation, 3 weeks before estimated due date.
    - Extremely preterm: < 28 weeks, 29–78% chance of survival, 50–80% chance of no disability at the age of 3 years.
    - Very preterm: 28 to < 32 weeks, 90–95% chance of survival.
    - Moderate to late preterm: 32 to < 37 weeks, infants born after 34 weeks have same survival rate as full-term infants.
  - Neonate: 44 weeks from conception, ≤ 28 days of corrected age.
  - Postterm infant: Born after 42 weeks.
  - Infant: Child up to 12 months.
  - Child: 1–12 years.
  - Adolescent: 13–16 years.
- Weight:
  - Small for gestational age: Babies < 10th percentile for gestational age.
  - Low birth weight: Baby < 2,500 g (5 lb, 8 oz) regardless of gestational age.
  - Very low birth weight: < 1,500 g (3 lb, 5 oz).
  - Extremely low birth weight: < 1,000 g (2 lb, 3 oz).
  - Prevalence of obesity overall (18.5%); 2–5-year-olds (14%), 6–11-year-olds (18%), 12–19-year-olds (20%).
  - Growth curves calculate norms for height, weight, and head circumference across ages, sexes, and special conditions (e.g., achondroplasia, Down syndrome).
- Neurological:
  - Pain can result in physiological findings (e.g., tachycardia, hypertension) and can be felt in all age groups; myth that babies do not feel pain due to undeveloped nervous systems.
  - Narcotic suppression of ventilation can increase $PaCO_2$.
  - Limited blood–brain barrier can result in prolonged action of drugs.
  - Cerebral blood vessels in the periventricular germinal matrix are susceptible to hemorrhage in premature infants.
  - Myelination occurs within 2 years in rostrocaudal fashion and completed by 7 years of age.
  - Brain has larger glucose requirement in children than in adults (6.8 vs. 5.5 mg glucose/100 mg brain per minute).
  - Gradual increase in cerebral blood flow as children develop; 42–49 mL/100 g brain per min in neonates to 110 mL/100 g brain per min in children aged 3–4 years before reducing into adults (30–90 mL/100 g brain per min).
  - More permeable blood–brain barrier to electrolytes and larger, lipid-soluble molecules.
  - Spinal cord terminates at L3 vertebral body in infants and retracts to L1/2 by 8 years of age.
- Psychological:
  - Infants < 6 months show limited separation anxiety.
  - Children up to 4 years show unpredictable separation anxiety.
  - Children up to 12 years upset by mutilating effects of surgery and possibility of pain.
  - Adolescents fear pain, medications, loss of control, and loss of ability to cope with illness; worsened by longer periods of hospitalization.
  - Developmental milestones show a large range of variability but can be helpful in identifying motor, psychological, and social development (▶ Table 10.1); red flags include loss of skills and parental concerns at any age.

- Airway:
  - Airway consideration differences from adults: Larger head, shorter trachea and neck, narrower nasal passages, larger tongue, high and anterior larynx, elongated epiglottis.
  - Neonatal airways are the most difficult and become easier as children grow.
  - Neonates and children aged 5 years are preferentially nasal breathers.
  - Primarily diaphragmatic breathing, 15% of oxygen consumption.
  - Airway narrowing at cricoid cartilage up to 5 years of age; small amounts of edema can occlude airway significantly in babies.
  - Larger occiput in infants and children; placement of small pillow under shoulders will improve sniffing position in children.
- Respiratory system:
  - Higher relative oxygen consumption (infant: 6 mL/kg/min, adult: 3 mL/kg/min) and minute ventilation in neonate than in adult.
  - More compliant chest wall than that of adults, poor negative intrathoracic pressure, minute ventilation is rate dependent, and positive end-expiratory pressure.
  - Functional reserve capacity decreases to small amount of total lung capacity (10–15%) at complete relaxation resulting in relatively easier airway closure, atelectasis, ventilation/perfusion imbalance, and hemoglobin desaturation.
  - Apnea is common in premature infants, significant if >15 seconds and associated with desaturation, cyanosis or bradycardia, irregular breathing (e.g., periodic breathing); common in both full-term and premature neonates; caffeine (10–20 mg/kg) can be used.
  - Hypoxic and hypercapnic ventilator drives not well develop in neonates and infants.

Table 10.1 Developmental milestones

Age	Motor	Speech/Language	Cognition/Social
Newborn	Primitive reflexes (e.g., step, Babinski, posture, grasp, root, suck)	Startles to sounds	Follows contrast and faces
2 mo	Head steady when held, head up 45° prone, bats at objects	Turns to voice, cooing	Social smile
4 mo	Sits with support, head up 90° prone, rolls front to back, palmar grasp	Laugh, squeal	Explores faces and objects
6 mo	Sits, raking grasp, transfers	Nonspecific babble	Stranger anxiety, looks for dropped objects, expresses emotion
9 mo	Pulls to stand, pincer grip	Mama, dada, gestures	Object permanence, separation anxiety
12 mo	Walks few steps, wide gait	1 word, responds to name	Points and gestures at wanted objects
15 mo	Walks well, uses spoon, tower 2 blocks	5 words	Looks for hidden objects, interested in items to show parents
18 mo	Stoops and recovers, runs, tower 4 blocks, scribbles, removes clothing	10–25 words	Symbolic play, parallel play
2 y	Jumps, up and down stairs, uses fork, tower 6 blocks	50 words, 50% intelligible, 2-word phases	Problem-solving, tantrums
3 y	Pedals trike, toilet training, draws circle, upstairs alternating feet	200 words, 75% intelligible, 3–4 words, asks why, states name, age, and sex	Simple time concept, counts, separates easily
4 y	Hops on 1 foot, draws square, down stairs alternating feet, cuts with scissors	Sentences, 100% intelligible, tells story	Preferred friend, identifies opposites and colors, fantasy play
5 y	Balance on 1 foot, skips, bicycle, draws person, tripod pencil grip, prints names	5,000 words, future tense, word play	Group of friends, games with rules

- Diaphragm and intercostal muscles show more type I muscle fibers that are not fatigue resistant; fatigable muscles then show early respiratory failure with increased work of breathing; muscle distribution approximates that of adults by 2 years of age.
- Postoperative apnea is more common in premature infants, within 12 hours postoperatively, infants with hematocrits < 30%, predisposition to airway obstruction, residual depressant medications, and central apnea.
- Cardiovascular:
  - More sensitive to hypovolemia because of lower contractility of cardiac muscle per g of tissue, reduced ventricular compliance; cardiac output is rate dependent, results in limited ability to increase stroke volume to increase cardiac output, limited Starling response, and afterload compensation.
  - Patent ductus arteriosus (PDA) closes within 2–4 weeks; increased arterial oxygen tension results in ductus constriction.
  - Foramen ovale begins closure after first breath, with increased pulmonary vascular resistance and left atrial pressure.
  - Sympathetic nervous system and baroreceptor reflexes not fully mature; infants show reduced catecholamine stores and response.
  - Neonate electrocardiogram shows right axis deviation compared with adults as myocardium develops.
  - Shock:
    - Volume status evaluated by examination (skin turgor, sunken anterior fontanelle, dry mucosa, edema), tachycardia, capillary refill.
    - Hepatomegaly can occur with extracellular volume overload.
    - Blood pressure changes occur late in children.
    - Dehydration categories: Mild (< 3% weight loss), moderate (3–10%), severe (> 10%).
    - Similar features and early goal-directed therapy options as in adults but lower reserve than adults resulting in rapid deterioration of compensated shock.
    - D50 glucose used early during resuscitation.
    - Corticosteroids considered in patients refractory to resuscitation or with adrenal suppression.
- Gastrointestinal:
  - Incomplete hepatic maturity in infants, hepatic blood flow increases over development; conjugation reactions are impaired in neonates.
  - Longer drug half-life in infants.
  - Reduced glycogen stores, albumin levels, ability to handle protein loads, and drug binding.
  - Increased risk of coagulopathy and higher free drug levels with reduced albumin.
  - Gastric pH alkalotic at birth and becomes acidic at 2 days; increased reflux due to decreased lower esophageal sphincter tone until 4–55 months.
- Blood and fluid volume composition in children:
  - Maintenance of fluid follows Holliday and Segar's rule of 4:2:1 (4 mL/kg for first 10 kg, 2 mL/kg for second 10 kg, 1 mL/kg for each kg after 20 kg).
  - Resuscitation:
    - Crystalloid: 10–20 mL/kg bolus, 1:1 fluid replacement every 4 hours with D5/0.5 NS + 20 mEq KCl with protracted fluid loss (e.g., vomiting, diarrhea).
    - Packed red blood cells: 10–15 mL/kg.
    - Fresh frozen plasma: 10–15 mL/kg.
    - Platelets: 1 unit/5 kg blood weight.
  - Neonates have higher total body water content (75%) compared with adults (60%); most content is extracellular compared with adults (40 vs. 20%).
  - Total body water approximates that of adults by 3 years of age.
  - Reduced muscle mass and fat content in children compared with adults; results in larger initial dose for water-soluble drugs and longer time until drug redistribution into fat or muscle.
  - Higher insensible losses for preterm infants, elevated respiratory rate, surgical malformations (e.g., gastroschisis, omphalocele, neural tube defects), increased body temperature, phototherapy/incubators, dryer environments, increased activity (e.g., crying).
  - Third spacing after trauma or major abdominal trauma can result in 1–20 mL/kg/hour of volume loss, after surgery for necrotizing enterocolitis can result in up to 50 mL/kg/hour volume loss.

Table 10.2 Blood volume for children

Age group	mL/kg
Premature neonates	95–100
Full-term neonates	85–90
Infants	80
Children	75–80
Adult men	75
Adult women	65

- ○ 4% dextrose added to fluid especially in younger children to prevent ketosis; hypoglycemia is common in stressed conditions and can result in neurological damage.
- ○ Blood volume varies by age (▶ Table 10.2), transitions from fetal hemoglobin to adult hemoglobin within 3 months; left-shifted oxyhemoglobin dissociation curve in infants, sharp drop in erythropoietin after birth.
- ○ Perioperative fluid goals: Urine output 1–3 mL/kg/hour, weight loss of 1–2%/day in first week; monitoring for edema, dehydration, and hepatomegaly.
- ○ Vitamin K given after birth to reduce hemorrhagic disease of newborn since vitamin K–dependent clotting factors and platelet function deficit for first few months after birth.
- • Renal function:
  - ○ 25% of adult function in infants, maturation by 2 years of age; results in elevated half-life of renally filtered drugs, reduced ability to excrete large sodium loads.
  - ○ Premature neonates show decreased creatinine clearance, impaired sodium retention, and poor concentrating ability.
- • Thermoregulation:
  - ○ Pediatric patients at higher risk for hypothermia because of larger body surface area to weight ratio, thin skin, limited fat, limited shivering, and nonshivering thermogenesis.

10.1.2 Anesthetic and Perioperative Considerations

- • Anesthesia workup[1]:
  - ○ History and physical exam obtained; attention to past experiences with anesthesia and postoperative nausea/vomiting (PONV), medications, family history (e.g., malignant hyperthermia, prolonged paralysis after succinylcholine, bleeding diathesis, PONV).
  - ○ No need for routine laboratory studies in healthy children.
  - ○ Patients with high-risk conditions may require preanesthesia clearance (▶ Table 10.3).
  - ○ Fasting guidelines vary by institution but are aimed to reduce the length of time patient cannot receive oral nutrition (▶ Table 10.4).
  - ○ Children with non-innocent murmurs, history of congenital heart disease, or pacemakers require workup by cardiology; plan for anticoagulation management required.
  - ○ Innocent murmur:
    - – 80% of children.
    - – Includes vibratory Still murmur, ejection murmur, cardiorespiratory murmur, murmur of physiologic peripheral pulmonary stenosis, venous hums, carotid bruits, and third heart sounds.
    - – Diastolic murmurs are pathologic.
  - ○ Upper respiratory tract infections with fevers, wheezing, or productive cough likely to cancel elective surgeries.
  - ○ Seizure disorders and neurological deficits are noted preoperatively to compare with postoperative examinations.
  - ○ Patients with hemoglobinopathies or coagulopathies require plans for coagulation depending on risk and extent of expected procedural blood loss; workup and coordination with hematology possible.
  - ○ Controlled hypertension and diabetes are recommended for elective surgery.

Table 10.3 Examples of high-risk patients potentially requiring preanesthesia clearance

Complex spine surgery

Airway reconstruction

Airway red flags: Difficulty with previous intubation or mask ventilation, Pierre–Robin syndrome, Treacher–Collins syndrome, Goldenhar syndrome, Down syndrome, Klippel-Feil syndrome, mucopolysaccharidosis, prior airway or cervical spine injury, prolonged neonatal intubation, stridor at rest

Major neurological, abdominal, or chest/cardiac surgery

Children with complex heart disease, heart failure, or pacemaker dependence

Children with severe or chronic respiratory disease (e.g., severe asthma, cystic fibrosis, ventilator-dependent, O_2-dependent)

Complex airway with craniofacial syndrome or history of difficult intubation

Obstructive sleep apnea

Muscular dystrophy, mucopolysaccharidosis, neuromuscular disorders

Cervical spine instability or children in neck braces

Hunter and Hurler syndrome

Morbidity obesity

Living-related organ donors

Transplant recipients

Patients with complex ethical (e.g., objections to blood transfusion, do-not-resuscitate orders), pain, or psychosocial issues

Table 10.4 Fasting time for children

Age (months)	Milk/solids	Clear liquids
<6	4 h	2 h
6–36	6 h	3 h
>36	8 h	3 h

- ○ Patients with renal impairment require evaluation of electrolytes, fluids status, and associated medical conditions.
- ○ Patients with active or treated tumors require specific consideration; mediastinal masses can cause airway or great vessel compression on induction; bleomycin or doxorubicin can result in pulmonary fibrosis and cardiomyopathy compromising anesthesia; radiation therapy can cause pulmonary and soft-tissue fibrosis.
- Fever in child:
  - ○ Fever defined as temperature of ≥ 100.4 °F (≥ 38 °C) in neonates, ≥ 100.4–102.2 °F (≥ 38.0–39.0 °C) in children 3–36 months, ≥ 100.0–103.0 °F (≥ 37.8–39.4 °C) in older children and adults; variation based on measurement type.
  - ○ Fever in neonates requires aggressive investigation (complete blood count, blood culture, urine culture, cerebrospinal fluid analysis and cultures, C-reactive protein/erythrocyte sedimentation rate), empiric treatment, and hospital admission.
  - ○ Fever in infants > 1–3 months should be investigated depending on clinical picture; those without unwell features can undergo close outpatient follow-up.
  - ○ Identification of the unwell child based on clinical examination (▶ Table 10.5).
  - ○ Individual dosing or alternation of weight-based dosing of acetaminophen and ibuprofen can be used to reduce fever and improve comfort; not used for young children until cause of fever evaluated.
    - – Acetaminophen: 10–15 mg/kg, max dose: 1 g, every 4–6 hours, max daily dose: 4 g, not used for children < 3 months.
    - – Ibuprofen: 10 mg/kg, max dose: 600 g, every 6 hours, max daily dose: 2.4 g, not used for children < 6 months.

Table 10.5 Signs/symptoms of unwell child

Color	Pallor, mottled or cyanotic skin
Activity	Agitated, appears ill, unarousable, weak cry/cough
Respiratory	Increased work of breathing
	Tachypnea
	Nasal flaring
	Drooling
	Grunting
	Wheezing, stridor
	Head bobbing
	Accessory muscles/retraction
	Cyanosis
	Irregular breathing/apnea
	Altered consciousness
	Agitation
	Diaphoresis
Circulation/hydration	Tachycardia
	Delayed capillary refill time
	Dry mucous membranes
	Reduced urine output
	Reduced skin turgor
Other	Rigors, limb swelling or disuse
	Bulging fontanelle
	Neck stiffness
	Seizure
	Focal neurological deficits

- Pediatric intubation:
  - Tube size:
    - Uncuffed: Age in years/4 + 4.
    - Cuffed: Age in years/4 + 3.
  - Depth: Endotracheal tube size × 3.
  - Complications:
    - Postintubation croup: 0.1–1%; risk with larger endotracheal tube, prone position, multiple attempts, traumatic intubation, patients aged 1–4 years, surgery > 1 hour, upper respiratory infection.
    - Laryngotracheal/subglottic stenosis: Risks with prolonged intubation, caused by laryngeal injury from large endotracheal tube, granulation tissue forms resulting in scarring.

10.2 Cardiopulmonary Abnormalities

Michael Karsy

10.2.1 Pulmonary Abnormalities

- Pulmonary sequestration:
  - Congenital nonfunctioning lung tissue with systemic but not pulmonary circulation, can have abnormal bronchial structure.
  - More common in males and on left side.

- Extralobar:
  - Separate tissue from lung.
  - Asymptomatic and found incidentally, 25% of sequestrations.
  - Associated with congenital diaphragmatic hernia, vertebral anomalies, and congenital heart disease.
  - Can become infected.
  - Treated with excision.
- Intralobar:
  - Incorporated tissue into normal lung, 75% of sequestrations.
  - Presents with recurrent pneumonia and abscess formation.
  - Treated with lobectomy.
- Diagnosed with prenatal ultrasound, prenatal magnetic resonance imaging (MRI), chest X-ray, or computed tomography (CT); CT angiography is used to identify blood supply prior to surgery.
- Congenital cystic pulmonary malformation/cystic adenomatoid.
  - Cystic proliferation of terminal bronchioles, results in proliferation of mucus-producing epithelium, smooth muscle cells, and elastic tissue and in incomplete gas exchange.
  - Presents with infection, pneumothorax, airway disease, or failure to thrive; occurs in 1:30,000 pregnancies.
  - Diagnosed on fetal ultrasound, MRI, or echocardiogram; infant chest X-ray, ultrasound, or CT.
  - Types:
    - I: 50% of cases, favorable outcome.
    - II: 40% of cases, smaller and numerous cysts, associated with birth defects (genitourinary, cardiac, skeletal, hydrocephalus, diaphragmatic hernia).
    - III: 10% of cases, large lesions, cause organ shift, can result in hydrops development (e.g., fluid in abnormal compartments), poor prognosis.
  - Treated with lobectomy:
- Congenital diaphragmatic hernia:
  - Failed fusion of transverse septum and pleuroperitoneal folds, associated with pulmonary hypoplasia, trisomy 18 and 21, cardiac malformations; incidence is 1:3,000.
  - Types:
    - Bochdalek: 90–95% cases, most common in left posterolateral location.
    - Morgagni: 5–10% cases, most common in right anterior midline.
    - Central hernia: Rare type, within center of diaphragm muscle.
  - Presents with respiratory distress, intrathoracic bowel compression within mediastinum, scaphoid abdomen, abnormally distended chest, or bowel sounds in chest; develops within 24 hours of life.
  - Diagnosed with prenatal ultrasound showing abnormal pulmonary findings or lung-to-head ratio; prenatal MRI used to evaluate liver position and lung volume; chest X-ray showing intestine within chest.
  - Treated initially with mechanical stabilization and may require inhaled nitric oxide and extracorporeal membrane oxygenation to manage pulmonary hypertension, arterial and venous access obtained, nasogastric tube used to decompress stomach.
  - Surgical repair involves subcostal or thoracotomy incision with primary repair or prosthetic closure.
- Tracheoesophageal fistula:
  - Failure of trachea separation from esophagus; incidence is 1:3,500; associated with VATER/VACTERL (vertebral, anal, cardiac, tracheoesophageal, renal, limb) syndrome or nonsyndromic anomalies.
    - V: vertebral; fused, missing, or extra vertebrae; 60–80% cases.
    - A: anorectal; anal atresia, genitourinary anomalies; 60–90% cases.
    - C: cardiac; 40–80% cases.
    - T: tracheoesophageal fistula; 50–80% cases.
    - R: renal agenesis; 50–80% cases.
    - L: radial limb hyperplasia; 40–50% cases.
  - Classified by Gross or Vogt systems (▶ Table 10.6, ▶ Fig. 10.1).
  - Presents with excessive salivation, feeding intolerance, gagging (types B, C, and D); respiratory difficulty with crying and gastric reflux into tracheobronchial tree (types C and D); delayed presentation with recurrent pneumonia, bronchospasm, or failure to thrive (type E).

Table 10.6 Tracheoesophageal fistula types

Gross classification	Vogt classification	Details
–	Type 1	Esophageal agenesis
Type A	Type 2	Proximal and distal EA
Type B	Type 3A	EA with proximal TEF
Type C	Type 3B	EA with distal TEF, 90% of cases
Type D	Type 3C	EA with proximal TEF and distal TEF
Type E or H	–	Variant of type D, TEF without EA, resembles H shape

Abbreviations: EA, esophageal atresia; TEF, tracheoesophageal fistula.

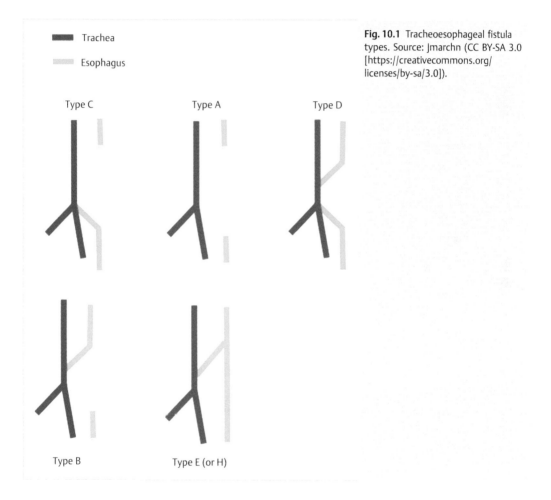

Fig. 10.1 Tracheoesophageal fistula types. Source: Jmarchn (CC BY-SA 3.0 [https://creativecommons.org/licenses/by-sa/3.0]).

- Workup:
  - Prenatal ultrasound can identify polyhydramnios.
  - Patient does not take oral nutrition until type of fistula can be identified.
  - Failure of Ryle feeding tube passage into stomach suggests esophageal atresia.
  - Chest X-ray shows dilated proximal pouch or coiled feeding tube.
  - Contrast esophagram with diluted barium can delineate pouch but risk of chemical pneumonitis.
  - Bronchoscopy and MRI preferred for identifying anatomy.
  - Evaluation of other congenital VACTER/VACTERL anomalies performed.

○ Treatment delayed 24–48 hours, feeding delayed until identification of fistula type and possible placement of feeding tube; open thoracotomy or thorascopic division performed for repair of fistula with esophageal dilation as needed; gastric transposition to cervical esophagus or colonic interposition used if unable to do primary anastomosis.

10.2.2 Congenital Heart Disease

Overview

- Most common congenital disorder in newborns, 6–13 per 1,000 live births; increased detection on prenatal screening.
- Cyanotic congenital heart disease: lesion allowing circulation of deoxygenated blood in systemic circulation by intra- or extracardiac shunting; may not be apparent unless with < 80% SpO_2 or anemia.
- Ductal-dependent congenital heart disease: PDA needed to supply lungs with right heart obstruction and for systemic supply with left heart obstruction.
- Critical congenital heart disease:
  ○ Defined by requirement for surgery or intervention within first year of life (e.g., ductal dependent and cyanotic lesions).
  ○ 25% of heart disease cases, 1% prevalence.
  ○ Most diagnosed prenatally.
  ○ Associated with prematurity, multifetal pregnancy, in utero infection (e.g., rubella, influenza), assistive reproductive technology, maternal comorbidities, and history of congenital heart disease.
  ○ Presents with shock, cyanosis, tachypnea, or pulmonary edema; some cases may not be apparent.
  ○ Requires urgent consultation with pediatric cardiologist.
- Newborn pulse oximetry screening: oximetry measured in right hand (preductal) and either foot (postductal) prior to discharge, positive if SpO_2 < 90% or < 95% in both upper and lower extremities on three measurements or > 3% difference between upper and lower extremities.
- Workup: Physical examination, pulse oximetry, chest X-ray, electrocardiography, and echocardiography; CT or MR angiography used to evaluate vascular anatomy; referral for angiography to delineate vascular connections, oxygenation, and pressures.
- Other clinical features requiring workup: Abnormal heart rate, heart location, S2 splitting, early- or midsystolic clicks, S3 gallop, pericardial friction rubs, non-innocent murmurs (▶ Table 10.7), hepatomegaly, diminished pulses in lower extremities, other congenital abnormalities.
- Indomethacin used to keep PDA open in cyanotic heart disease.
- Initial treatment involves oxygenation and hemodynamic support; treatment plans can use temporizing procedures and definitive procedures with immediate consultation from pediatric cardiology.

Table 10.7 Features of innocent murmurs

	Cardiac disease	Innocent murmur
Clinical history	• Family history of congenital heart disease • Abnormal ultrasound or ECG • Maternal risk • Age < 1 y • Respiratory difficult, cyanosis, poor growth, poor feeding, chest pain, syncope, diaphoresis	• Negative family history • Normal ultrasound or ECG • Age > 2 y • Nonsyndromic • Asymptomatic
Murmur	• Grade ≥ 3 • Holosystolic or diastolic • Abnormal S2, gallop rhythm with S3 or S4, friction rub	• Grade ≤ 2 • Short systolic, not diastolic, musical • Normal S2 and splitting, no gallop rhythm
Other	• Abnormal vital signs, hepatomegaly, extracardiac congenital anomalies • Abnormal pulse oximetry, chest X-ray, ECG, or ultrasound	• Normal vitals

Abbreviation: ECG, electrocardiogram.

Types of Congenital Heart Conditions

- Bicuspid aortic valve: Most common, 0.5–2%; isolated defect rarely diagnosed in infancy.
- Hypoplastic left heart syndrome:
  - 2–3% of congenital heart disease; results in cyanosis.
  - Small left ventricle unable to support systemic circulation.
  - Variation in mitral and aortic atresia defines types.
  - Right heart supports pulmonary and systemic circulation via PDA and atrial septal defect; can result in honeymoon period after birth where patient appears normal.
  - Staged surgeries:
    - Norwood procedure: First 2 weeks of life, allowed right ventricle supply of systemic circulation, main pulmonary artery connected to aorta, subclavian artery connected to pulmonary artery via shunt (e.g., modified Blalock-Taussig shunt), or ventricle connected to pulmonary artery via shunt (e.g., Sano shunt).
    - Bidirectional Glenn shunt procedure: 4–6 months of life; pulmonary artery connected to superior vena cava allowing oxygen-poor blood return to the heart and reducing right heart work to pump blood to lungs.
    - Fontan procedure: 1.5–3 years; pulmonary artery connected to inferior vena cava, oxygen-poor blood returned to lungs, oxygen-rich and oxygen-poor blood no longer mix in heart.
- Pulmonary atresia with intact ventricular septum:
  - 1–3% of congenital heart disease.
  - Complete obstruction of right ventricular outflow tract, varying right ventricular and tricuspid valve hypoplasia, blood returned to systemic circulation via patent foramen ovale and coronary circulation.
  - Surgical repair includes biventricular repair, univentricular palliation, 1.5 ventricle hybrid repair, and cardiac transplantation.
- Tetralogy of Fallot:
  - Most common cyanotic congenital heart disease type, 7–10% of congenital heart disease.
  - Associated with genetic conditions (e.g., Down, Alagille, DiGeorge, and velocardiofacial syndromes).
  - Features: Ventricular septal defect, right ventricle outflow obstruction (e.g., pulmonary valve, subvalvar obstruction, muscular hypertrophy), overriding aorta (aorta displaced to right with blood flow from both ventricles), right ventricle hypertrophy, associated with other cardiac defects (e.g., atrial septal defect, abnormal coronary artery branching).
  - Right ventricle outflow obstruction distinguishes severity of condition.
  - Tet spells: Episodic cyanotic spells, unclear mechanism but from occlusion of right ventricular outflow tract; results from agitation, feeding or bowel movement; can progress to loss of consciousness and cardiac arrest; reduced with squatting in older children.
  - Treatment may involve indomethacin treatment to keep PDA open; most repairs completed in infancy.
  - Surgical treatment involves combinations of closure of ventricular septal defect, dilation or patching of pulmonary obstruction, resection of infundibular muscle, and/or bypassing pulmonary obstruction via a conduit.
- Total anomalous pulmonary venous connection:
  - 0.7–1.5% of congenital heart disease; results in cyanosis.
  - All four pulmonary veins fail to connect to left atrium and drain into systemic circulation.
  - Subdivided (e.g., supracardiac, cardiac, infracardiac, mixed) based on location of pulmonary vein drainage into systemic circulation and obstructed versus unobstructed pulmonary veins.
  - Treatment depends on the subtype of venous anomaly and involves reconstruction of a normalized venous inlet.
- Transposition of great arteries:
  - 3% of congenital heart disease; results in cyanosis.
  - Most common dextro or D type; results in cyanotic heart disease with right heart supplying systemic circulation and left heart supplying pulmonary circulation; intracardiac or extracardiac connection allows mixing of blood.

- Associated with ventricular septal defects, dynamic or anatomical left ventricular outflow tract obstruction, mitral and tricuspid valve abnormalities, coronary artery abnormalities.
- Double-outlet right ventricle: defines pulmonary artery and aorta arising off right ventricle; can be seen with transposed great arteries.
- Difficult to detect by ultrasound prenatally but detected via workup for cyanotic congenital heart disease.
- Treated initially with balloon atrial septostomy followed by later vessel switch, reimplantation of coronary arteries, and closure of septal defects.
- Tricuspid atresia:
  - Third most common cyanotic heart disease.
  - Congenital agenesis or absence of tricuspid valve; blocks communication of right atrium and ventricle.
  - Subtypes include muscular, membranous, valvular, and Ebstein atresia.
  - Classified by malposition of associated vessels.
  - Associated with septal defects, right ventricular hypoplasia, pulmonary outflow obstruction, transpositions of the great arteries, pulmonary artery hypoplasia, aortic or subaortic stenosis, aortic coarctation, and coronary abnormalities.
  - Treated with modified Blalock-Taussig shunt connecting innominate artery to pulmonary artery with pulmonary artery banding to reduce pulmonary blood flow, followed by bidirectional Glenn procedure and Fontan procedure; other associated procedures performed depending on patient.
- Truncus arteriosus:
  - 4% of critical congenital heart disease; results in cyanosis.
  - Common arterial trunk supplying aorta and pulmonary arteries; cyanotic congenital heart defect.
  - Associated with a single semilunar truncal valve, aortic arch abnormalities, septal defects, coronary abnormalities, aberrant subclavian, and superior vena cava vessels.
  - Classified by Society of Thoracic Surgeons depending on origin and branches of vessels.
  - Temporization with pulmonary artery banding can be used; definitive treatment with pulmonary artery reattachment to right ventricle via conduit, repair of the truncus with a patch, closure of the ventricular septa defect.
- Coarctation of the aorta:
  - 4–6% of congenital heart disease.
  - Narrowing of descending aorta at insertion of ductus arteriosus just distal to the left subclavian artery; results in cardiac strain resulting in hypertrophy or failure.
  - Associated with Turner syndrome, single ventricle disorders, transposition of the great vessels, valvular abnormalities, septal defects, or patent foramen ovale.
  - Can be undiagnosed in adults; increased risk of cerebral aneurysms, spinal subarachnoid hemorrhage, aortic aneurysms, and aortic dissection.
  - Asymmetry of upper and lower extremity blood pressures, pulses, and oximetry can be seen.
  - Treated with balloon angioplasty, stent placement, or surgical repair (e.g., end-to-end anastomosis, subclavian flap aortoplasty, bypass graft).
- Ebstein anomaly:
  - Can result in cyanosis.
  - Abnormalities of tricuspid valve and right ventricle, variable morphology; results in displacement of annular attachments; variable degrees of tricuspid regurgitation are seen; reduced right ventricle function.
  - Associated with patent foramen ovale, septal defects, pulmonary outflow obstruction, PDA, accessory conduction pathways, and left ventricular dysfunction.
  - Treated with repair or replacement of the tricuspid valve, repair of septal defects, or cardiac ablation of accessory conduction pathways.
- Interrupted aortic arch:
  - Absence or discontinuation of the aortic arch; can occur distal to the left subclavian artery (type A), between the left carotid and subclavian (type B), or between the left innominate and carotid artery (type C).
  - Associated with ventricular septal defects.

- Treated with reconnection of the discontinued segment, closure of septal defects, and repair of a PDA.
- PDA:
  - 3–8:10,000 live births.
  - Vascular connection between the pulmonary artery and aorta, which does not obliterate into the ligamentum arteriosum.
  - Classified based on variation of anatomy; sized depending on flow rates.
  - Rise in systemic arterial oxygen tension and decrease in circulating prostaglandin E2 promote closure within 10–15 hours of delivery, complete closure at 2–3 weeks of age.
  - Associated with prematurity and genetic factors (e.g., Down syndrome, CHARGE, Cri-du-chat, Holt-Oram syndrome, and Noonan syndrome).
  - Rare risk of infective endocarditis.
  - High risk for pulmonary hypertension with larger untreated shunts.
  - Treated with indomethacin or ibuprofen for small defects, percutaneous interventional closure, or open ligation.

10.3 Gastrointestinal Abnormalities

Katie W. Russell and Stephen J. Fenton

10.3.1 Congenital Gastrointestinal Anomalies

- Anorectal malformations:
  - Needs vertebral, anal, cardiac, tracheoesophageal, renal, limb (VACTERL) workup of other organ systems during the presentation of anorectal malformations due to high rate of associated anomalies.
  - Multiple anatomic variations.
  - Female patients.
    - 85% of cases are low-lying lesions.
    - Rectovestibular fistula.
    - Rectovaginal fistula.
    - Perineal fistula.
    - Anal atresia without fistula.
    - Anal stenosis.
    - Cloaca (single opening for the vagina, urethra, and rectum).
  - Male patients:
    - 85% of cases are high-lying lesions.
    - Rectourethral fistula (bulbar).
    - Rectoprostatic fistula.
    - Anal atresia without fistula.
    - Anal stenosis.
  - Repair depends on anatomy:
    - Low-lying lesions are typically repaired via primary posterior sagittal anorectoplasty (PSARP).
    - High-lying or complicated lesions may require a colostomy followed by PSARP often with laparoscopic assistance.
  - Long-term bowel management with enemas, laxative, or a combination is essential for function.
- Hirschsprung disease.
  - Most common cause of colonic obstruction in neonates.
  - 85% of cases in neonates occur at the rectosigmoid junction.
  - Pathophysiology is failure of neural crest ganglion cells to progress in a craniocaudal fashion.
  - Most common sign is failure to pass meconium in the first 48 hours of life.
  - Explosive, watery stool after rectal examination is a classic examination finding but not always present.
  - Rectal biopsy is diagnostic, showing an absence of ganglion cells and hypertrophic nerves in the myenteric plexus.

- Contrast enema can also be helpful showing the transition point from normal to abnormal bowel.
- Irrigations are often needed to bridge to surgery and sometimes after surgery.
- Treatment is colonic resection to the level of ganglion cells and an anorectal pull-through.
- Hirschsprung-associated enterocolitis is a deadly complication.
  - Admit patient and administer intravenous (IV) fluids, IV antibiotics, and rectal irrigations.
- Small left colon syndrome:
  - Colonic caliber change usually at the splenic flexure causing obstruction in the neonate.
  - At least half of the cases are associated with maternal diabetes.
  - Contrast enema typically both diagnostic and therapeutic.
- Meconium plug syndrome (occurs in the colon):
  - Inspissated meconium within the colon that causes neonatal obstruction.
  - Treatment by water-soluble contrast enema with evacuation of cast-like plugs from the colon; may need to be repeated.
  - Spontaneous stools usually follow enema.
  - Consider rectal biopsy to rule out Hirschsprung disease if unable to follow-up closely.
- Meconium ileus (occurs in the ileum):
  - Bowel obstruction that occurs because the consistency of the meconium is thicker than normal within the ileum.
  - Most affected children have cystic fibrosis and need gene testing and confirmatory sweat testing.
  - Water-soluble contrast enema is the first line of treatment; may need to be repeated.
  - Some infants will require an operation to clear the obstruction. Most often it is done by opening bowel and flushing out meconium. Others require ostomy with mucus fistula to flush out downstream intestine.
  - DIOS (distal intestinal obstructive syndrome):
    - Similar disease that occurs in older children with cystic fibrosis; due to thickened stool from lack of pancreatic enzymes.
    - Treatment includes water-soluble contrast enemas, oral Mucomyst, and pancreatic enzyme replacement.
- Jejunoileal atresia:
  - In utero vascular accident causes interruption of the blood supply to the small intestine and resulting atresia.
  - Treatment is resection and primary anastomosis at the time of resection or ostomy and delayed anastomosis depending on patient status.
  - The length of bowel missing from the prenatal vascular compromise determines the severity of disease; if a large amount of bowel is gone, short gut syndrome may occur.
- Alimentary duplications:
  - Duplications can occur anywhere along the enteric tract, but are most common within the small bowel.
  - Presentation can be incidental or a variety of symptoms depending on location including obstruction, bleeding, and infection.
  - Resection is recommended in most instances to prevent complication of malignant transformation.
- Malrotation:
  - Bilious emesis in a neonate is a surgical emergency until proven otherwise.
  - Malrotation is the failure of the intestine to complete the normal counterclockwise 270-degree rotation with fixation of the mesentery to the retroperitoneum.
  - Patients with malrotation are also at risk for midgut volvulus because of the narrow-based mesentery.
  - Volvulus is twisting of the intestine around the superior mesenteric artery (SMA) leading to infarction of the entire midgut (distal duodenum to distal transverse colon, including all of the small bowels). Most affected children present within the first month of life and almost all present with the first year.
  - Bilious emesis should be worked up with an upper gastrointestinal series to the ligament of Treitz, looking for normal positioning of the duodenum (characteristic C loop that crosses midline with fourth portion rising to the level of the pylorus).

- ○ Symptomatic children with malrotation need surgery, and a patient with midgut volvulus needs emergent surgery.
- ○ Treatment is through a Ladd procedure: reduce volvulus, resect abnormal attachments to the right upper quadrant (Ladd bands), broaden the mesentery, straighten out the duodenum, place the colon on the patient's left side, place the small bowel on the patient's right side, appendectomy.
- ○ Delay in operative treatment of midgut volvulus can lead to loss of midgut with significant resection resulting in short gut syndrome or death.
- Duodenal atresia:
  - ○ Annular pancreas, duodenal web, or preduodenal portal vein causing obstruction in the duodenum.
  - ○ Associated with Trisomy 21 and cardiac defects.
  - ○ Prenatal diagnosis is made by seeing polyhydramnios and a double bubble sign (fluid in the stomach and duodenum).
  - ○ Postnatal abdominal X-ray with a double bubble sign is confirmatory (air in the stomach and duodenum).
  - ○ Treatment is duodenoduodenostomy typically using a double diamond technique.
- Gastroschisis:
  - ○ Protrusion of abdominal viscera through the abdominal wall to the right of the umbilicus.
  - ○ The viscera, usually small bowel, colon, and stomach, is not covered by a membrane, but instead are bathed in the amniotic fluid, sometimes leading to matting of the bowel.
  - ○ Typically not associated with other anomalies, not including malrotation.
  - ○ Initial treatment involves placing the infant in a plastic bag from the nipples down with moisture to keep organs moist; fluid resuscitation is used to reduce insensate fluid loss.
  - ○ Closure techniques range from primary reduction and sutureless closure to gradual reduction in a Silastic silo followed by abdominal wall closure in the operating room.
  - ○ 20% will be complicated by atresia, perforation, or in the worst circumstance midgut volvulus and bowel death before or after delivery.
- Omphalocele:
  - ○ Midline defect in which the abdominal wall is not fully formed and viscera are covered with the amniotic sac.
  - ○ Consider giant omphalocele when the liver is contained in the sac or the fascial defect is greater than 5 cm. These children are born with underdeveloped lungs (pulmonary hypoplasia) and varying degrees of pulmonary hypertension.
  - ○ Highly associated with other anomalies (50%), most often a congenital heart defect. All children with an omphalocele, including small defect, should undergo echocardiogram.
  - ○ Pentalogy of Cantrell includes cardiac defects, pericardial defects, sternal absence, diaphragmatic hernia, and omphalocele.
  - ○ Depending on how the infant is doing, small omphaloceles are typically closed during the initial hospitalization.
  - ○ Increasingly, pediatric surgeons are managing giant omphaloceles with nonoperative management with initial wound care of the omphalocele, allowing it to epithelialize, followed by closure at 1 year of age, a strategy called "paint and wait."

10.3.2 Acquired Gastrointestinal Conditions

- Necrotizing enterocolitis (NEC):
  - ○ Inflammation and infection of the intestine that occurs usually in premature infants.
  - ○ Risk factors include prematurity, small for gestational age, hypoxia, hypotension, anemia, ventilation, and sepsis.
  - ○ The classic presentation is bloody stool after enteric feedings.
  - ○ Diagnosis is made by abdominal X-ray or abdominal ultrasound with a finding of pneumatosis of the bowel.
  - ○ Treatment is either bowel rest and antibiotics or surgery.
  - ○ Indications for surgery include pneumoperitoneum, portal venous gas, or progressive peritonitis despite bowel rest and antibiotics.

- Spontaneous intestinal perforation.
  - A single perforation of the intestine of a neonate without underlying NEC.
  - Also common in premature infants and can be difficult to differentiate from NEC.
  - Can be associated with indomethacin used for closure of the PDA.
  - Treatment is surgery with bowel resection and ostomy creation.
  - In a very small birthweight baby (< 1,000 g), peritoneal drainage may be effective in evacuating the infection.
- Pyloric stenosis:
  - Gastric outlet obstruction that occurs in infants typically between 3 and 8 weeks.
  - Presents with projectile nonbilious emesis.
  - Diagnosis is made with ultrasound showing a thickened (> 4 mm) and elongated (> 14 mm) pylorus.
  - Electrolyte abnormalities include hypochloremic, hypokalemic metabolic alkalosis.
  - Resuscitation is crucial to correct electrolytes before patient undergoes general anesthesia.
  - Treatment is by laparoscopic or open pyloromyotomy.
- Ileocecal intussusception:
  - Intussusception is a type of bowel obstruction that usually occurs in children between 3 months and 3 years of age.
  - The terminal ileum invaginates into the cecum.
  - An antecedent viral or bacterial upper respiratory or gastrointestinal illness is common and likely incites lymphoid hyperplasia that acts as a lead point for the intussusception.
  - In older children (> 4 years), one needs to be suspicious of a pathologic lead point such as a Meckel diverticulum, polyp, or lymphoma.
  - Treatment is typically done by a radiologist performing an air or contrast enema to reduce the intussusception.
  - Surgical intervention is required in the case that radiologic reduction is unsuccessful after multiple attempts or if the patient is septic, has peritoneal signs on examination, or evidence of pneumoperitoneum on imaging. Surgery includes manual reduction of the intussusception. Ileocecectomy rarely required.
- Appendicitis:
  - By far the most common abdominal surgical urgency in children.
  - Likely caused by obstruction of the appendiceal lumen by lymphoid tissue or a fecalith leading to inflammation and infection.
  - In the United States, laparoscopic or open appendectomy is the standard of care, but there is some evidence that nonoperative therapy with antibiotics is also effective in some early cases of simple appendicitis.
  - Perforated appendicitis with large abscess formation is often treated with a draining procedure and antibiotics.
  - Interval appendectomy is indicated if there is a fecalith.
- Meckel diverticulum:
  - A Meckel diverticulum is the most common anomaly of the gastrointestinal tract, occurring in at least 2% of the population.
  - It results from the incomplete obliteration of the omphalomesenteric duct.
  - Most are asymptomatic but can cause obstruction, bleeding, or diverticulitis, all of which require a Meckel diverticulectomy.
  - Bleeding usually occurs from ectopic gastric tissue that secretes acid and causes ulcers in the ileum distal to the diverticulum. A "Meckel" scintigraphy scan is sometimes helpful in diagnosis.
  - The diverticulum can adhere to the anterior abdominal wall or other structures, causing a lead point for intussusception or for the bowel to twist or kink, causing obstruction.
  - Inflammation of the diverticulum can mimic appendicitis.
- Foreign body ingestion:
  - This is a common problem seen by pediatric surgeons.
  - Button battery ingestion is a surgical emergency because they can erode into the esophagus, leading to tracheoesophageal fistula or vascular injury.
  - Ingestion of multiple magnets may also require surgery because the magnets can connect through multiple loops of bowel, forming fistulae, or result in a bowel obstruction.

Table 10.8 Choledochal cysts

Type	%	Description	Treatment
I	85%	Fusiform dilation of CBD, normal intrahepatic ducts	Resection with hepaticoduodenostomy or hepaticojejunostomy
II	3%	A true diverticulum off the CBD	Resection; may be able to save CBD; may need reconstruction similarly to type I cysts
III	1%	Involvement of intraduodenal duct and sphincter of Oddi	Resection, possible reconstruction vs. sphincteroplasty
IV	10%	Multiple cysts both extra- and intrahepatic	Resection of CBD and possible lobectomy if cysts confined to only part of the liver with reconstruction
V	1%	Caroli disease with multiple intrahepatic cysts leading to hepatic fibrosis	May need liver transplant

Abbreviation: CBD, common bile duct.

- Most foreign bodies that pass the pylorus will pass all the way through the intestinal tract, rarely there will be obstruction at the ileocecal valve that requires operative intervention.
- Foreign bodies that are retained in the stomach can usually be removed endoscopically.
- Older patients with recurrent foreign body ingestion may need psychiatric evaluation.

10.3.3 Hepatobiliary

- Choledochal cysts (▶ Table 10.8):
  - Dilation of the common bile duct (CBD) and/or hepatic ducts thought to be related to anomalous junction of the CBD and pancreatic duct leading to reflux of pancreatic enzymes.
  - These need to be resected because of risk of cholangiocarcinoma, pancreatitis, cholangitis, and obstructive jaundice.
- Biliary atresia:
  - Progressive jaundice persisting > 2 weeks after birth is concerning.
  - The cause is unknown, but the bile ducts become inflamed and obliterated causing biliary obstruction and hepatic fibrosis.
  - Treatment includes a Kasai portoenterostomy.
    - After Kasai, one-third of patients recover, one-third require a transplant within the first year, and one-third require a liver transplant after 1 year.
  - Outcomes are improved if surgery is done before 3 months of age.

10.3.4 Hernias

- Umbilical:
  - Failure of closure of the umbilical ring.
  - Even large umbilical hernias will become smaller within the first year of life.
  - Incarceration is very uncommon.
  - The majority is closed spontaneously by 4 years of age.
  - Umbilical hernia repair is typically delayed until 4–5 years of age and includes a primary closure of the umbilical defect.
- Epigastric:
  - Small defect in the fascia above the umbilicus but below the sternum usually containing preperitoneal fat.
  - Because of fat-containing falciform ligament, the risk of intestinal incarceration is extremely small.
  - Repair is required if the child is symptomatic or the bulge is unsightly.
  - Treatment is primary repair, taking care to mark the spot before anesthesia because it can be difficult to find when the patient is anesthetized.
- Inguinal:
  - Inguinal hernia occurs in approximately 3–5% of term male infants and 10–15% of premature male infants.

○ The testicles descend into the scrotum around 30 weeks' gestation, after which the patent processus vaginalis should involute and obliterate. Incomplete obliteration results in an indirect inguinal hernia.

○ Repair is recommended to prevent incarceration of bowel and growth of the defect from constant stretching.

○ The timing of repair is somewhat controversial but typically occurs when the child is able to safely undergo general anesthesia.

○ Laparoscopic and open techniques are used with comparable results.

10.4 Pediatric Neoplasms

Michael Karsy

10.4.1 Overview

- Overall, neoplasms in children are rare compared with adults; 13,500 cases and 1,500 deaths in children age 0–14 years compared with 1.4 million cases and 575,000 deaths in adults.
- 2nd leading cause of death after trauma.
- Leukemia (33%), brain tumors (25%), lymphomas (8%), soft-tissue sarcomas (7%), and primary malignant bone tumors (4%) are most common (% of pediatric tumors).
- 350,000 adult survivors of pediatric cancer; therapy results in infertility, stunted development, cardiotoxicity, secondary cancers (3–12% of survivors).

10.4.2 Specific Pediatric Tumors

- Neuroblastoma:
  ○ Tumors of neural crest origin.
  ○ Most common malignant pediatric abdominal tumor, most common tumor in infants, most common extracranial solid tumor in children.
  ○ Can be identified prenatally in some cases.
  ○ 800 cases/year in the United States.
  ○ 90% cases diagnosed by the age of 5 years, 50% of cases diagnosed by the age of 2 years, 66% of cases spread to lymph nodes by the time of diagnosis.
  ○ 80% overall 5-year survival.
  ○ Presents: Catecholamine excess resulting in hypertension (25% of cases), vasoactive intestinal peptide excess, retroperitoneal abdominal mass, less commonly cervicothoracic mass causing respiratory distress, spinal cord compression. or Horner syndrome.
  ○ Diagnosis: Urinary catecholamine assay, abdominal X-ray shows tumor calcification, ultrasound delineates solid and cystic components, computed tomography (CT) and magnetic resonance imaging (MRI) to outline size and location of tumor, metaiodobenzylguanidine (MIBG) nuclear imaging can evaluate primary tumor and metastatic bone involvement.
  ○ Treatment depends on Children's Oncology Group risk category depending on age, *MYCN* gene copies, and histology.
    – < 6 months of age with small tumor: Observation.
    – Low risk (stage 1, 2A/B): Surgical excision alone, 95% 5-year survival.
    – Intermediate risk (stage 3): Surgery and chemotherapy, 90–95% 5-year survival.
    – High risk (stage 3 with amplified *MYCN*, stage 4): Chemotherapy followed by > 90% resection, radiotherapy, autologous hematopoietic stem cell rescue, biological therapies; 40–50% 5-year survival.
  ○ International Neuroblastoma Risk Group classification based on age, histology, *MYCN* gene amplification, 11q aberration, and DNA ploidy used to delineate four risk categories.
  ○ Poor prognosis for stage 3 and 4 tumors.
- Wilms tumor/nephroblastoma:
  ○ Most common primary malignant pediatric renal tumor, 2nd most common abdominal tumor.
  ○ 500 cases/year.

- ○ Most cases diagnosed before the age of 10 years, two-thirds diagnosed before the age of 5 years.
- ○ 5–10% show multiple or bilateral tumors.
- ○ Differential diagnosis includes mesoblastic nephroma, which is most common benign renal neoplasm in infants with 60% diagnosed before 6 months and nephrectomy being curative.
- ○ Presents: Mean age 36 months, abdominal or flank pain (33%) or asymptomatic abdominal mass, hematuria, hypertension (50%), associated congenital abnormalities (15%; WAGR syndrome: Wilms tumor, aniridia, genitourinary malformation, mental retardation; Beckwith–Wiedemann syndrome, Denys–Drash syndrome).
- ○ Diagnosis: Ultrasound initially used to determine tumor size, vascular and renal involvement; CT to determine renal origin, evaluate for bilateral tumors, and metastatic spread to liver or lungs.
- ○ Treatment: Resection (e.g., nephrectomy), staging with hilar and regional lymph node sample, renal vein thrombus removal, followed by neoadjuvant chemotherapy and radiation; National Wilms Tumor Study Group provides recommendations.
- ○ Overall 90% survival, 5–15% risk of recurrence mostly within the first 2 years.
- ○ National Wilms Tumor Study staging delineates five stages depending on tumor spread before chemotherapy treatment; Societe Internationale d'Oncologie Pediatrique (SIOP) staging used in Europe after chemotherapy treatment.
- ○ Improved prognosis with younger age, less anaplasia or sarcomatous changes, less spread to lymph nodes and other organs, lower tumor stage, better response to treatment, loss of heterozygosity of 1p and 16q.
- Brain and spine tumors:
  - ○ See Chapter 14.4 Neurosurgical Neoplasms.
- Rhabdomyosarcoma (RMS):
  - ○ 50% of soft-tissue sarcomas, 350 cases/year.
  - ○ Two-thirds of cases diagnosed before the age of 6 years.
  - ○ Associated with neurofibromatosis (*NF1* mutation) and Li–Fraumeni (*p53* mutation), Beckwith–Wiedemann (*IGF-2* mutation), and Costello (*HRAS* mutation) syndromes.
  - ○ Histological types:
    - – Embryonal: Intermediate prognosis, most common, occurs in young children and head/neck and genitourinary tract.
    - – Botryoid and spindle cell: Less common, favorable prognosis, grape-like gross appearance, occurs in bladder or vagina of infants or nasopharynx of older children.
    - – Sclerosing and spindle cell: Less common, poor prognosis.
    - – Alveolar: Poor prognosis.
    - – Anaplastic: Poor prognosis.
  - ○ Presents most commonly in head/neck (35–40% cases), genitourinary tract (25% cases), and extremities (20%); results in painful mass with swelling; 25% of cases have distant metastasis at the time of diagnosis.
  - ○ Diagnosis: Diagnostic biopsy performed when possible including enlarged lymph nodes but coordinated with surgical planning to reduce risk of tract seeding, genetic subtyping and karyotyping important for prognosis and treatment identification; CT or MRI staging performed; lumbar puncture rarely used for parameningeal RMS.
  - ○ Treatment involves resection and reconstruction, chemotherapy, and radiation; clinical group and TNM staging system used to assign treatment and predict prognosis.
- Retinoblastoma:
  - ○ Most common intraocular tumor.
  - ○ 10–15% of infant cancers; 95% 5-year survival with treatment otherwise uniformly fatal; limited eye salvage.
  - ○ Associated with retinoblastoma (*RB1*) gene mutation; 15% of cases familial.
  - ○ Enlarging tumor shows exophytic, endophytic (e.g., vitreal), and diffuse-infiltrating patterns.
  - ○ At-risk children with familial history of retinoblastoma face frequent screening through childhood or genetic testing.
  - ○ Trilateral retinoblastoma: Unilateral or bilateral retinoblastoma with pineal, suprasellar, or parasellar tumors; 44% 5-year survival for pineal trilateral retinoblastoma; 57% 5-year survival for nonpineal trilateral retinoblastoma.

- Leukocoria in children < 2 years, strabismus, nystagmus; less likely decreased visual acuity, inflammation, family history of disease, iris heterochromia; most present with advanced intraocular disease.
  - Diagnosis: Prompted ophthalmological follow-up required including physical examination, ophthalmological examination under anesthesia, ocular ultrasound, optic coherence tomography, and MRI of brain/orbits; metastatic workup performed if clear evidence of extraocular tumor invasion, otherwise low yield.
  - Treatment: Biopsy contraindicated because of tumor seeding; vision-sparing therapy initially considered including chemotherapy (intravitreous, intraocular, periocular, systemic), cryotherapy, laser photoablation, and I-125 brachytherapy; external beam radiation therapy or enucleation used for higher risk tumors or salvage therapy.
  - Patients monitored closely after enucleation because of risk of recurrence within 12–24 months.
  - Classified via International Classification for Intraocular Retinoblastoma or other systems, divided into five groups (A–E).
  - Metastatic disease shows poor prognosis (50% 1-year survival); multimodal therapy, external beam radiotherapy, and autologous hematopoietic stem cell rescue may be used.
  - 30–40% risk of secondary malignancy with heritable retinoblastoma compared with 2% risk for sporadic disease; secondary diseases include trilateral pineal retinoblastoma, osteogenic and soft-tissue sarcoma among others; continued MRI screening recommended.
- Sacrococcygeal teratoma:
  - Most common overall pediatric germ cell tumor and pediatric extragonadal germ cell tumor; rare in adults.
  - Tumor contains cells from all three germ layers; mature versus immature teratomas determined by degree of cellular differentiation; malignant teratomas contain malignant features (e.g., yolk sac component or alpha-fetoprotein production, embryonal carcinoma, primitive neuroectodermal tumor).
  - Presents: *In utero* mass off caudal end of fetus, obstruction of the rectum or bladder.
  - Altman classification describes degree of externally versus internally visible tumor.
  - Currarino triad: Autosomal dominant condition with (1) sacral malformation, (2) presacral mass (e.g., teratoma, anterior sacral meningocele), and (3) anorectal malformation; 20% of cases have all three abnormalities.
  - Diagnosis: Ultrasound can identify mass position, track size *in utero*, and distinguish solid versus cystic components; evaluation of bladder outlet obstruction, hydronephrosis, rectal stenosis/atresia, and high output cardiac failure can be performed by ultrasound; MRI evaluates extent of tumor and distinguishes distal neural tube defect (e.g., myelomeningocele, myelocystocele).
  - Overall survival is 73%; worse prognosis with larger tumors, hydrops, and higher solid tumor components; high risk of recurrence with inability to resect all tumors.
  - Treatment: Observation for smaller tumors, delivery after 36 weeks, resection and reconstruction used postnatally; incompletely resected tumors can be treated with chemotherapy, *in utero* laser ablation; bladder drainage and cyst aspiration have been trialed; *ex utero* resection has been evaluated in high-risk patients (e.g., high-output cardiac failure, tumor hemorrhage, nonreassuring fetal testing, impending labor due to tumor).
  - Risk of fecal/urinary incontinence and lower limb weakness with or without treatment.

10.5 Craniofacial Anomalies

Fatma Betul Tuncer and Faizi Siddiqi

10.5.1 Cleft Lip and/or Palate

- Epidemiology[2]:
  - Cleft lip:
    - Incidence varies with ethnicity: Asian (1:500) > Caucasian (1:1,000) > Black (1:2,000).
    - Left:right:Bilateral = 6:3:1.

- Risk factors: Family history; maternal use of ethanol, steroids, barbiturates, diazepam, isotretinoin, maternal smoking, advanced paternal age.
      - < 15% of cases are syndromic: Van der Woude syndrome (lower lip pits), trisomy 21.
   ○ Cleft palate:
      - The third most common congenital abnormality following club foot and cleft lip.
      - Can be associated with cleft lip (cleft lip and palate) or isolated (isolated cleft palate).
      - Cleft lip with palate is more common than the isolated cleft palate.
   ○ Isolated cleft palate:
      - 1 in 2,000, no ethnic variation in incidence.
      - More common in females.
      - 50% of cases are associated with syndromes compared with < 15% of cleft lip and palate cases.
      - Associated syndromes: Velocardiofacial syndrome, DiGeorge syndrome, Stickler syndrome.
- Diagnosis:
   ○ Made by clinical examination.
   ○ Prenatal ultrasound and magnetic resonance imaging (MRI) have increased the prenatal diagnosis of cleft lip and palate (especially of cleft lip), allowing families to meet with plastic surgeon before the delivery.
   ○ Cleft may be seen at the lip level, alveolar line, and/or palatal level. It can be unilateral or bilateral. Any combination of cleft lip and/or palate is possible.
   ○ Types of cleft lip (▶ Fig. 10.2):
      - Complete cleft lip: Cleft of the upper lip, nasal sill, and alveolar line. Has greater nasal deformity than other types.
      - Incomplete cleft lip: Cleft of the upper lip, intact nasal sill.
      - Microform cleft lip: Notched vermillion–cutaneous junction, elevated cupid's bow < 3 mm.[3]
   ○ Nasal deformity in cleft lip: When there is a cleft lip, varying degrees of the following findings in nose may occur on the affected side: alar flattening; inferior, posterior, and lateral displacement of the alar base; hypoplastic maxilla; shortened columella; deviation of nasal septum (to the nondeviated side).
   ○ Types of cleft palate:
      - Complete cleft palate: Cleft of the primary and secondary palates, which are separated at the level of incisive foramen.
      - Incomplete cleft palate: Cleft of the secondary palate, does not extend to incisive foramen.
      - Submucous cleft palate: Specific subtype of cleft palate that appears intact in physical examination, but muscles and bone are separated as in cleft palate; bony notch in the hard palate, zona pellucida (bluish mucosa in the midline that trans-illuminates), and bifid uvula can be seen.
   ○ Another classification system for cleft lip and palate is Veau classification (▶ Fig. 10.3):
      - Veau type I: Incomplete cleft, soft palate only.
      - Veau type II: Hard and soft palate, secondary palate only.
      - Veau type III: Complete unilateral cleft lip and palate.
      - Veau type IV: Complete bilateral cleft lip and palate.
- Clinical manifestations of cleft palate:
   ○ Difficulty feeding: Specialized bottles (Habermann, Dr. Brown's) are often needed.
   ○ Velopharyngeal insufficiency: The inability to generate intraoral pressure because of nasal air emission in cleft palate patients frequently manifests as articulation difficulties.

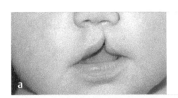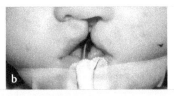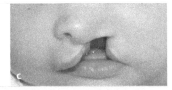

Fig. 10.2 (a–c) Types of cleft lip based on severity.

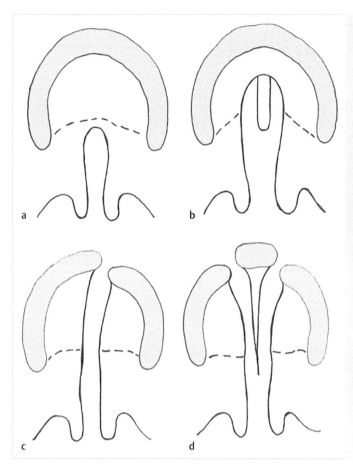

Fig. 10.3 (a–d) Veau classification of cleft lip and palate.

- ○ Hypernasality: Excessive nasal resonance during the production of vowels.
- ○ Hearing disorders: Chronic otitis media due to Eustachian tube dysfunction. Tensor veli palatine muscle that functions to open up Eustachian tube and normalize pressure fail to do so; thus, fluid builds up in the middle ear, causing recurrent otitis media, inflammation, and scarring.
- ○ The consequences of orofacial cleft are not limited to cosmetic deformities but also speech problems, hearing loss, dental anomalies, swallowing defects, and growth disturbance.
- Treatment of cleft lip[4]:
  - ○ Usually undertaken around 3 months of age (rules of 10: > 10 weeks old, > 10 pounds, Hb > 10 mg/dL).
  - ○ Preoperative molding can be used starting after birth to bring cleft segments together and to minimize tension across cleft after the surgery. It can be in the form of lip taping, nasoalveolar molding (NAM), orthodontic appliance (Latham), or surgical lip adhesion.
  - ○ Goals of treatment: Achieving symmetry, reconstruction of orbicularis oris, and correction of nasal deformity.
  - ○ Surgical techniques:
    - – Millard repair and its modifications: Rotation and lengthening of medial lip segment (noncleft side) and advancement of lateral lip segment (cleft side).
    - – Fisher anatomical subunit repair.
  - ○ Revision surgeries for lip (hypertrophic scarring, short lip, vermilion notching) or nose (cleft septorhinoplasty) may be needed before school age or at adolescent period.

- Treatment of cleft palate:
  - Timing varies from one center to another; can be done at one or two stages. Soft palate should be ideally repaired between 8 and 12 months of age for optimal speech production. Some centers delay hard palate repair until 2 years of age to minimize negative effects of surgery on maxillary growth.
  - Goals of treatment: Separation of oral and nasal cavities, speech (velopharyngeal competence), hearing, and prevention of recurrent otitis media (ear tubes may be inserted at the time of repair).
  - Surgical techniques:
    - Straight line repair with intravelar veloplasty: Identification of abnormally inserted palatal muscles and repositioning posteriorly in the transverse fashion.
    - Furlow's double opposing Z-plasty: Lengthening of palate and overlapping of palatal muscles by performing reverse Z-plasties on the oral and nasal mucosa.
  - Secondary surgeries for palate: Palatal fistula repair, speech surgeries (sphincter pharyngoplasty, pharyngeal flap), orthognathic surgeries for midface hypoplasia (LeFort I advancement, mandibular setback, double jaw, etc.).
  - Alveolar bone grafting:
    - Alveolar cleft and commonly associating nasolabial fistula can be repaired and grafted with bone or bone substitute before eruption of the canine teeth. Timing of this surgery varies between centers. Grafting of the alveolus at the time of cleft lip and palate repair is known as primary bone grafting and grafting at a later stage is known as secondary bone grafting.
    - Goals of surgery: Achieving enough bone support for canine tooth eruption, orthodontic movement, and stable dental arch; prevention of maxillary collapse on the cleft side; elevation of alar base; separation of antrum and nasal cavity.
    - Autologous iliac crest cancellous bone graft is the most common technique for alveolar bone grafting. Bone morphogenetic protein-2 (off-label use) and demineralized bone matrix have been shown to have equal results with autologous bone grafting.[5]

10.5.2 Craniosynostosis

- Etiology:
  - Premature fusion of one or more of the cranial sutures causing abnormal head shape.
  - Virchow's law: Growth of skull is restricted perpendicular to the affected suture. Compensatory growth occurs parallel to the affected suture.
- Epidemiology:
  - Incidence is 1 in 2,500 live births.
- Normal physiology:
  - Brain size triples by 1 year of age.
  - Posterior fontanelle closes around 3–6 months and anterior fontanelle closes at 9–12 months.
  - Metopic suture fuses the earliest at 5–9 months; may show ridging during closure. This condition should be differentiated from trigonocephaly, where deformity is present at birth.
- Classification of synostoses:
  - Single- versus multisuture synostosis.
  - Syndromic versus nonsyndromic synostosis.
  - Single-suture synostosis (▶ Fig. 10.4). From the most common to the rarest form:
    - Sagittal: Scaphocephaly (long and narrow head shape), increased anteroposterior diameter, decreased width, decreased cephalic index (< 75), frontal bossing, and occipital coning.
    - Metopic: Trigonocephaly (triangular head), supraorbital retrusion, bitemporal narrowing, hypotelorism.
    - Unicoronal: Anterior plagiocephaly, flattening of ipsilateral forehead and supraorbital rim, bossing of contralateral forehead, nasal tip deviated to the affected side, shallow orbit, harlequin deformity, and chin deviated to the contralateral side.
    - Bicoronal: Recession of supraorbital ridges, brachycephaly (short in anteroposterior distance), turribrachycephaly (tall and short skull).
    - Lambdoid: Posterior plagiocephaly, flattening of ipsilateral occiput, mastoid bulge; the rarest form of single-suture synostosis.

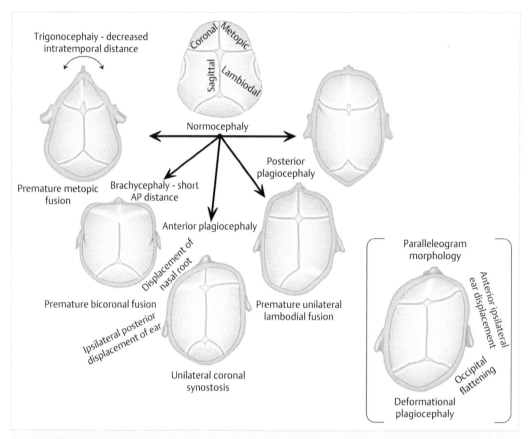

Fig. 10.4 Single-suture synostoses.

- Syndromic synostoses (Apert, Crouzon, Pfeiffer syndromes, etc.):
  - Often linked to an autosomal dominant mutation (*FGFR2* gene in Crouzon and Pfeiffer and *TWIST-1* gene in Saethre–Chotzen) and may be associated with dysmorphisms of the face, trunk, and extremities: exorbitism (Crouzon, Apert, Pfeiffer), parrot beak (Apert), cleft palate (Apert), complex syndactyly of hands and feet (Apert), broad thumbs and halluces (Pfeiffer), low frontal hairline (Saethre–Chotzen).
  - Commonly associated with bicoronal synostosis.
  - Higher risk of increased intracranial pressure than single-suture synostoses.[6]
  - Other considerations: Midface hypoplasia, malocclusion, and obstructive sleep apnea are very common in this patient population. LeFort III advancement and other orthographic surgeries may be needed in early childhood or at skeletal maturity.
- Diagnosis and evaluation:
  - Primarily done by physical examination; computed tomography (CT) scans can be used for confirmation of diagnosis, surgical planning, and/or evaluation of syndromic synostosis.
  - Physical examination shows palpable ridge and abnormal cranial morphology based on the affected suture.
  - Funduscopic examination may be warranted, especially in syndromic or multisuture synostosis for increased signs of intracranial pressure.
- Treatment:
  - Goals of treatment are expanding intracranial volume, reducing risk of increased intracranial pressure, and normalizing the head shape.
  - Timing and choice of treatment are highly variable.

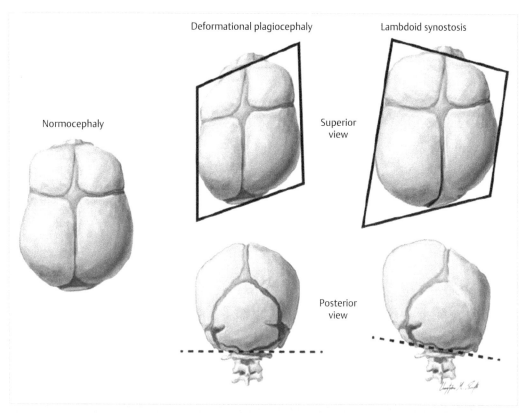

Fig. 10.5 Deformational plagiocephaly.

- ○ Major risk of surgery is blood loss and risks of transfusion in younger patients given their small circulating blood volume.
- ○ Endoscopic strip craniectomy.
  - – Done between 2 and 6 months.
  - – Mainly used for single-suture synostoses; requires postoperative helmet therapy for 3–12 months.
  - – Duration of helmet therapy depends on age at the time of surgery and the involved suture.
  - – Less risk of blood transfusion and shorter hospitalization than cranial vault remodeling.
- ○ Cranial vault remodeling:
  - – Typically performed between 6 and 12 months, but earlier if elevated intracranial pressure or multisuture synostosis.
  - – Although bones are more malleable and dura can spontaneously heal bone defects when surgery is performed at a younger age, the likelihood of recurrence increases.
  - – One to two nights of observation in intensive care unit needed postoperatively.
  - – Could be anterior, posterior, or total cranial vault remodeling based on the deformity.
  - – Fronto-orbital advancement is a type of anterior cranial vault remodeling.
- ○ Posterior vault expansion with distraction osteogenesis[7]:
  - – Recently popularized for treatment of multisuture or syndromic synostosis, or elevated intracranial pressure.
  - – Requires two-staged operation; expands intracranial volume more than single-stage operation.
- • Deformational plagiocephaly (▶ Fig. 10.5):
  - ○ Not a synostosis but deformation of skull secondary to external forces (supine positioning as a result of "Back to Sleep" campaign, musculoskeletal problems such as torticollis).
  - ○ Frequently mistaken for lambdoid or unicoronal synostosis.

○ Head assumes a parallelogram shape with occipital flattening and ipsilateral frontal bossing. Ear is displaced anterolaterally on the same side, whereas in synostotic plagiocephaly head is in trapezoid shape, ear is displaced posteriorly and inferiorly, facial asymmetry is common, and mastoid bulge is present in lambdoid synostosis.

○ Diagnosis: Physical examination.

○ Treatment:
  – Observation, head positioning, and increase tummy time for mild to moderate deformities.
  – Custom-made molding helmet therapy for moderate to severe deformities.
  – Treatment of any associating torticollis.

10.6 Genitourinary Abnormalities

Michael Karsy

10.6.1 Common Pediatric Genitourinary Issues

- Pediatric urinary tract infection (UTI):
  ○ Cause:
    – Similar but distinct workup compared with adults (see Chapter 11.2 Urinary Tract Infection and Inflammation).
    – Incidence is 3%; childhood risk is 8% in girls versus 2% in boys, uncircumcised boys 10 times higher risk than circumcised boys.
    – Can present with more nonspecific symptoms than adults (e.g., poor feeding, irritability, abdominal distension, fever, flank pain) and requires higher clinical suspicion.
    – Recurrent infection results in renal scarring, renal failure, and hypertension.
    – Most common serious complication of pediatric UTI is pyelonephritis.
  ○ Special considerations in pediatric patients:
    – Bacterial UTI more likely due to dysfunctional voiding, congenital anomalies, stones, or sexual abuse.
    – Fungal UTI associated with immunosuppression, congenital anomalies, or invasive lines; significant risk in neonatal intensive care unit.
    – Viral cystitis associated with immunosuppression (e.g., organ transplantation) or chemotherapy.
    – Congenital anomalies and obstruction (see Chapter 10.6.2 Congenital Anomalies).
    – Sexual abuse: Considered in children with external bruising, fear of examination, prolonged incontinence.
  ○ Stones and infection:
    – More commonly due to metabolic abnormalities.
    – Presents with fever, dysuria, urgency, and UTI.
    – Flank pain possible but not as common in children < 5 years.
    – Similar workup as in adult stones (see Chapter 11.5 Nephrolithiasis/Urolithiasis, Ureter Injuries, and Renal Cysts).
  ○ Dysfunctional voiding syndrome and infection:
    – Lack of coordination between detrusor muscle and external sphincter; due to lazy/high-capacity or overactive bladders.
    – Can result in vesicoureteral reflux.
    – Treatment: Behavioral modification/timed voids, bowel regimen, anticholinergic medications, and prophylactic antibiotics.
  ○ Diagnosis:
    – Urethral or suprapubic catheterization most accurate; colony-forming units/mL suggesting infection (10^5 voided specimens or 10^3 catheterized specimens).
    – Radiological examination of renal and bladder ultrasound with voiding cystourethrogram if ultrasound abnormal recommended by the American Academy of Pediatrics for febrile child from ages 2 months to 2 years with first UTI.

- Imaging can be used for older children with possible structural abnormalities, atypical organisms, failure to improve with treatment, or unclear infection source.
  - Treatment: Short-term antibiotics commonly used but tailored to culture results; local resistance rates; and treatment of cystis, pyelonephritis, and anatomical abnormalities; trimethoprim with sulfonamide commonly used for prophylaxis.
- Enuresis:
  - Definition: Intermittent incontinence during sleep in child ≥ 5 years old.
  - Combination of inability to wake with full bladder, excessive nighttime urine production, or decrease bladder capacity.
  - 5–10% U.S. prevalence by the age of 7 years.
  - Workup: History, physical, evaluation of comorbidities (e.g., diabetes, constipation, UTI, obstructive sleep apnea, dysfunctional voiding, psychiatric or neurological issues), urinalysis, imaging used for additional evaluation in select cases.
  - Treatment:
    - Bed alarm therapy, behavioral modification (e.g., limited fluid, waking at night, bladder raining, reward system), and/or desmopressin used as first-line therapy for 6–8 weeks.
    - Secondary medications can be considered (e.g., tricyclic antidepressants, diclofenac, indomethacin, and anticholinergics).
    - Referral to pediatric urologist with failure of standard therapy, anatomical abnormalities, recurrent UTI, or neurological disorders.
  - Red flags: Daytime incontinence, urgency, frequency, dribbling, incomplete emptying, straining, weak stream, leakage, voiding excessively during day, dysuria, history of UTIs.

10.6.2 Congenital Anomalies

- Bladder anomalies:
  - Bladder diverticulum:
    - Rare herniation of bladder mucosa through bladder wall close to insertion of ureter due to weakness in the fascial sheath.
    - Increases risk of UTIs, incidentally found during workup for UTI in young children.
    - May coexist with vesicoureteral reflux, recurrent UTI, hydronephrosis, and other congenital malformations or syndromes; stasis of urine can result in stone formation.
    - Diagnosis: Voiding cystourethrogram.
    - Treatment: Resection with reconstruction of bladder.
  - Bladder exstrophy–epispadias–cloacal exstrophy complex:
    - Failure of midline closure from umbilicus to perineum; spectrum of severity; 1:10,000–50,000 births, more common in males.
    - Epispadias: Opening in dorsal urethra.
    - Bladder extrophy: Bladder, urethra, and penis mucosa open to abdominal skin; urine drips from bladder; more common in males.
    - Cloacal extrophy: Severe defect; omphalocele covering of abdominal contents, bladder, penis/clitoris/vagina split in halves, rectal opening missing or atretic.
    - Associated with separation of public symphysis and bifid genitalia.
    - Diagnosis: Prenatal ultrasound, physical examination.
    - Treatment: Staged bladder reconstruction and management of vesicoureteral reflux; first treatment closes bladder to hold urine and places bladder inside pelvis; reconstruction of the genitalia occurs at the age of 2 years, bladder neck reconstruction with ureter repositioning occurs at the age of 5 years.
  - Prune belly/Eagle-Barrett/triad syndrome.
    - Wrinkled abdominal wall of neonates; mostly in males; unclear cause.
    - Results in absence of abdominal wall musculature, hydronephrosis, ureter dilation, bilateral undescended testes, vesicoureteral reflux, and urethral abnormalities.
    - Associated with renal failure, bronchopulmonary dysplasia, and fetal death.
    - Diagnosed on prenatal or postnatal ultrasound.

- Treatment: Surgical reconstruction with orchiopexy, ureter reconstruction, and abdominoplasty; management of urinary obstruction, renal dysplasia, and possible hydronephrosis.
  - Megacystis syndrome:
    - Large, thin-walled, smooth bladder without obstruction forms; occurs mostly in females; overfilling of fetal bladder resulting in poor myoneural function.
    - Presets with UTI, vesicoureteral reflux into upper tract.
    - Associated with posterior urethral valves, Ehlers-Danlos, urethral diverticulum, microcolon hypoperistalsis syndrome, sacral meningomyelocele, sacrococcygeal teratoma, and pelvic neuroblastoma.
    - Diagnosis: Voiding cystourethrogram shows reflux and upper tract dilation.
    - Treatment: Ureteral reimplantation.
  - Bladder duplication/septation:
    - Rare bladder division into halves; complete or partial types.
    - Associated with single or duplicated urethras; duplication of genitalia, lumbar vertebrae, and bowels; fibromuscular fistulas between rectum, vagina, and urethra.
    - Treatment: Anatomical reconstruction depending on anomalies and bladder drainage.
  - Bladder ears:
    - Lateral extensions of bladder through inguinal canal; rare in adults.
    - Must be recognized during herniorrhaphy to not be mistaken for herniation sac.
    - Diagnoses: Voiding cystourethrogram, intravenous pyelogram, abdominopelvic computed tomography (CT).
  - Bladder agenesis:
    - Rare, fewer than 20 cases, always in females.
    - Incompatible with life.
    - Ureters enter into abnormal structures.
    - Associated with hydroureteronephrosis, renal dysplasia, other associated anomalies.
  - Urachal anomalies:
    - Urachal sinus that drains to umbilicus, results in abdominal inflammation and cyst formation.
    - Associated with bladder outlet obstruction, stone formation, recurrent UTI by the age of 2–4 years.
    - Presents with wet umbilicus, granulation tissue, or asymptomatic; can be incidentally found; drainage seen with straining.
    - Diagnosis: Voiding cystourethrogram.
    - Treatment: Excision of abnormality.
- Penile anomalies:
  - Chordee:
    - Ventral, lateral, or rotational curvature of the penis, apparent with erection, due to fibrosis along corpus spongiosum.
    - Associated with hypospadias.
    - Can be due to scar tissue from a circumcision.
    - Treatment: 6–18 months with penoplasty/scar release.
  - Epispadias:
    - Urethral opening on glans, penile shaft, penopubic junction, between clitoris and labia, or abdomen.
    - 1:120,000 males and 1:500,000 females.
    - Associated with bladder exstrophy.
    - Presents with incontinence, reflux, and UTIs.
    - Partial epispadias shows better control of continence.
    - Complete epispadias requires bladder outlet reconstruction for urinary control.
    - Treatment: Cantwell–Ransley technique commonly used for repair.
  - Hypospadias:
    - Failure of tabularization and formation of urethral groove; occurs commonly in males at penoscrotal junction, scrotal folds, or perineum; rare in females.
    - Associated with chordee, failed foreskin development, and cryptorchidism.
    - 1:250 births in males.

- Treatment: Preputioplasty (use of foreskin for repair) at 3–6 months of life, hormone injection can increase penis size to aid in repair, distal versus proximal hypospadias shows differing repair strategies, tubularized incised plate repair used for distal repair.
  - Phimosis and paraphimosis:
    - Phimosis: Most common penile abnormality; constriction of foreskin not allowing retraction over glands; treated with topical steroids.
    - Paraphimosis: Inability of retracted foreskin to return to normal position; can be treated with relaxing incision followed by circumcision or topical steroids.
- Urethral anomalies:
  - Ureteropelvic junction obstruction:
    - Most common cause of congenital hydronephrosis; affects males more than females; can result from abnormal muscle development at ureteropelvic junction.
    - Associated with other congenital abnormalities (e.g., VATER).
    - Diagnosis: Fetal and postnatal ultrasound show hydronephrosis, can be incidentally identified during workup for UTI, diuretic-enhanced radionucleotide scan or magnetic resonance (MR) urogram used to evaluate obstruction location.
    - Treatment: Pyeloplasty, removal of blockage and reconnection of ureter to renal pelvis, stenting can be used to decompress the kidney.
  - Ureterovesical junction obstruction:
    - 2nd most common cause of congenital hydronephrosis; can result from abnormal development of ureter and be incidentally identified during workup for UTI.
    - Diagnosis: Prenatal or postnatal ultrasound show hydronephrosis, MR urogram shows ureterocele (outpouching of ureter where it enters the bladder) without dilation of ureteropelvic junction, voiding cystourethrogram.
    - Treatment: Ureteroplasty, removal of blockage and reconnection of ureter to bladder; may require stent; 10% risk of recurrence.
  - Vesicoureteral reflux:
    - 25–30% of antenatal and 1% of newborn hydronephrosis.
    - Increase risk of UTI and renal scarring.
    - 5 grades of severity outlining dilation of ureter and renal pelvis.
    - Presents: UTI, hydronephrosis, other genitourinary anomalies (30%); presents earlier in males.
    - Treatment: Observation as mild cases resolve over time, antibiotic prophylaxis controversial, surveillance ultrasound to follow hydronephrosis, voiding cystourethrogram, open versus endoscopic Deflux procedure (hyaluronic acid injection to increase resistance of reflux).
  - Urethral stricture or urethral meatal stenosis:
    - Urethral meatal stenosis most common after circumcision.
    - Urethral stricture most common after crush or saddle injury.
    - Congenital stricture diagnosed prenatally by ultrasound and postnatally by retrograde urethrography.
    - Treated with meatotomy and endoscopic versus open urethroplasty.
  - Urethral valves:
    - Most common cause of obstruction in males, does not affect females.
    - Folds in posterior urethra causing obstruction of urinary flow, results in hesitancy, decreased urinary stream, increased risk of UTI, overflow incontinence, myogenic bladder, vesicoureteral reflux, and hydronephrosis.
    - Diagnosis: Prenatally by bilateral hydroureteronephrosis or oligohydramnios, postnatally detected with voiding cystourethrography, distended bladder and poor urinary stream, eventually results in renal failure.
    - Potter's sequence: Severe cases of valve obstruction resulting in oligohydramnios, pulmonary hypoplasia, uterine molding.
    - Treated with immediate placement of Foley and bladder decompression, endoscopic urethroplasty, fetal therapy with vesicoamniotic shunt.
  - Ectopic ureteral orifices:
    - Opening of single or duplicated ureters on lateral bladder, along trigone, in the bladder neck, distal to sphincter, on genital system, or externally.

- Associated with incontinence when beyond sphincter control and vesicoureteral reflux.
- Treated with urethroplasty.
- Retrocaval ureter:
  - Rare, abnormal vena cava or iliac vessel development usually on right resulting in compression and obstruction of the ureter; presents in 30 and 40 seconds with hydronephrosis.
  - Treated with ureteroureteral anastomosis anterior to vena cava or iliac vessel.
- Ureter duplication:
  - Partial or complete duplication of one or both ureters, duplication of renal pelvis; can cause reflux in portions of the kidney depending on urine flow.
  - Associated with ureter ectopia, ureter stenosis, vesicoureteral reflux, and ureterocele.
  - Treated when there is obstruction, reflux, or incontinence; incomplete duplication typically asymptomatic.
- Ureter stenosis:
  - Narrowing of ureter, more common at ureteropelvic junction then ureterovesical junction.
  - Associated with recurrent infection, hematuria, obstruction, reflux, and hydronephrosis.
  - Treated with ureteroplasty or pyeloplasty.
- Ureterocele:
  - Dilation of ureter, occurs due to prolapse at ureterovesical junction, associated with renal dysplasia at ureteropelvic junction, can cause bladder neck obstruction or intralabial mass in females.
  - Associated with recurrent infection, reflux, hydronephrosis, and stone formation.
  - Treated with reconstruction or resection of affected ureter and kidney.
- Genital anomalies:
  - Congenital hydrocele:
    - Fluid collection in scrotum between layers of tunica vaginalis, noncommunicating or communicating with abdominal cavity via processus vaginalis.
    - Secondary to epididymitis, orchitis, testicular torsion, epididymis torsion, trauma, or tumor in children and adolescents.
    - Presents as painless, enlarged scrotum; enlarges with Valsalva maneuver in communicating types.
    - Diagnosis: Physical examination, transillumination shows cystic collection, ultrasound used to rule out primary causes.
    - Treatment: Spontaneously resolves; treated if present beyond 2 years, symptomatic, or injured skin integrity.
  - Cryptorchidism:
    - Undescended testes commonly within inguinal canal and rarely in peritoneal or retroperitoneal cavity; 80% diagnosed at birth, 20% diagnosed at early adolescence after growth spurt.
    - 3% of term infants, 30% of preterm infants; 60% of undescended testes descend within first 4 months, 0.8% infant treatment rate.
    - Associated with subfertility, testicular carcinoma (three times increased risk), testicular torsion with acute abdomen, and testicular trauma in inguinal canal.
    - Reposition reduces but does not eliminate testicular carcinoma risk.
    - 90% associated with patent processes vaginalis and inguinal hernia.
    - 10% bilateral and evaluation for congenital adrenal hyperplasia considered.
    - Ectopic testis: Testis exiting external inguinal ring but lying in abnormal location (e.g., suprapubic, inguinal pouch, perineum, inner thigh).
    - Diagnosis: Physical examination to rule out retracted testis; no treatment for hypermobile testis as it resolves with testicular hypertrophy during puberty; diagnostic laparoscopy or open inguinal exploration performed between 4 and 12 months.
    - Treatment: Orchiopexy with return of testis to normal position or orchiectomy performed; surgery at 6 months reduces infertility and cancer risk but can be done later.
    - Hormonal treatment with gonadotropin-releasing hormone analogs and human chorionic gonadotropin controversial.
  - Atypical genitalia/disorders of sex development:
    - Congenital discrepancy between external genitalia and gonadal and chromosomal sex.

- – 1:1,000–1:4,500 births.
- – Includes bilateral cryptorchidism, scrotal/perineal hypospadias, clitoromegaly, posterior labial fusion, phenotypic female with palpable gonad, discordant genitalia and sex chromosomes, female virilization (e.g., congenital adrenal hypoplasia).
- – Diagnosis: History and physical examination with criteria for length measurements of external genitalia; early referral to medical genetics or endocrinology; karyotyping, hormonal and genetic testing focused depending on examination; ultrasound and MR imaging used to evaluate internal organs; cystoscopy/vaginoscopy used to evaluate urethral and vaginal anatomy.
- – Three broad karyotype categories: 46, XX DSD; 46, XY DSD; and mixed sex chromosome DSD.
- – Treatment involves sex assignment therapy and long-term follow-up for hormonal and fertility issues.
- • Renal anomalies:
  - ○ Autosomal recessive polycystic kidney disease.
    - – Cystic renal disease that presents in infant and children (1:20,000 births), autosomal dominant disease more often presents in adults.
    - – Kidney enlargement with small cysts and renal failure can be seen; liver enlargement with periportal fibrosis, bile duct proliferation, and cysts can be seen; pulmonary hypoplasia, renal dysfunction, and oligohydramnios seen in infants.
    - – 30% of newborns die within the first few weeks; most who survive may require renal and hepatic transplantation, placement of portacaval or splenorenal shunts.
    - – Diagnosis: Ultrasound, MR imaging, or CT used postnatally; *PKHD1* genetic testing used for those meeting clinical criteria.
  - ○ Duplication anomalies:
    - – Duplication of renal pelvis, ureters, calyx, or ureteral orifice possible unilaterally or bilaterally.
    - – Single renal parenchyma unit.
    - – Treatment of ureteral ectomy, ureterocele, and vesicoureteral reflux may be necessary.
  - ○ Fusion anomalies:
    - – Fusion of renal parenchyma with separate ureters entering the bladder; increased risk of reflux, obstruction, and congenital renal cystic dysplasia.
    - – Horseshoe kidney: Most common fusion abnormality; fusion of lower poles of bilateral kidneys by fibrous isthmus; obstruction of ureter treated with pyeloplasty if necessary.
    - – Crossed fused renal ectopia: 2nd most common fusion abnormality; both kidneys located ipsilaterally and one ureter crosses midline; obstruction of ureter treated with pyeloplasty if necessary.
    - – Fused pelvic kidney/pancake kidney: Single pelvic kidney serves two collecting systems and ureters; treated with reconstruction if necessary.
  - ○ Renal malformation:
    - – Renal agenesis: Failure of renal formation; results in Potter syndrome (oligohydramnios, pulmonary hypoplasia, extremity and facial dysmorphisms); uniformly fatal.
    - – Unilateral renal agenesis: Absent renal parenchyma and ureter formation; contralateral kidney hypertrophies to maintain homeostasis.
    - – Renal dysplasia: Abnormality of renal vasculature, tubules, scollecting ducts, or drainage on histology; treatment based on degree of renal impairment.
    - – Renal ectopia: Abnormal renal location of one or both kidneys due to failure of cephalic migration of kidneys; associated with obstruction, reflux, renal dysplasia, and anomalies of other renal anatomy; can be located in thorax, pelvis, or fused.
    - – Crossed fused renal ectopia: Kidneys fused ipsilaterally, 90% show some fusion.
    - – Pelvic kidney: Most common form of renal ectopia; obstruction from infection or stone can mimic appendicitis or pelvic inflammatory disease; associated with other urogenital anomalies.
    - – Renal hypoplasia: Small, underdeveloped kidney due to inadequate embryological formation.
  - ○ Renal vein thrombosis:
    - – Unilateral or bilateral thrombosis of intrarenal vein, life-threatening.
    - – 90% of cases are in patients < 1 year of age; 75% of cases are in patients < 1 month of age.
    - – More common in males and on left side.
    - – Treated with anticoagulation therapy; most kidneys with involvement show atrophy.

References

[1] Goldschneider KR, Cravero JP, Anderson C, et al. Section on Anesthesiology and Pain Medicine. The pediatrician's role in the evaluation and preparation of pediatric patients undergoing anesthesia. Pediatrics. 2014; 134(3):634–641

[2] Kosowski TR, Weathers WM, Wolfswinkel EM, Ridgway EB. Cleft palate. Semin Plast Surg. 2012; 26(4):164–169

[3] Yuzuriha S, Mulliken JB. Minor-form, microform, and mini-microform cleft lip: anatomical features, operative techniques, and revisions. Plast Reconstr Surg. 2008; 122(5):1485–1493

[4] Monson LA, Kirschner RE, Losee JE. Primary repair of cleft lip and nasal deformity. Plast Reconstr Surg. 2013; 132(6):1040e–1053e

[5] Hammoudeh JA, Fahradyan A, Gould DJ, et al. A comparative analysis of recombinant human bone morphogenetic protein-2 with a demineralized bone matrix versus iliac crest bone graft for secondary alveolar bone grafts in patients with cleft lip and palate: review of 501 cases. Plast Reconstr Surg. 2017; 140(2):318e–325e

[6] Renier D, Sainte-Rose C, Marchac D, Hirsch JF. Intracranial pressure in craniostenosis. J Neurosurg. 1982; 57(3):370–377

[7] Derderian CA, Bastidas N, Bartlett SP. Posterior cranial vault expansion using distraction osteogenesis. Childs Nerv Syst. 2012; 28(9):1551–1556

11 Genitourinary

Michael Karsy

11.1 Urological Basics and Testing

11.1.1 Foley Catheter Placement

- 15–70% of catheter-associated urinary tract infections (UTIs) can be prevented with proper infection control measures.
- Repeated or blind catheter insertion can result in patient discomfort, urethral trauma, and subsequent stricture.
- Consideration of alternatives should be performed including condom catheters, suprapubic catheterization, and other methods; prior urological history (e.g. prostate surgery, strictures) should be considered.
- Absolute contraindication: Confirmed or suspected urethral injury (e.g., meatal blood, high-riding prostate, distended urinary bladder, associated pelvic or saddle injuries).
- Relative contraindications: Urethral stricture, recent urological surgery, uncooperative patient.
- Blind catheterization:
  - Patient initial positioning (e.g., females in frog-leg position), equipment laid out, urogenital area cleaned thoroughly then prepped, one contaminated hand and one clean hand used, balloon inflated after catheter positioned and secured.
  - Injection of 10–15 mL of a water-soluble lubricant-anesthetic (e.g., Urogel) can improve patient comfort and facilitate catheter insertion.
  - Penis elongated at 60 degrees without compressing urethra, retracted foreskin replaced at end of procedure.
  - Typically 16–18 Fr catheter used for males, 12–14 Fr catheter used for stricture, 20–24 Fr catheter used for enlarged prostate to prevent catheter kinking during insertion.
  - Catheter insertion to Y-hub ensures tip in bladder before balloon to prevent urethral rupture; flushing of catheter if no flow can help unclear blocked gel.
  - Pain can signify a false passage and should be reevaluated; pain during balloon inflation can suggest balloon is within the urethra and should be reevaluated.
  - Males: After first failed attempt, 18-Fr coude catheter can help overcome an acute angle in the prostate urethra; 12-Fr silicone catheter and can be used for medium-sized strictures and bladder neck contractures.
  - Females: After first failed attempt, catheter usually left within vagina and to help guide next catheter into proper position; alternative positioning can include bilateral straight leg raising to improve anatomical visualization; speculum or fingers can help guide catheter.
- Assistive catheterization technologies: DirectVision System (microendoscopy on a three-way Foley catheter) used for high-risk patients (e.g., enlarged prostate, stricture, difficult insertions, false passages, anticoagulation therapy), fiberoptic camera assisted placement can be used as last resort.
- Urological consultation suggested after initial failed attempt despite good technique or in high-risk situations, goal to reduce urethral trauma with multiple attempts.

11.1.2 Urological Evaluation

- Urinalysis interpretation:
  - pH can vary between 4.5 and 8, average: 5.5–6.5.
  - Blood: Normally < 3 red blood cells/high-powered field.
  - Protein: Normally 80–150 mg/day; proteinuria indicates renal disease or multiple myeloma; can be seen after strenuous exercise.
  - Leukocyte esterase: Detects neutrophils; not always seen during bacteriuria.
  - Nitrite: Suggests gram-negative bacteria converting nitrates to nitrites; sensitivity 35–85%, less accurate with urine containing fewer bacteria.

- Cytology:
  - Red blood cells: Dysmorphic cells suggest passage through glomerulus versus normal structure from tubular and lower urinary tract bleeding.
  - Casts:
    - Red blood cell casts arise from glomerular bleeding and glomerulonephritis.
    - White blood cell casts arise from acute glomerulonephritis, pyelonephritis, and tubulointerstitial nephritis.
    - Hyaline casts are composed of protein arise from tubular epithelial cells (e.g., Tamm–Horsfall mucoprotein).
  - Crystals: Evaluation of urinary stones can evaluate cause.
  - Obtained after voiding or bladder wash; used to evaluate transitional cell carcinoma or treatment; sensitivity and specificity for malignancy diagnosis depends on morphology and types of cells evaluated.
- Prostate-specific antigen (PSA):
  - Glycoprotein secreted by prostatic epithelial cells and used to liquefy the ejaculate for fertilization; 75% bound to plasma proteins, 25% free and excreted in urine.
  - Prostate biopsy recommended in men with PSA >2.5 ng/mL; age-specific normal levels vary by race and prostate volume; 5% risk of cancer in screened men but notable level of false positives resulting in biopsy with risks.
  - Indications: Patient request, lower urinary tract symptoms, abnormal digital rectal examination, progressive bone/back pain, unexplained symptoms suggesting malignancy, spontaneous thromboembolism, or deep vein thrombosis in men, monitoring of prostate cancer.
  - PSA level: Direct level in blood (ng/mL).
  - PSA density: PSA level divided by size of prostate on transrectal ultrasound.
  - PSA velocity: Change of PSA level over period of time.
  - PSA doubling time: Time for PSA level to double.
- Urodynamic testing:
  - Testing to evaluate bladder and urethra.
  - Commonly used to evaluate men with prostate hypertrophy, females with incontinence failing conservative management, and neuropathy/spinal cord injury.
  - Helpful adjunct in patients with unclear or unreliable symptoms (e.g., urge incontinence).
  - Types:
    - Cystometry: Bladder pressure measurement during filling.
    - Pressure-flow study: Recording of bladder pressure during voiding; valuates bladder and urethral sphincter behavior; detrusor pressure determined by difference between intra-abdominal pressure and intravesicular/bladder pressure, recorded in pressure of ($P_{det} = P_{abd} - P_{ves}$; cm H_2O) and flow (Q_{max}, mL/second).
    - Videocystometry: Fluoroscopic evaluation during pressure-flow study.
    - Uroflowmetry: Evaluates urine flow rate and volume, compared with standardized curves (e.g., Bristol flow rate nomogram); used to evaluate suspected prostatic obstruction; limited accuracy in women.

11.1.3 Radiological Evaluation

- X-ray: Used for evaluation of renal calculi (sensitivity: 50–70%).
- CT imaging: Used to evaluate renal masses, staging of renal and bladder cancer, assessment of stone size and location, evaluation of perirenal collections, renal trauma, and evaluation of hydronephrosis.
- Magnetic resonance imaging: Used to stage bladder and prostate cancer, localization of undescended testes; evaluation of stones in patients unable to receive radiation.
- Ultrasound:
  - Indications: Hematuria, renal tumor, renal stones, hydronephrosis, post-void bladder residuals, ultrasound placement of nephrostomy tube and suprapubic catheter, urethral strictures, testicular torsion, testicular descent, testicular blood flow and ischemia/infarction, varicoceles, and testicular atrophy.

- ○ Transrectal ultrasound used to measure prostate size, assist in prostate biopsy, and investigate azoospermia.
- ○ Bladder volume (mL) = bladder height (cm) × width (cm) × depth (cm) × 0.7.
- Intravenous pyelography/intravenous urography:
  - ○ Intravascular contrast agent administered before X-rays of urinary system.
  - ○ Indications: Evaluation of hematuria, renal masses, filling defects in collecting system and ureters, localization of calcification, investigation of ureteric colic, congenital urinary tract abnormalities (e.g., duplication, malrotation, horseshoe kidneys), follow-up for postureteric surgery/strictures.
  - ○ 1–5% of patients have side effects, including rare anaphylaxis; 1:40,000–1:200,000 risk of death with anaphylaxis.
  - ○ Phases:
    - – Plain films: Evaluate calcifications over kidneys, ureters, and bladder.
    - – Nephrogram phase: Proximal convoluted tubules imaged as contrast filtered.
    - – Pyelogram phase: Distal tubule imaged as water absorbed and contrast is not absorbed, images of ureter and bladder performed.
- Voiding cystourethrography:
  - ○ Retrograde contrast filling of bladder via catheter followed by X-rays during normal voiding; used to detect bladder dysfunction, bladder outlet, and urethral obstruction.
  - ○ Indications: Evaluation of urination with neuropathic bladder problems or obstruction.
- Cystography:
  - ○ Retrograde contrast filling of bladder via catheter.
  - ○ Indications: Vesicocolic and vesicovaginal fistulas, bladder rupture.
- Urethrography:
  - ○ Retrograde contrast filing of urethra.
  - ○ Indications: Urethral strictures or injury.
- Ileal loopogram:
  - ○ Retrograde contrast filling of ileal conduit.
  - ○ Indications: Evaluates free reflux into ureters versus obstruction at ureteroileal junction from stenosis or transitional cell carcinoma.
- Retrograde pyelography:
  - ○ Retrograde contrast filling of ureters via cystoscope.
  - ○ Indications: Evaluates ureters and renal pelvis for stones, ureteric injury, or transitional cell carcinoma.
- Nuclear medicine studies:
  - ○ ^{99m}Tc-mercapto-acetyl-triglycine, ^{99m}Tc-dimercaptosuccinic acid, and ^{99m}Tc-methylene-disphosphonate.
  - ○ Indications: Evaluate renal function of each kidney, renal obstruction, response to Lasix, metastatic disease.

11.2 Urinary Tract Infection and Inflammation

11.2.1 Urinary Tract Infection

- Inflammatory response of urothelium to bacterial infection consistent with clinical symptoms and laboratory studies.
- Represents 10–15% of healthcare-associated infections, 1–5% of postoperative infections; accounts for 13,000 deaths annually in the United States.
- Cystitis: Infection of the bladder; includes frequency, urgency, small voiding volumes, and suprapubic pain.
- Dysuria: Urethral burning and pain with voiding.
- Bacteriuria:
  - ○ Bacteria in urine; can be asymptomatic colonization or symptomatic.
  - ○ Bacteria ascend urethra mostly from large bowel; bloodstream spread is rare.
  - ○ Risk factors include female sex, older age, menopause, pregnancy, diabetes mellitus, prior UTI, catheters, urolithiasis, genitourinary malformations, urinary obstruction.
  - ○ Up to 20–30% elderly females and 10% elderly males.

- Pyuria: White blood cells in urine or sedimented urine; indicates inflammatory reaction to bacteria.
- Diagnosis:
  - Urinary dipstick: Sensitivity 35–85%, best performance with leukocyte esterase and with high bacterial load; < 2% risk of infection if protein, leukocyte esterase, and nitrate negative.
  - Urinary microscopy: Diagnostic of > 3 white blood cells/high-powered field in centrifuged sample.
  - Urine culture: Diagnostic with ≥ 10^2 colony-forming units (CFU)/mL with symptoms, positive criterion depends on sample type (▶ Table 11.1).
- Recurrent UTI: > 2 infections in 6 months or ≥ 3 infections in 12 months; can be due to bacterial persistence or reinfection; arises from underlying functional or anatomical problem.
  - Evaluation: Kidney, ureter, and bladder X-ray to detect renal calculi; renal ultrasound to detect hydronephrosis or radio-opaque stones; identification of post-void residuals; intravenous (IV) pyelogram, or computed tomography (CT) urogram, flexible cystoscopy to evaluate anatomical problems.
- Complicated UTI: Patients with underlying abnormality, pregnant women, with obstruction or immunosuppression, and often men; longer treatment required.
  - Evaluation required for complicated UTI, patients with urosepsis, pyelonephritis, perinephric abscess, recurrent UTI, pregnant patients, unusual organisms (e.g., *Proteus* from infected urolith).
- Catheter-associated UTI: Presence of ≥10^3 CFU/mL with single catheterized sample or within 48 hours of catheter removal.
- Treatment depends on specific patient infection pattern and bacteria (▶ Table 11.2).

Table 11.1 Probability of urinary tract infection based on culture results

Collection type	Colony-forming units (/mL)	Infection probability
Suprapubic	Gram negative	> 99%
	Gram positive > 1,000	> 99%
Catheterization	> 10^5	95%
	$10^{4–5}$	Likely
Clean catch male	> 10^4	Likely
Clean catch female	> 10^5	80–95% depending on number of positive specimens

Table 11.2 Urinary tract infection organisms and treatment

Infection type	Common causative bacteria	Treatment options[a]
Uncomplicated UTI, cystitis and pyelonephritis	*Escherichia coli, Staphylococcus saprophyticus, Enterococcus* spp., *Klebsiella pneumonia, Proteus mirabilis*	Nitrofurantoin, amoxicillin, amoxicillin/clavulanate, cephalexin, cefpodoxime, fosfomycin, trimethoprim/sulfamethoxazole, fluoroquinolones
Complicated UTI, urosepsis	Uncomplicated UTI bacteria, antibiotic-resistant *E. coli, Pseudomonas aeruginosa, Acinetobacter baumannii, Staphylococcus* spp., *K. pneumonia*	Ceftriaxone, ceftazidime, cefepime, piperacillin/tazobactam, aztreonam, meropenem, ertapenem, doripenem, colistin, fluoroquinolones
Catheter-associated UTI	*P. mirabilis, Morganella morganii, Providencia stuartii, Corynebacterium urealyticum, Candida* spp.	
Recurrent UTI	*P. mirabilis, K. pneumonia, Enterococcus* spp., *Enterobacter* spp., antibiotic-resistant *E. coli, Staphylococcus* spp.	Prevention: Nitrofurantoin, trimethoprim/sulfamethoxazole
Acute bacterial prostatitis	*E. coli, P. aeruginosa, Serratia marcescens, Enterococcus* spp.	Fluoroquinolone, trimethoprim/sulfamethoxazole

[a] Antibiotics should be narrowed based on sensitivities of cultured bacteria and institutional/local rates of bacteria resistance.

11.2.2 Acute Pyelonephritis

- Involves fever, flank pain, tenderness, urgency, elevated white count; accompanies lower UTI, vesicoureteric reflux, obstruction, malformations, pregnancy, and indwelling catheters.
- Differential includes cholecystitis, pancreatitis, diverticulitis, appendicitis.
- Diagnosis: Bacterial culture with possibly $< 10^5$ CFU/mL, workup for anatomical issues can include imaging studies.
- Treatment: Oral antibiotics can be started for patients who are not systemically ill, patients with systemically ill patients treated with IV antibiotics; pyelonephrosis or perinephric abscesses may require drainage, especially if not responding to antibiotics.
- Emphysematous pyelonephritis: Rare form of acute pyelonephritis caused by gas-forming organisms, mostly *Enterobacter* spp. including *Escherichia coli*.
- Xanthogranulomatous pyelonephritis: Severe renal infection associated with renal calculi and obstruction; can result in renal tissue necrosis, calcification, and dysfunction.
- Chronic pyelonephritis: Renal scarring occurring from radiological or pathological findings of infection.

11.2.3 Urosepsis

- 25% of all sepsis cases; develops from community- and hospital-acquired UTIs.
- Most commonly from urinary catheters, urinary tract surgery, and urinary tract obstruction.
- Treatment: Early recognition; evaluation of urinary function and urinary culture; treatment of sepsis with broad-spectrum, empiric antibiotics; resuscitation of potential septic shock.

11.2.4 Prostatitis

- Infection with or without inflammation of the prostate; associated with UTI and urinary tract anomalies.
- Classified by National Institutes of Health.
  - I: Acute bacterial prostatitis.
  - II: Chronic bacterial prostatitis.
  - III: Chronic pelvic pain syndrome.
  - IIIA: Inflammatory chronic pelvic pain syndrome.
  - IIIB: Noninflammatory chronic pelvic pain syndrome.
  - Asymptomatic inflammatory prostatitis.
- Diagnosed with clinical features, boggy prostate, Meares–Stamey or 4-glass test of segmented urine cultures which allows evaluation of different parts of urinary stream (first 10 mL [urethritis or prostatitis], midstream [cystitis], first 10 mL after prostate massage [bacterial prostatitis], or end prostate massage [bacterial prostatitis]).
- Treatment: Antibiotics, short-term catheterization to treat urinary retention, antiandrogenic treatments.

11.2.5 Other Infections/Inflammatory Conditions

- Fournier gangrene: Necrotizing fasciitis of genitalia and perineum; commonly from polymicrobial organisms, predisposition from diabetes, local trauma, urine extravasation, and surgical procedures.
- Epididymitis: Inflammation of epididymis and testis from bacterial infection; associated with history of UTI or sexually transmitted diseases; differential diagnosis includes testicular torsion.
- Periurethral abscess: Infection associated with urethral stricture, urethral catheterization, and gonococcal infection.
- Interstitial cystitis: Bladder disorder with urgency and suprapubic pain; unclear etiology; predominantly in women; diagnosed by criteria from National Institute of Diabetes, Digestive and Kidney Diseases (NIDDK): (1) cystoscopic evidence of Hunner bladder ulcer or petechial hemorrhages, (2) bladder/pelvic pain or urinary urgency, (3) does not meet multiple exclusion criteria.
- Balanitis: Inflammation of glans penis, associated with poor hygiene.

- Paraphimosis: Urological emergency with penile foreskin retracted behind gland and unable to be repositioned.
- Phimosis: Inability to retract foreskin.

11.3 Lower Urinary Tract Disorders

11.3.1 Lower Urinary Tract Symptoms (LUTS)

- General term describing symptoms from urological and nonurological causes of urinary obstruction.
- Bladder outlet obstruction: Combination of functional or anatomic causes inhibiting normal voiding patterns; can result in LUTS or other signs/symptoms.
- LUTS defined by six factors: Hesitancy, poor flow, frequency, urgency, nocturia, and terminal dribbling; evaluated using International Prostate Symptom Score.
- Causes: benign prostatic hyperplasia (BPH), anatomical disruption, neoplasms, inflammatory disorders, infection, neurological disorders (e.g., multiple sclerosis, Parkinson disease, spinal cord/cauda equina compression, detrusor sphincter dyssynergia), bladder functional impairment.
- Sex-based differences:
  - Commonly caused by BPH in men, less commonly urethral stricture and malignant prostate enlargement.
  - Less common in women; due to pelvic prolapse, urethral stricture, urethral diverticulum, postsurgery for stress incontinence, impaired relaxation of external sphincter, pelvic masses, Fowler syndrome.

11.3.2 Benign Prostatic Hyperplasia

- Combination of epithelia and stromal cells in periurethral prostate with reduced programmed cell death.
- Affects 50% of men in 60 s and 90% of men in 80 s.
- Testosterone and dihydrotestosterone (DHT) regulate BPH by direct and paracrine effects; DHT is the most potent effector of BPH.
- Evaluation:
  - Specific evaluation of bed wetting, enlarged bladder, bladder pain, hematuria, back pain, and neurological symptoms included.
  - Assessment of International Prostate Symptom Score.
  - Digital rectal examination with prostate-specific antigen testing.
  - Serum creatinine evaluates renal function, followed up with renal ultrasound.
  - Post-void residual, uroflowmetry, and pressure studies used depending on clinical situation and provider.
- Treatment:
  - Monitoring, antiandrogenic medications.
  - Transurethral resection of the prostate (TURP).
  - Transurethral radiofrequency needle ablation.
  - Transurethral microwave thermotherapy.
  - High-intensity focused ultrasound.
  - Transurethral electrovaporization of the prostate.
  - Laser prostatectomy.
  - Open prostatectomy.
- α_1-Adrenoceptor blockers:
  - Used to reduce prostatic smooth muscle contraction; 30–40% rate of improvement of symptoms by > 25%, 80% show some improvement in symptoms.
  - Nonselective: Phenoxybenzamine, prazosin; effective but increased side effects.
  - Long-acting: Terazosin, doxazosin.
  - α_{1a}-Subtype selective: Tamsulosin, alfuzosin, silodosin.
  - Side effects: Weakness (5%), dizziness (6%), headache (2%), postural hypotension (1%), retrograde ejaculation (8%).

- 5α-Reductase inhibitors:
  - Used to inhibit conversion of testosterone to dihydrotestosterone, shrinks prostate epithelium over several months, low reduction in risk of urinary retention, may reduce hematuria from BPH.
  - Finasteride blocks type II isoenzyme, dutasteride blocks type I and II isoenzymes.
  - Side effects: Loss of libido (5%), impotence (5%), reduced ejaculate volume (< 3%).
- Surgical treatment:
  - TURP used for patients with failure of medical therapy, recurrent acute retention, high-pressure chronic retention, renal impairment from obstruction, recurrent hematuria, bladder stones.
  - Other transurethral procedures can be an alternative.
  - Open surgery used for patients with large prostates, limited ability to undergo TURP, failed TURPs, long urethra, presence of bladder stones that cannot be treated.

11.3.3 Acute Urinary Retention

- Painful inability to void, diagnosed with large volume of urine (e.g., 500–800 mL).
- Mechanisms: Increased urethral resistance, low bladder pressure, interruption of bladder innervation, or poor coordination of central voiding center with external sphincter relaxation.
- Types: Spontaneous/primary (e.g., BPH) versus precipitated/secondary (e.g., anticholinergic) to a specific disease or event.
- Causes:
  - BPH.
  - Hematuria.
  - Sacral cord injury or compression.
  - Spinal cord injury with detrusor–sphincter dyssynergia.
  - Pelvic surgery with injury to pelvic parasympathetic plexus.
  - Pelvic fracture with urethral disruption.
  - Anesthetic drug, anticholinergics, sympathomimetic agents.
  - Abdominal surgery, perineal surgery, immobility postoperatively, pain.
  - S2–4 neurotropic virus.
  - Multiple sclerosis, transverse myelitis, diabetic cytopathy.
  - Pelvic prolapse.
  - Urethral stricture/diverticulum.
  - Fowler syndrome.
- Treatment:
  - Urethral or suprapubic catheterization with recording of volume, intermittent self-catheterization.
  - Reevaluation of patient medications.
  - Prostate antiandrogenic treatments.
  - Prostate stent, long-term catheter.
  - Sacral neuromodulation.
  - Repair of strictures, treatment of other causes.
- Trial without catheter: 50% of patients with spontaneous retention experience another episode within the next week, 70% in 1 year.
- High-pressure chronic retention: Bladder volumes > 800 mL, bladder pressures > 30 cm H_2O, and hydronephrosis; can result in renal failure; patients unaware if voiding spontaneously without need to void; patients presenting with bed-wetting and distended bladder.

11.3.4 Urinary Incontinence

- Loss of voluntary control of urination, demonstrated objectively, social and/or hygienic concern.
- Affects 12–43% of adult women and 3–11% of adult men.
- Categories:
  - Stress incontinence: Urine loss with increased intra-abdominal pressure; due to bladder neck/urethral hypermobility (e.g., childbirth, uterine prolapse) and neuromuscular defects (e.g., radical prostatectomy).

- Urge incontinence: Sudden, uncontrollable urination, bladder overactivity, or bladder irritation (e.g., infection, tumor, neuropathy).
- Overactive bladder: Urinary urgency with or without urge incontinence; associated with increased frequency and nocturia.
- Overflow incontinence: Urinary leakage from bladder overdistension; seen with increased residual urine or chronic retention.
- Total incontinence: Continuous leakage of urine; can be due to fistulous communication between bladder and vagina, ectopic ureter, or total disruption of internal and external sphincters.
- Functional incontinence: Loss of urine due to cognitive deficits or poor mobility.
- Mixed urinary incontinence: Combination of stress and urinary incontinence, patients show urgency.
- Nocturnal enuresis: Involuntary loss of urine in sleep; 0.5% prevalence in adults, common in children up to 7 years old.
- Postmicturition dribble: Pooling of urine in bulbous urethra after voiding; affects 20% of healthy adult males.
- Workup:
  - History and physical, pelvic examination.
  - Urethral hypermobility can be assessed with Q-tip; Bonney test evaluates continence by repositioning of urethra and bladder neck, urodynamic testing, cystometrogram; Valsalva leak point pressure, evaluates pressure where half-full bladder leaks, videourodynamics, sphincter electromyography.
- Differential for urinary incontinence in the elderly ("DIAPPERS"):
  - Evaluate *d*ementia/*d*elirium, *i*nfection, *a*trophic vaginitis, *p*harmaceutical drugs, *p*sychological disease, *e*xcessive fluid input/output, *r*estricted mobility, *s*tool impaction.
- Treatment for stress incontinence:
  - Pelvic floor exercises, restricted fluid consumption, weight loss, bladder training, Duloxetine treatment (off-label).
  - Injection of polymers into bladder neck and periurethral muscles.
  - Retropubic suspension procedures for females.
  - Urethral inserts, pessary placement, or pubovaginal slings.
  - Artificial urinary sphincter, pressure-regulated balloon placed extraperitoneally.
- Treatment for overactive bladder/urge incontinence.
  - Behavioral modification, pelvic floor exercises, biofeedback.
  - Sacral, anticholinergic agents (e.g., oxybutynin, tolterodine, trospium, solifenacin, darifenacin, fesoterodine).
  - Tricyclic antidepressants (e.g., imipramine).
  - Baclofen.
  - Intravesical botulinum toxin A injection.
  - TURP for BPH.
  - Pelvic neuromodulation, augmentation enterocystoplasty.
  - Conduit diversion of ureters to ileum and stoma.
  - Ileocystoplasty to divert bladder to ilium, detrusor myectomy.
- Treatment for mixed incontinence: Combination of treatments for stress and urge incontinence depending on patient.

11.3.5 Nocturia

- Nocturia: Frequent needing to get up and urinate at night, not same as enuresis (e.g., bedwetting).
- Nocturnal polyuria: > 1/3 of 24-hour output at night, normal total 24-hour output.
- Polyuria: >3 L urine output in 24 hours.
- Found in 40% of men aged 60–70 years, associated with increased risk of death likely from endocrine and cardiovascular disease.
- Causes:
  - Urological: BPH, overactive bladder, incomplete bladder emptying.

- Nonurological: Renal failure, diabetes mellitus or insipidus, polydipsia, hypercalcemia, medication use (e.g., diuretics), autonomic dysfunction, obstructive sleep apnea, idiopathic.
- Workup: Voiding diary over 7-day period to evaluate nocturia and polyuria, evaluation of urine and serum electrolytes, and osmolality.
- Treatment:
  - Fluid restriction, diuretics before bedtime.
  - Desmopressin therapy.
  - Treatment of obstructive sleep apnea.
  - Prostate antiandrogenic medications, URP.
  - Sacral neuromodulation.

11.3.6 Vesicovaginal Fistula (VVF) and Ureterovaginal Fistula (UVF)

- Abnormal communication between bladder and vagina or ureter and vagina.
- Associated with prolonged childbirth, pelvic surgery, neoplasm, endometriosis, inflammatory bowel disease, pelvic fracture, infection, or congenital abnormality.
- Workup: Pelvic exam, oral phenazopyridine/vesicular methylene blue test distinguishes VVF from UVF, cystoscopy, intravenous pyelogram, bilateral retrograde pyelogram.
- Treatment: Catheterization and anticholinergics for small VVF, electrocoagulation of fistula, stenting of fistula closed, surgical repair within 2–3 weeks for simple cases, and 3–6 months for complicated cases.

11.3.7 Urethral Stricture

- Narrowing of urethra due to scar tissue.
- Anterior urethra: Scar in corpus spongiosum; due to inflammatory conditions, infection, straddle injury, iatrogenic injury (e.g., traumatic catheterization).
- Posterior urethra: Scar in the urethra from traumatic distraction injuries.
- Presents with hesitancy, poor flow, post-micturition dribbling, urinary retention, and recurrent infection.
- Identified on failed catheterization, requires further workup and urological consultation to identify type injury pattern and potential treatment.
- Treatment: Urethral dilatation without creating more scar, endoscopic stricture lysis, open excision, and reconstruction.

11.4 Reproductive and Sexual Function

Also see Chapter 12.3 Obstetrics Overview.

11.4.1 Common Conditions Affecting Sexual Health

- Scrotal pain:
  - Can be due to epididymitis, orchitis, epididymo-orchitis, testicular torsion, neoplasm, referred ureteric colic, inguinal hernia, or nerve root (e.g., ilioinguinal or genitofemoral) irritation/entrapment.
  - Broad differential requires detailed history/physical to localize imaging and other testing.
- Priapism:
  - Painful, prolonged erection.
  - Low-flow/ischemic priapism: Hematological disease (e.g., hemoglobinopathy), infiltration of corpora cavernosa with malignancy, pharmacological.
  - High-flow/nonischemic priapism: Perineal trauma with arteriovenous fistula.
  - Workup: Digital rectal examination used to examine prostate; corporal blood gas can distinguish ischemic versus nonischemic priapism.

- Hematospermia:
  - Blood in semen:
  - Causes:
    - Iatrogenic from prostate biopsy or treatment cystoscopy.
    - Prostate brachytherapy.
    - Inflammatory causes (e.g., prostatitis, urethritis, epididymo-orchitis).
    - Urological cancers.
    - Benign prostatic hypertrophy.
    - Infection or idiopathic.
  - Workup: Urine culture, digital rectal examination; transrectal ultrasound, flexible cystoscopy, and renal ultrasound for recurrence; evaluation of upper tract for concurrent hematuria.
  - Treatment: Directed at cause, observation, empiric antibiotics.
- Male infertility:
  - Affects 15% of couples globally, 20–30% of infertility cases.
  - Semen analysis for volume, liquefaction time, pH, sperm concentration, morphology and motility; leukocyte presence suggests infection.
  - Oligospermia: Sperm concentration < 20 million/mL; commonly due to varicoceles, cryptorchidism, idiopathic causes, drug/toxin exposure, fever, or cancer.
  - Azoospermia: Absence of sperm in ejaculate; can be due to obstruction or abnormalities of spermatogenesis.
  - Retrograde ejaculation: Due to neurological dysfunction (e.g., spinal cord injury) or anatomical disruption.
  - Workup:
    - Evaluation of follicle-stimulating hormone, luteinizing hormone, testosterone, and prolactin performed to rule testicular failure or pituitary dysfunction.
    - Additional workup includes chromosomal analysis, fructose concentration, testicular biopsy, evaluation of sperm penetration into cervical mucus.
    - Scrotal ultrasound to evaluate varicocele and testicular abnormalities.
    - Transrectal ultrasound to evaluate ejaculate volume and anatomical abnormalities.
    - Vas deferens vasography with injection of scrotum to evaluate anatomy.
    - Venography to evaluate and embolize varicoceles.
  - Medical treatments:
    - Antiestrogens (e.g., clomiphene citrate) used to increase luteinizing hormone-releasing hormone, human chorionic gonadotrophin used if pituitary axis intact, testosterone replacement, dopamine agonists for hyperprolactinemia.
    - Electroejaculation used via rectal probe to postganglionic sympathetic nerves for patients with spinal cord injury.
    - Treatment of erectile dysfunction.
    - Retrograde ejaculation treated with oral adrenergic agents to increase bladder neck smooth muscle tone, oral sodium bicarbonate to optimize urine pH, or assisted contraception.
  - Surgical treatments:
    - Transurethral resection of ejaculatory ducts, epididymovasostomy, vasovasostomy: Used to improve blockage of various structures with normal testis.
    - Microsurgical epididymal sperm aspiration: Used in the setting of vas deferens agenesis.
    - Artificial insemination with donor sperm or in vitro fertilization.
    - Testicular sperm extraction: Used during testicular failure with atrophy.
  - Assisted contraception:
    - Intrauterine insemination: Ovarian stimulation with sperm placement into uterus.
    - In vitro fertilization: Ovarian stimulation with retrieval, fertilization in petri dish, and reimplantation of embryos to uterus.
    - Gamete intrafallopian transfer: Oocyte and sperm mixed and placed into fallopian tube.
    - Intracytoplasmic sperm injection: Direct sperm injection into oocyte.
  - Erectile dysfunction:
    - Affects 10% of men mostly between the age of 40 and 70 years.

Table 11.3 Common causes of erectile dysfunction using mnemonic "IMPOTENCE"

Mnemonic	Characterization	Cause
I	Inflammatory	Prostatitis
M	Mechanical	Peyronie disease
P	Psychological	Depression/anxiety, stress
O	Occlusive vascular	Hypertension, smoking, diabetes, veno-occlusive mechanisms
T	Trauma	Pelvic fractures, spinal cord injury, penile trauma
E	Extra	Iatrogenic from pelvic surgery, old age, renal failure, cirrhosis
N	Neurogenic	Spinal cord injury, degenerative conditions, peripheral neuropathy
C	Chemical	Antihypertensives, antiarrhythmics, antidepressants, anxiolytics, antiandrogens, anticonvulsants, anti-Parkinson drugs, statins, alcohol, LHRH analogs
E	Endocrine	Hypogonadism, pituitary dysfunction

Abbreviation: LHRH, luteinizing hormone-releasing hormone.

– Divided into psychogenic and organic causes (▶ Table 11.3).
– Parasympathetic stimulation via S2–4 nerves controls erection, sympathetic stimulation via T11–L2 sympathetic plexus controls ejaculation, and detumescence.
– Vasoocclusive mechanism of sinusoidal spaces against tunic albuginea with contraction of ischiocavernosus muscles produces erection, mediated by nitric oxide and cyclic GMP.
– Ejaculation: Alkaline prostatic secretion followed by spermatozoa and seminal vesicles.
– Evaluated via blood tests of hormonal function, lipids, glucose, and prostate-specific antigen; nocturnal penile tumescence testing; color Doppler evaluates blood flow before and after intercavernosal injection of prostaglandin E1; cavernosometry and cavernosography evaluate flow of vasoactive drugs and blood flow; penile arteriography used to evaluate blood flow disruption due to trauma.
– Treated with therapy if psychological, oral phosphodiesterase inhibitors (e.g., sildenafil/Viagra, tadalafil/Cialis, vardenafil/Levitra), testosterone replacement, intraurethral therapy, intracavernosal injections (e.g., alprostadil/Caverject, papaverine, and phentolamine), vacuum erection device, penile prosthesis.

• Varicocele:
  ○ Dilation of pampiniform plexus of spermatic cord and results in correctable cause of infertility, due to incompetent venous valves, more likely on left side.
  ○ Identified with Valsalva maneuver or when standing; can cause pain in scrotal area.
  ○ Associated with oligospermia and abnormal sperm function.
  ○ Surgical approaches: Retroperitoneal near anterosuperior iliac spine, inguinal near inguinal canal, subinguinal below the external ring, and laparoscopic with goals to ligate veins.
  ○ Embolization via femoral vein can be performed with coils or sclerosing agents.
• Peyronie disease:
  ○ Benign disease resulting in curvature of penis from fibrotic plaques of the tunica albuginea due to repetitive minor trauma; prevalence of 1% in men aged 40–60 years.
  ○ Results in painful erections and penile deformity.
  ○ Evaluated by examination, color Doppler ultrasound can evaluate vascular abnormalities, MRI used for evaluation of complex fibrosis.
  ○ Early active inflammation treated with vitamin E, tamoxifen, or colchicine.
  ○ Surgical treatments: Nesbit procedure (degloving and ellipse of deformity), penile plication (sutures along convex side), plaque incision and grafting, penile implant.
• Priapism:
  ○ Erection > 4–6 hours, low-flow veno-occlusive and urological emergency with erection > 4 hours, high-flow from trauma does not require emergent intervention.
  ○ Causes: Intracavernosal injection therapy, medications, thromboembolic (e.g., sickle cell disease, leukemia), spinal cord injury, trauma, infection.

○ Cavernous arterial blood sampling can determine low-flow priapism due to low pH, low pO_2, and elevated PCO_2.

○ Color Doppler used to evaluate ruptured artery with blood extravasation.

○ Treated with blood aspiration and injection of α_1-adrenergic agonist, fluid hydration, and ice packs.

11.5 Nephrolithiasis/Urolithiasis, Ureter Injuries, and Renal Cysts

11.5.1 Nephrolithiasis/Urolithiasis

- Flank pain/urinary colic.
  - ○ Flank pain with waxing and waning of pain severity, radiates to groin; flank pain does not correlate with stone position; no comfortable reposition.
  - ○ Acute pain more likely to be due to ureter obstruction, chronic pain suggests disease in kidney or renal pelvis.
  - ○ Nonnephrolithiasis causes of flank pain:
    - – Clot from renal neoplasm.
    - – Urethral obstruction, ureteropelvic junction obstruction.
    - – Infection.
    - – Renal infarction or vessel injury, renal bleeding.
    - – Calyceal diverticulum, renal cystic disease.
    - – Testicular torsion.
    - – Abdominal aortic aneurysm, myocardial infarction, pneumonia.
    - – Muscle spasm, gynecological pathology (e.g., ovarian cyst, ectopic pregnancy, ovarian vein syndrome).
    - – Appendicitis, diverticulitis, bowel disease or obstruction, pancreatitis, nerve root impingement.
    - – Vertebral body fracture, degenerative spine disease.
  - ○ Workup: History and examination are key, abdominal palpation used to identify tender and nontender areas, pregnancy test in women, urinalysis.
  - ○ Chronic flank pain: Urological or abdominal neoplasms, kidney stones, infection, testicular trauma, ureteric reflux, degenerative spine disease.
- Nephrolithiasis:
  - ○ 8–10% prevalence, 70% of cases asymptomatic.
  - ○ 50% of patients with urinary colic fail to show a nephrolith on imaging or stone passage.
  - ○ More common in Caucasians, men, ages 20–60 years, 10% incidence by the age of 70 years.
  - ○ Nephrolith formation (▶ Table 11.4) occurs when concentrations of calcium and oxalate are higher than solubility product, lowered concentrations of inhibitors (e.g., magnesium, glycosaminoglycans, Tamm–Horsfall protein) promote nephrolith formation.
  - ○ Presentation: Colicky flank pain, location of pain, and associated history help delineate other causes.
  - ○ Differential includes:
    - – Peritonitis, urinary tract infection (UTI).

Table 11.4 Incidence of nephroliths

Stone type	% of nephroliths	Risk factors/causes
Calcium oxalate	85	Hypercalciuria, hypercalcemia from primary hyperparathyroidism, hyperoxaluria, hypocitraturia, hyperuricosuria
Uric acid	5–10	Gout, myeloproliferative disorders, idiopathic
Calcium phosphate and calcium oxalate	10	Renal tubular acidosis
Pure calcium phosphate	Rare	
Struvite/infected nephrolith	2–20	Urease-producing bacteria
Cystine	1	Inherited cystinuria

- Pregnancy, ectopic pregnancy, ovarian torsion, ovarian cysts/masses, testicular torsion.
  - Aortic dissection, renal or splenic infarction.
  - Bowel ischemia or obstruction, diverticulitis, appendicitis, cholecystitis.
  - Pulmonary embolism, pneumonia.
  - Retroperitoneal hematoma, iliopsoas abscess.
- Evaluation:
  - Low risk: Urea, electrolytes, complete blood count, calcium, uric acid, urine culture, urine pH.
  - High risk (e.g., previous history of stone, family history, gastrointestinal disease, gout, chronic UTI, nephrocalcinosis): Low-risk evaluation; 24-hour urine for calcium, oxalate, uric acid, and cystine; workup of renal tubular acidosis.
  - Staghorn calculi can result in renal failure and urosepsis, temperature evaluated.
- Imaging:
  - Renal ultrasound: 95% sensitive for diagnosis.
  - X-ray diagnosis/radio-opacity decreases in order: Calcium phosphate, calcium oxalate > cystine, magnesium ammonium phosphate (struvite) > uric acid, triamterene, xanthine, indinavir.
  - Intravenous (IV) pyelogram used for patients with radiolucent stones, specifically indinavir stones.
  - Computed tomography (CT) urography useful for all types of nephroliths except for indinavir types, 95% specificity and 97% sensitivity for diagnosing nephroliths.
  - Magnetic resonance imaging (MRI) used to evaluate hydronephrosis if relevant; can evaluate location of nephroliths.
- Treatment:
  - Treatment may not alleviate all pain or infection.
  - Earlier treatment favored for younger patients, larger stones, more clinical symptoms, or struvite staghorn calculi.
  - Observation for stones < 4 mm because 90% will pass within 3 weeks, monitored with weekly X-rays, stones > 5 mm referred for urological evaluation.
  - Urgent urological consultation required in cases of urosepsis, anuria, or renal failure.
  - Pain control with nonsteroidal anti-inflammatory agents and opiates; calcium channel antagonists reduce ureteric contractions; α-blockers may improve distal nephrolith obstruction; increased fluid intake is unhelpful in flushing stones because of reduced renal blood flow and urine output with obstruction.
  - Medical dissolution therapy can be used for uric acid and cysteine nephroliths.
  - Extracorporeal lithotripsy (ESWL): Electrohydraulic, electromagnetic, or piezoelectric methods; most effective for stones < 2 cm in diameter in favorable locations (e.g., renal collecting system) of nonobese patients, less effective for cystine or calcium oxalate stones; side effects involve hematuria (0.5%), acute renal injury in patients with previous hypertension.
  - Intracorporeal lithotripsy: Electrohydraulic, pneumatic, ultrasonic, and laser methods using fluoroscopic guidance.
  - Flexible uteroscopy: Uses stone baskets and graspers for renal stones more than ureter stones; commonly combined with laser lithotripsy; used in patients with lithotripsy failure, lower pole stones, cystine stones, obesity, stones in calyceal diverticulum, patient with high risk of bleeding, horseshoe, or pelvic kidneys.
  - Percutaneous nephrolithotomy: Uses dilation of the renal collecting system using cystoscopically and percutaneously placed fluid followed by percutaneous lithotripsy; used for stones >3 cm, staghorn calculi, and those failing ESWL or flexible uteroscopy; 1% risk of hemorrhage.
  - Laparoscopic ureterolithotomy.
  - Open surgery: Used for complex stones, failure of endoscopic surgery, gross obesity, kyphoscoliosis, or where multiple percutaneous approaches would be needed.
  - Ureter JJ stenting or nephrostomy tube can relieve stone pain from obstruction.
- Stone prevention: High fluid intake, adequate calcium and potassium intake, reduced sucrose, sodium, animal protein intake.
- Bladder stones mostly consist of struvite or uric acid, treated cystoscopically or by open surgery.

11.5.2 Urethral Injury

- External causes from trauma; internal causes from abdominal surgery.
- Intravenous pyelography shows limited diagnosis, direct inspection with retrograde or anterograde injection preferred for diagnosis, CT urography used for delayed diagnosis.
- Presents with ileus, urosepsis, elevated fluid from abdominal drains, flank pain, urinoma (breach of urinary tract causing urine collection in perirenal fat), pelvic pain.
- Treatment:
  - Direct, tension-free repair with 4–0 or 5–0 absorbable suture at the time of injury or within 2 weeks of injury.
  - Percutaneous nephrostomy placed with IV antibiotics until repair.
  - JJ stenting for 3–6 weeks if ureter ligated with absorbable suture.
  - Primary ureteroureterostomy used for < 2-cm injuries.
  - Ureteroneocystostomy: Reimplantation of ureter into bladder directly, with psoas hitch or Boari bladder flap for lower injuries.
  - Transureteroureterostomy: Ipsilateral to contralateral ureter anastomosis.
  - Ileum replacement or autotransplantation of kidney into pelvis used with long-segment damage.
  - Permanent cutaneous ureterostomy tube or nephrectomy used during poor life expectancy or extensive damage.

11.5.3 Renal Cysts

- Simple cysts:
  - Single or multiple cysts; confined to renal cortex; filled with simple fluid.
  - 20% of adults have cysts by the age of 40 years, 50% of adults aged > 50 years have simple cysts.
  - Present asymptomatically and incidentally, rarely rupture or get infected.
  - Diagnosed by ultrasound; calcification, septation, irregular margins, concern for malignancy or clusters of cysts require further workup with CT-guided aspiration or MRI.
  - Treatment:
    - Bosniak classification helps predict malignancy (▶ Table 11.5).
    - Asymptomatic cysts do not require treatment.
    - Cysts causing pain are treated with percutaneous aspiration with or without injection of a sclerosing agent, or resection.
    - Infected cysts require drainage.
- Calyceal diverticulum:
  - Dilation of pericalyceal system, associated with nephrolith formation.
- Medullary sponge kidney:
  - Multiple dilations of distal collecting ducts; incidence between 1:5,000 and 20,000.
  - Commonly presents asymptomatically; can present with renal stone disease, UTI, or hematuria.
  - Diagnosed by IV pyelogram, evaluation of hypercalciuria.
  - Treatment: Asymptomatic disease requires no treatment, reduction of hypercalciuria and thiazide diuretics can reduce nephrolith production.

Table 11.5 Bosniak classification of cysts

Type	Features	% malignant	Treatment
I	Simple, smooth margins, no enhancement, no septations, no calcification	0	None, no follow-up
II	Smooth margins, thin septa, minimal calcifications, no enhancement	10	Observation with repeat ultrasound
III	Irregular margins, moderate calcification, > 1-mm septation	40–50	Surgical exploration with or without partial nephrectomy
IV	Cystic malignant lesion, irregular margin, enhancing areas	90	Radical nephrectomy

- Renal cystic disease:
  - Acquired type:
    - Associated with chronic end-stage renal failure, develops in one-third of patients after 3 years of dialysis.
    - Can cause pain and increases risk of renal tumors three to six times.
    - Multiple, bilateral cysts.
  - Autosomal dominant adult polycystic kidney disease:
    - Multiple, bilateral cysts, hereditary disposition with positive family history in 50% of cases.
    - Incidence: 0.1%.
    - Accounts for 10% of renal failure, which is inevitable in this disease.
    - Treatments aim to preserve renal function, treatment of hypertension, infected cysts, hematuria controlled with embolization and nephrectomy, eventually requires dialysis and renal transplantation.

11.6 Genitourinary Neoplasms

11.6.1 Presentation of Neoplasms

- Hematuria:
  - Macroscopically visible to naked eye, microscopically defined as three or more red blood cells (RBCs) per high-power centrifuged specimen; normal < 1 million RBC/24 hours.
  - No urological issues found in 50% of patients with gross hematuria and 70% with microscopic hematuria.
  - False positive: Menstruation, uterine bleeding, myoglobinuria, free hemoglobin from transfusion reaction, bacterial peroxidases, povidone.
  - False negative: Rare.
  - Medical causes: Glomerulonephritis (30% of pediatric cases), renal parenchymal diseases (e.g., IgA nephropathy, postinfectious glomerulonephritis, Henoch–Schönlein purpura), Alport syndrome, thin basement membrane disease, Fabry disease), vasculitis, coagulation disorders, anticoagulation use, sickle cell disease/trait, renal papillary necrosis, hypercalciuria, vascular disease with infarction of kidney.
  - Surgical causes: Cancer (30% of causes; urothelial or squamous cell carcinoma, renal cell carcinoma, prostate cancer), urolithiasis, infection, inflammation, trauma, renal cystic disease, congenital anatomical abnormalities, benign prostate hyperplasia, urinary tract stricture.
  - Hematuria workup depending on patient's risk.
    - Low risk (asymptomatic patients aged < 40 years): Treatment of urinary tract infection (UTI) and repeat urinalysis in 4–6 weeks; evaluation of upper tract (e.g., ultrasound, computed tomography [CT], intravenous pyelography), cell cytology, cystoscopy on case-by-case basis, magnetic resonance imaging (MRI) is of limited benefit; retrograde pyelography used as second-line imaging.
    - High risk: Full evaluation with flexible cystoscopy, upper tract evaluation with retrograde pyelogram and ureteroscopy.
- Differential diagnosis of lumps: Inguinal or femoral hernia, enlarged lymph node, saphena varix (e.g., dilation of proximal saphenous vein), hydrocele of cord or vagina, undescended testis, lipoma, femoral aneurysm, psoas abscess, tumor or malignancy (e.g., testicular, epididymis, paratesticular), testicular torsion, traumatic testicular rupture, benign cysts, infection, epididymitis/epididymo-orchitis, epididymal cyst, inguinal hernia, sebaceous cyst.
- Radiological evaluation of renal masses:
  - Renal ultrasound: Used as first-line investigation for flank pain or renal mass, detects cysts or masses > 1.5 cm.
  - CT scan with and without contrast used to evaluate real mass, Bosniak classification of renal cysts used (see Chapter 11.5 Nephrolithiasis/Urolithiasis, Ureter Injuries, and Renal Cysts).
  - MRI with contrast used to evaluate advanced diseases.
  - Fine-needle aspiration less useful for renal masses; used for renal abscess, cysts, or diagnosis of lymphoma or metastatic lesions.

11.6.2 Prostate Cancer

- 1:6 lifetime risk of prostate cancer in men, incidence of 164,000 cases annually in the United States, 2% risk of 5-year death.
- Prostatic intraepithelial neoplasia and atypical small acinar proliferation are premalignant lesions.
- Clinical TNM staging defines tumor extension, lymph node invasion, and metastasis.
- Transrectal ultrasound with biopsy:
  - Used with abnormal digital rectal examinations and elevated prostate-specific antigen (PSA), patients with biopsies of premalignant lesions, patients undergoing transurethral resection of the prostate, and reevaluation of treatment effect.
  - Small risk of infection, urosepsis, rectal bleeding, and hematuria.
  - 10–12 core biopsy obtained.
  - Gleason score (▶ Table 11.6): Pathological grading of biopsy specimen differentiation, individual score ranges from 1 to 5, primary grade given to cells in largest area of tumor and secondary grade given to next largest area (i.e., scores written as $3+4=7$); predictive of tumor spread, risk of metastasis, and risk of death.
    - ≤ 6: Suggests cancer likely to grow slowly.
    - 7: Intermediate risk.
    - ≥ 8: Dedifferentiated tumor.
- National Comprehensive Cancer Network (NCCN) classification uses TNM staging (▶ Table 11.7), Gleason score, and PSA levels to delineate treatment and predict survival by dividing patient into risk categories (▶ Table 11.8).
- Treatment:
  - Observation, surveillance, prostatectomy with adjuvant therapy.
  - Radical prostatectomy: Involves excision of prostate, prostatic urethra, and seminal vesicles with rebuilding of the vesicourethral junction; can be performed open, laparoscopically, or robotically; used in men with localized prostate cancer, life expectancy of > 10 years, and goals for cure; 40% reduction in death compared with observation but depends on tumor grade.
  - Complications of radical prostatectomy:
    - Injury to obturator nerve, urethra, or rectum managed intraoperatively.
    - Postoperative catheter displacement treated with replacement using cystoscopy and guidewire, catheter maintained for up to 2 weeks.
    - Lymphatic leaks or lymphocele treated with continued wound drains and possible sclerotherapy.
    - Erectile dysfunction (> 50% patients) treated medically or with rehabilitation.
    - Incontinence (5% of patients) treated with pelvic floor exercises, biofeedback, and urethral slings.
    - Bladder neck stenosis (5–8% patients) treated endoscopically.
  - Antiandrogenic therapy:
    - Used postoperatively especially for advanced tumors, tumors can dedifferentiate into androgen-independent/castration-resistant disease, results in need for cytotoxic chemotherapy and androgen receptor blockade.
    - Surgical castration involves bilateral orchiectomy.
    - Medical castration involves luteinizing hormone-releasing hormone (LHRH) agonist (e.g., leuprolide, goserelin, buserelin, triptorelin), LHRH antagonists (e.g., degarelix, abarelix).

Table 11.6 Natural history of localized prostate cancer

Gleason biopsy grade	% risk of metastasis within 10 y	% risk of death within 15 y
2–4	19%	4–7%
5	42%	6–11%
6	42%	18–30%
7	42%	42–72%
8–10	74%	56–87%

Table 11.7 TNM staging prostate adenocarcinoma

TNM staging	Findings
T0	T0: no primary tumor
T1	T1a: nonpalpable tumor, present < 5% TURP specimens
	T1b: nonpalpable tumor, present > 5% TURP specimens
	T1c: nonpalpable tumor, present on needle biopsy
T2	T2a: palpable tumor < 1/2 of one lobe
	T2b: palpable tumor > 1/2 of one lobe
	T2c: palpable tumor both lobes
T3	T3a: palpable tumor, advanced into periprostatic tissue
	T3b: palpable tumor, advanced into seminal vesicles
T4	T4a: palpable tumor, advanced into adjacent structures, fixed
	T4b: palpable tumor, advanced into pelvic side-wall, fixed
N	N0: no regional node
	N1: tumor of regional nodes
M	M0: no metastasis
	M1a: non regional lymph node metastasis
	M1b: bone metastasis
	M1c: other site metastasis with or without bone metastasis

Table 11.8 Prostate adenocarcinoma National Comprehensive Cancer Network (NCCN) group staging

NCCN group stage	Findings
Very low risk	T1c, PSA < 10 ng/mL, Gleason ≤ 6, cancer ≤ 50% core samples
Low risk	T1a, T1b, T1c, T2a, PSA < 10 ng/mL, Gleason ≤ 6
Intermediate risk	T2b, T2c, PSA 10–20 ng/mL, Gleason 7
High risk	T3a, PSA > 20 ng/mL, Gleason 8–10
Very high risk	T3b, T4, Gleason 8–10

Abbreviation: PSA, prostate-specific antigen.

- – Androgen receptor blockade (e.g., flutamide, bicalutamide, nilutamide, enzalutamide).
- – Maximal androgen blockade involves medical or surgical castration with antiandrogenic therapy.
- – CYP17 receptor blockers (e.g., ketoconazole, abiraterone acetate) aim to reduce androgen hormone production.
- ○ PSA recurrence involves consecutively rising values, managed with digital rectal examination and biopsy if palpable mass; PSA values can be predictive of postoperative treatment response to radiation.
- ○ Radiation treatment involves external beam radiotherapy, hypofractionated radiotherapy, and brachytherapy seeds or wires.
- ○ Salvage treatment involves radical prostatectomy, cryotherapy, high-intensity focused ultrasound, cytotoxic chemotherapy, and other treatments.

11.6.3 Bladder Cancer

- Second most common urological cancer, 80,000 annual cases in the United States, 75% 5-year survival overall.
- Benign tumors rare, > 90% transitional cell carcinoma/urothelial carcinoma, 1–7% squamous cell carcinoma, 2% adenocarcinoma, rarely other types.
- Graded into well, moderately, and poorly differentiated.
- Clinical TNM staging (► Table 11.9) defines tumor extension, lymph node invasion, and metastasis.

Table 11.9 TNM staging of bladder carcinoma

TNM staging	Findings	5-y survival[a]
T0	T0: no primary tumor, noninvasive papillary carcinoma	
	Tis: carcinoma in situ	
	Ta: noninvasive papillary carcinoma	
T1	Invades subepithelial connective tissue	90%
T2	T2a: invades inner half of muscularis propria	63–88%
	T2b: invades outer half of muscularis propria	
T3	T3a: microscopic invasion of perivesicular structures	63–88%
	T3b: macroscopic invasion of perivesicular structures	37–61%
T4	T4a: invasion of prostate, uterus, vagina, bowel	10%
	T4b: invasion of pelvis or abdominal wall	
N	N0: no regional nodes	30%
	N1: single node < 2 cm	30%
	N2: single node 2–5 cm or multiple nodes < 5 cm	
	N3: multiple nodes > 5 cm	
M	Distant metastasis	

[a] Survival involving first-time radical cystectomy.

- Urothelial carcinoma in situ defines a premalignant lesion.
- Commonly presents with asymptomatic hematuria, pain signifies advanced stage obstructive disease or malignant cystitis.
- Diagnosed with CT urography before and after intravenous (IV) contrast; cytology and MRI can be used to evaluate tumor extension.
- Treatment:
  - Transurethral resection of bladder tumor (TURBT) for early-stage tumors.
  - Staging lymphadenectomy performed if imaging suggestive of local tumor spread.
  - Frequent follow-up for evaluation of recurrence, transurethral fulguration used for small recurrences.
  - Adjuvant intravesicular chemotherapy and Bacillus Calmette–Guerin strain *Mycobacterium bovis* can be used.
- Muscle-invasive bladder cancer has poor prognosis; treated with combination of radical TURBT, radical cystectomy with urinary diversion, partial cystectomy, systemic chemotherapy, palliative therapy, or external beam radiotherapy depending on patient.
- Urinary diversion:
  - Ureterosigmoidostomy: Ureter drainage into sigmoid colon, patients may be prone to UTI, long-term risk of colon cancer with diversion.
  - Ileal conduit: Ureter drainage to an isolated ileal segment, which makes a neobladder, and then to a stoma; an ileoileostomy reapproximates ileum; neobladder emptied by catheterized stoma or anastomosed to urethra.

11.6.4 Renal Cell Carcinoma

- Adenocarcinoma arising from proximal convoluted tubule; accounts for 85% of renal malignancies, 65,000 cases annually, 75% 5-year survival.
- Associated with von Hippel–Lindau mutation, chromosome 7 and 17 mutation.
- Fuhrman grade divides into four grades: Well (1), moderate (2), and poorly (3, 4) differentiated.
- TNM staging important for prognostication (▶ Table 11.10).
- Present with hematuria (50%), mass (30%), constitutional symptoms (25%, i.e., night sweats, fatigue, weight loss), acute varicocele (5%), paraneoplastic syndromes (10–40%).

Table 11.10 TNM staging of renal cell carcinoma

TNM staging	Findings	5-y survival
T1	T1a: <4 cm	90–100%
	T1b: 4–7 cm	80–90%
T2	>7 cm but within kidney	70–80%
T3	T3a: invades perinephric tissue	60–70%
	T3b: invades renal veins or subdiaphragmatic IVC	50–80%
	T3c: invades right atrium, vena cava, or supradiaphragmatic IVC	
T4	Invades beyond perinephric/Gerota fascia	5–30%
N	N1: single nodes	
	N2: ≥2 node	
M	Distant metastasis	5–100%

Abbreviation: IVC: inferior vena cava.

- Evaluated by ultrasound and CT imaging, urine cytology and culture, laboratory studies; staging chest CT and bone scan can be performed; renal vain or inferior vena cava involvement evaluated by MRI; biopsy not routinely performed because of tract seeding.
- Treatments:
  - Surveillance for small, localized tumors.
  - Radiofrequency ablation for localized tumors.
  - Open or laparoscopic radical nephrectomy versus partial nephrectomy.
  - Hormonal and cytotoxic therapy has a limited role.
  - Radiotherapy used for metastatic bone lesions.
  - Immunotherapy (e.g., interleukin-2, interferon A-2b) and molecular therapy (e.g., sunitinib, sorafenib, temsirolimus, everolimus, bevacizumab) are potential options.

11.6.5 Testicular Cancer

- Most common solid tumor in men aged 20–45 years; 9,000 annual cases in the United States with 95% 5-year survival.
- Presents with painless scrotal lump; acute scrotal pain from tumor hemorrhage is rare (5%).
- 90% malignant germ cell tumors; divide into seminomatous (e.g., seminoma), non-seminomatous (e.g., teratoma, yolk sac tumor, choriocarcinoma), and mixed germ-cell/non-germ cell tumors; rarely other types of tumors, metastasis to the testis, or sex cord stroma tumors.
- Evaluated with scrotal ultrasound; differential includes infection, trauma, hernia, torsion, and tumor; abdominal and chest CT obtained for staging, serum tumor markers (e.g., α-fetoprotein, β-human chorionic gonadotropin, lactate dehydrogenase, placental alkaline phosphatase, CD30, γ-glutamyl transferase) measured before treatment.
- Treatment:
  - Radical orchiectomy, curative in 80% of patients.
  - Retroperitoneal lymph node dissection surgery can be performed after radical orchiectomy for reducing risk of relapse but has 5–25% morbidity rate.
  - Contralateral testis biopsies performed for high-risk patients with intratubular germ cell neoplasm (IGCN)/carcinoma in situ.
  - Cytotoxicity therapy used for germ cell, non–germ cell, and other tumors.
  - Radiotherapy used for seminomas, IGCN, and lymphoma.
- TNM staging performed for risk categorization and treatment (▶ Table 11.11); International Germ Cell Cancer Collaborative Group (IGCCCG) staging divides germ cell tumors based on tumor spread and tumor markers into good, intermediate, and poor risk categories.

Table 11.11 TNM staging of testicular cancer

TNM staging	Findings
T0	T0: no primary tumor
	Tis: carcinoma in situ
T1	Testis and epididymis, invades tunica albuginea
T2	Testis and epididymis, invades tunica vaginalis
T3	Spermatic cord with or without vascular invasion
T4	Scrotum with or without vascular invasion
N	N1: node ≤ 2 cm or multiple nodes > 2 cm
	N2: node 2–5 cm or multiple nodes summed 2–5 cm
	N3: node > 5 cm
M	Distant metastasis

Table 11.12 TNM staging of renal pelvis/ureter urothelial carcinoma

TNM staging	Findings	5-y survival
T0	T0: no primary tumor	
	Tis: carcinoma in situ	
	Ta: noninvasive papillary carcinoma	
T1	Invades subepithelial connective tissue	60–100%
T2	Invades muscularis propria	
T3	Invades perinephric structures	20–50%
T4	Invades adjacent organs	
N	N0: no regional nodes	15%
	N1: single node < 2 cm	
	N2: single node 2–5 cm or multiple nodes < 5 cm	
	N3: single or multiple node > 5 cm	
M	Distant metastasis	10%

11.6.6 Other Urological Neoplasms

- Renal pelvis and ureter:
  - 90% of transitional cell carcinoma/urothelial carcinoma, also includes benign inverted papilloma, fibroepithelial polyp, squamous cell carcinoma, adenocarcinoma, and rare sarcoma.
  - 10% of renal tumors; presents with hematuria and flank pain; 50% develop bladder urothelial carcinoma.
  - Evaluated via cytology, ultrasound, intravenous pyelogram, or CT urogram.
  - TNM staging (▶ Table 11.12) performed and treatment with nephroureterectomy, percutaneous or ureteroscopic resection, systemic chemotherapy, palliative surgery, or arterial embolization for hematuria; radiotherapy is ineffective.
- Penile tumors:
  - Benign noncutaneous lesions: Cysts, syringoma (sweat gland tumor), neurilemoma, angioma, lipoma, pseudotumor, or granuloma from injections, Behcet disease.
  - Benign cutaneous lesions: Pearly penile papules, zoon balanitis, lichen planus.
  - Infection: Chancroid, genital herpes, granuloma inguinale, lymphogranuloma venereum, syphilis.
  - Viral lesions: Condyloma acuminatum, bowenoid papulosis, molluscum contagiosum.
  - Premalignant lesions.

- o Penile cancer: Squamous cell carcinoma (95% of penile lesion, TNM staging and Broder grading for tumor aggressiveness used for risk stratification and treatment); others include Kaposi sarcoma, basal cell carcinoma, melanoma, sarcoma, and Paget disease; metastatic lesions to the penis are rare.
- Urethral cancer:
  - o Commonly squamous cell carcinoma (75%); rarely adenocarcinoma (8%), sarcoma, and melanoma.
  - o TNM staging used to guide risk stratification and treatment.
- Wilms tumor:
  - o See Chapter 10.4 Pediatric Neoplasms.
- Neuroblastoma:
  - o See Chapter 10.4 Pediatric Neoplasms.

12 Obstetrics/Gynecology

Edited by Erol Arslan

12.1 General Gynecology

Erol Arslan, Fulya Gokdagli, and Cigdem Akcabay

12.1.1 Genital Tract Infections

- Bacterial vaginosis (BV):
  - Vaginal flora normally composes from multiple aerobic and anaerobic species.
  - All conditions that disturb the vaginal flora cause vaginal infections.
  - *Lactobacillus* species are the most common microorganism causes of BV and they form the acidic environment of vagina (normal vaginal pH is between 4 and 4.5) by producing lactic acid.
  - Other causes include *Gardnerella vaginalis, Ureaplasma urealyticum, Mycoplasma hominis.*
  - BV is one of the most common causes of vaginitis seen in all ages.
  - Complex clinical syndrome with increased vaginal secretion, bacterial accumulation, and lower polymorphonuclear leukocyte count than an infectious process.
  - Risk factors: Oral sex, douching, cigarette smoking, intrauterine devices, intercourse during menstruation.
  - Diagnosis is based on at least showing three of the followings which are known as the Amsel criteria[1]:
    - Positive amine or "whiff" test (adding 10% KOH to a fresh sample of discharge results with fishy odor).
    - Vaginal pH > 4.5.
    - Presence of 20% per HPF of "clue cells."
    - Non-viscous, milky-white, homogenous adherent vaginal discharge.
  - Treatment: Oral and/or vaginal metronidazole or clindamycin, no need for partner therapy as it is not a sexually transmitted disease (STD).
  - Complications: Pelvic inflammatory disease (PID), premature rupture of membranes (PROM), preterm delivery, chorioamnionitis.
- Trichomoniasis vaginalis:
  - Most common cause of protozoal infections and most prevalent nonviral STD in the United States.
  - Acquired by direct sexual contact.
  - Diagnosed mostly in women; men are generally asymptomatic.
  - Symptoms: Foul-smelling yellow or green vaginal discharge, dyspareunia, urinary symptoms, vaginal and vulvar itching, or erythema.
  - Vaginal pH is > 4.5.
  - Diagnosis: Motile organisms by wet prep microscopy; nucleic acid amplification tests (NAATs) have been gaining importance in diagnosis with its sensitivity and specificity.
  - 2015 Center for Disease Control (CDC) STD treatment guidelines recommended two strategies; a single 2-g dose of metronidazole or tinidazole, or 7-day course of 500 mg metronidazole twice daily.
- Vulvovaginal candidiasis:
  - Most common cause is *Candida albicans.*
  - Risk factors: Obesity, pregnancy, diabetes mellitus, broad-spectrum antibiotic use.
  - Symptoms: Cottage cheese-like, odorless discharge, pruritus, erythema due to itching.
  - Vaginal pH is < 4.5.
  - Diagnosis: History and direct inspection, microscopically identification of yeast might be done by adding saline and 10% KOH to vaginal discharge, culture is limited to cases that do not respond to treatment or in those having infection but yeast cannot be seen in microscopy.
  - Treatment: Single oral dose of 150 mg fluconazole, or vaginal form of butoconazole, clotrimazole, miconazole, and nystatin.
- Chlamydia trachomatis[2]:
  - Cervicitis is characterized by a purulent cervical discharge or cervical bleeding due to any manipulation to cervix (e.g., coitus, performing examining swab).

○ *C. trachomatis* is the most common STD (1.6 million annual cases in the United States in 2015) followed by *Neisseria gonorrhea* (470,000 annual cases in the United States in 2015).

○ Usually asymptomatic, when getting symptomatic mucopurulent discharge, edematous and hyperemic endocervical tissue as well as dysuria due to urethritis are the common findings.

○ While it affects a large population, CDC recommends its screening annually for all sexually active women < 25 years old as well those ≥ 25 years with increased risk for infection.

○ Diagnosis: Microscopic inspection of > 20 leukocyte per HPF in secretions after adding saline and more specifically culture, NAAT, and enzyme-linked immunosorbent assay.

○ If *C. trachomatis* is diagnosed, screening for other STDs is indicated.

○ Primary treatment: Azithromycin 1 g orally once or 2 × 100 mg doxycycline for 7 days.

○ Alternative treatment: 4 × 500 mg erythromycin, 2 × 300 mg ofloxacin, or 1 × 500 mg levofloxacin for 7 days.

- Neisseria gonorrhea[2]:
  ○ Gram-negative coccobacillus that invade columnar and transitional cells and therefore do not affect the vagina.
  ○ Can cause cervicitis, infection of Bartholin and Skene glands, upper genital tract by ascending and invading endometrium or fallopian tube.
  ○ After a decline in 2009 in the United States, there has been a slight increase.
  ○ Second most common notifiable disease in the United States.
  ○ Generally asymptomatic but if being symptomatic a nonirritating, white-to-yellow discharge is the main finding.
  ○ Diagnosis: Culture, NAATs.
  ○ Recommended treatment by CDC for uncomplicated gonococcal infection of cervix, urethra, or rectum is single dose 125 mg IM ceftriaxone, or orally used of 400 mg cefixime, 500 mg ciprofloxacin, 400 mg ofloxacin, 250 mg levofloxacin.[3]
  ○ Like chlamydia, if gonorrhea is diagnosed, screening is recommended for other STDs.

12.1.2 Genital Infections with Mass Lesions

- Human papillomavirus (HPV)[2]:
  ○ According to the CDC, HPV is the most common STD in the United States.
  ○ Genital warts are the typical lesion, generally asymptomatic.
  ○ More than 100 types:
    – Types 6 and 11 are known as the source of genital warts (condyloma acuminata).
    – Types 16, 18, 31, and 45 cause cervical intraepithelial neoplasia and thus squamous cell carcinoma.
  ○ Diagnosis: Direct inspection for genital wart and colposcopy for vaginal or cervical lesions.
  ○ Treatment for warts is varied including surgical excision, imiquimod 5% cream, podofilox 0.5% gel, topical trichloroacetic acid, CO_2 laser excision.
  ○ For prevention, there is a vaccine against four types of HPV (types 6, 11, 16, and 18).
- Molluscum contagiosum:
  ○ Poxvirus infection.
  ○ Typical lesions are dome-shaped papules with central umbilication with a diameter between 2 and 5 mm.
  ○ Diagnosis is made by direct inspection of typical lesion.
  ○ Lesion diameter is larger in immunosuppressed patients like human immunodeficiency virus (HIV)/acquired immunodeficiency syndrome (AIDS).
  ○ Generally self-limited but if needed cryo-freezing and laser ablation can be used.

12.1.3 Genital Infections with Ulcerative Lesions

Herpes Simplex Infection

- DNA virus with two types, Herpes Simplex Virus 1 (HSV-1) and HSV-2.[2]
- HSV-1 mostly causes orolabial herpes and HSV-2 is known as genital herpes; it has to be recognized that HSV-1 is the cause of 15% of genital herpes cases.
- Only one-third of patients who acquired genital herpes become symptomatic.
- The virus enters sensory nerve endings and becomes latent.

- Risk of transmission is greatest during recurrences, sexual contact is not advised during this time; viral shedding can allow transmission outside of recurrences also.
- Primary infection symptoms are generally vague like fever, fatigue, and painful lymphadenopathy.
- After prodromal symptoms, classical genital herpes can be recognized by typical papular lesions that progress to vesicles and ulcers.
- Laboratory diagnosis:
  - Directly demonstrates the virus in genital lesions; take the swabs from the base of the lesion (unroofed the vesicles with a needle).
  - At the first episode of genital herpes, HSV typing is recommended.
  - Culture.
  - HSV DNA detection is the gold standard for diagnosis.
  - Serological testing is recommended in the following conditions:
    - History of recurrent or atypical genital disease when virus cannot be detected.
    - First-episode of genital herpes; to distinguish between acute and older infection.
    - For patients who have partners with genital herpes.
    - Asymptomatic pregnant women who have a history of genital herpes in the partner.
- Treatment is indicated in the first episode of genital herpes but does not change the natural history of infection, reduces severity and duration of episodes.
- Treatment within 5 days includes oral antiviral therapy for 5–10 days:
  - Acyclovir 400 mg three times a day or 200 mg five times a day.
  - Famciclovir 250 mg three times a day.
  - Valacyclovir 500 mg two times a day.
- Recurrences are generally self-limiting and treatment is individualized; supportive therapy is generally sufficient for most patients.
- More than six recurrences per 1 year, support suppressive treatment, acyclovir (total dose of 800 mg daily; whether four times of 200 mg or two times of 400 mg) or valacyclovir (250 mg twice daily).

Syphilis

- Bacterial STD caused by *Treponema pallidum*.[2]
- Transmitted via sexual contact with infectious lesions, blood transfusion, or transplacentally.
- Classified as early (primary, secondary, and early latent) and late (late latent and tertiary syphilis).
- The first sign of the disease is a painless, solitary lesion which is known as chancre (primary syphilis) that may not be recognized by the patient.
- Disease is not treated until progress to secondary syphilis, characterized by generalized mucocutaneous lesion mostly on palms and soles.
- Untreated syphilis can resolve or enter latent stage.
- Latent syphilis is a phase in which patient is asymptomatic while serological tests are positive.
- If the infection has persisted < 2 years, it is termed "early latent"; if more than > 2 years, it is termed "late latent syphilis."
- During primary, secondary, and early latent stage, the disease is sexually transmitted.
- Transplacental transmission may be after several years of initial maternal onset.
- Congenital syphilis is one of the most devastating conditions that result with adverse pregnancy outcomes.
- Diagnosis is primarily based on history, physical examination, and laboratory testing.
- Multiple laboratory tests are used for diagnosing syphilis (▶ Table 12.1).
- *T. pallidum* cannot be cultured in vitro and the definitive diagnosis can be made by identifying the spirochete by dark field microscopy.

Table 12.1 Laboratory tests that have been using for the diagnosis of syphilis

Treponemal tests	Nontreponemal tests
Treponema pallidum hemagglutination assay (TPHA)	Rapid plasma reagin (RPR)
Treponema pallidum particle agglutination assay (TPPA)	Venereal diseases research laboratory (VDRL)
Fluorescent treponemal antibody absorbed (FTA-ABS)	Toluidine red unheated serum test (TRUST)

- If syphilis is detected in a patient, it is recommended to search for other STDs.
- WHO STD treatment guidelines: Benzathine penicillin G (2.4 million units of IM once for early syphilis; 2.4 million units IM weekly for 3 weeks for late syphilis or unknown stage in pregnant and nonpregnant adults).
- Alternative treatments for early syphilis: Procaine penicillin (1.2 million units 10–14 days IM), doxycycline (100 mg twice daily orally for 14 days), ceftriaxone (1 g IM once daily for 10–14 days), azithromycin (2 g once orally).
- Pregnant women: Benzathine penicillin G (2.4 million units IM once), alternative treatments with erythromycin (500 mg orally four times daily for 14 days) rather than doxycycline in pregnancy, otherwise alternative treatment same as above.
- Alternative treatments for late syphilis: IM procaine penicillin (1.2 million units once daily for 20 days), doxycycline (100 mg twice daily orally for 30 days for nonpregnant women), erythromycin (500 mg four times daily orally for 30 days for pregnant women).

12.1.4 Pelvic Inflammatory Disease

- PID is known as upper genital tract infection which includes endometritis, salpingitis, parametritis, oophoritis, tubo-ovarian abscess, and pelvic peritonitis.[4]
- Most common infectious agents: *Neisseria gonorrhea*, *Chlamydia trachomatis* followed by *Mycoplasma genitalium* and other organisms including anaerobes and vaginal flora microorganisms.
- Risk factors: Young age, multiple partners, new partner, IUDs, any intervention to uterine cavity.
- The symptoms of PID: Lower abdominal pain, deep dyspareunia, abnormal bleeding, and abnormal vaginal or cervical discharge.
- Physical signs: Lower abdominal tenderness, adnexal tenderness on bimanual vaginal examination, and cervical motion tenderness on bimanual vaginal examination.
- Diagnosis: Positive test results (*N. gonorrhea*, *Chlamydia*, and *M. genitalium*), high levels of infection markers (C-reactive protein [CRP], erythrocyte sedimentation rate, leukocyte count), fever (> 38 °C).
- Tubo-ovarian abscess diagnosis: ultrasound CT, and MRI.
- Diagnosis of salpingitis by laparoscopy is highly sensitive finding for the diagnosis of PID.
- The treatment regimens are presented in ▶ Table 12.2.

Table 12.2 Treatment regimens of PID both for outpatient and inpatient management

Outpatient regimens	Inpatient regimen
IM ceftriaxone 500 mg single dose *followed by* 14 d of treatment with oral doxycycline 100 mg twice daily	IM/IV ceftriaxone 1 g once daily
plus	*plus*
Metronidazole 500 mg twice daily	IV doxycycline 100 mg twice daily
	followed by oral doxycycline 100 mg twice daily
	plus
	metronidazole 500 mg twice daily
	to complete 14 d
Oral ofloxacin 400 mg twice daily	IV clindamycin 900 mg three times daily
or	*plus*
Levofloxacin 500 mg once daily	IM/IV gentamicin (3–6 mg/kg once daily)
plus	*followed after complete 14 days by either*
Oral metronidazole 500 mg twice daily *for 14 d*	Oral clindamycin 450 mg four times daily
	or
	Oral doxycycline 100 mg twice daily
	plus
	Metronidazole 500 mg twice daily
Oral moxifloxacin 400 mg once daily *for 14 d*	
Abbreviation: PID, pelvic inflammatory disease.	

- Conditions that required inpatient managements are uncertainty in diagnosis, failure with oral therapy, severe symptoms or signs, presence of tubo-ovarian abscess, not able to tolerate oral therapy, pregnancy.

12.1.5 Uterine Leiomyomas

- Background:
  - Known as fibroids and myomas.
  - Most common pelvic tumors in women and they are composed from smooth muscle cells and fibrous connective tissue.
  - Monoclonal tumors of the uterine muscular layer and in benign character.
  - Estimated incidence is 20–50%.
  - Malign transformation is extremely rare (< 0.5%).
  - The submucosal myomas were classified due to myometrial relation and revised in 2011 by FIGO adding other types (▶ Table 12.3).[5]
- Diagnosis:
  - Most are asymptomatic and diagnosed incidentally during pelvic examination or in autopsy.
  - Most common symptoms: Abnormal uterine bleeding, low back pain, pelvic pain and/or pressure, dyspareunia, urinary symptoms (frequency, urgency, and urinary retention), digestive symptoms (constipation and bowel dysfunction).
  - Bimanual pelvic examination may reveal a firm, irregular pelvic mass.
  - First-line imaging method is ultrasound (preferably transvaginal ultrasound [TVUSG]), highly sensitive for initial diagnosis and monitoring changes.
  - Sonohysterography is especially used in differential diagnosis of submucosal myomas from polyps, minimally invasive, cost-effective compared with hysteroscopy.
  - Hysterosalpingography used to evaluate tubal patency and uterine cavity contour in infertile women.
  - Hysteroscopy: Gold standard method, advantage of being performed in an office setting even for small submucosal myomas < 1 cm without anesthesia.
  - MRI: most sensitive for diagnosis and localization, provides info on degeneration, used before embolization to evaluate vasculature, used after treatment to evaluate complications.
- Medical treatment[3]:
  - Expectant management is common, individualized treatment for patients.
  - Nonsteroidal anti-inflammatory drugs (NSAIDs) can be used for dysmenorrhea; combined oral contraceptives improve the symptoms of dysmenorrhea, dyspareunia, and abnormal uterine bleeding.
  - Levonorgestrel-releasing intrauterine devices treat menorrhagia and is a contraceptive.
  - Gonadotropin-releasing hormone (GnRH) analogs decrease uterine volume, fibroid volume, and bleeding; risk of adverse effects for long-term use; fibroids regrow after stopping treatment within 8 to 12 months.
  - Mifepristone (RU486) is an antiprogestin agent that decreases fibroid volume, side-effects of endometrial hyperplasia.

Table 12.3 Classification of myomas

Type	Description
0	Pedunculated intracavitary
1	< 50% intramural
2	≥ 50% intramural
3	Contacts endometrium but 100% intramural
4	Intramural
5	Subserosal with a ≥ 50% intramural component
6	Subserosal with a < 50% intramural component
7	Subserosal pedunculated
8	Other (cervical, parasitic, etc.)

○ Other treatments: Progestins, estrogens, selective estrogen receptor modulators (SERMs), androgens, and aromatase inhibitors.
- Surgical treatment:
  ○ Used after failure of medical management, patient symptoms, or desires for fertility.
  ○ Treatment options depend on size, location, and number of fibroids; treatments include myomectomy, hysterectomy, endometrial ablation, myolysis, uterine artery, or uterine fibroid embolization.

12.1.6 Endometriosis

- Definition and background[6]:
  ○ Presence of endometrium out of uterine cavity, first described in 1860, poorly understood etiology but most commonly accepted theory is of retrograde menstruation.
  ○ Affects 10–15% of reproductive age women.
  ○ Risk factors: Infertility history, early menarche, family history of endometriosis, intercourse during menses, low body weight, prolonged menstrual flow, short cycle interval.
- Presentation:
  ○ Symptoms: Chronic pelvic pain, dyspareunia, dysmenorrhea, menorrhagia, uterosacral ligament nodularity, adnexal mass, infertility.
  ○ Diagnosis: Bimanual pelvic exam for nodularity in uterosacral ligaments and pouch of Douglas, imaging laparoscopy with biopsy (risk of false-positive lesions).
  ○ Imaging: Ultrasound (cysts with low-level homogenous internal echoes consistent with old blood), TVUSG preferred (detects deeply infiltrating rectovaginal endometriosis); CT and MRI studies can be useful for deep-seated lesions.
  ○ CA-125 can be useful for diagnosis but is more beneficial for follow-up.
  ○ Endometriosis may increase risk of ovarian cancer especially the endometrioid and clear cell types.
- Treatment:
  ○ Depends on symptom type and severity, goals of treatment, and fertility preservation; treatment improves pain but does not improve infertility.
  ○ Pain management:
    – NSAIDs.
    – Progestins (first-line treatment, oral norethindrone, DMPA-SC, intrauterine levonorgestrel).
    – Combined oral contraceptives.
    – Danazol: Androgenic, severe side-effects.
    – GnRH analogs: Side-effects of osteopenia and menopause, second-line treatment.
    – Aromatase inhibitors: Anastrozole and letrozole, combined with GnRH analogs for 12 months, second-line treatment.
  ○ Surgery: Used for endometrioma, infertility (e.g., assistive reproductive technology), and medically refractory pain treatment; goal to ablate visible disease, laparoscopic methods preferred, treatment may reduce ovarian reserve, combined with medical therapy to reduce recurrence risk.
  ○ Medical and surgical treatments for chronic pelvic pain are limited.

12.1.7 Adenomyosis

- Epidemiology[7]:
  ○ Definition: Presence of endometrial glands and stroma in myometrium.
  ○ Risk factors: Multiparity, early menarche, short menstrual cycles.
  ○ Accompanied by leiomyoma (50%), endometrial hyperplasia (25%), and endometriosis (10%).
  ○ Presentation: Mostly asymptomatic; classical triad of enlarged, soft, and tender uterus; menorrhagia; and dysmenorrhea.
- Diagnosis: Ultrasound limited, MRI more sensitive, histopathology from hysterectomy is definitive.
- Treatment: Depends on age and fertility, treatments include NSAIDs, combined oral contraceptives, progestins, and GnRH analogs; curative treatment from hysterectomy.

12.1.8 Abnormal (Dysfunctional) Uterine Bleeding

- Epidemiology[8]:
  - Definition: Bleeding from uterine corpus in reproductive age nonpregnant women with abnormal features in duration, volume, frequency, and/or regularity which has been present for the majority of last 6 months.
  - Regular menstrual cycle is defined as 28 ± 7 days, with blood flow lasting 4 ± 2 days and an average blood loss of 20–60 mL.
  - Common chief complaint in gynecological visits, occasionally patients present with acute bleeding requiring emergent intervention and blood transfusion.
  - Incidence of 14–25% in reproductive age women.
  - Terms:
    - Menorrhagia: Prolonged (> 7 days) or heavy cyclic (blood loss > 80 mL) menstruation.
    - Metrorrhagia: Intermenstrual bleeding, generally accompanied to menorrhagia.
    - Hypomenorrhea: Shortening of menses or diminished blood flow.
    - Oligomenorrhea: Cycles with intervals of > 35 days.
    - Polymenorrhea: Cycles with intervals of < 21 days.
    - Withdrawal bleeding: Predictable bleeding due to sudden decline in progesterone level.
    - Postcoital bleeding: Bleeding occurs due to vaginal intercourse.
  - Classification with multiple causes; can use acronym PALM-COEIN (▶ Table 12.4).[5]
- Diagnosis:
  - History (acute vs. chronic bleeding), history of bleeding (pattern, symptoms of anemia, reproductive history, sexual history, association of fever or pelvic pain, systemic diseases, medications), physical exam, labs (complete blood count, pregnancy test, β-human chorionic gonadotropin (β-hCG), thyroid stimulating hormone, prolactin, coagulation tests).
  - TVUSG is the preferred first-line diagnostic tool; evaluates endometrial thickness, adnexal leiomyomas, and adenomyosis; color Doppler distinguishes myomas from polyps, saline uterine infusion improves resolution.
  - Hysteroscopy: Diagnostic and can obtain biopsy; biopsy is especially important in women > 40 years old.
  - CT and MRI are utilized as second-line imaging.
- Treatment:
  - Treatment of other medical conditions (e.g., coagulation disorders).
  - NSAIDs: Improves dysmenorrhea symptom.
  - Tranexamic acid: Antifibrinolytic agent.
  - Progestins: Especially indicated in anovulatory cycles to reduce endometrial proliferation.
  - Combination oral contraceptive pills: Results in endometrial atrophy, decreases dysmenorrhea and improves fertility, and uses short or long term.
  - Estrogens: Mostly used during acute bleeding.
  - Dilatation and curettage: Used to control acute bleeding.
  - Hysteroscopic resection: Uses for endometrial polyps, can be outpatient.
  - Hysterectomy: Gold standard.
  - Radiofrequency or laser ablation.

Table 12.4 PALM–COEIN classification system for abnormal uterine bleeding in reproductive-age women

PALM (structural causes)	COEIN (nonstructural causes)
Polyp	Coagulopathy
Adenomyosis	Ovulatory dysfunction
Leiomyoma	Endometrial
Malignancy and hyperplasia	Iatrogenic
	Not yet classified

Source: 2011 FIGO classification "PALM-COEIN."

12.1.9 Gynecologic Causes of Acute Abdomen

- Distinct causes from male patients, considered in all women with acute abdominal and/or pelvic pain (▶ Table 12.5), see Chapter 4.1, Acute Abdomen and Chapter 12.4.9, Obstetric and Gynecologic Causes of Acute Abdomen During Pregnancy.
- Adnexal torsion[9]:
  - Partial or complete rotation of the adnexa (ovary, fallopian tube, or both) on its vascular pedicle; isolated tubal torsion is rare.
  - Mostly affects children, adolescents, and reproductive age women; can occur in any age group,
  - Most adults have adnexal masses which are generally benign; pediatric cases involve normal ovaries in up to 50%.
  - Cystic teratomas: Most common cause of adnexal torsion in pregnancy.
  - Cystadenomas: Majority of benign neoplasms.
  - Malignant neoplasms and inflammatory lesions less likely torsion.
  - Venous blood is impaired first followed by arterial flow.
  - Presentation: Acute, unilateral, sharp pain; pain can be intermittent due to partial torsion; nausea/vomiting (70%) and fever (10%) can be seen.
  - Diagnosis: Abdominal tenderness, rebound, palpable mass (90% adults, 40% children); nonspecific leukocytosis and elevated CRP, ultrasound (first-line imaging, enlarged ovary, lack of Doppler flow not always seen), CT and MRI with contrast (second-line imaging).
  - Treatment: Surgical treatment without delay to prevent ovarian necrosis, laparoscopic treatment with detorsion initially used, cystectomy used for adnexal masses.
- Ovarian cyst rupture:
  - Benign ovarian cystic masses: Functional cysts (follicular, corpus luteal, and theca lutein cysts), benign cystic teratomas, endometriomas.
  - Functional cysts are the most common ones.
  - Most are asymptomatic and diagnosed incidentally; most ruptures show only vague symptoms but can have acute, severe abdominal pain; most show history of intercourse or trauma.

Table 12.5 Differential diagnosis for acute abdomen in females

Common causes

- Urinary tract infection and cystitis
- Pelvic inflammatory disease
- Dysmenorrhea
- Labor

Uncommon causes

- Ectopic pregnancy
- Appendicitis
- Biliary colic
- Ovarian syndromes (adnexal torsion, ovarian cyst rupture)
- Miscarriage

Rare

- Ovarian hyperstimulation syndrome
- Curtis–Fitz-Hugh syndrome
- Toxic shock syndrome

Other causes not specific to women

- Gastroenteritis
- Appendicitis
- Abdominal aortic aneurysm
- Peptic ulcer
- Biliary colic, acute cholecystitis
- Acute pancreatitis
- Acute intestinal obstruction
- Renal colic
- Small bowel/mesenteric infarction

- Diagnosis: Abdominal ultrasound or TVUSG showing free fluid around ovary and pouch of Douglas.
- Treatment: Expected management, follow-up of hemoglobin/hematocrit, pain medications, various surgical treatments if bleeding or pain continue.
- Ectopic pregnancy[10]:
  - Pregnancy outside the uterine cavity.
  - 2% of all reported pregnancies, major cause of morbidity and mortality, 2.7% pregnancy-related deaths, prevalence of 18% in pregnant women with first trimester bleeding or pain.
  - Most commonly located in ampulla of fallopian tube (97% cases), other locations include cornual, cervical, abdominal, ovarian, cesarean scar, heterotopic, and a pregnancy unknown location.
  - Risk factors: Previous history of ectopic pregnancy, history of tubal damage (infection, tubal surgery), assistive reproductive technology pregnancies, smoking, intrauterine devices, tuberculosis.
  - Presents with secondary amenorrhea, vaginal bleeding/spotting, abdominal/pelvic pain, or tenderness.
- Diagnosis: TVUSG, serum β-hCG:
  - Early intrauterine gestational sac may be visualized as early as fifth week of gestation; hypoechoic sac (double decidual sign) may be intrauterine pregnancy or pseudogestational sac seen in an ectopic pregnancy.
  - Heterotopic pregnancy: Rare, simultaneous intrauterine, and ectopic pregnancies.
  - β-hCG level ≥ 2,000 mIU/mL without a visualized gestational sac on TVUSG suggests ectopic pregnancy.
  - β-hCG values increase by two-thirds in 48 hours of intrauterine pregnancies, 1% of patients show slower rate of rise.
- Treatment:
  - Methotrexate: Treatment of choice, folate antagonist, effects proliferative tissues like trophoblasts, may take 3–6 weeks until full effect.
  - Surgical treatment indications: Hemodynamic instability, > 4 cm adnexal mass with positive fetal cardiac activity, ruptured ectopic pregnancy; laparoscopy preferred over laparotomy; salpingectomy most common approach.
  - Dilatation and curettage can be used in accessible, nonviable pregnancies.
  - Repeated β-hCG level with expectation to see a 15% decrement within 24 hours.

12.1.10 Other Gynecologic Causes of Pelvic Pain Imitating Acute Abdomen

- Primary dysmenorrhea:
  - Definition: Painful menstruation.
  - Starting 1–2 years after the first menstrual period, always happens in ovulatory cycles, pain starts with menstrual cycle and continues for 48–72 hours.
  - Due to increased endometrial prostaglandin secretions, not due to organic pelvic pathology.
  - Treatment: NSAIDs, oral contraceptives, nonpharmacological methods.
- Secondary dysmenorrhea:
  - Starting in advanced ages (years after the first menstruation), pain starts 1–2 weeks before cycles and persists for days.
  - Due to other reason (e.g., endometriosis, adenomyosis, intrauterine devices).
  - Treatment: Management of main pathology.
- Mittelschmerz:
  - Reaction from follicular fluid and blood entering peritoneal cavity during ovulation, occurs during cycles with acute onset with short duration.
  - Generally unilateral.
  - Treatment: Self-limited, expected management.

12.2 Gynecologic Oncology

Cem Yalçinkaya

12.2.1 Red Flags for Gynecological Malignancies

- Background:
  - Most common malignancies: Cervical, ovarian, endometrial, vulvar cancer.

- Rare malignancies: Cancer of the vagina, gestational trophoblastic tumors, and fallopian tube cancer.
- Some gynecological malignancies are preventable and some can be diagnosed during the preinvasive period.
- Early diagnosis of a malignancy is usually associated with better outcomes and increased survival.
- Early diagnosis is not easy; many of the symptoms of gynecological cancers are nonspecific.
- Early referral to a gynecologist or gynecological oncologist is recommended during presentation of abnormal imaging findings, elevated tumor markers, or evidence of abdominal/distant metastases.
- Ovarian cancer:
  - Red flags:
    - Vague signs/symptoms.
    - Abdominal distention and bloating.
    - Pelvic and abdominal pain, pressure in pelvis and lower back.
    - Feeling full sooner, indigestion, nausea, constipation.
    - Fatigue, weight loss.
    - Ascites.
    - Abdominal or pelvic mass on examination.
    - CA125 > 35 IU/mL (especially in postmenopausal women).
  - Malignant imaging features of adnexal mass[11]: Size > 10 cm, mural nodules, papillary projections, presence of ascites, bilaterality, presence of solid component, hypervascularity on color Doppler ultrasound, irregular shape.
- Endometrial cancer:
  - Improved survival for stage I (95%) versus stage IV (14%), early diagnosis warranted.[12]
  - Red flags:
    - Postmenopausal bleeding (major red flag).
    - Abnormal menstrual cycles (intermenstrual bleeding or heavily menses).
    - Endometrial thickness > 4 mm on ultrasound for postmenopausal women.
    - Atypical endometrial cells on Pap smear.
- Cervical cancer[13]:
  - Preventable by effective screening and vaccination programs.
  - Premalignant lesions and most early-invasive lesions are asymptomatic.
  - Red flags:
    - Intermenstrual, postcoital, and postmenopausal bleeding.
    - Persistent vaginal discharge.
    - Positive high-risk HPV and cytological abnormalities on Pap test.
    - Symptoms despite normal cervical cytology (low sensitivity).
- Vulvar cancer:
  - Commonly identified by patient directly but can present after delay (poor examination, patient or physician reluctant for examination).
  - Pruritus common; other features include ulceration, pigmentation, warts, or nodules.
  - Red flags:
    - Pruritus and tenderness.
    - Pain or burning.
    - Lymphadenopathy in inguinal region or leg edema (usually suggestive of advanced disease).

12.2.2 Ovarian, Fallopian Tube and Primary Peritoneal Cancer

- Background[14]:
  - Majority (about 90%) arise from surface epithelium, and are called epithelial carcinomas; germ cell tumors and sex-cord stromal tumors less likely (10% of cases).
  - Epithelial ovarian, fallopian tube, and peritoneal cancers are considered a single entity and treated the same way.
  - 10% of epithelial carcinomas have a genetic origin.
  - About 70% of patients are in advanced stage at the time of diagnosis, with poor 5-year survival rates of only about 20%.

○ Removal of the tumor and through surgical staging is the basic treatment for early ovarian cancer.
○ The aim of surgery for advanced stages is removal of all macroscopic tumoral implants, if possible.
- Epidemiology[13]:
  ○ Second most common gynecological malignancy in the United States, major cause of cancer death, fifth most common malignancy in women.
  ○ Mean age of diagnosis is 63 years but can be seen in younger women.
- Etiology[14]:
  ○ Risk factors: Caucasian; family history of ovarian, breast, or colon cancer; late menopause; nulliparity; BRCA1/BRCA2 mutations; Lynch syndrome.
  ○ Recommended that all patients with epithelial ovarian cancer undergo genetic risk evaluation.
- Screening and prevention[14]:
  ○ Routine screening is not feasible or recommended.
  ○ Patients with BRCA1/BRCA2 can be offered risk-reducing salpingo-oophorectomy.
  ○ High-risk women (e.g., strong family history of ovarian cancer or breast cancer survivors) may benefit from annual TVUSG and serum CA125 measurements.
  ○ Oral contraceptives reduce the risk of ovarian cancer.
- Presentation and diagnosis:
  ○ Nonspecific symptoms, bloating, abdominopelvic pain, early satiety, swelling, ascites, irregular fixed pelvic mass on exam.
  ○ CA125 elevated in advanced disease but normal in 50% of stage I patients.
  ○ Differential diagnosis: Tubo-ovarian abscess, endometrioma, uterine fibroids, functional cysts, benign neoplasms.
  ○ Early referral recommended.
- Staging:
  ○ Staging via International Federation of Gynecology and Obstetrics (FIGO) and TNM systems[15] (▶ Table 12.6).
  ○ Workup: Pelvic exam and transvaginal ultrasound are the first-line evaluation; diagnosis requires laparoscopic or open surgical exploration; ovarian biopsy not recommended due to spillage of malignant cells; abdominopelvic CT and MRI can assess extent of disease and create surgical plan.
  ○ Paracentesis, thoracentesis, image-guided peritoneal biopsy or omental cake biopsy used for diagnosis if unclear or if neoadjuvant chemotherapy considered.
  ○ Breast and gastrointestinal tumors can metastasize to the ovaries and mimic ovarian cancer.
  ○ Mammography performed to evaluate suspicious breast masses.
- Treatment[14]:
  ○ Surgical management with gynecology oncology recommended; laparotomy preferred but laparoscopic exploration used in selected patients.
  ○ Tumor limited to ovary or fallopian tube: Total hysterectomy, bilateral salpingo-oophorectomy, infracolic omentectomy, pelvic and para-aortic lymphadenectomy, and thorough surgical staging with visualization of peritoneal surfaces and biopsies from suspicious areas.
  ○ Advanced disease: Cytoreduction surgery (debulking) with or without three to four cycles of neoadjuvant chemotherapy.
  ○ Upper abdominal disease: Can involve bowel resection, appendectomy, cholecystectomy, stripping of diaphragm and peritoneal surfaces, splenectomy, partial cystectomy or gastrectomy with reconstruction, distal pancreatectomy, omentectomy, partial hepatectomy.
  ○ Postoperative adjuvant therapy used in most patients.

12.2.3 Endometrial Cancer

- Background[16]:
  ○ Most common type of uterine corpus cancer is endometrial cancer (adenocarcinoma of endometrial lining).
  ○ Uterine sarcomas are rare (3% of all uterine cancers).
  ○ About 80% of cases of endometrial cancer are stage I at the time of diagnosis, with 5-year survival rates of over 95%.

Table 12.6 FIGO staging of ovary, fallopian tube, and peritoneum cancer (FIGO 2017)

TNM (FIGO stage)	Definition
T1(I)	Tumor limited to ovaries or fallopian tubes
• T1a(IA)	Tumor limited to one ovary (capsule intact) or fallopian tube surface; no malignant cells in ascites or peritoneal washings
• T1b(IB)	Tumor limited to one or both ovaries (capsules intact) or fallopian tubes; no tumor on ovarian or fallopian tube surface, no malignant cells in ascites or peritoneal washings
• T1c(IC)	Tumor limited to one or both ovaries or fallopian tubes with any of the following
• T1c1(IC1)	Surgical spill
• T1c2(IC2)	Capsule ruptured before surgery or tumor on ovarian or fallopian tube surface
• T1c3(IC3)	Malignant cells in ascites or peritoneal washings
T2(II)	Tumor involves one or both ovaries or fallopian tubes with pelvic extension below pelvic brim or primary peritoneal cancer
• T2a(IIA)	Extension and/or implants on uterus and/or fallopian tubes and/or ovaries
• T2b(IIB)	Extension to other pelvic intraperitoneal tissues
T3(III)	Tumor involves one or both ovaries or fallopian tubes, or primary and/or peritoneal cancer, with cytologically or histologically confirmed spread to the peritoneum outside the pelvis and/or metastasis to the retroperitoneal lymph nodes
• T3a(IIIA1)	Positive retroperitoneal lymph nodes only (cytologically or histologically proven)
• T3a(IIIA 1i)	Metastasis up to 10 mm in greatest dimension
• T3a(IIIA 1 ii)	Metastasis more than 10 mm in greatest dimension
• T3a(IIIA2)	Microscopic extrapelvic (above the pelvic brim) peritoneal involvement with or without positive retroperitoneal lymph nodes
• T3b(IIIB)	Macroscopic peritoneal metastasis beyond pelvis up to ≤ 2 cm in greatest dimension or less in greatest dimension with or without retroperitoneal lymph node metastasis
• T3c(IIIC)	Macroscopic peritoneal metastasis beyond pelvis more than 2 cm in greatest dimension with or without retroperitoneal lymph node metastasis (excludes extension of tumor to capsule of liver and spleen without parenchymal involvement of either organ)
T4(IV)	Distant metastasis excluding peritoneal metastases
• T4a(IVA)	Pleural effusion with positive cytology
• T4b(IV4B)	Liver, splenic, or parenchymal metastases and metastases to extra-abdominal organs (including inguinal lymph nodes and lymph nodes outside of the abdominal cavity)

Note: Tx, T0, NX, and M categories are not shown.

- Epidemiology[13]:
  - Most common gynecological malignancy in the United States and developed countries.
  - Fourth most common malignancy after breast, colorectal, and lung cancer in American women.
  - Mean age of diagnosis is 63 years; 4% of endometrial cancer patients are younger than 40 years.
- Etiology:
  - Inherited risk factor: Lynch syndrome (LS)/hereditary nonpolyposis colon cancer (HNPCC) syndrome (5% of all endometrial cancers, 40–60% lifetime risk of endometrial cancer).
  - Modifiable risk factors: Unopposed estrogen, high body mass index, polycystic ovarian syndrome, early menarche and late menopause, nulliparity, infertility, estrogen-producing tumors, and estrogen replacement without a progestin for menopausal symptoms.
- Screening and prevention[16]:
  - Presents with postmenopausal bleeding and can be diagnosed early by endometrial biopsy.
  - Screening asymptomatic women for endometrial cancer is not recommended, annual endometrial biopsy for LS carriers after age 35 may be acceptable.
  - Risk factor reduction: Overweight or obese women should be encouraged to lose weight; oral contraceptive pill usage is also associated with a decrease in endometrial cancer.

Table 12.7 FIGO staging of endometrial cancer

FIGO stage	Definition
I	Tumor confined to the corpus uteri, including endocervical glandular involvement
• IA	Tumor limited to the endometrium or invading less than half of the myometrium
• IB	Tumor invading one half or more of the myometrium
II	Tumor invading the stromal connective tissue of the cervix but not extending beyond the uterus. Does *not* include endocervical glandular involvement
III	Tumor involving serosa, adnexa, vagina, or parametrium
• IIIA	Tumor involving the serosa and/or adnexa (direct extension or metastasis)
• IIIB	Vaginal involvement (direct extension or metastasis) or parametrial involvement
• IIIC1	Cancer is growing in the body of the uterus, spread to pelvic lymph nodes
• IIIC2	Cancer is growing in the body of the uterus, spread to aortic lymph nodes
IV	
• IVA	Tumor invading the bladder mucosa and/or bowel mucosa
• IVB	Distant metastasis (includes metastasis to inguinal lymph nodes, intraperitoneal disease, lung, liver, or bone)

Note: Tx, T0, NX, and M categories are not shown.

- Presentation and diagnosis[17]:
  - Presents with abnormal uterine bleeding (irregular menses and intermenstrual bleeding) or postmenopausal bleeding.
  - Advanced disease can present with abdominal pain, abdominal distention. and changes in gastrointestinal function.
  - Any vaginal bleeding in a postmenopausal woman must be investigated to exclude malignancy.
  - Postmenopausal bleeding should be assessed with transvaginal ultrasonography; endometrial thickness is > 4 mm; endometrial sampling is necessary; persistent or recurrent postmenopausal bleeding with endometrial thickness > 5 mm also requires endometrial sampling.
- Staging:
  - Staged using FIGO and TNM systems[15] (▶ Table 12.7).
  - Pelvic examination, pelvic ultrasonography, pathology necessary.
  - CT or MRI of chest, abdomen, and pelvis may be helpful.
  - No clear benefit for serum tumor markers[16] (e.g., CA125).
- Treatment[16]:
  - Total hysterectomy and bilateral salpingo-oophorectomy (removal of the cervix, uterus, fallopian tubes, and ovaries) is the mainstay of the surgery, unless there are absolute medical contraindications; performed using the open, laparoscopic, robotic, or vaginal approach.
  - Ovarian preservation can be considered in young patients with early-stage low-grade tumor and no obvious ovarian disease.
  - Comprehensive surgical staging, including lymphadenectomy, should be performed on high-risk patients, including nonendometrioid histology, grade 3 tumor, deep myometrial invasion, or cervical invasion.
  - In medically unfit patients, radiation therapy or hormone therapy may be appropriate.
  - For advanced disease, treatment must be individualized; total hysterectomy, bilateral salpingo-oophorectomy, and, if possible, cytoreductive surgery should be performed.
  - Fertility-preserving therapy could be considered in young patients with a histological diagnosis of grade 1 endometrial carcinoma.
  - Myometrial invasion and ovarian metastasis should be excluded by MRI for these patients. These patients must be referred to specialized centers. They should be informed that this is a nonstandard approach. Fertility-preserving medical treatment for endometrial cancer is based on progestins with medroxyprogesterone acetate (400–600 mg/day) or megestrol acetate (160–320 mg/day). The levonorgestrel-releasing intrauterine device can be use instead of oral progestins.
  - The adjuvant treatment with radiotherapy or chemotherapy after surgery is related to the stage or grade of the disease.

12.2.4 Cervical Cancer

- Background:
  - Leading cause of death from cancer in women from developing countries.
  - Caused by infection with certain types of human papillomavirus (HPV).
  - HPV initially causes a preinvasive lesion which can be detected by screening and treated before becoming invasive cancer.
  - Vaccination significantly decreases the incidence of preinvasive lesions and, thus, cervical cancer.
  - Common histologic types are squamous cell (80%) and adenocarcinoma (20%).
- Epidemiology[18]:
  - > 500,000 new annual cases and > 250,000 death worldwide.
  - 80% of cases in developing countries.
  - Most common gynecological malignancy in the world, but third in the United States.
  - Mean age of diagnosis is about 47 years.
- Etiology:
  - Risk factor is persistent HPV infection.
  - Other risk factors[19]: Early onset of first coitus, multiple partners, high-risk partner, history of sexually transmitted infections, high parity, immunosuppression, smoking, and oral contraceptives.
- Screening and prevention[20]:
  - Cervical cytology (often combined with HPV test) detects preinvasive lesion.
  - All women should undergo an annual physical examination, including Pap smear, within 3 years of first coitus, or by the age of 21 years.
  - All women should undergo liquid-based cytology every 3 years from 21 to 30 years.
  - Vaccination is most effective if performed before becoming sexually active.
- Presentation and diagnosis:
  - Early cervical cancer may be asymptomatic or presents with irregular bleeding (postcoital, intermenstrual, or postmenopausal).
  - Persistent vaginal discharge, pelvic or lower back pain, and urinary frequency are suggested advanced diseases.
  - Diagnosed by cervical biopsy if grossly visible.
  - Colposcopic evaluation used if abnormal Pap smear without a visible lesion.
  - Physical examination (with rectovaginal touch) can reveal the extent of tumor and parametrial involvement; may be irregular, ulcerated. or exophytic; lesion may involve upper vagina.
- Staging:
  - TNM classification and revised FIGO clinical staging systems used[15] (▶ Table 12.8).
  - CT, MRI, or positron emission tomography can be used for tailoring treatment plans, but their results do not change the FIGO stage.
- Cytological abnormalities and preinvasive lesions[19,20]:
  - Atypical squamous cells of undetermined significance (ASCUS), atypical squamous cells cannot exclude high-grade squamous intraepithelial lesions (ASC-H), low-grade squamous intraepithelial lesion (LSIL), high-grade intraepithelial lesion (HSIL), and carcinoma in situ are epithelial cell abnormalities of cytology.
  - Adenocarcinoma in situ is glandular cell abnormality of cytology.
  - For patients with ASCUS smear, HPV testing is preferred, but repeating the cytology is also acceptable. For all other cytological abnormalities, colposcopic evaluation should be done.
  - Colposcopy: Examination of the cervix magnification; punch biopsy can be taken from the suspected areas.
  - LGSIL (formerly called CIN I) and HGSIL (formerly called CIN II and III) are premalignant histological lesions of cervix.
  - HSIL (CIN II and III) should be treated by ablative or excisional procedures. LSIL (CIN I) lesions often regress spontaneously; therefore, observation is preferred.
- Treatment[21]:
  - The choice of therapy depends on disease stage and patient factors.

Table 12.8 FIGO staging and TNM classification system for cervical cancer

TNM category	FIGO stage	Definition
T1	I	
• T1a	• IA	Invasive carcinoma that can be diagnosed only by microscopy, with maximum depth of invasion <5 mm
• T1a1	• IA1	Measured stromal invasion <3 mm in depth
• T1a2	• IA2	Measured stromal invasion ≥3 mm and <5 mm in depth
• T1b	• IB	Invasive carcinoma with measured deepest invasion ≥5 mm (greater than stage IA), lesion limited to the cervix uteri
• T1b1	• IB1	Invasive carcinoma ≥5 mm depth of stromal invasion and <2 cm in greatest dimension
• T1b2	• IB2	Invasive carcinoma ≥2 cm and <4 cm in greatest dimension
–	• IB3	Invasive carcinoma ≥4 cm in greatest dimension
T2	II	Carcinoma beyond uterus but not pelvic wall or lower 1/3 of vagina
• T2a	• IIA	Involvement limited to the upper two-thirds of the vagina without parametrial involvement
• T2a1	• IIA1	Invasive carcinoma <4 cm in greatest dimension
• T2a2	• IIA2	Invasive carcinoma ≥4 cm in greatest dimension
• T2b	• IIB	With parametrial involvement but not up to the pelvic wall
T3	III	Tumor extension to pelvic sidewall, invasion lower 1/3 vagina, and/or causes hydronephrosis or non-functioning kidney and/or involves pelvic and/or paraaortic lymph nodes
• T3a	• IIIA	Lower 1/3 vagina, not extending to pelvic wall
• T3b	• IIIB	Extension to pelvic wall and/or hydronephrosis or non-functioning kidney
–	IIIC1	Pelvic lymph node metastasis only
–	IIIC2	Paraaortic lymph node metastasis
T4	IVA	And/or hydronephrosis or non-functioning kidney
	IVB	Invasion of distant organs

Note: Tx, T0, NX, and M categories are not shown.

- ○ Treatment options for early-stage include surgery or primary radiation therapy.
- ○ Surgical management should be chosen to avoid radiotherapy side effects for early-stage disease and small tumor volumes (IA, IB1, and selected IIA1).
- ○ For stage IA disease, conization or simple hysterectomy could be appropriate.
- ○ Stage IB1 and IIA1 lesions are usually treated with radical hysterectomy and pelvic lymphadenectomy.
- ○ For stage IB2 and IIA2 lesions, chemoradiotherapy is the preferred treatment.
- ○ For stage IIB, III, and IVA lesions, chemoradiotherapy is recommended.
- ○ Patients with distant metastases are treated palliatively.

12.2.5 Vulvar Cancers

- Background[13,22]:
  - ○ 90% squamous cell, 6,000 annual cases, and 1,000 annual deaths in the United States, mean age 68 years.
- Epidemiology:
  - ○ Two pathways for formation: (1) HPV infection and smoking result in vulvar intraepithelial neoplasia, (2) HPV infection and chronic disease (e.g., lichen sclerosis).
  - ○ Risk factors: Vulvar intraepithelial neoplasia, prior history of cervical cancer, smoking, and vulvar lichen sclerosis.
- Etiology: Presents with vulvar lesion that may be ulcerated, raised, nodular, or warty; prolonged pruritus; lesions commonly on labium majus but can be in other sites as well.
- Staging:
  - ○ Staged using FIGO and TNM systems[15] (▶ Table 12.9).

Table 12.9 FIGO staging and TNM of squamous vulvar cancer

TNM category	FIGO stage	Definition
T1		
• T1a	IA	Lesions ≤ 2 cm, confined to vulva or perineum, stroma invasion ≤ 1.0 mm, no nodal metastasis
• T1b	IB	Lesions > 2 cm size or stroma invasion > 1.0 mm, confined to vulva or perineum, negative nodes
T2	II	Tumor of any size, extension to perineal structures, 1/3 lower urethra, 1/3 lower vagina, or anus, negative nodes
T3	IVA	Tumor of upper urethra and/or vaginal mucosa, bladder mucosa, rectal mucosa, or fixed to pelvic bone
N1		1–2 regional nodes
• N1a	IIIA	1–2 nodes, ≤ 5 mm
• N1b	IIIA	1 node, > 5 mm
N2	IIIB	
• N2a	IIIB	≥ 3 nodes, ≥ 5 mm
• N2b	IIIB	≥ 2 nodes, > 5 mm
• N2c	IIIC	Metastasis with extracapsular spread
N3	IVA	Fixed/ulcerated nodes
—	IVB	Distant metastasis (including pelvic lymph node metastasis)

Note: Tx, T0, NX, and M categories are not shown.

- ○ Evaluation of cervix, vagina, and anus performed by physical exam; imaging can include ultrasound, PET, CT, or MRI to evaluate metastasis.
- ○ Suspected lesions undergo biopsy.
- Treatment:
  - ○ Primary lesion and groin nodes managed independently.
  - ○ Early stages: Excision of primary vulvar lesion, radical local excision.
  - ○ Later stages: Large, central, or multicentric lesions treated with modified radical vulvectomy, goal for free margins.
  - ○ Groin lymphadenectomy performed for tumors greater than stage T1a, superficial and deep femoral nodes removed.
  - ○ Postoperative radiotherapy used for patients with more than one metastatic lymph node and/or extracapsular lymph node involvement.

12.3 Obstetrics Overview

Erol Arslan

12.3.1 Preconceptional Counseling

- Preconceptional care: "a set of interventions that aim to identify and modify biomedical, behavioral, and social risks to a woman's health or pregnancy outcome through prevention and management."[23,24]
- Up to 50% of pregnancies in the United States are unplanned.
- Gynecologists, internists, family practitioners, and pediatricians consider first line for preconceptional care.
- Give information and provide the most suitable contraception method to those who do not want another pregnancy.
- Folic acid:
  - ○ Planning for pregnancy: Prescribe 400 µg folic acid starting at least 1 month (preferably 3 months) before attempting conception and continue until 12th gestational week for neural tube defect (NTD) prophylaxis.

○ Prescribe 4–5 mg (10 times higher than normal dosage) starting 3 months before attempting conception to 12th gestational week to women who have a history of NTD children.
○ Prescribe 1–4 mg folic acid at preconception/first trimester in the following conditions:
  – Epilepsy.
  – Pregestational diabetes.
  – Coeliac disease, inflammatory bowel disease.
  – History of children with oral facial cleft, structural heart disease, limb defect, urinary tract anomaly, and hydrocephalus.

• Discuss the adverse effects of obesity on pregnancy outcomes to overweight woman and offer weight loss as well medications to them.
• Pregestational diabetes: one of the most common medical condition that affects both mother and fetus; increases the risk of miscarriage, congenital anomalies, perinatal death, and neonatal problems; explain the relation between higher A_{1C} levels and congenital anomalies; encourage good glycemic control before conception.
• Discuss the adverse effects of thyroid disease on conception rates and pregnancy outcomes and offer medication if needed.
• Inform the epileptic patients about teratogenicity of antiepileptic medications and change the medications to less teratogenic ones like lamotrigine; prescribe higher dose of single-drug regimen instead of multiple-drug regimens; consult a neurologist to assist with medications.

12.3.2 Prenatal Care

• Initial visit[25]:
  ○ Assessment of obstetric risk factors (including the history of preterm birth, preeclampsia, gestational diabetes).
  ○ Assessment of smoking and substance abuse.
  ○ Immunizations; influenza (annually) and Tdap (27–36 weeks).
  ○ Family history of congenital defects and disorders.
  ○ Depression and domestic violence screening.
  ○ Discuss weight gain recommendations.
  ○ Discuss first trimester aneuploidy screening.
  ○ Laboratory tests (▶ Table 12.10).
• Second trimester assessment:
  ○ Fetal anatomic assessment at 17–22 gestational week.
  ○ MSAFP and aneuploidy screening at 15–20 gestational week.
  ○ At 24–28 gestational week: hemoglobin (Hb)/hematocrit (Hct), gestational diabetes screening with 50 g oral glucose tolerance test (OGTT) if it is abnormal 100 g OGTT for diagnosis; Rh antibody screen if Rh negative; Rh-immune prophylaxis if indicated.
  ○ At 27–36 gestational week: Tdap.
  ○ Repeat depression and domestic violence assessment.
  ○ Counseling for cessation of smoking and substance abuse.
  ○ Provide breastfeeding encouragement, education, and support.

Table 12.10 Laboratory test that hast to be run during initial prenatal visit

Blood type and Rh factor	Gonorrhea and chlamydia
Antibody screening	VDRL/RPR
Hemoglobin/hematocrit	Urine culture
Pap smear at age 21 and up in every 3 y	HbsAg
Rubella and varicella	HIV

Other screening tests which are indicated due to risk factors: drug screen, TB skin test, hemoglobin electrophoresis, Tay-Sachs, cystic fibrosis, familial dysautonomia

- Third trimester assessment:
  - At 32–34 gestational week: VDRL/RPR, gonorrhea and chlamydia tests, Hb/Hct, and HIV.
  - At 35–37 gestational week: Group B streptococcal (GBS) culture, ultrasound if clinically indicated.
  - Provide breastfeeding encouragement, education, and support.
  - Repeat depression and domestic violence assessment.
  - Counseling for cessation of smoking and substance abuse.
- Frequency of prenatal care visits:
  - Up to 20 weeks, every 4–6 weeks (6 weeks for lower risk women).
  - 20–28 weeks, every 4 weeks.
  - 28–36 weeks, every 2–3 weeks (3 weeks for lower risk women).
  - 36 weeks to delivery, every week.
- Subsequent prenatal care visits:
  - Weight gain.
  - Urine dipstick for protein, glucose, and ketones.
  - Fetal heart rate present/absent.
  - Blood pressure.
  - Fetal movement present/absent.
  - Fundal height.
  - Signs and symptoms of labor.

12.3.3 Gestational Age Assessment and Imaging Risks

- The first step in the evaluation of a pregnant woman is assessing the gestational age in order to determine the timing of screening tests and assessment of fetus and mother.[26]
- Laboratory assessment:
  - hCG can be detected as early as 6 days after ovulation.
  - Not reliable for determining gestational age.
  - Doubles every 29–53 hours during the first 30 days.
  - hCG peaks at 8–10 weeks of gestation.
  - When it reaches a level of 1,500–2,000 IU/L, the gestational sac has to be seen by transvaginal ultrasound. If cannot be seen, consider the ectopic pregnancy.
- Physical examination:
  - After 4 weeks of conception, the uterus will increase 1 cm/per week.
  - At 12 weeks, uterus is palpable above the pubic symphysis.
  - At 16 weeks, uterus is palpable between the umbilicus and the pubic symphysis.
  - At 20 weeks, the uterine fundus is palpable on the umbilicus.
  - After 20 weeks, the pubic symphysis to fundal height in centimeters is correlated with the weeks of gestation.
- Ultrasound examination:
  - Between 4.5 and 5th gestational week, an intrauterine gestational sac (fluid filled collection) is seen.
  - Between 5 and 6th gestational week, yolk sac is seen.
  - Between 5.5 and 6th gestational week, a fetal pol with cardiac activity is seen.
  - For the first trimester, crown-rump length is the most accurate measurement for gestational age.
  - For the second trimester, measurement of biparietal diameter, head circumference, femur length, and abdominal circumference (AC) can be used with less accuracy.
  - No adverse fetal effects have been shown with ultrasound (including Doppler studies) so far and it can be used safely; should utilize as low as reasonably achievable (ALARA) principles for minimizing dose.[27]
- Magnetic resonance imaging:
  - Safe during pregnancy.
  - Gadolinium-based agents can cross the placenta into the fetal circulation and amniotic fluid, used only if benefits outweigh risks.
  - In lactating women, breastfeeding may continue after gadolinium use.
- Ionizing radiation including X-rays:
  - The risk depends on dose of radiation and the gestational age (▶ Table 12.11 and ▶ Table 12.12).

Table 12.11 Adverse effects of ionizing X-ray due to gestational age and dose

	Age	Fetal impact	Teratogenic doses
Gestational Period	Before implantation (0–2 wk after fertilization)	Death of embryo or no consequence (all or none)	50–100 mGy
	Organogenesis (2–8 wk after fertilization)	Congenital anomalies	200 mGy
		Growth restriction	200–250 mGy
Fetal period	8–15 wk	Severe intellectual disability (high risk)	60–310 mGy 25 IQ-point loss/1,000 mGy
		Intellectual deficit	200 mGy
		Microcephaly	
	16–25 wk	Severe intellectual disability (low risk)	250–280 mGy

Table 12.12 Classification of imaging modalities due to their radiation doses

Very low dose examinations (<0.1 mGy)	Low to moderate dose examinations (0.1–10 mGy)	High-dose examinations (10–50 mGy)
Cervical spine X-ray	Abdominal X-ray	Abdominal CT
Head or neck CT	Lumbar spine X-ray	Pelvic CT
X-ray of any extremity	IV pyelography	PET/CT whole body scintigraphy
Mammography (2 views)	Double-contrast barium enema	
Chest X-rays (2 views)	Chest CT	
	CT pulmonary angiography	
	Low-dose perfusion scintigraphy	
	Technetium-99 m bone scintigraphy	
	Pulmonary digital subtraction angiography	

- ○ Extremely high dosages (> 1 Gy) during early embryogenesis will be lethal to the embryo.
- ○ In addition to the teratogenesis, theoretically it has a very small risk of carcinogenesis (10–20 mGy fetal exposure increases the risk of leukemia 1.5–2 times) in fetal exposure.
- Computed tomography:
  - ○ Clinical use depends on risks/benefits (▶ Table 12.11 and ▶ Table 12.12).
  - ○ Iodinated media passes fetal circulation and amniotic fluid, not shown to be teratogenic in animal studies but risk/benefits weighted for clinical use.
  - ○ Breastfeeding can be continued after use of IV iodinated contrast.
- Nuclear medicine imaging:
  - ○ Most common indication in pregnancy is using ventilation–perfusion lung scanning for detection of pulmonary embolism. Fetal exposure is supposed to be < 5 mGy in this procedure.
  - ○ Most common used radioisotope is technetium 99 m and its half-life is 6 hours, can be used during pregnancy, and not all radioisotopes are as safe.
  - ○ Radioactive iodine (iodine 131) crosses placenta and its half-life is 8 days and therefore cannot be used during pregnancy.
  - ○ For lactating women, decision of breastfeeding status has to be made with an expert on nuclear medicine.
- Teratogens and fetotoxic agents:
  - ○ Any agent that has effects during embryonic and fetal period by causing permanent changes in structural and functional features.
  - ○ While birth defects affect 2–3% pregnancies, less than 1% of all birth defects are caused by medications.
  - ○ The teratogenic effects of drugs are based on time and dose.
  - ○ The most sensitive period is first trimester.
  - ○ FDA categorized the drugs due to their potential risk of teratogenicity (▶ Table 12.13).

Table 12.13 FDA classification of drugs due to their potential effects of teratogenicity

Category	Definitions	Examples
A	Well-controlled studies in humans show no risk to the fetus	Levothyroxine, potassium
B	No well-controlled studies have been conducted in humans; animal studies show no risk to the fetus	Penicillins, macrolides
C	No well-controlled studies have been conducted in humans; animal studies have demonstrated an adverse effect on the fetus	2/3 of drugs are in this category; Ca-channel blockers, zidovudine
D	There is evidence that can cause fetal harm; but in certain situation, benefits overweigh the hazardous effect	Azathioprine, carbamazepine, corticosteroid
X	Controlled studies in both animals and humans demonstrate fetal abnormalities, fetal harm overweighs any possible benefit	Bosentan, aminopterin, ribavirin, radioisotopes, isotretinoin

12.3.4 Early Pregnancy Loss

- Definition[28]:
  - Early pregnancy loss (EPL): Nonviable intrauterine pregnancy with either an empty gestational sac or a gestational sac containing an embryo or fetus without fetal heart activity within the first $12^{6/7}$ weeks of gestation.
  - 10% of all clinically recognized pregnancies.
  - Most common risk factors are advanced maternal age and prior EPL.
  - Most known cause is chromosomal abnormalities with a 50% probability.
- Diagnosis: Physical examination (vaginal bleeding uterine cramping), ultrasound (with guidelines from the Society of Radiologists in Ultrasound Multispecialty Panel on Early First Trimester Diagnosis of Miscarriage and Exclusion of a Viable Intrauterine Pregnancy), β-hCG follow-up.
- < 70% rise in β-hCG levels suggestive of ectopic pregnancy.
- Medical management[29]: Higher rate of expulsion medically than expectant management and as effective as surgery in late first trimester; combined drug regimens (800 µg misoprostol following 24 hours after 200 mg of mifepristone) or repeated doses of misoprostol (oral or vaginally) may be used; abortion rates of 78.6–94.6%.
- Surgical management: May be preferred in women with hemorrhage, hemodynamic instability, anemia, coagulopathy, cardiovascular disease, or infection; suction curettage commonly used.

12.4 Obstetrical Emergencies

Erol Arslan

12.4.1 Hypertensive Diseases in Pregnancy

- One of the main causes of maternal and perinatal mortality worldwide.
- Complication in up to 10% of pregnancies.
- Increasing incidence due to increased obesity rate, multiple pregnancies related to assistive reproductive technology, delaying childbirth, and advanced maternal age.
- Diagnosis: Physical examination (evaluation of headache, visual symptoms, abdominal pain, nausea/vomiting), lab tests (complete blood count, serum aminotransferases, lactate dehydrogenase [LDH], blood urea nitrogen, creatinine, urine analysis), fetal evaluation (ultrasound, amniotic fluid index, nonstress testing, biophysical profile).

Gestational Hypertension

- Definition: New-onset hypertension with two measured value of systolic blood pressure (SBP) ≥140 mm Hg and/or diastolic blood pressure (DBP)≥ 90 mm Hg *and* no proteinuria after 20 weeks of gestation.[1]
- Resolves after delivery (important for distinguishing from chronic hypertension).

- If SBP ≥160 mm Hg or DBP ≥110 mm Hg it is scored as severe, and closer postdelivery follow-up is needed.
- Generally good prognosis except in severe cases.
- Up to 50% of women with gestational hypertension (especially that diagnosed before 32th gestational weeks) will develop preeclampsia.

Preeclampsia

- Incidence is estimated to be 2–8% globally, maternal mortality is 15–20% in developed countries.[30]
- A major cause of maternal mortality and morbidity, perinatal deaths, preterm birth, and intrauterine growth restriction.
- Risk factors: Multifactorial, obesity, nulliparity, pregestational diabetes, history of previous preeclampsia.
- Most preeclampsia cases do not have any risk factors.
- Pathophysiology: Multiple theories; abnormal trophoblastic invasion during placentation, maladaptive immunological tolerance between maternal and fetal tissues, abnormal maternal inflammation and cardiovascular adaptation from pregnancy, genetic and epigenetic factors.
- Diagnosis: New-onset hypertension (SBP ≥ 140 mm Hg or DBP ≥ 90 mm Hg) *and* proteinuria (≥ 300 mg/dL in 24-hour urine collection *or* ≥ 0.3 mg/dL of protein/creatinine ratio in spot urine analysis *or* dipstick reading of 2 + proteinuria) after 20 weeks of gestation.
- Criteria in absence of proteinuria (as well markers of severe preeclampsia): Thrombocytopenia (platelet < 100,000/mm^3), high serum creatinine level (> 1.1 mg/dL or two times normal values in the absence of other renal diseases), liver transaminases (two times normal values), pulmonary edema, new-onset headache that is unresponsive to the medication with visual symptoms.
- SBP ≥ 160 mm Hg or DBP ≥ 110 mm Hg apart 4 hours without treatment is another criterion for severe preeclampsia.

Eclampsia

- Diagnosis: Hypertension, new-onset tonic-clonic, focal, or multifocal seizures.[30]
- Rule out: Other potential causes of seizures (e.g., epilepsy, intracranial hemorrhage, sinuses vein thrombosis, or drug use).
- 1:2000 pregnancies in developed countries, 2.7% incidence in developing countries, 2% of severe preeclamptic patients without magnesium prophylaxis.
- Seizures follow headache, visual disturbance or epigastric pain in 80% of cases; seizures may present before preeclampsia diagnosis.
- Eclamptic convulsions can be antepartum, intrapartum, or postpartum.
- Postpartum convulsions can be early (< 48 hours after delivery) or late.
- Mortality low in Western countries by up to 14% than that in developing countries.
- Associated eclampsia conditions with maternal morbidity: Abruptio placentae, disseminated intravascular coagulopathy, Hemolysis, Elevated Liver enzymes, Low Platelets (HELLP) syndrome, renal failure, pulmonary edema or acute respiratory distress syndrome, cerebrovascular accident, cardiac arrest.

HELLP Syndrome

- Definition[31]:
  - **H**emolysis: Abnormal peripheral blood smear, increased bilirubin > 1.2 mg/dL, increased lactic dehydrogenase > 600 IU.
  - **E**levated **l**iver enzymes: Two times of normal range of asparate aminotransferase and alanine transaminase.
  - **L**ow **p**latelet (thrombocytopenia): Platelet count < 100,000/mm.[32]
- Incidence: 0.5–0.9% of pregnancies, often in third trimester, 30% of cases are postpartum.
- Presents with right upper quadrant or epigastric pain, nausea/vomiting.
- Differential diagnosis: Thrombotic thrombocytopenic purpura (TTP), hemolytic uremic syndrome (HUS), acute fatty liver of pregnancy, viral hepatitis, cholangitis.

Table 12.14 Conditions that required immediate delivery independent from the gestational age

Maternal	Fetal
• Uncontrolled severe hypertension (persistent BP ≥ 160/110) • Persistent headache, refractory to treatment • Epigastric or right upper quadrant pain • Visual disturbance, altered mental status • Stroke • Myocardial infarction • HELLP syndrome • New or worsening renal dysfunction (creatinine > 1.1 mg/dL or twice baseline) • Pulmonary edema • Eclampsia • Suspected acute placental abruption	• Fetus without expectation for the survival (lethal anomaly or extreme prematurity) • Fetal death • Abnormal fetal testing • Persistent reversed end-diastolic flow in the umbilical artery

Management of Hypertension in Pregnancy

- Delivery if at $37^{+0/7}$ weeks or considered earlier if impending maternal or fetal demise (▶ Table 12.14), expectant management used for < $34^{0/7}$ weeks of pregnancies if possible with close monitoring and delivery if necessary, outpatient management can be utilized for mothers without impending demise with frequent fetal monitoring assessments.[30]
- Delaying delivery for 48 hours to administer corticosteroids preferred.
- Magnesium sulfate (MgSO$_4$) treatment initiated early and maintained for 24 hours postdelivery.
- HYPITAT trials demonstrated earlier delivery improved maternal outcome but increased risk of neonatal respiratory distress syndrome.[3]
- Seizure prophylaxis: Magnesium sulfate as first-line treatment (4–6 g IV load diluted in 100 mL and delivered over 15–20 min, followed by 1–2 g/hour maintenance), phenytoin, benzodiazepine, nimodipine.
- Magnesium toxicity: Concerning in patients with renal impairment and dose adjusted, risk of respiratory depression, emergency correction of toxicity with calcium gluconate, and/or IV furosemide.
- Hypertension treatment goal to reduce cardiac, renal, and cerebral injury; treated with IV hydralazine, IV labetalol, or oral nifedipine.
- Regional anesthesia preferred over general anesthesia in eclampsia.

Management of Eclampsia

- Initial supportive steps: Call for help, try to prevent maternal injury, placement in lateral decubitus position, prevention of aspiration, administer oxygen, monitoring vital signs including oxygen saturation.
- Most eclamptic seizures are self-limited and nonstress test findings improve once seizures stop.
- Eclampsia is not an absolute indication for delivery.
- If convulsions recur, an additional 2–4 g of IV MgSO$_4$ should be administered over 5 minutes.
- In refractory seizures to MgSO$_4$ (e.g., lasting 20 minutes after the bolus or > 2 recurrences), further treatments have to be considered:
  - Sodium amobarbital (250 mg IV in 3 minutes).
  - Thiopental, or phenytoin (1,250 mg IV at a rate of 50 mg/minutes).
  - Endotracheal intubation and assisted ventilation.
  - Head imaging.

Management of HELLP Syndrome

- Immediate delivery advocated with goals to optimize fetal outcomes (e.g., 48 hours of corticosteroids), maternal supportive care.

- Close monitoring during labor and postpartum period is mandatory, laboratory testing at least at 12-hour interval, thrombocytopenia can worsen 1 day postdelivery, and disease intensity can worsen up to 2 days postdelivery.
- Continued thrombocytopenia and elevated liver enzymes 4 days postpartum should prompt reevaluation of HELLP syndrome diagnosis.
- 90% of patients with HELLP syndrome have improvement in laboratory findings (platelet count and liver enzymes) in 7 days.

12.4.2 Acute Fatty Liver of Pregnancy

- Incidence: 1/10,000–1/15,000.[33]
- Mostly seen in third trimester, nulliparous women, and multiple gestation.
- Etiology: Mitochondrial abnormalities of fatty acid oxidation.
- Presents with persistence vomiting/nausea, malaise, anorexia, progressive jaundice over 1–2 weeks, rarely with hepatic encephalopathy, 15–20% without clear symptoms.
- Diagnosis:
  - Findings depend on disease severity: Hypoglycemia, bilirubin (< 10 mg/dL), liver transaminases (elevated but < 1,000 U/L), hemolysis, thrombocytopenia, elevated LDH, leukocytosis, hematocrit (elevated due to hemoconcentration), coagulopathy (serious; due to disseminated intravascular coagulopathy [DIC]).
  - Ultrasound, CT, and MRI can be used for diagnosis, but the gold standard is liver biopsy.
- Differential diagnosis: Preeclampsia, HELLP, DIC, hepatitis, Budd–Chiari syndrome, adult-onset Reye syndrome, and cholestasis.
- Treatment: Early delivery, supportive care.
- Maternal mortality: 15% due to a variety of reasons, still high morbidity; hepatic dysfunction can resolve postpartum.

12.4.3 Intrahepatic Cholestasis of Pregnancy

- Incidence: 0.2–5.6% depending on geography.
- Presents: Pruritus worse at night affecting palms and feet, usually in the second or third trimester.
- Diagnosis: Liver function testing (aspartate aminotransferase, alanine aminotransferase, gamma-glutamyl transferase, bilirubin, and bile acids elevated; repeated weekly if pruritus present but initial lab results are normal).
- Differential diagnosis: Hepatitis, hyperemesis gravidarum, HELLP, acute fatty liver of pregnancy.
- Treatment: Topical lotions, cholestyramine, and ursodeoxycholic acid (no evidence of improvement of fetal or neonatal outcomes), early delivery (37 weeks) offered due to higher risk of meconium and stillbirth.
- Liver function generally normalizes postpartum.

12.4.4 Obstetrical Hemorrhage

- Hemorrhage, hypertension, and infections are primary global causes of maternal death; 50% of maternal deaths and 13% of pregnancy-related deaths are due to hemorrhage.[34]
- Estimated blood loss typically underestimated due to hypervolemia of pregnancy:
  - Vaginal delivery (500 mL) vs. C-section (1,000 mL) + 500 mL for per 3% decrement in hematocrit level.
- Treatment:
  - Call for help, airway/breathing/circulation (ABC) assessment, supplemental oxygen, supportive care, large bore IV with resuscitation with crystalloids, type and cross with evaluation of Rh antibody status, evaluation of transfusion need and coagulation factors, urinary catheterization, and transfer to higher level facility if necessary.
- Antepartum hemorrhage[35]:
  - Definition: Hemorrhage from/into genital tract from 24 weeks to delivery.
  - Affects 3–5% of pregnancy.

- Commonly due to placenta previa and abruption; > 50% have unknown causes.
- Placenta previa:
  - Placental attachment to uterus near or overlying internal os.
  - Placenta previa totalis: Internal os is covered totally by placenta.
  - Placenta previa partialis: Internal os is partially covered by placenta.
  - Marginal placenta previa: Placenta ending at the edge of internal os but did not overlie it.
  - Low-lying placenta: Placenta implanted in lower uterine segment but ended at 2 cm far from internal os.
  - Incidence: 0.3%, 20% of vaginal bleeding cases between 22 and 28 weeks.
  - Usually resolves by term due to migration of placenta from low uterine segment to upper parts of uterus.
  - Risk factors: History of previous placenta previa and cesarean section.
  - Placental invasion (e.g., accreta, increta, percreta) considered with previous placenta previa and higher risk.
  - Present with painless vaginal bleeding after second trimester.
  - Diagnosis: Abdominal or TVUSG.
  - Treatment: History of placenta previa solicited during emergency evaluations and prior to vaginal examinations that can cause heavy bleeding, speculum exam otherwise done; referral to tertiary care center recommended; bed rest with close follow-up; delivery by cesarean section at 37–38 weeks.
- Abruptio placenta:
  - Premature separation of placenta from its normally implanted site before delivery.
  - Incidence: 0.5%, comprises 40% of second trimester bleeding.
  - Risk factors: Prior abruption, preeclampsia, chronic hypertension, polyhydramnios, chorioamnionitis, cocaine use, smoking.
  - Presents with sudden-onset abdominal pain, vaginal bleeding, and uterine tenderness; not all symptoms seen at initial presentation.
  - Diagnosis: Physical examination, nonstress testing (shows decelerations or bradycardia), ultrasound.
  - Early diagnosis may preclude major morbidities (e.g., acute kidney injury, fetal loss, fetal hypoxia, DIC, hypovolemic shock, and Sheehan syndrome).
  - Vaginal examination and nonstress test (NST) distinguish placenta abruptio from labor and/or threatened premature labor.
  - Divided as partial and total abruption.
  - Treatment: Delivery dependent on partial vs. total abruption, cervical dilation, fetal heart tracings, and maternal hemodynamic stability.
  - Delayed diagnosis results in high maternal and fetal mortality due to fetal loss, consumptive coagulopathy, and hypovolemic shock.
- Vasa previa:
  - Fetal vessels are localized in fetal membranes instead of placenta and umbilical cord; fetal vessels can be near to internal cervical os.
  - Extremely rare condition (1 in 5,000 pregnancies), 70% mortality.
  - Increased risk with low-lying placentas.
  - Presents with acute, painless, frequently heavy bleeding due to rupture of membranes.
  - Diagnosis: TVUSG.
  - Treatment: Immediate delivery.
- Postpartum hemorrhage[36]:
  - Definition: Blood loss of ≥1,000 mL, ≥10% decrease in hemoglobin/hematocrit *or* with signs of hypovolemia within 24 hours of delivery.
  - Higher blood loss necessary in pregnant women for symptoms due to hypervolemia of pregnancy, goal for early recognition of blood loss prior to vital sign changes.
  - Common causes are known as "the 4 Ts," also divided into early versus late causes (▶ Table 12.15):
    - Tonus (uterine atony, composed 70–80% of postpartum hemorrhage).
    - Trauma (vaginal or cervical lacerations, uterine rupture).
    - Tissue (placental retention).
    - Thrombin (coagulopathy, abruption).

Table 12.15 Etiology of postpartum hemorrhage

Early (within 24 h)	Late (between 24 h after delivery and postpartum 12th weeks)
• Uterine atony • Lacerations • Retained placenta • Placental invasion anomalies (accreta) • Coagulation defects • Uterine inversion	• Subinvolution of the placental site • Retained products of conception • Infection • Inherited coagulation defects (e.g., von Willebrand factor deficiency

 ○ Treatment: Management of hemorrhage, initiation of IV oxytocin infusion, additional considerations (uterine massage, bimanual uterine compression, external aortic compression, balloon or condom tamponade, uterine compression sutures, uterine artery ligation or embolization, iliac artery ligation, hysterectomy).

12.4.5 Preterm (Premature) Labor and Birth

• Definition: Delivery between 20 and 37th gestational weeks.[37]
• Early preterm delivery: Delivery between 20 and 34th gestational weeks.
• Late preterm delivery: Delivery between 34 and 36th + gestational weeks.
• Leading cause of neonatal mortality and most common indication for antepartum hospitalization, 70% of neonatal and 36% of infant deaths, 25–50% of long neurological impairment.
• Annual incidence of 12% in the United States.
• Presents with frequent abdominal cramping, back pain, lower pelvic pain, vaginal spotting/light bleeding, rupture of membranes.
• Risk factors: History of previous preterm birth, multiparity, smoking, uterine or cervical abnormalities (e.g., fibroids, unicorn uterus, cervical conization), vaginal bleeding during pregnancy, polyhydramnios, short duration between pregnancies, urinary tract infection (UTI) or sexually transmitted disease (STD), periodontal disease.
• Diagnosis: Pelvic exam, ultrasound (evaluation of cervical length), evaluation of uterine contractions (tocodynamometer), and fetal fibronectin or vaginal pH (assessment of premature rupture of membranes).
• Treatment: Corticosteroids (from 23rd to 34th gestational weeks), magnesium sulfate (from 24th to 32nd gestational weeks, neuroprotective), tocolytics (stop contractions to allow corticosteroids to take effect; indomethacin, nifedipine, magnesium sulfate, and β-mimetics).
• Prevention: Prophylactic progesterone (cervical length < 25 mm between 16 and 24 weeks), prophylactic cervical cerclage (cervical length < 25 mm, history of preterm premature rupture of membranes, or cervical trauma).

12.4.6 Premature Rupture of Membranes (PROM)

• Rupture of membranes before the onset of labor.[38]
• Preterm PROM: Rupture of membranes before 37 weeks.
• PROM affects 3% of all pregnancies in the United States.
• Risk factors: Previous history of PROM, intra-amniotic infections, and same risk factors of preterm labor.
• Preterm PROM: 50% of cases have birth within 1 week, 15–25% cases have clinically evident intra-amniotic infection, 15–20% have postpartum infection, 2–5% have abruptio placenta, most common complication is prematurity.
• Diagnosis: Vaginal exam deferred for speculum exam to avoid infection risk unless patient has contractions, visualization of amniotic fluid in cervical canal or vagina most sensitive, pH test, ferning test.

- Treatment: Evaluation of gestational age and fetal exam, delivery indicated if fetal compromise, clinical chorioamnionitis or abruption placenta.
  - ≥ 34 weeks: Delivery, GBS prophylaxis as indicated.
  - $24^{0/7}$–$33^{6/7}$ weeks: Expectant management, antibiotic prophylaxis, corticosteroids, GBS prophylaxis as indicated, magnesium sulfate if ≤ 32 weeks.
  - ≤ 24 weeks: Patient counseling, labor induction, antibiotics if ≥ 20 weeks; GBS prophylaxis, corticosteroids, or tocolysis not recommended.

12.4.7 Nausea and Vomiting of Pregnancy, Hyperemesis Gravidarum

- Nausea and vomiting of pregnancy (NVP): Symptoms in first trimester without other causes.
- Hyperemesis gravidarum (HG): Severe NVP with triad of > 5% prepregnancy weight loss, dehydration, electrolyte imbalance.
- Common cause of hospital admission; NVP affects 80% of pregnant women; HG affects 0.3–3.6% of pregnant women.
- Primarily cause from rising β-human chorionic gonadotropin (β-hCG) level.
- Treatment: First-line antiemetics (H_1 receptor antagonists, phenothiazines); second-line antiemetics (metoclopramide, ondansetron); rehydration with normal saline and KCl; outpatient IV rehydration therapy if tolerating some oral intake, inpatient treatment if not tolerating oral intake, ketonuria, > 5% weight loss, or comorbidities (UTI).

12.4.8 Surgery during Pregnancy

- No current anesthetic agents have teratogenic effects in standard dosages at any gestational age.[39]
- Fetal heart rate monitoring important for hemodynamic management and delivery decision making.
- Urgent surgery should be performed regardless of trimester.
- Elective surgery should be postponed until after delivery.
- Second trimester ideal for surgery; abortion risk highest during first trimester; preterm contractions and birth highest risk during third trimester.
- Nonobstetric surgery should be done in a facility where neonatal, pediatric, and obstetric care is available.
- Previable fetus: Document heart rate by Doppler pre-op and post-op.
- Viable fetus: Monitor fetal heart rate and uterine contractions pre-op and post-op.
- Intraoperative electronic fetal monitoring uses: Viable fetus, obstetric surgeon available to intervene, informed consent available for possible emergency cesarean delivery.

12.4.9 Obstetric and Gynecologic Causes of Acute Abdomen During Pregnancy

- Abruptio placenta, miscarriage, ectopic pregnancy, and adnexal torsion are well-known causes of acute pelvic pain during pregnancy and have been previously discussed; also see Chapters 4.1 Acute Abdomen and 12.1.9 Gynecological Causes of Acute Abdomen.
- Uterine Rupture:
  - Complete separation of all uterine layers with extrusion of fetal parts to the peritoneal cavity.
  - In uterine dehiscence, despite the disruption of uterine muscle, the serosa is intact.
  - Overall incidence is 2/10.000.
  - The most known risk factor is previous uterine surgery, including cesarean section, and the incidence is increased to 0.2% in those women.
  - Despite its rarity, it is the one of the most catastrophic conditions in pregnancy both for mother and fetus which may cause hemorrhagic shock, need for hysterectomy for mother, hypoxic ischemic encephalopathy for fetus, and maternal and fetal death.
  - Other risk factors include external trauma, placenta percreta, grand multiparity, and obstructed labor

- Signs and symptoms: Acute onset severe abdominal pain, vaginal bleeding, cessation of uterine contractions, peritoneal irritation, and abnormal fetal heart rate pattern.
- Diagnosis: History (cessation of uterine contractions, following severe abdominal pain) is highly informative. For confirmation, use USG (empty uterine cavity with fetal parts in abdominal cavity).
- Management: Emergent laparotomy following ABC protocol.
- Degeneration of Leiomyoma[40]:
  - Most fibroids are asymptomatic.
  - Pain is the most common complication of fibroids in pregnancy.
  - Degeneration of fibroids (which is called red or carneous) is a well-known cause of severe abdominal pain during pregnancy.
  - Risk factors are pedunculated and >5cm fibroids.
  - The mechanisms of pain are thought to be due to rapid growth of fibroids that result in ischemia, necrosis, changing uterine architecture, and release of prostaglandins from cellular damage within the fibroid.
  - The incidence of degeneration in a pregnant woman with leiomyoma is estimated to be 10%.
  - Diagnosis is mostly based on clinical history and physical examination; also, heterogeneous appearance of fibroids by ultrasound is supportive in nature.
  - The most important point is to consider fibroid degeneration in acute abdomen cases before any invasive procedure.
  - Treatment includes hydration and analgesic treatment comprising NSAIDs
- Chorioamnionitis:
  - Affects 10% of the patients with preterm labor.
  - Signs and symptoms: uterine tenderness, pain, fever, vaginal and/or cervical discharge, and maternal and fetal tachycardia:
  - Management includes broad-spectrum antibiotics and termination of pregnancy.
- Rupture of subcapsular hematoma of the liver:
  - Complication of hemolysis, elevated liver enzymes, low platelet count (HELLP) syndrome.
  - Extremely rare but highly mortal for both mother and fetus.
  - Emergent laparotomy is needed by a general surgeon.
  - Massive transfusion of blood and blood products are essential.
- Torsion of the uterus[41]:
  - In more than 80% of pregnancies, the uterus is dextrorotated due to left location of sigmoid colon.
  - It is defined as rotation more than 45 degrees around the long axis of the uterus.
  - Symptoms include abdominal pain, urinary retention, and even shock.
  - Diagnosis is made by laparotomy.
  - Treatment involves rotating the uterus back to his normal position

References

[1] Amsel R, Totten PA, Spiegel CA, Chen KC, Eschenbach D, Holmes KK. Nonspecific vaginitis. Diagnostic criteria and microbial and epidemiologic associations. Am J Med. 1983; 74(1):14–22

[2] Centers for Disease Control and Prevention. Sexually Transmitted Diseases Surveillance. 2016. Available at: https://www.cdc.gov/std/stats16/default.htm. Accessed February 27, 2019

[3] Sabry M, Al-Hendy A. Medical treatment of uterine leiomyoma. Reprod Sci. 2012; 19(4):339–353

[4] Ross J, Guaschino S, Cusini M, Jensen J. 2017 European guideline for the management of pelvic inflammatory disease. Int J STD AIDS. 2018; 29(2):108–114

[5] Munro MG, Critchley HO, Broder MS, Fraser IS, FIGO Working Group on Menstrual Disorders. FIGO classification system (PALM-COEIN) for causes of abnormal uterine bleeding in nongravid women of reproductive age. Int J Gynaecol Obstet. 2011; 113(1):3–13

[6] Practice bulletin no. 114: management of endometriosis. Obstet Gynecol. 2010; 116(1):223–236

[7] Taran FA, Stewart EA, Brucker S. Adenomyosis: epidemiology, risk factors, clinical phenotype and surgical and interventional alternatives to hysterectomy. Geburtshilfe Frauenheilkd. 2013; 73(9):924–931

[8] Committee on Practice Bulletins—Gynecology. Practice bulletin no. 136: management of abnormal uterine bleeding associated with ovulatory dysfunction. Obstet Gynecol. 2013; 122(1):176–185

[9] Kives S, Gascon S, Dubuc É, Van Eyk N. No. 341-diagnosis and management of adnexal torsion in children, adolescents, and adults. J Obstet Gynaecol Can. 2017; 39(2):82–90

[10] Barash JH, Buchanan EM, Hillson C. Diagnosis and management of ectopic pregnancy. Am Fam Physician. 2014; 90(1):34–40

[11] American College of Obstetricians and Gynecologists' Committee on Practice Bulletins—Gynecology. Practice Bulletin No. 174: Evaluation and management of adnexal masses. Obstet Gynecol. 2016; 128(5):e210–e226

[12] UK CR. Uterine Cancer survival statistics. 2016. Available at: http://www.cancerresearchuk.org/health-professional/cancer-statistics/statistics-by-cancer-type/uterine-cancer/survival. Accessed July 26, 2017

[13] Siegel RL, Miller KD, Jemal A. Cancer statistics, 2017. CA Cancer J Clin. 2017; 67(1):7–30

[14] National Comprehensive Cancer Network. NCCN Clinical Practice Guidelines in Oncology: Ovarian Cancer, Including Fallopian Tube Cancer and Primary Peritoneal Cancer. NCCN Clinical Practice Guidelines in Oncology. 2018. Available at: https://www.nccn.org/. Accessed January 2, 2019

[15] FIGO Cancer Reports. Int J Gynaecol Obstet. 2018; 2018(143) Suppl 2:i–iv, 1–158

[16] Colombo N, Creutzberg C, Amant F, et al. ESMO-ESGO-ESTRO Endometrial Consensus Conference Working Group. ESMO-ESGO-ESTRO Consensus Conference on Endometrial Cancer: diagnosis, treatment and follow-up. Int J Gynecol Cancer. 2016; 26(1):2–30

[17] Practice Bulletin No. Practice Bulletin No. 149: endometrial cancer. Obstet Gynecol. 2015; 125(4):1006–1026

[18] American College of Obstetricians and Gynecologists.. ACOG practice bulletin. Diagnosis and treatment of cervical carcinomas. Number 35, May 2002. Int J Gynaecol Obstet. 2002; 78(1):79–91

[19] Cibula D, Pötter R, Planchamp F, et al. The European Society of Gynaecological Oncology/European Society for Radiotherapy and Oncology/European Society of Pathology guidelines for the management of patients with cervical cancer. Int J Gynecol Cancer. 2018 May;28(4):641–655

[20] Curry SJ, Krist AH, Owens DK, et al. US Preventive Services Task Force. Screening for cervical cancer: US Preventive Services Task Force Recommendation Statement. JAMA. 2018; 320(7):674–686

[21] Koh WJ, Abu-Rustum NR, Bean S, et al. Cervical cancer, version 3.2019, NCCN Clinical Practice Guidelines in Oncology. J Natl Compr Canc Netw. 2019; 17(1):64–84

[22] National Comprehensive Cancer Network. NCCN Clinical Practice Guidelines in Oncology: Vulvar Cancer (Squamous Cell Carcinoma). NCCN Clinical Practice Guidelines in Oncology. 2018. Available at: https://www.nccn.org/. Accessed January 2, 2019

[23] Farahi N, Zolotor A. Recommendations for preconception counseling and care. Am Fam Physician. 2013; 88(8):499–506

[24] Johnson K, Posner SF, Biermann J, et al. CDC/ATSDR Preconception Care Work Group, Select Panel on Preconception Care. Recommendations to improve preconception health and health care–United States. A report of the CDC/ATSDR Preconception Care Work Group and the Select Panel on Preconception Care. MMWR Recomm Rep. 2006; 55 RR-6:1–23

[25] Routine prenatal care summary 2017. Available at: http://apecguidelines.org. Accessed January 15, 2020

[26] Naidu K, Fredlund KL. Gestational Age Assessment. StatPearls. 2018. Available at: https://www.ncbi.nlm.nih.gov/books/NBK526000/. Accessed January 15, 2020

[27] Committee on Obstetric Practice. Committee Opinion No. 723: Guidelines for diagnostic imaging during pregnancy and lactation. Obstet Gynecol. 2017; 130(4):e210–e216

[28] ACOG Practice Bulletin No. ACOG Practice Bulletin No. 200 Summary: early pregnancy loss. Obstet Gynecol. 2018; 132(5):1311–1313

[29] Kapp N, Eckersberger E, Lavelanet A, Rodriguez MI. Medical abortion in the late first trimester: a systematic review. Contraception. 2019; 99(2):77–86

[30] ACOG Practice Bulletin No. ACOG Practice Bulletin No. 202 Summary: gestational hypertension and preeclampsia. Obstet Gynecol. 2019; 133(1):211–214

[31] Dusse LM, Alpoim PN, Silva JT, Rios DR, Brandao AH, Cabral AC. Revisiting HELLP syndrome. Clin Chim Acta. 2015; 451(Pt B):117–120

[32] Broekhuijsen K, van Baaren GJ, van Pampus MG, et al. HYPITAT-II study group. Immediate delivery versus expectant monitoring for hypertensive disorders of pregnancy between 34 and 37 weeks of gestation (HYPITAT-II): an open-label, randomised controlled trial. Lancet. 2015; 385(9986):2492–2501

[33] Sibai BM. Imitators of severe pre-eclampsia. Semin Perinatol. 2009; 33(3):196–205

[34] Khan KS, Wojdyla D, Say L, Gülmezoglu AM, Van Look PF. WHO analysis of causes of maternal death: a systematic review. Lancet. 2006; 367(9516):1066–1074

[35] The Royal College of Obstetricians and Gynaecologists. Antepartum Haemorrhage (Green-top Guideline No. 63). 2014. Available at: https://www.rcog.org.uk/en/guidelines-research-services/guidelines/gtg63/. Accessed January 15, 2017

[36] Committee on Practice Bulletins-Obstetrics. 183: Postpartum hemorrhage. Obstet Gynecol. 2017; 130(4):e168–e186

[37] American College of Obstetricians and Gynecologists' Committee on Practice Bulletins—Obstetrics. Practice Bulletin No. 171: Management of preterm labor. Obstet Gynecol. 2016; 128(4):e155–e164

[38] Committee on Practice Bulletins-Obstetrics. ACOG Practice Bulletin No. 188: Prelabor rupture of membranes. Obstet Gynecol. 2018; 131(1):e1–e14

[39] Committee on Obstetric Practice and the American Society of Anesthesiologists. Committee Opinion No. 696: Nonobstetric surgery during pregnancy. Obstet Gynecol. 2017; 129(4):777–778

[40] Lee HJ, Norwitz ER, Shaw J. Contemporary management of fibroids in pregnancy. Rev Obstet Gynecol. 2010; 3(1):20–27

[41] Jensen JG. Uterine torsion in pregnancy. Acta Obstet Gynecol Scand. 1992; 71(4):260–265

13 Dermatology

Rachel Elizabeth Ward and Nasreen Bowhan

13.1 Skin Cancer

13.1.1 Basal Cell Carcinoma

- Epidemiology:
  - The most common cancer in the United States.
  - 2 million new cases of basal cell carcinoma (BCC) per year.[1]
  - Mean age is 64.9 ± 13.8 years.
  - 0.04% had metastatic disease.[2]
  - Most closely linked to episodes of high sun exposure.
- Diagnosis:
  - Most commonly presents as a pearly telangiectatic papule or nodule (▶ Fig. 13.1). Often ulcerated and/or pigmented. Predilection for sun-exposed skin on patients with light skin type. Spares glabrous skin.
  - Biopsy for confirmation and to identify aggressive histologic subtypes.
  - The National Comprehensive Cancer Guideline (NCCN) version 1.2019 stratifies tumors into a high-risk or low-risk category based on the risk of recurrence.[3]
- High-risk anatomic location and size:
  - Area "H," any size: Central face, eyelids, nose, lips, chin, ear, periauricular area, temple; genitals, nipples/areola; hands, feet, ankles, nail unit.

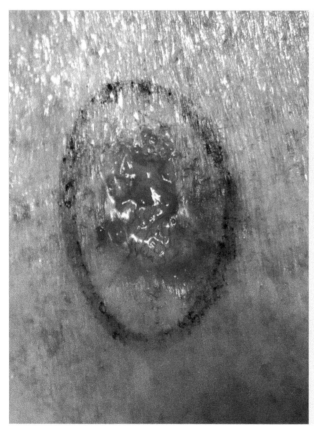

Fig. 13.1 Basal cell carcinoma. An ulcerated pearly telangiectatic nodule. Notice pigmentation at 4 o' clock.

- Area "M" > 10 mm: Cheeks, forehead, scalp, neck, jawline; pretibial.
- Area "L" > 20 mm: Trunk, extremities (excluding pretibial surface, hands, feet, nail units, ankles.
  - Clinical features: Poorly defined borders, recurrent, history of immunosuppression, site of prior radiation.
  - Histology: Aggressive growth pattern, perineural invasion.
- Imaging: Imaging rarely indicated unless locally advanced and deep structure involvement is suspected.
- Surgical management: First-line therapy for low-risk tumors.
  - American Academy of Dermatology working group recommends standard excision with 4-mm margins and postoperative margin assessment.[4]
  - Standard excision on nodular or superficial BCC on low-risk location has a 2–4% recurrence rate after 3–5 years.
  - Excision is superior to curettage and electrodessication plus cryotherapy on the head and neck of nonaggressive subtypes based on higher recurrence rates 8.2 and 17.6%.[5]
  - Curettage and electrodessication generates a scar and not commonly used on terminal hair-bearing sites such as the scalp, axillae, pubic region, beard area in men.
  - Radiation for patients in whom surgery is contraindicated.
- First-line therapy for high-risk tumors:
  - Mohs micrographic surgery (MMS) or excision with complete margin evaluation.
  - Systematic reviews of the literature show 1 and 5.6% 5-year recurrence rate for primary and recurrent BCC, respectively.
  - Recurrence rate is superior to all other treatment modalities.[6]
  - RCT showed 10-year recurrence rate for MMS is 4.4% as compared to 12.2% for standard excision.[7]
  - Standard excision with wide margins, postoperative margin evaluation, linear closure, or delayed closure.
  - Immediate closure via tissue rearrangement makes a positive margin very difficult to manage.[3,4]
  - Radiation considered for patients in whom surgery is contraindicated.[3]
- Medical and nonsurgical management:
  - Topical monotherapy can be considered for some small tumors in low-risk locations when surgery is not feasible.[4]
  - Imiquimod 5% cream is Food and Drug Administration (FDA) approved for the treatment of superficial BCC on the trunk, neck, and extremities.
  - Efudex 5% cream.
  - Photodynamic therapy: Topical application and incubation of a photosensitizer followed by exposure to light—red light, blue light, or broad band.
  - Radiation is often used as adjuvant therapy, although data are limited.[4]
  - Vismodegib is the first systemic medication approved by FDA for metastatic BCC, for locally advanced BCC that has recurred following surgery, or for those who are surgery or radiosurgery non-candidates.

13.1.2 Squamous Cell Carcinoma

- Epidemiology:
  - Cutaneous squamous cell carcinoma (cSCC) is the second most common form of human cancer.
  - 200,000–400,00 new cases each year in the United States.[8]
  - Most closely linked to cumulative sun exposure.
    - Higher incidence in certain immunosuppressed patients such as solid-organ transplant recipients.[9]
- Diagnosis:
  - Often presents as an indurated hyperkeratotic papule or nodule. May have a raised erythematous base (▶ Fig. 13.2).
  - Biopsy is necessary to rule out benign and precancerous mimickers of cSCC such as seborrheic keratoses and actinic keratoses.
  - Also guides management based on high-risk features and depth of invasion.
  - Acceptable biopsy methods include punch, shave, excision.[10]

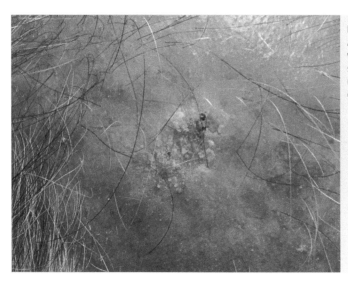

Fig. 13.2 Squamous cell carcinoma. An indurated hyperkeratic plaque. It was treated with liquid nitrogen on several occasions. Shave biopsy revealed invasive squamous cell carcinoma.

- ○ NCCN stratifies cSCC into a high-risk and low-risk category to guide clinicians' management strategies. They define a tumor as high risk if it satisfies any of the following criteria:
  - – Size and location: Area L ≥ 20 mm, area M ≥ 10 mm, area H, all sizes.
  - – Clinical features: Poorly defined borders, recurrent, history of immunosuppression, site of prior radiation or chronic inflammation, rapidly growing, neuro symptoms.
  - – Histologic features: Poorly differentiated, high-risk histologic subtype (acantholytic, adenosquamous/mucin producing, desmoplastic, metaplastic), depth ≥ 2 mm (Clark level IV, V), perineural/lymphatic/vascular involvement.
- • Imaging:
  - ○ Imaging is indicated when there is suspicion of extensive disease such as involvement of bone, perineural or deep soft tissue.
  - ○ MRI with contrast preferred for suspected perineural or deep soft-tissue involvement.
  - ○ CT with contrast preferred for suspected bony involvement.
  - ○ Imaging can be utilized to assess deep structure involvement if advanced localized disease.
  - ○ Fine needle aspiration or core biopsy for palpable regional nodes or abnormal nodes identified by imaging studies.[11]
- • Surgical management:
  - ○ Majority are successfully treated with standard treatment modalities such as excision. Consider recurrence rate, preservation of function, patient desire/expectation, and potential complications.
  - ○ First-line therapy for low-risk tumors:
    - – Standard excision with 4–6 mm margins and postoperative margin assessment; 5-year local recurrence rate is 5.4%.
    - – Curettage and electrodessication, excluding terminal hair-bearing sites such as the scalp, axillae, pubic region, beard area in men, shows a 5-year local recurrence rate of 1.7% (only small, low-risk tumors were treated).
    - – Radiation for patients in whom surgery is contraindicated; 5-year local recurrence rate is 6.4%.[12]
  - ○ First-line therapy for high-risk tumors[11]:
    - – MMS or excision with complete margin evaluation; 5-year local recurrence rate is 3.0%.
    - – For cSCC, local recurrence 5-year rates for MMS and excision are 10 and 23.3%, respectively.
    - – Standard excision with wide margins, postoperative margin evaluation, linear closure or delayed closure; clearance rate of 95% when excised with a margin of at least 6 mm.[13]
    - – Radiation for patients in whom surgery is contraindicated.
    - – Management of lymph node metastases: Based on location and number of nodes, whether ipsilateral or bilateral, superficial parotidectomy indicated when parotid is involved.[11]

- Medical and nonsurgical management:
  - Available data do not support the use of topical treatments except for squamous cell carcinoma in situ.
  - Radiation and cryotherapy can be considered when surgery is not feasible/practical, contraindicated, undesired.
  - Radiation—primary or adjuvant treatment.
  - Cryotherapy can be considered for low-risk tumors. Target tumor with equal depth and margin as standard excision.[11]
  - For locally advanced and metastatic disease, coordination with surgical, medical, and radiation oncologists may be necessary.

13.1.3 Cutaneous Melanoma

- Epidemiology:
  - In 2018, there were an estimated 91,270 new cases of melanoma and 9,320 melanoma-related deaths in the United States[16]; many early melanomas were likely not reported.[14]
  - Risk factors: Ultraviolet light exposure; skin type, hair color, eye color; personal or family history of melanoma; multiple dysplastic nevi; certain inherited genetic mutations.
- Diagnosis:
  - Classically presents as a mostly brown or black macule with irregular pigment distribution and atypical shape or outline. It can lack pigment or be nodular.
  - Can be found on any cutaneous surface.
  - Dermoscopy: Helpful for identifying high-risk lesions; guide for sampling biopsy of very large lesion or those in cosmetically or functionally sensitive areas.[15]
  - Biopsy: Critical for diagnosis and staging; ideal biopsy is excisional with 1–3 mm margins to a depth where the lesion is not transected at the base; acceptable methods include fusiform ellipse, punch, deep shave/saucerization to at least the deep reticular dermis.[15]
  - TNM-based pathologic staging:
    - Stage 1: IA < 0.8 mm, no ulceration; IB < 0.8 mm with ulceration, 0.8–1.0 mm with or without ulceration.
    - Stage II: > 1.0.
    - Stage III: Node positive, satellite/in-transit metastasis.
    - Stage IV: Metastatic.
  - Prognosis is most closely linked to depth of invasion, the Breslow depth. Histologic ulceration is also associated with worse prognosis.
  - Elevated LDH levels associated with worse prognosis for stage IV disease.[15]
- Imaging:
  - Not indicated for stage IA, IB, or IIA without signs or symptoms of metastasis.
  - Surveillance imaging is useful for stage IIB or higher.
  - Routine imaging not recommended beyond 3–5 years for any stage.
  - Stage IIB, IIC, or III developed metastatic disease in a median of 1.4 years.
  - CT or PET can be considered if sentinel lymph node study is positive.[14]
- Surgical management:
  - Excision with negative histologic margins is first-line therapy for all tumors including melanoma in situ.
  - Margin size is determined by Breslow depth:
    - In situ: 0.5–1.0 mm margin.
    - Breslow < 1 mm: 1.0 cm margin.
    - Breslow 1–2 mm: 1.0–2.0 cm margin.
    - Breslow 2 mm or more: 2.0 cm margin.
    - Excise to (but not including) underlying muscular fascia.[15]
  - MMS or staged excision with complete margin assessment can be considered for lentigo maligna on the face, ear, scalp.[15]
  - Sentinel lymph node biopsy: Used for tumors > 1.0 mm thickness, thinner tumors with ulceration, high mitotic rate, lymphovascular invasion, or patients younger than 40 years.

- Sentinel lymph node biopsy allows for accurate staging, crucial for decision making in adjuvant systemic therapy and may qualify patients for clinical trial enrollment.
- If sentinel node study is positive, acceptable options include lymph node dissection or surveillance with serial ultrasound every 4 months for the first 2 years followed by every 6 months for years 3 through 5.
- Lymph node biopsy might not impact survival.[14,15]
- Medical and nonsurgical management:
  - Imiquimod 5% cream.
  - Adjuvant radiation can be considered in some high-risk desmoplastic tumors (Breslow > 4 mm, extensive perineural invasion, head and neck location, narrow deep margin).
  - Systemic interferon, chemotherapy, and immunotherapy often used for stage III and IV diseases.[17]

13.2 Skin Flaps

- See Chapter 9, Plastic Surgery.
- Flaps are most often used in dermatologic surgery after the surgical removal of tumors, commonly using the Mohs technique.
- The most important use of any flap is to preserve function of the surgical area.
  - Often accomplished by changing a tension vector or avoiding functional anatomic borders.

13.2.1 Anesthesia

- Local.
  - The most commonly used technique to deliver anesthesia is via intradermal and/or subcutaneous injection.
  - Slower speed of injection and smaller caliber needle, and the addition of a buffering agent helps mitigate pain and discomfort for the patient.
- Regional nerve block:
  - Anesthesia of proximal sensory nerves allows for a wider area of anesthesia using a smaller volume of anesthetic.
  - Knowledge of anatomic landmarks and the course of sensory and motor nerves is essential.
  - Vasoconstriction at the site of surgery is significantly diminished with nerve blocks compared with local infiltration.
- Anesthetic compounds:
  - Most commonly used anesthetic in dermatologic surgery is lidocaine 1–2%.
  - Bupivacaine can be added for prolonged duration of anesthesia (240–480 minutes with epinephrine vs. lidocaine: 60–400 minutes with epinephrine).[18]
  - Epinephrine 1:1,000,000 can be added to any anesthetic for vasoconstrictive effects. Use with caution in patients with peripheral vascular disease.

13.2.2 Antibiotic Use

- American Academy of Dermatology provides advisory statements on the use of antibiotic prophylaxis in dermatologic surgery.[19]
- Purpose is to prevent surgical-site infections, hematogenous total joint infection, and/or infective endocarditis.
- The majority of dermatologic surgeries and patients do not require antibiotic prophylaxis.
- If performing surgery on an infected skin site, tailor antibiotic choice based on culture results. All patients undergoing surgery on an infected skin site should be treated aggressively with proper antibiotics.

13.2.3 Prevention of Infective Endocarditis and/or Hematogenous Total Joint Infection

- High-risk patients:
  - Cardiac: History of prosthetic cardiac valve, previous infective endocarditis, congenital heart disease, cardiac transplant patients.

○ Orthopaedic: < 2 years after joint replacement, previous prosthetic joint infection, immunocompromised/immunosuppressed patients, type 1 diabetes, HIV infection, malignancy, malnourishment, hemophilia.
- Low-risk patients:
  ○ Cardiac: Pacemaker, defibrillator, peripheral vascular or coronary artery stents, vascular grafts, breast implants, penile prostheses, CNS shunts.
  ○ Orthopaedic: Orthopaedic pins, plates, screws, most healthy patients with total joint prostheses (> 2 years after joint replacement).

13.2.4 Prophylaxis

- Indications: Undergoing dermatologic surgery on infected skin (high- and low-risk patients), if surgical site breaches oral mucosa (only high-risk patients) or high-risk surgical sites (below).
- Medications given 60 minutes prior to procedure.
- Non–oral site antibiotics:
  ○ Cephalexin or dicloxacillin 2 g PO.
  ○ If penicillin (PCN) allergy, clindamycin 600 mg PO or azithromycin/clarithromycin 500 mg PO.
- Oral site antibiotics:
  ○ Amoxicillin 2 g PO.
  ○ If PCN allergy, clindamycin 600 mg PO or azithromycin/clarithromycin 500 mg PO.
- If site is not infected nor in the oral mucosa, prophylaxis is *not* indicated, even in patients considered "high risk."

13.2.5 Prevention of Surgical-Site Infections

- High-risk surgical sites: Lower extremity (especially below knee), groin, wedge excision of lip or ear, skin flaps on nose, skin grafts, extensive inflammatory skin disease.
- Prophylaxis indications: Recommended for surgery on any of the aforementioned sites.
- Medications given 60 minutes prior to procedure.
- Wedge excision of lip/ear, flaps on nose, and all grafts antibiotics:
  ○ Cephalexin or dicloxacillin 2 g PO.
  ○ If PCN allergy, clindamycin 600 mg PO or azithromycin/clarithromycin 500 mg PO.
- Lower extremities and groin antibiotics.
  ○ Cephalexin 2 g PO or trimethoprim-sulfamethoxazole-double strength (TMP-SMX-DS) 1 tablet PO or levofloxacin 500 mg PO.
  ○ If PCN allergy, TMP-SMX-DS 1 tablet PO or levofloxacin 500 mg PO.

13.2.6 Use of Blood Thinners

- Although antiplatelet and anticoagulant medications will cause increased intraoperative and sometimes postoperative bleeding (and thus complications), the standard of care is to continue all medically necessary agents for dermatologic surgeries, as the risk of catastrophic thromboembolic event outweighs the benefit of stopping medications prior to cutaneous surgery.[20]
- It is recommended that INR is checked prior to surgery in patients taking warfarin. Consider delaying surgery if INR > 3–4.
- Consider stopping prophylactic/nonmedically indicated use of NSAIDs (3 days), aspirin (10 days), and vitamin/herbal supplements (7 days) prior to surgery. Can resume 3–7 days postprocedure.[20]
- Avoid alcohol consumption for 3 days before and 3 days after surgery.

13.2.7 Flap Techniques

- Sliding flaps: Main tension vector is in the opposite direction of flap movement.
- Advancement flaps:
  ○ Does not redirect primary tension vector.

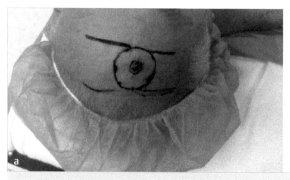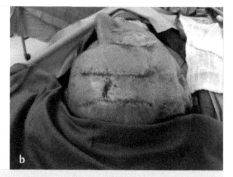

Fig. 13.3 H-plasty. (a, b) A 2-cm squamous cell carcinoma excised leaving a 6-cm defect approximated with an H-flap under local anesthesia. (Source: Forehead. In: Gastman B, ed. Cutaneous Malignancies: A Surgical Perspective. 1st ed. Thieme; 2017.)

- ○ Burow wedge flap (east-to-west): Laterally displaces one standing cone to an area of donor tissue.
- ○ Crescentic flap: Laterally displaces one standing cone (similar to the Burow advancement flap), but this cone is shaped in a crescent shape to conform to curved areas, such as the alar crease or lateral eyebrow; the crescentic shape elongates one arm of the standing cone, which often eliminates the need for dog-ear redundancy revision.[21]
- ○ V to Y (island pedicle or kite) flap: Used in repair of the nasal ala, nasal tip, nasolabial fold, or upper cutaneous lip[22]; the elongated standing cone is separated from the surrounding skin; the area under the flap is undermined incompletely to develop a myocutaneous pedicle; the flap is advanced over the defect and sutured into place; length:width ratio = 2–3:1; disadvantages include mobility constrained by length of myocutaneous pedicle, pincushioning.[22]
- ○ U-plasty (O to U): Laterally displaces two standing cones, thus moving cones to areas of preferred donor tissue.
- ○ H-plasty (O to H): Bilateral advancement flap; similar to a bilateral U-plasty, wherein each side displaces two standing cones laterally, advancing the flap from both sides to cover the defect (▶ Fig. 13.3).
- ○ T-plasty (A to T): Bilateral advancement flap; used for small defects, especially near mental crease.
- ○ Mucosal flap: Used for large defects on mucosal lip.
- ○ Helical rim flap: Large defects on superior helix.
- • Rotation flaps:
  - ○ Redirects primary tension vector.
  - ○ Should be oversized to overcome pivotal/rotational restraint at the flap's pivot point.
  - ○ Unilateral:
    - – Use: Scalp, cheek (especially medial), temple, infraorbital.[21]
    - – Arc originates from superior portion of defect.
    - – Elevating arc above the height of the defect allows for compensation of pivotal/rotational restraint. This decreases the secondary gravitational pull of the flap, which may lead to ectropion.[23]
    - – Standing cones are removed from the inferior distal portion of the defect and at any location along the superior arc of the flap.
  - ○ Bilateral (O to Z): Especially useful on the scalp where there is decreased inherent tissue laxity; flap elevated in the subgaleal space.
  - ○ Dorsal nasal (Rieger or Hatchet) flap: Nasal root and glabellar skin as donor site and rotates flap inferiorly to cover defects on the nasal dorsum, tip, and bridge.
  - ○ Cervicofacial (Mustarde): For large cheek defects.
  - ○ Lower eyelid (Tenzel): For larger lower lateral eyelid defects.
  - ○ Peng: Larger defects (> 1.5 cm) on distal nasal tip and nasal bridge.[24]
- • Lifting flaps:
  - ○ Are lifted over normal skin and set into place.

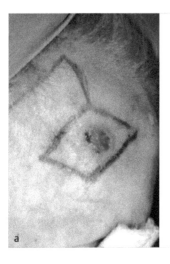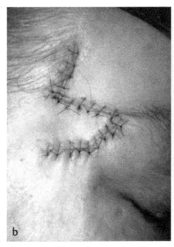

Fig. 13.4 Rhombic flap, before and after. (a) This patient had a basal cell carcinoma involving the lateral eyebrow and temporal area. **(b)** During forehead reconstruction, a rhombic flap reconstruction was performed. The defect is closed without tension or undue distortion of natural anatomic landmarks. (Source: Forehead Reconstruction. In: Jackson I, ed. Local Flaps in Head and Neck Reconstruction. 2nd ed. Thieme; 2007.)

- ○ Have both pivotal (rotational) and linear movements.
- ○ Redirects primary tension vector.
- ○ Transposition flaps:
  - – Used mostly for medium-to-large flaps on head and neck.[22]
  - – Rhombic (rhomboid) flap: Angle of flap tip can be modified (60 degrees = Limberg; 30–60 degrees = Dufourmentel; 30 degrees = Webster); used near free margins (lower eyelid, medial canthus, proximal nose, temple, peripheral cheek; ▶ Fig. 13.4).[21]
  - – Bilobed flap: Pedicle can be medially or laterally based; the addition of a second lobe facilitates greater flap movement; used for smaller defects (< 1.5 cm) on distal nasal tip, lateral nasal ala, temporal forehead. Modifications can be used for larger neck, cheek, and postauricular defects; disadvantages include pin cushioning, trapdoor defect, and alar retraction.[25]
  - – Banner flap: Long, thin flaps with high length:width ratio (3–5:1); used for upper and lower eyelid, medial canthus, superior helical rim, proximal nasal bridge, nasal sidewall.[21]
  - – Melolabial/nasolabial flap: Flap is extended down melolabial fold and transposed over the inferolateral nasal ala; ideal for larger defects covering the nasal ala and/or nasal sidewall; disadvantage includes potential blunting of the alar crease.
  - – Z-plasty: Mainly used in scar revision surgery to correct eclabium, ectropion, or other contracted scars.
- ○ Interpolation flaps:
  - – Typically two stages: Flap harvesting and insetting over the defect, then pedicle takedown and debulking 2–3 weeks later where the pedicle is divided.
  - – Paramedian forehead flap: Blood supply from supratrochlear artery; used for large defects (> 1.5 cm) on the distal nose and ala.
  - – Lip-switch (Abbe) flap: Blood supply from labial artery, used for full-thickness defect at least 40% of the length of the lip.
  - – Cheek-to-nose/melolabial flap: Used larger defects encompassing most of the nasal ala.
  - – Retroauricular flap: Use for large helical rim and anterior auricular defects.

References

[1] Asgari MM, Moffet HH, Ray GT, Quesenberry CP. Trends in basal cell carcinoma incidence and identification of high risk subgroups. 1998–2012. JAMA Dermatol. 2015; 151(9):976–981

[2] Goldenberg G, Karragiannis T, Palmer JB, et al. Incidence and prevalence of basal cell carcinoma (BCC) and locally advanced BCC (LABCC) in a large commercially insured population in the United States: a retrospective cohort study. J Am Acad Dermatol. 2016; 75 (5):957–966.e2

[3] National Comprehensive Cancer Network. Basal cell skin cancer (version 1.2019). Available at: https://www.nccn.org/professionals/physician_gls/pdf/nmsc.pdf. Accessed January 28, 2019

[4] Kim JYS, Kozlow JH, Mittal B, Moyer J, Olencki T, Rodgers P, Work Group, Invited Reviewers. Guidelines of care for the management of basal cell carcinoma. J Am Acad Dermatol. 2018; 78(3):540–559

[5] Kuijpers DI, Thissen MR, Berretty PJ, Ideler FH, Nelemans PJ, Neumann MH. Surgical excision versus curettage plus cryosurgery in the treatment of basal cell carcinoma. Dermatol Surg. 2007; 33(5):579–587

[6] Rowe DE, Carrol RJ, Day CL, Jr. Long term recurrence rates in previously untreated (primary) basal cell carcinoma implications for patient follow-up. J Dermatol Surg Oncol. 1989; 15(3):315–328

[7] van Loo E, Mosterd K, Krekels GA, et al. Surgical excision versus Mohs' micrographic surgery for basal cell carcinoma of the face: a randomised clinical trial with 10 year follow-up. Eur J Cancer. 2014; 50(17):3011–3020

[8] Karia PS, Han J, Schmults CD. Cutaneous squamous cell carcinoma: estimated incidence of disease, nodal metastasis, and deaths from disease in the United States, 2012. J Am Acad Dermatol. 2013; 68(6):957–966

[9] Kim C, Cheng J, Colegio OR. Cutaneous squamous cell carcinomas in solid organ transplant recipients: emerging strategies for surveillance, staging, and treatment. Semin Oncol. 2016; 43(3):390–394

[10] Kim JYS, Kozlow JH, Mittal B, Moyer J, Olenecki T, Rodgers P, Work Group, Invited Reviewers. Guidelines of care for the management of cutaneous squamous cell carcinoma. J Am Acad Dermatol. 2018; 78(3):560–578

[11] National Comprehensive Cancer Network. Basal cell skin cancer (version 2.2019). Available at: https://www.nccn.org/professionals/physician_gls/pdf/squamous.pdf. Accessed January 28, 2019

[12] Lansbury L, Bath-Hextall F, Perkins W, Stanton W, Leonardi-Bee J. Interventions for non-metastatic squamous cell carcinoma of the skin: systematic review and pooled analysis of observational studies. BMJ. 2013; 347f:6153

[13] Rowe DE, Carroll RJ, Day CL, Jr. Prognostic factors for local recurrence, metastasis, survival rates in squamous cell carcinoma of the skin, ear, lip. Implications for treatment modality. J Am Acad Dermatol. 2013; 149(5):541–547

[14] National Cancer Institute. Surveillance, epidemiology and end results program. Cancer stat facts: Melanoma of the skin. Available at: https://seer.cancer.gov/statfacts/html/melan.html. Accessed January 31, 2019

[15] Swetter SM, Tsao H, Bichakjian CK, et al. Guidelines of care for the management of primary cutaneous melanoma. J Am Acad Dermatol. 2019; 80(1):208–250

[16] National Comprehensive Cancer Network. Cutaneous melanoma (version 1.2019). Available at: https://www.nccn.org/professionals/physician_gls/pdf/cutaneous_melanoma.pdf. Accessed January 28, 2019

[17] Strom T, Caudell JJ, Han D, et al. Radiotherapy influences local control in patients with desmoplastic melanoma. Cancer. 2014; 120(9):1369–1378

[18] Kouba DJ, LoPiccolo MC, Alam M, et al. Guidelines for the use of local anesthesia in office-based dermatologic surgery. J Am Acad Dermatol. 2016; 74(6):1201–1219

[19] Wright TI, Baddour LM, Berbari EF, et al. Antibiotic prophylaxis in dermatologic surgery: advisory statement 2008. J Am Acad Dermatol. 2008; 59(3):464–473

[20] Brown DG, Wilkerson EC, Love WE. A review of traditional and novel oral anticoagulant and antiplatelet therapy for dermatologists and dermatologic surgeons. J Am Acad Dermatol. 2015; 72(3):524–534

[21] Cook JL, Goldman GD, Holmes TE. Random pattern cutaneous flaps. In: Robinson JK, Hanke CW, Siegel DM, Fratila A, Bhatia A, Rohrer T, eds. Surgery of the Skin, Procedural Dermatology. Elsevier Health Sciences; 2014:252–285

[22] Martinez-Diaz GJ, Gladstone H. Reconstruction: flaps, grafts, and other closures. In: Alam M, ed. Evidence-Based Procedural Dermatology. Springer; 2011:133–146

[23] Chen TM, Wanitphakdeedecha R, Nguyen TH. Flaps. In: Vidimos AT, Ammirati CT, Poblete-Lopez C, eds. Dermatologic Surgery: Requisites in Dermatology. Elsevier Health Sciences; 2009:163–180

[24] Ahern RW, Lawrence N. The Peng flap: reviewed and refined. Dermatol Surg. 2008; 34(2):232–237

[25] Cho M, Kim DW. Modification of the Zitelli bilobed flap: a comparison of flap dynamics in human cadavers. Arch Facial Plast Surg. 2006; 8(6):404–409, discussion 410

14 Neurosurgery

Edited by Michael Karsy, Hussam Abou-Al-Shaar, and Jian Guan

14.1 Traumatic Brain Injury

Michael Karsy and Gregory W. J. Hawryluk

14.1.1 Assessment and Treatment

- Traumatic brain injury (TBI): An alteration in brain function, or other evidence of brain pathology caused by an external force to the head.
- Initial injury is classified as *primary* traumatic brain injury (e.g., contusion, laceration, bone fragments, diffuse axonal injury). Delayed injury is termed *secondary injury* and occurs at the molecular level. *Secondary insults* occur at the level of the patient (e.g., hypoxia, hypotension) and can be treated by physicians.
- Assessment begins with Advanced Trauma Life Support (ATLS) primary and secondary surveys.
- Information evaluated by a neurosurgeon includes age and mechanism of injury; neurological status is examined including Glasgow Coma Scale (GCS; ▸ Table 14.1 and ▸ Table 14.2), pupils, brainstem reflexes (e.g., cough, gag, corneal), stigmata of cranial injury (e.g., raccoon's eyes, Battle sign, CSF rhinorrhea or otorrhea, hemotympanum), associated traumatic injuries with prioritization of diagnostic studies and interventions.
- Facial injuries should be stabilized if able; ocular injuries can be assessed and treated by immediate lateral canthotomy; scalp lacerations can be immediately cleansed and stapled; intubation should be performed for airway protection prior to neurosurgical interventions.
- TBI severity can be divided by GCS:
  - GCS 15: Minimal/concussion.
  - GCS 13–15: Mild.
  - GCS 9–12: Moderate.
  - GCS ≤ 8: Severe, requires intubation.

Table 14.1 Glasgow coma scale (GCS)

Score	Eyes	Verbal	Motor
6			Follows commands
5		Oriented	Localizes to pain
4	Spontaneous	Confused	Withdraws from pain
3	To command	Inappropriate words	Flexor/decorticate posturing
2	To pain	Incomprehensible sounds	Extensor/decerebrate posturing
1	None	None	None

Notes: GCS reported with total score and subcomponents (e.g., GCS 15 and E4V5M6); motor subcomponent is most predictive of 30-day outcome. Patients assigned 1 point for verbal subscore if intubated and a T is placed after the GCS score to communicate that the patient is intubated (e.g., GCS 8T).

Table 14.2 Pediatric Glasgow coma scale

Score	Eyes	Verbal	Motor
6			Follows commands or spontaneous
5		Appropriate words/phrases; smiles/coos	Localizes to pain
4	Spontaneous	Inappropriate words; consolable crying	Withdraws from pain
3	To command or shout	Persistent and inappropriate crying	Flexor/decorticate posturing
2	To pain	Incomprehensible sounds, grunts, restlessness	Extensor/decerebrate posturing
1	None	None	None

Table 14.3 Canadian and New Orleans head CT rules

Canadian head CT rule	New Orleans head CT rule
Applies to patients GCS 13–15, age > 16, no blood thinners, and no postinjury seizures	Applies to patients GCS 15 and normal neurological exam
CT obtained if any of the following is positive: • GCS < 15 at 2 h postinjury • Suspected open or depressed skull fracture • Signs of basilar skull fracture • Episodes ≥ 2 of vomiting • Age ≥ 65 • Retrograde amnesia to event ≥ 30 min • Dangerous mechanism (e.g., pedestrian struck by motor vehicle, occupant ejected from motor vehicle, fall > 3 feet, fall > 5 stairs)	CT obtained if any of the following is positive: • Headache • Vomiting • Age > 60 • Alcohol or drug intoxication • Persistent anterograde amnesia • Visible trauma above the clavicle • Seizure

- GCS communicates severity of injury rapidly, has good interobserver reliability, and is predictive of discharge and long-term outcome especially motor score.
- CT evaluation of head includes soft-tissue and bone windows, Canadian CT rule or New Orleans trauma rule helps avoid unnecessary CT scans (▶ Table 14.3).
  - Low risk for intracranial injury: CT head not indicated, linear nondisplaced skull fractures not required, overnight observation considered.
  - Moderate or high risk for intracranial injury: CT imaging indicated, further clinical follow-up may be necessary.
- Concussion[1]:
  - Disturbance of brain function from direct or indirect force to the head.
  - Multiple grading systems were created but have been abandoned because of lack of validity.
  - American Academy of Neurology has guidelines emphasizing individual evaluation.
  - Sports concussion assessment tool 5 (SCAT5)[1]: Standardized method for evaluating concussion in athletes ≥ 13 years, child SCAT involved for children 5–12 years, involves a standardized form of multiple sections of questions, used to evaluate concussion severity and track change over time, recommends removal from play on the same day of injury with later medical clearance before returning to play.
  - Patients returned to full activity over six tiers of incremental increased activity with 24-hour increments as long as asymptomatic.
  - Postconcussive syndrome: Persistent headache, dizziness, exercise intolerance, memory dysfunction, emotional dysregulation, or intractable headaches that persist after a concussion; may require long-term rehabilitation.
  - Second impact syndrome: Rare condition with formation of malignant vasogenic edema resulting in coma and 50–100% mortality rate; occurs after second head injury while symptomatic from primary concussion.
- Radiological evaluation:
  - CT imaging indicated for head trauma; skull X-rays lack sensitivity.
  - Acute blood, bone, or bullets (e.g., fragments) show up as bright/hyperdense on CT scans; subacute blood is isointense; chronic blood is hypodense.
  - Scalp edema can help localize site of impact; contrecoup injury refers to a brain contusion remote from the site of impact as a result of brain movement within the skull.
  - Follow-up CT head utilized to rule out worsening of contusions; timing of repeat imaging varies on institution.
  - Marshall CT classification predicts outcome from injury severity:
    - I: No visible pathology on CT scan.
    - II: Cisterns present, midline shift 0–5 mm, no lesion > 25 cc.
    - III: Cisterns compressed, midline shift 0–5 mm, no lesion > 25 cc.
    - IV: Midline shift > 5 mm, lesion > 25 cc.
    - V: Any surgically evacuated lesion.
    - VI: Nonsurgically evacuated lesion, lesion > 25 cc.

Table 14.4 Utah blunt cerebrovascular injury score[2]

Utah score (higher scores predict increased probability of injury)	
GCS ≤ 8	1
Focal neurological deficits	2
Carotid canal fracture	2
Petrous temporal bone fracture	3
Cerebral infarction on head CT	3

- ○ CT angiography of head and neck vessels can be indicated to rule out blunt cerebrovascular injury seen in 1–2% of blunt trauma (▶ Table 14.4)[2]; particularly indicated in the context of fractures in proximity to major cerebral vessels (see Chapter 14.2.4 Medical management).
  - ○ Delayed MRI can be helpful during hemorrhages, evaluation of diffuse axonal injury, and diagnosis of stroke.
- Radiological findings and treatment (▶ Fig. 14.1):
  - ○ Epidural hematoma (EDH): Biconvex, may cross dural barriers, usually due to arterial bleeding from the middle meningeal artery, associated with temporal bone fractures (pterion) and lucid interval, surgically treated if ≥ 1 cm or progressively worsening. Better prognosis as often less direct brain injury.
  - ○ Subdural hematoma: Crescent-shaped, does not cross dural barriers, most commonly found over the convexity but may also be found in tentorial or parafalcine areas, usually due to venous or bone bleeding. Correlates with higher impact trauma and marked brain injury; surgically treated if ≥ 1 cm thickness or ≥ 5 mm of midline shift.
  - ○ Subarachnoid hemorrhage (SAH): A poor prognosticator; high-density blood typically over the convexity; when voluminous and near basal cisterns, strongly consider aneurysm rupture as an antecedent to the severe TBI.
  - ○ Intracerebral hemorrhage (ICH): High-density blood within the parenchyma.
  - ○ Hemorrhagic contusion: High-density blood adjacent to bony prominences (frontal and occipital poles, sphenoid wing, temporal lobe).
  - ○ Intraventricular hemorrhage (IVH): Less likely in trauma.
  - ○ Skull fractures: Linear, nondisplaced fractures can be conservatively managed; stellate, comminuted fractures, or injury to vascular structures may require surgical treatment; temporal bone fractures may require additional thin-cut views to evaluate facial nerve and otologic bones.
  - ○ Depressed skull fractures generally require operative repair when depressed more than the width of the skull or when cosmetically sensitive. Open skull fractures require surgical debridement.
  - ○ Pneumocephalus can often be managed conservatively; CSF otorrhea or rhinorrhea can be treated with observation or CSF diversion and rarely requires surgical treatment; must watch these patients for meningitis!
- Medical treatments:
  - ○ Intracranial pressure monitor placed for patients who meet criteria (see Chapter 2.2, Neurological Monitoring) and patients treated in intensive care settings with experience in head trauma.
  - ○ Antiseizure medications:
    - – Levetiracetam 20 mg/kg IV once followed by 10 mg/kg BID for 1 week; generally being used instead of Dilantin in contemporary practice.
    - – Utilized to reduce risk of early posttraumatic seizure occurring within 1 week for moderate-to-severe TBI, no impact on late (>2 weeks after injury) posttraumatic seizures or epilepsy, level 2 evidence.
    - – Other agents (e.g., phenytoin, valproate, carbamazepine) have been utilized.
  - ○ Level I evidence that steroids are associated with harm after head injury.[3]
  - ○ Gastrointestinal prophylaxis with proton pump inhibitors or H2 blockers recommended to reduce risk of Cushing gastric ulcers in severe TBI.
  - ○ Permissive hypertension with systolic blood pressure from 100 to 200 allowed to encourage cerebral perfusion.
- Surgical treatments[4,5]:
  - ○ Decompressive hemicraniectomy: Remove or large cranial bone flap typically performed as a last resort to reduce ICP; can be unilateral or bifrontal; effective at reducing mortality but is associated with

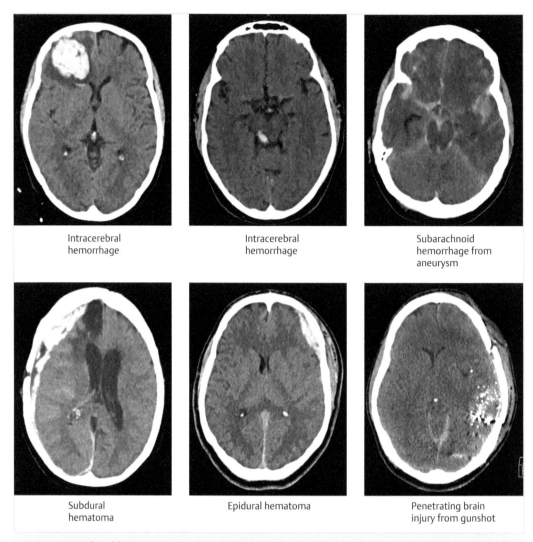

Intracerebral hemorrhage	Intracerebral hemorrhage	Subarachnoid hemorrhage from aneurysm
Subdural hematoma	Epidural hematoma	Penetrating brain injury from gunshot

Fig. 14.1 Examples of findings seen in traumatic brain injury. Note basal cistern subarachnoid hemorrhage pattern due to an aneurysm and should not be mistaken for trauma.

increased risk of vegetative outcome; requires second surgery to replace bone flap; overall 30% overall complication rate including hemorrhage, seizure, infection, bone flap absorption, and hydrocephalus.[4,5]

○ Posterior fossa decompression can be used for evacuating hemorrhages causing brainstem compression and obstructive hydrocephalus.

○ Evacuation of ICH controversial for improving outcome, data better evaluated for spontaneous ICH.[6]

○ Penetrating brain injury (e.g., bullets, knives) requires debridement of bone and shrapnel; hard-to-access fragments are left alone unless infected[7].

14.1.2 Guidelines

• Guidelines for the Management of Severe Traumatic Brain Injury—4th Edition and Guidelines for the Management of Penetrating Brain Injury in 2001 by the Brain Trauma Foundation synthesize the literature and provide recommendations for care (with levels of evidence; ► Table 14.5)[8].

Table 14.5 Guidelines from the Brain Trauma Foundation[8]

Level of evidence	Recommendations
2A	Bifrontal decompressive hemicraniectomy does not improve 6-mo postinjury outcome in severe TBI with ICP levels > 20 mm Hg for more than 15 min within a 1-h period that are refractory to first-tier therapies; decompression reduces ICP and ICU days
	Frontotemporoparietal decompression measuring 12 × 15 cm or 15 cm diameter recommended
2B	Early (within 2.5 h) and short-term (48 h postinjury) prophylactic hypothermia not recommended to improve outcomes
None	Hyperosmolar therapy may lower intracranial pressure but insufficient evidence to support specific recommendation
3	EVD system with continuous drainage can lower ICP more effectively than intermittent use
	CSF drainage to lower ICP with GCS < 6 during the first 12 h can be considered
2B	Prolonged prophylactic hyperventilation ($PaCO_2 \leq 25$ mm Hg) not recommended
2B	Barbiturates to induce burst suppression as prophylaxis against the development of elevated ICP not recommended
	Barbiturate administered to control elevated ICP refractory to maximal medical and surgical treatment recommended, hemodynamic stability essential before and after barbiturate therapy
	Propofol recommended for control of ICP but does not improve mortality or 6-mo outcome, high-dose propofol can produce morbidity
1	Steroids not recommended for improving outcome or reducing ICP
2A	Basal caloric replacement by 5th day recommended to reduce mortality
2B	Transgastric jejunal feeding recommended to reduce incidence of ventilator-associated pneumonia
2A	Early tracheostomy reduces mechanical ventilation days but no evidence that it reduces mortality or rates of pneumonia
	Povidone-iodine does not reduce ventilator-associated pneumonia and may increase risk of acute respiratory distress syndrome
3	Antimicrobial-impregnate catheters may reduce catheter-related infections during EVD
3	Low-molecular-weight heparin or low-dose unfractionated heparin with mechanical prophylaxis may reduce risk of deep vein thrombosis; however, there is an increased risk for intracranial hemorrhage expansion
2A	Prophylactic phenytoin or valproate not recommended for preventing late posttraumatic seizures
	Phenytoin decreases risk of early posttraumatic seizures (within 7 d of injury); early posttraumatic seizures have not been associated with worse outcomes
	Insufficient evidence to recommend levetiracetam over phenytoin for efficacy and safety
2B	ICP monitoring reduces in-hospital and 2-wk postinjury mortality in severe TBI
2B	Guideline-base recommendations for CPP monitoring decrease 2-wk mortality
3	Jugular bulb monitoring of arteriovenous oxygen content difference may reduce mortality and improve outcomes 3 and 6 mo postinjury
	Jugular venous saturation of < 50% may be a threshold to reduce mortality and improve outcomes
3	Systolic blood pressure ≥ 100 mm Hg for patients 50–69 y or ≥ 110 mm Hg for patients 15–49 y or over 70 y may decrease mortality and improve outcomes
2B	Treatment of ICP ≥ 22 mm Hg recommended to reduce mortality
3	Combination of ICP and clinical CT findings used to make management decisions
2B	CPP between 60 and 70 associated with favorable outcome but depends on patient's autoregulatory status
3	Avoidance of CPP > 70 mm Hg recommended to reduce risk of adult respiratory failure

Abbreviations: CPP, cerebral perfusion pressure; GCS, Glasgow coma scale; ICP, intracranial pressure; TBI, traumatic brain injury.

- Brain Trauma Foundation (BTF) guidelines cover medical and surgical treatments, neurological monitoring, and treatment thresholds.[8]

14.1.3 Brain Death Examination

- Guidelines from the American Academy of Neurology aimed to determine criteria that could be utilized to determine brain death (▶ Table 14.6)[9]; no case report of spontaneous functional recovery or recovery after maximal treatment has been seen for patients meeting such criteria.
- Difficult but not impossible to perform brain death testing immediately in the trauma bay due to requirements for normothermia, negative toxicology, and blood gas testing.

14.1.4 Outcome/Rehabilitation

- After initial treatment, rehabilitation is individualized to patient's needs.
- Involves treatment with physical, occupational, speech/language, physical medicine, psychology/psychiatry, and social support.
- Goals to return patients to society while managing injuries and deficits.
- Guidelines from the Ontario Neurotrauma Foundation[10] and Brain Injury Association of America[11] have discussed the role for rehabilitation after TBI.
- International Mission for Prognosis and Analysis of Clinical Trials in TBI (IMPACT)[12] calculator useful as prognostic tool in adults with TBI and GCS ≤ 12; predicts 6-month mortality and 6-month unfavorable outcome; inputs include patient age, GCS motor score, pupillary exam, presence of hypoxia, presence of hypotension, Marshall brain injury CT classification, traumatic SAH on CT, epidural mass on CT, glucose and hemoglobin.

14.2 Spinal Injury

Michael Karsy and Erica F. Bisson

14.2.1 Epidemiology

- Spinal cord injury (SCI): Injury to the spinal cord from trauma, infection, vascular anomalies, neoplasm (▶ Fig. 14.2), or a degenerative process.[13]
- 54 cases per million in the United States; 17,000 new hospitalizations/year + 4,000 patients who die on the scene.
- Average age at injury: 42 years; males account for 80% of new cases; younger patients are associated with trauma and older patients are associated with falls.
- Causes: 38% vehicular trauma, 30.5% falls, 13.5% violence, 9% sports, 5% medical/surgical, 4% other.
- 30% rate of rehospitalization one or more times after SCI.

14.2.2 Diagnosis

- Initial hemodynamic stabilization and CT imaging can be performed by the first-responding provider with early spine surgeon consultation for further imaging or clinical management (▶ Fig. 14.3). Stabilization of airway, breathing, and circulation (ABCs) takes precedence prior to further SCI workup.
- High-energy mechanisms, associated polytrauma, or cervical vertebral trauma should suspect SCI and associated vascular injuries.
- SCI classification aids in tracking neurological recovery and predicting outcome. The American Spinal Injury Association (ASIA) International Standards for Neurological Classification of Spinal Cord Injury, commonly referred to as the AIS, is used to communicate about injury location and severity (▶ Table 14.7). Numeric AIS scores are calculated by identifying the sensory level by pin prick and light touch for each side, the motor level for each side, and then a letter grade is assigned. Preserved sacral function is a key prognostic factor suggesting delayed improvement and thus key to an incomplete SCI.

Table 14.6 Brain death testing[9]

Prerequisites	Irreversible coma present and cause is known
	Neuroimaging explains coma
	CNS depressant drugs are absent, toxicology screen completed
	No evidence of residual paralytics
	Absence of severe acid–base, electrolyte, or endocrine abnormalities
	Normothermia or mild hypothermia (core temperature > 36 °C)
	Systolic blood pressure ≥ 100 mm Hg
	No spontaneous respirations
Examination (all must be checked)	Pupils nonreactive
	Corneal reflex absent
	Oculocephalic reflex absent, tested if C-spine stable
	Oculovestibular/cold caloric reflex absent
	No facial movement to stimulation at supraorbital or temporomandibular joint seen
	Gag reflex absent
	Couch reflex absent to tracheal suctioning
	Absent of motor response to noxious stimuli in all four extremities
Apnea testing (all must be checked)	Patient is hemodynamically stable
	Ventilator adjusted to provide normocarbia ($PaCO_2$ 34–45 mm Hg)
	Patient preoxygenated with 100% FiO_2 for > 10 min to PaO_2 > 200 mm Hg with a PEEP of 5 cm H_2O
	Oxygen provided via suction catheter at the level of the carina at 6 L/min or via a T-piece with continuous positive airway pressure (CPAP) at 10 cm H_2O
	Ventilator disconnected and spontaneous respirations are absent
	Arterial blood gas shows PCO_2 ≥ 60 mm Hg or rise of 20 mm Hg from baseline, draws at 8–10 min or serial draws every 2 min can be performed
	Apnea test aborted if patient fails above or becomes hemodynamically unstable
Ancillary testing (needs to be performed only in patients who cannot undergo apnea testing)	
Cerebral angiography	Contrast should be injected in the aortic arch under high pressure and reach both anterior and posterior circulations
	No intracerebral filling should be detected at the level of entry of the carotid or vertebral artery to the skull
	External carotid circulation should be patent
	Filling of superior sagittal sinus may be delayed
Electroencephalography (EEG)	Minimum of eight scalp electrodes used
	Interelectrode impedance should be between 100 and 10,000 Ohm
	Integrity of recording system should be tested
	Distance between electrodes should be at least 10 cm
	Sensitivity should be increased to at least 2 μV for 30 min with inclusion of appropriate calibrations
	High-frequency filter should not be set below 30 Hz; low-frequency filter should not be set above 1 Hz
	EEG should demonstrate a lack of reactivity to intense somatosensory or audiovisual stimuli
Transcranial Doppler ultrasonography (TCD)	TCD must have a reliable signal, may be less reliable in patients with a prior craniotomy
	Abnormalities include reverberating flow, small systolic peaks in early systole
	Bilateral insonation of anterior and posterior circulation should be performed using the suboccipital transcranial window (temporal lobe, above the zygomatic arch and vertebrobasilar arteries)

(Continued)

Table 14.6 (*Continued*) Brain death testing[9]

Cerebral scintigraphy (technetium Tc 99 m hexametazime [HMPAO])	Isotope should be injected within 30 min of reconstitution
	Anterior and lateral planar image counts (500,000) of the head should be performed immediately, 30–60 min postinjection, and 2 h postinjection
	Optional to confirm injection with imaging of the liver
	No radionucleotide localization in the middle cerebral, anterior cerebral, or basilar artery territories should be seen
	No tracer in the superior sagittal sinus should be seen, minimal tracer from the scalp may be seen

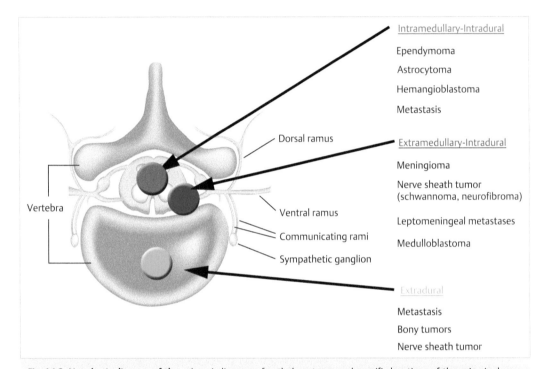

Intramedullary-Intradural

Ependymoma

Astrocytoma

Hemangioblastoma

Metastasis

Dorsal ramus

Extramedullary-Intradural

Meningioma

Nerve sheath tumor (schwannoma, neurofibroma)

Vertebra

Ventral ramus

Communicating rami

Sympathetic ganglion

Leptomeningeal metastases

Medulloblastoma

Extradural

Metastasis

Bony tumors

Nerve sheath tumor

Fig. 14.2 Neoplastic diseases of the spine. A diagram of pathology types and specific locations of the spine is shown. Tumors can be characterized by their location, namely, extradural (typically metastatic cancer), intradural extramedullary (meningiomas and schwannomas), or intradural intramedullary (ependymomas and astrocytomas) tumors. Additional lesions of the spine include lymphoma, multiple myeloma, chordoma, and a variety of primary bone tumors.

- Injury types: 45% incomplete tetraplegia, 21.3% incomplete paraplegia, 20% complete paraplegia, 13.3% complete tetraplegia, 0.4% normal.
- Spine injury patterns (▶ Fig. 14.4) may be due to trauma or other injury mechanisms:
  ○ Tetraplegia: Injury of arms and legs.
  ○ Paraplegia: Injury of legs only.
  ○ Central cord syndrome: Characterized by injury to the traversing anterolateral spinothalamic tract, results in a cape-like distribution of numbness commonly at the level of the shoulder blades with weakness and/or numbness in the hands (distal > proximal) and possibly legs (proximal > distal).
  ○ Brown–Sequard syndrome: Hemisection of the spinal cord (i.e., bullet or knife injury); results in ipsilateral paralysis (corticospinal tract), ipsilateral loss of proprioception and vibration (dorsal columns), and contralateral loss of pain and temperature sensation (anterolateral spinothalamic).

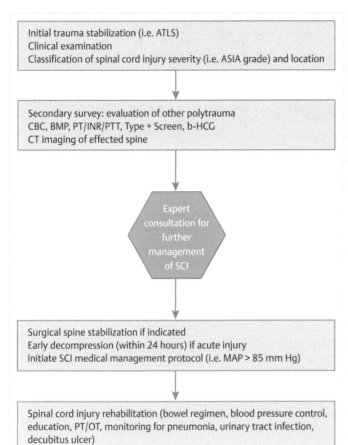

Fig. 14.3 Flow diagram of spinal cord injury management. ASIA, American Spinal Injury Association; ATLS, Advanced Trauma Life Support; BMP, basic metabolic panel; CBC, complete blood count; CT, computerized tomography; INR, international normalized ratio; MAP, mean arterial blood pressure; PT, prothrombin time; PT/OT, physical therapy/occupational therapy; PTT, partial thromboplastin time; SCI, spinal cord injury.

Table 14.7 American spinal injury association (ASIA) scale

Type	Injury	Description
A	Complete	No motor or sensory function in sacral segments S4–S5
B	Incomplete	Sensory but not motor function below injured level, sacral sparing at S4–S5
C	Incomplete	Motor function with < 3 strength in more than half of key muscle groups below injured level
D	Incomplete	Motor function with ≥ 3 strength in more than half of key muscle groups below injured level
E	Normal	Return of motor and sensory function after injury

○ Anterior spinal artery infarction: Deficits of the ventral horns and motor weakness.
○ Posterior spinal artery infarction: Injury of the dorsal horns resulting in deficits of proprioception and vibration.

14.2.3 Imaging

- CT scans have supplanted X-rays to image any presumed fracture of the spine due to improved sensitivity and wide availability. Allows improved classification of fracture pattern depending on location in spine.
- Rapid CT interpretation: Misalignment of anterior and posterior marginal lines, spinolaminar line, and interspinous line can allude to injury (▶ Fig. 14.5).
- Excessive prevertebral swelling (normal: < 7 mm at C2/3 or < 21 mm at C6/7) can allude to injury.

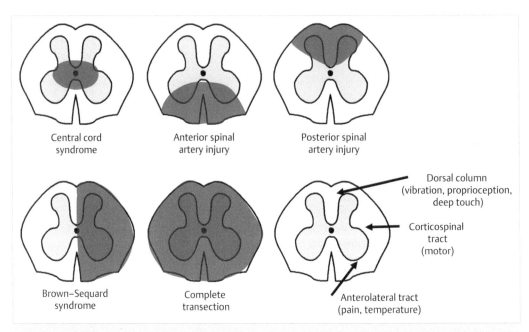

Fig. 14.4 Spinal cord injury patterns.

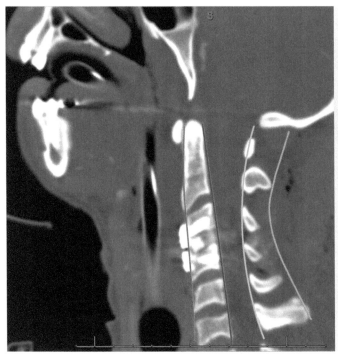

Fig. 14.5 Rapid CT assessment of spine instability. Assessment of the anterior marginal line (*red*), posterior marginal line (*blue*), spinolaminar line (*green*), and interspinous line (*orange*) can be a rapid method to evaluate spine malalignment and potential instability. Bone cortical surfaces evaluated for fragments and breaks. Soft-tissue swelling assessed (6 mm at C2 and 22 mm at C6 within normal limits).

- MRI used to evaluate ligamentous injury (anterior longitudinal ligament, posterior longitudinal ligament, ligamentum flavum), herniated disks, epidural hematoma, and spinal cord T2/STIR signal change.
- Cervical fractures with possible vertebral artery injury are evaluated with CT angiograms of the head/neck. Diagnostic cerebral angiograms are used for severe injuries or if requiring endovascular treatment.
- Isolated spinous and transverse process fractures do not necessitate expert consultation and are managed with pain control.

14.2.4 Medical Management

- Injury pathophysiology[14]:
  - Primary injury: Initial traumatic injury to the spinal cord via shear, laceration, contusion, and compression; not treatable.
  - Secondary injury: Subsequent neurological injury from molecular mechanisms (i.e., oxidative stress); optimized with medical treatment.
  - SCI → spine shock (areflexia/hyporeflexia and autonomic dysfunction) → neurogenic shock (disconnected sympathetic innervation, decreased heart rate, blood pressure, cardiac output, and systemic vascular resistance) → spasticity (hyperreflexia, increased muscle tone).
- Medical management[14]:
  - Immobilization of the level of injury until definitive decompression and/or stabilization.
  - Augmentation of mean arterial blood pressure (MAP) > 85 mm Hg for 3–7 days (with dopamine or norepinephrine).
  - Initiation of a SCI protocol (e.g., bowel regimen to prevent constipation and ileus).
  - Lower extremity compression stockings to reduce deep vein thrombosis (DVT) and pulmonary embolism (PE) risk.
  - Abdominal binder to improve MAP; cough assistance to reduce risk of pneumonia.
  - Nutritional support to prevent muscle atrophy and catabolism; peptic ulcer prophylaxis.
  - Rehabilitation consultation for subsequent care.
  - Early mobilization to improve recovery and reduce risk of DVT, PE, pneumonia, and pressure ulcers.
  - No specific medical drug exists for SCI currently.[14]
  - Bracing (cervical thoracic orthosis, thoracolumbosacral orthosis, Jewett brace, Minerva) aims to reduce motion and improve pain control, limited efficacy, stability checked with upright X-rays in brace compared to initial supine imaging.
  - Dissection injuries to the vertebral artery are graded using the Biffl grade (▶ Table 14.8).[15] Grade 1 and 2 dissections are treated with aspirin to prevent stroke formation as these heal well.[16] Grade 3, 4, and 5 injuries are treated with a combination of anticoagulation, endovascular, or open treatments to either repair or sacrifice the vessel.
- Corticosteroid[17,18,19]:
  - Controversial and not recommended by the 2013 American Association of Neurological Surgeons/Congress of Neurological Surgeons (AANS/CNS) Joint Taskforce guidelines statement.[20]
  - National Acute Spinal Cord Injury Studies (NASCIS) were a series of three large randomized clinical trials evaluating methylprednisolone sodium succinate, NASCIS III demonstrated a 5-point improvement in motor score when treated between 3 and 8 hours; concern for higher rates of wound infection, pulmonary embolism, and pneumonia with steroid treatment.

Table 14.8 Carotid or vertebral artery blunt injury (Biffl grade)

Type	Description	Treatment
I	Luminal irregularity or dissection with < 25% narrowing	Anticoagulation (e.g., aspirin) or carotid stenting if progression of injury
II	Dissection or intramural hematoma with > 25% luminal narrowing or intimal flap	
III	Pseudoaneurysm	Carotid stenting
IV	Occlusion	Anticoagulation or endovascular vessel sacrifice
V	Transection with free extravasation	Open repair, bypass, or sacrifice

14.2.5 Surgical Management

- Injury classification has evolved the surgical decision-making process, but much of the criteria for surgery continues to depend on expert opinion.[20]
  - Denis model: Spine instability with disruption in two of three spine compartments.
  - AOSpine classification: Categorizes fractures by mechanism of injury, more commonly used by spine surgeons; compression (type A), extension (type B), translation/rotation (type C); fractures of type B and C patterns more commonly need surgical fixation while fractures of type A patterns can be often managed conservatively.
  - Thoracolumbar Injury Classification and Severity (TLICS) scale and the Subaxial Cervical Spine Injury Classification (SLIC) system (▶ Table 14.9) suggest surgery with score ≥ 5, easy to use.
- Fracture types:
  - Atlantooccipital dissociation: Separation of C1 from the occipital condyle (> 2.5 mm suggests dissociation on CT scan more accurately than cervical X-rays) due to disruption of the alar and capsular ligaments, highly unstable, and requires occipitocervical fusion.
  - Occipital condyle avulsions: Type 1 (impacted fracture, treated with collar), type 2 (basilar skull fracture extending into condyle, treated with collar), type III (avulsion injury, potentially unstable, and may require occipitocervical fusion).
  - C1/Jefferson fractures: Fractures of both the anterior and posterior tubercle of C1, treated with collar if minimally displaced with intact transverse ligament, C1–C2 fusion if significant fracture displacement or disrupted transverse ligament.
  - C2/Hangman fractures: Fracture with or without angulation of the C2 pars interarticularis, type 1 (< 3 mm displacement, treated with collar), type II (> 3 mm displacement and > 11-degree angulation, hard collar if reducible, C1–C2 or C2–C3 fusion if disrupted disk), type IIa (< 3 mm displacement and > 11-degree angulation, same treatment as type II), type III (associated facet dislocation, requires C1–C3 fusion).
  - Atlantoaxial rotatory subluxation: Hyperflexibility of cervical spine resulting in C1–C2 dislocation, often in children with trauma, can be reduced but often requires fixation.

Table 14.9 TLICS or SLICS for prediction of surgical need

	TLICS		SLICS	
Category	Characteristic	Score	Characteristic	Score
Fracture morphology	None	0	None	0
	Compression	1	Compression	1
	Burst	2	Burst	2
	Translation/rotation	3	Distraction	3
	Distraction	4	Rotation/translation	4
Integrity of posterior ligamentous complex	Intact	0	Intact	0
	Suspected injury	2	Indeterminate	1
	Injured	3	Disrupted	2
Neurological status	Intact	0	Intact	0
	Nerve root injury	2	Nerve root injury	1
	Complete injury	2	Complete injury	2
	Incomplete injury	3	Incomplete injury	3
	Cauda equina	3	Continuous cord compression with neurodeficit	+1

Score: ≤ 3, nonoperative treatment; 4, nonoperative or operative at clinician discretion; ≥ 5, operative.

Abbreviations: SLICS, Subaxial Cervical Spine Injury Classification system; TLICS, Thoracolumbar Injury Classification and Severity.

- Dens fracture: Type I (fracture at superior tip, hard collar), type II (fracture at base of dens, controversial treatment in hard collar, halo fixation or C1–C2 fusion depending on patient age and risk for malunion), type III (fracture through base and body of C2, hard collar or halo).
  - Jumped or perched cervical facets: Injury from flexion and axial load, often associated with SCI, urgent traction performed at bedside or in operating room with need for fixation due to instability.
  - Spinous or transverse process fractures: Often nonoperative even when extends into facets or found at multiple contiguous levels.
  - Teardrop fracture: Hyperflexion injury with anteroinferior bone chip and sagittal split fracture, highly unstable and requires fixation, can be mistaken for avulsion fracture which is stable.
  - Compression fracture: Disruption of the superior or inferior vertebral endplate, usually treated nonoperatively with or without bracing.
  - Burst fracture: Disruption of the superior and/or inferior vertebral endplate with posterior displacement of a bone fragment into the spinal canal; can be treated nonoperatively in the setting of mild pain, no progressive deformity and no neurological symptoms; symptomatic lesions treated with spine fusion.
  - Chance fracture: Fracture across the bony elements extending from the posterior lamina through the vertebral bodies; can be managed nonoperatively if fragments are well apposed, otherwise requires surgical treatment.
  - Fraction/dislocation: Disruption, displacement, and malrotation of a spine fracture; almost always unstable and requires operative fixation.
- Various anterior and posterior surgical approaches possible with goal of bony fusion over 3–6 months; hardware can be removed for some fractures after healing (e.g., burst fractures, pediatric fractures).
- Timing of surgical decompression remains controversial, some evidence that surgery within 24 hours of injury shows improved outcomes after cervical cord injury.[21]
- Sports-related fractures are more controversial and have limited data, thus require the use of expert opinion, evaluation of injury and anatomy, and regard to level of activity to determine return-to-play.[22]

14.2.6 Additional Topics

- Cauda equina syndrome (CES):
  - Neurological emergency but rare; significant morbidity or potential for recovery depending on treatment; earlier onset of symptoms and earlier treatment predicts improved recovery.
  - Occurs in 1–2% of herniated disks.
  - CES results from compression of the lumbosacral nerve roots below L1, and most often presents with asymmetric lower extremity weakness, perineal or saddle numbness (S3–S5 distribution), and bladder/bowel dysfunction, along with back pain and potential gait dysfunction.
  - Can mimic conus medullaris compression syndrome (compression of distal tip of the spinal cord; ▶ Table 14.10).
  - Up to 20% of patients can have continued urological or sexual dysfunction after treatment.
  - Treated with lumbar decompression.
- Malignant spinal cord compression (MSCC):
  - Causes (▶ Fig. 14.2):
    - Epidural disease directly results in cord compression.
    - Tumor causes pathological fractures resulting in spinal canal compromise.
    - Tumor hemorrhage or vascular insult results in acute neurological decline causing a spinal emergency.
  - Patients with a known history of aggressive primary cancer are counseled on monitoring for malignant spinal cord compression MSCC by evaluating changes in neurological symptoms.
  - Patients with known cancer and new-onset back pain should have MR imaging.
  - Surgical decompression followed by radiation shows improved outcomes than radiation alone for preservation of neurological function.[23]
  - Surgery for MSCC follows the same general principles as for traumatic SCI, including rapid decompression of the spinal cord and nerves followed by stabilization if necessary.

Table 14.10 Comparison of cauda equina and conus medullaris syndrome

Clinical feature	Cauda equina syndrome	Conus medullaris syndrome
Level	L2 sacrum compression	L1–L2 compression
Presentation	Sudden and unilateral	Sudden and bilateral
Reflexes	Knee and ankle impacted	Ankle impacted
Radicular pain	More severe	Less severe
Lower back pain	Less	More
Impotence	Absent	Frequent
Numbness	Asymmetrical	Symmetrical
Motor strength	Asymmetric, a reflexive paraplegia	Symmetric, hyperreflexive, distal paresis of lower limbs
Sensory	Asymmetrical saddle anesthesia	Symmetrical saddle anesthesia
Sphincter	Urinary retention, presents later	Urinary and fecal incontinence, presents earlier

Table 14.11 C-spine clearance

NEXUS criteria for C-spine imaging	Canadian C-spine rule
Focal neurological deficit + 1	Age ≥ 65 y, extremity paresthesias or dangerous mechanism (fall ≥ 3 feet/5 stairs, axial loading injury, high-speed motor vehicle collision, bicycle collision, motorized recreational vehicle)
Midline spinal tenderness present + 1	
Altered level of consciousness present + 1	Absence of low-risk factors (sitting position in ED, ambulatory at any time, delayed neck pain, midline tenderness, simple rear end motor vehicle collision)
Intoxication present + 1	Inability to rotate neck 45 degrees left and right
Distracting injury present + 1	*Yes to any factor suggests inability to clear patient without imaging*
Score ≥ 1 suggests inability to clear patient without imaging	

- ○ Surgical approach to the cervical, thoracic, and lumbar spine varies based on tumor location, tumor type, and response to prior treatment (including radiation). For patients with back pain without neurologic symptoms, bracing, radiation, and kyphoplasty are potential treatment strategies.
  - ○ Partial tumor resection with the goals of separating tumor from the spinal cord (i.e., separation surgery) can be useful for later stereotactic radiosurgery.
- Cervical spine clearance[20]:
  - ○ NEXUS criteria (▶ Table 14.11) can be used to reducing imaging for spine clearance, 83–100% sensitivity for detecting cervical SCI.
  - ○ Canadian C-spine Rule (▶ Table 14.11) shows improved sensitivity (99.4 vs. 90.7%) from NEXUS for detecting cervical SCI.
  - ○ CT imaging better for evaluating fractures than X-rays. Normal CT has a high likelihood ratio of ruling out unstable cervical injury.[24,25]
  - ○ Clinical clearance attempted after normal CT imaging without pain.
  - ○ Clearance in the setting of pain can be performed using flexion/extension films, MRI of the neck, or physician preference.

14.2.7 Rehabilitation

- SCI rehabilitation requires interdisciplinary inpatient and outpatient care over long time periods.[26]
- Airway clearance: Ventilator dependence decreases survival and pneumonias are the leading cause of death after SCI; secretion clearance by cough assist, vest therapy, mucolytics (sodium bicarbonate, acetylcysteine); diaphragmatic stimulators can aid in high cervical SCI; early tracheostomy reduces ventilator time, sedation requirements, and ICU stay and improves suctioning.

- Venous thromboembolism: Occurs in 50–100% of SCI patients, greatest incidence between 3 and 14 days; prevented with pneumatic compression stockings, heparin, screening ultrasounds, and inferior vena cava filters.
- Autonomic dysreflexia: Occurs with T6 or higher lesions, normal noxious stimuli generates uncontrolled hypertension due to an absent feedback mechanism; risk of stroke; treated by removing noxious stimuli (e.g., urinary catheterization, bowel movement, reducing pressure ulcers).
- Nutrition: Generally poor in acute postinjury period, continued muscle atrophy over time.
- Gastric motility: Reduced bowel motility due to hypotonic bowel and hypertonic sphincter; treated with bowel regimen.
- Neurogenic bladder: Bladder overdistension without feedback about fullness along with sphincter spasticity; treated with anticholinergics (e.g., oxybutynin, tolterodine, Botox) for bladder and alpha-adrenergics (e.g., terazosin, tamsulosin, Botox) for sphincter.
- Pressure ulcers: Occur in 20–30% of patients in rehab; most common in sacrum (39%), heels (13%), ischium (8%), occiput (6%); treated with early mobilization and wound care.
- Depression: Occurs in 30% of SCI patients compared to 10% in general population.
- Heart disease: Increased risk compared to general population.
- Orthostatic hypotension: Occurs with injuries above T6, treated with blood pressure augmenting agents.
- Heterotopic ossification: Bone deposits in soft tissue around hips and knees, difficult to treat.
- Hypo/hyperthermia.
- Chronic pain.
- Spasticity: Treated with baclofen, diazepam, Zanaflex, physical therapy, Botox.
- Sexual and reproductive health.

14.3 Vascular Diseases

Jeyan Kumar, Yashar Kalani, and Min Park

14.3.1 Anatomy/Physiology

- The brain receives roughly 20% of the cardiac output with normal cerebral blood flow of 50 mL/100 mg/min.
- Paired carotid and vertebral arteries provide the majority of the vascular supply to the brain.
- Common carotid artery bifurcates at C4 into the internal carotid artery (ICA) and external carotid artery (ECA).
- ECA provides blood to the face and neck.
  - Can have multiple anastomoses with the ICA and vertebral arteries.
  - Seven branches (proximal to distal from bifurcation): Superior thyroid, ascending pharyngeal, lingual, facial, occipital, posterior auricular, superficial temporal, and internal maxillary arteries.
- Internal carotid artery:
  - Divided into seven segments, C1–C7. Becomes intradural at C5 (clinoidal) segment.
  - Terminates into two main branches: anterior cerebral artery and middle cerebral artery.
- Vertebral artery (VA):
  - Arises from the subclavian artery bilaterally and enters the foramen transversarium of the cervical vertebrae at C6, exits the foramen at C2 and crosses laterally on C1 prior to entering the dura at the foramen magnum.
  - Divided into four segments (V1–V4) and becomes intradural at V4. VAs combine to form the basilar artery.
  - Left VA dominant 50%, right VA 25%, and no dominance 25%.
- Circle of Willis:
  - Circulatory anastomoses of the anterior and posterior circulation via the anterior communicating and posterior communicating arteries with the internal carotid and posterior cerebral arteries.
  - Can maintain cerebral perfusion in situations of stenosis or occlusion.

14.3.2 Subarachnoid Hemorrhage

- Epidemiology:
  - Subarachnoid hemorrhage (SAH): Bleeding between the arachnoid membrane and pia mater (▶ Fig. 14.6).
  - Incidence of aneurysmal SAH in the United States: 9.7–14.5 per 100,000 persons.[27]
  - Aneurysmal SAH incidence peaks at 55–60 years of age, 1.24 times more common in women, higher in African Americans and Hispanics compared to Caucasians.[28]
  - Smoking, hypertension, and excessive alcohol consumption are important risk factors for the development of SAH.[29]
- Etiology:
  - Major classification: Spontaneous versus traumatic.
  - Spontaneous causes: Aneurysmal (most common, 75–85%), cerebral arteriovenous malformation (AVM), CNS vasculitis, tumor, vessel dissection, coagulopathies (i.e., thrombocytopenia), dural sinus thrombosis, spinal AVM, illicit drug use (e.g., cocaine), sickle cell anemia, pituitary apoplexy, pretruncal aneurysmal SAH, no cause determined (14–22%).[30]
  - SAH can be accompanied with intracerebral hemorrhage (ICH).
- Diagnosis (▶ Fig. 14.7):
  - Spontaneous SAH classically described as sudden, thunderclap headache. Described as the "worst headache of my life" and often accompanied with nausea, vomiting, AMS, HTN, nuchal rigidity (meningismus), and/or photophobia.

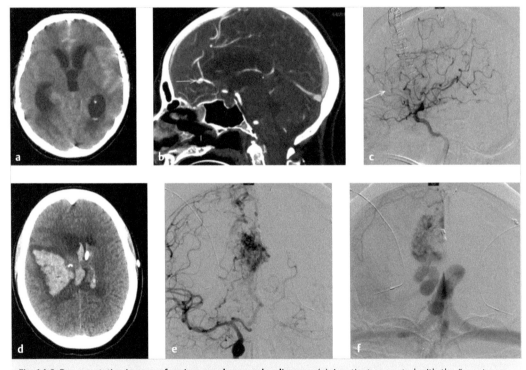

Fig. 14.6 Representative images of various cerebrovascular diseases. (a) A patient presented with the "worst headache of their life" and modified Fisher Grade 4 subarachnoid hemorrhage (SAH) and **(b)** a CT angiography (CTA) demonstrating a ruptured left pericallosal aneurysm. **(c)** A diagnostic cerebral angiography following surgical clipping of the ruptured aneurysm. **(d)** A second patient with a spontaneous intracerebral hemorrhage presented with the "worst headache of their life" and acute onset of left-sided hemiparesis. The patient had an intracerebral hemorrhage (ICH) score of 1. **(e)** Arterial phase diagnostic cerebral angiography demonstrating a Spetzler–Martin grade 5 arteriovenous malformation (AVM) with ruptured Spetzler–Martin grade 5 AVM and **(f)** a late phase arterial angiography demonstrated the markedly enlarged deep venous drainage.

○ Hunt-Hess Grade[31]: symptom-based classification of aneurysmal SAH. Grades 1–5 in order of increasing mortality (▶ Table 14.12).

○ World Federation of Neurological Societies (WFNS) grading of aneurysmal SAH[32]: Glasgow Coma Scale score with absence/presence of major neurologic deficit. Grades 0–5 in order of increasing mortality (▶ Table 14.13).

○ Fisher classification[33] and modified Fisher classification[34]: imaging-based grading of aneurysmal SAH with severity predicting symptomatic vasospasm. Grades 1–4 in order of increasing risk of vasospasm (▶ Fig. 14.6a, ▶ Table 14.14).

○ Computed tomography (CT) and CT angiography (CTA) of the head to identify a possible vascular source for the SAH (▶ Fig. 14.6b).

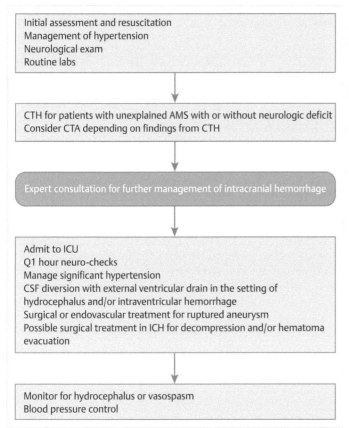

| Initial assessment and resuscitation |
| Management of hypertension |
| Neurological exam |
| Routine labs |

| CTH for patients with unexplained AMS with or without neurologic deficit |
| Consider CTA depending on findings from CTH |

Expert consultation for further management of intracranial hemorrhage

| Admit to ICU |
| Q1 hour neuro-checks |
| Manage significant hypertension |
| CSF diversion with external ventricular drain in the setting of hydrocephalus and/or intraventricular hemorrhage |
| Surgical or endovascular treatment for ruptured aneurysm |
| Possible surgical treatment in ICH for decompression and/or hematoma evacuation |

| Monitor for hydrocephalus or vasospasm |
| Blood pressure control |

Fig. 14.7 Flow diagram of patient with intracranial hemorrhage. CTH, computed tomography of the head; AMS, altered mental status; CTA, computed tomography angiography; ICU, intensive care unit; Q1, every one hour; CSF, cerebrospinal fluid; ICH, intracerebral hemorrhage.

Table 14.12 Hunt/Hess Score for aneurysmal SAH

Symptoms	Grade
Slight headache or nuchal rigidity, asymptomatic, alert, and oriented	1
Moderate to severe headache, nuchal rigidity, no neurologic deficits other than cranial nerve palsies	2
Lethargy or confusion, mild focal neurological deficit	3
Stupor, moderate to severe neurologic deficit	4
Comatose, showing signs of severe neurologic deficit (decerebrate posturing)	5

Abbreviation: SAH, subarachnoid hemorrhage.

Table 14.13 World Federation of Neurological Surgeons grading system for SAH

Glasgow Coma Scale	Motor deficit	Grade
15	Absent	1
13–14	Absent	2
13–14	Present	3
7–12	Present or absent	4
3–6	Present or absent	5

Abbreviation: SAH, subarachnoid hemorrhage.

Table 14.14 Modified Fisher Scale for subarachnoid hemorrhage

Grade	Description
0	No SAH and no IVH
1	Focal or diffuse, thin SAH, no IVH
2	Focal or diffuse, thin SAH, IVH present
3	Focal or diffuse, thick SAH, no IVH
4	Focal or diffuse, thick SAH, IVH present

Abbreviations: IVH, intraventricular hemorrhage; SAH, subarachnoid hemorrhage.

- ○ Digital subtraction angiography (DSA) is the gold standard for imaging of CNS vasculopathies and is used to identify a vascular source for the SAH if the CT/CTA is negative. It may be used to better define the anatomy in preparation of surgical treatment or as a modality for intervention (see later).
- ○ Lumbar puncture can be used if clinical suspicion of SAH exists with a negative CT scan. Assesses for xanthochromia (yellow color of supernatant) and presence of red blood cells (compare tubes 1 and 4 for decreasing number of RBCs to differentiate traumatic tap vs. SAH).
- ○ MRI of the brain not routinely used for the initial assessment of SAH.
- • Treatment (▶ Fig. 14.6):
  - ○ Medical management:
    - – Admission to an ICU.
    - – Intubation, if required to protect the airway.
    - – Blood pressure control to avoid significant hypertension (i.e., systolic blood pressure [SBP] < 140 or SBP < 160).
    - – Correction of coagulopathies or thrombocytopenia.
    - – Initiate deep vein thrombosis (DVT) prophylaxis with SCDs on admission and prophylactic subcutaneous low-molecular-weight heparin/heparin when appropriate.
    - – Management of acute elevations in intracranial pressure (ICP) with hyperosmotic agents (i.e., mannitol, hypertonic saline).
    - – Physical, occupational, and speech therapy for assessment and treatment.
  - ○ Surgical management:
    - – CSF diversion with external ventricular drain or lumbar drain (not common) in the presence of hydrocephalus and/or for elevated ICP management.
    - – Endovascular intervention for embolization of the aneurysm and/or intra-arterial treatment of vasospasm.
    - – Craniotomy for clipping of ruptured aneurysms.
    - – Possible craniectomy for surgical treatment of brain swelling.
- • Complications:
  - ○ Cerebral vasospasm:
    - – Symptomatic narrowing of arterial vessels following subarachnoid hemorrhage. Remains a significant cause of morbidity and mortality in this patient population.

- Radiographic vasospasm is found in 43% of all aneurysmal SAHs and symptomatic vasospasm in 32.5%. There is a 30% mortality with symptomatic vasospasm and 34% of symptomatic vasospasm results in permanent neurologic deficits.[35]
- Radiographic evidence as early as day 4, peak incidence between days 10 and 17; mean time to symptomatic vasospasm is 7.9 days.[35]
- Potentially reversible with increasing blood pressure or vasodilation by intra-arterial treatment with calcium channel blockers (e.g., verapamil) or balloon angioplasty. Oral nimodipine is used as a neuroprotective agent for vasospasm.
  - Hydrocephalus:
    - Reported incidence between 6 and 67% for acute and chronic hydrocephalus.
    - Acute/subacute (days 0–13): Treated with external ventricular drain and potential ventriculoperitoneal shunt placement.
    - Chronic: Can present in a delayed fashion following SAH. 21.2% of patients required shunting after external ventricular drain, 26% of shunted patients received shunts after discharge.[36]

14.3.3 Spontaneous Intracerebral Hemorrhage

- Epidemiology:
  - Second most common cause of stroke comprising 10–15% of all strokes.[37]
  - Worldwide incidence of 10–20 per 100,000 population. High incidence of mortality with 38% of patients passing away within the first year.[38]
  - Increased incidence with age, gender (male > female), and ethnicity (African Americans > Caucasians).[37]
- Causes/risk factors:
  - Hypertension: Cerebrovascular damage to small arteries and arterioles from long-standing hypertension (chronic) versus acute crisis such as with certain drugs (e.g., cocaine).
  - Alcohol consumption: Moderate to heavy consumption of alcohol within 24 hours or 1 week presents an increased risk of ICH in a dose-dependent manner.[39]
  - Anticoagulant therapy increases the risk of ICH by seven- to ten-fold.[37,40]
  - Liver disease or coagulopathy (e.g., leukemia or thrombocytopenia).
  - Neoplasm: Can be the initial presentation of a cerebral neoplasm:
    - Primary tumors: Most commonly glioblastoma multiforme and oligodendroglioma.
    - Most common hemorrhagic metastatic tumors: Renal cell, melanoma, prostate, or lung.[37]
  - Hemorrhagic conversion of an ischemic stroke.
  - Vascular malformations: Cavernoma, AVM, or aneurysm (generally in conjunction with SAH).
  - Cerebral amyloid angiopathy, deposition of beta-amyloid within vessel walls. Can present with repeated lobar hemorrhages in the elderly.
  - Dural or venous sinus thrombosis.
- Diagnosis:
  - Can present with gradual progressive onset of neurological deficit versus ischemic stroke where deficits are maximal at onset, but can also present acutely.
  - CT of the head is used for the initial diagnosis and allows for measurement of clot volume, presence of intraventricular hemorrhage, and/or the presence of hydrocephalus.
  - CTA of the head and neck to evaluate for underlying vascular sources.
  - MRI of the brain to evaluate for underlying lesions. May need to be repeated in a delayed setting following resorption of the hematoma for suspicious lesions (suspected neoplasm) obscured by the hemorrhage.
  - DSA, if suspicion for underlying vascular lesion, such as AVM or aneurysm, that was not identified by the CTA of the head.
  - ICH score (▶ Table 14.15), five-point scale that evaluates 30-day mortality.[41]
- Treatment:
  - Medical management:
    - Admission to a monitored unit (intensive care unit).
    - Intubation, if required, to protect the airway.
    - Blood pressure control to avoid significant hypertension (i.e., SBP < 140 or SBP < 160).

Table 14.15 Intracerebral hemorrhage (ICH) score

Description	Score
Glasgow coma scale	GCS 3–4: +2
	GCS 5–12: +1
	GCS 13–15: 0
Age ≥ 80	+1
ICH volume ≥ 30 mL	+1
Intraventricular hemorrhage	+1
Infratentorial location of hemorrhage	+1

Note: 30 day mortality for scores: 1 (13%), 2 (26%), 3 (72%), 4 (97%), 5 (100%).

- Correction of coagulopathies or thrombocytopenia.
- Initiate DVT prophylaxis with SCDs on admission and prophylactic subcutaneous low-molecular-weight heparin/heparin when appropriate.
- Management of acute elevations in intracranial pressure (ICP) with hyperosmotic agents (i.e., mannitol, hypertonic saline).
- Prophylactic antiepileptic drug treatment is controversial; 8% of patients with ICH will develop seizures within 30 days.[42]
- Physical, occupational, and speech therapy for assessment and possible treatment.
  ○ Surgical management:
- External ventricular drain placement for treatment of hydrocephalus and/or intraventricular hemorrhages.
- Craniectomy for infratentorial hemorrhages: Brainstem compression may cause rapid neurologic decline requiring surgical intervention.
- Craniectomy for supratentorial hemorrhage: Role of surgical intervention remains controversial; Surgical Trial in Traumatic Intracerebral Haemorrhage (STICH) and STICH II demonstrated no significant benefits with surgery; Minimally Invasive Surgery with Thrombolysis in Intracerebral Haemorrhage Evacuation (MISTIE) III trial demonstrated that surgery did not improve outcomes after a year for moderate to large hemorrhages.[43,44,45]
- Clot location, size, presence of midline shift, persistently elevated ICP, pathology (e.g., tumor, AVM), and neurologic exam (GCS) used to determine candidacy for surgical evacuation.
- Trials for minimally invasive evacuation of ICH are ongoing.

14.3.4 Stroke:

- Epidemiology:
  ○ Third leading cause of death in the United States; results in 140,000 annual deaths; leading cause of long-term disability in the United States.
  ○ Affects 795,000 people annually with 600,000 being first strokes; roughly every 40 seconds; affects 15 million people worldwide.
  ○ 75% of strokes occur in patients > 65 years of age.
  ○ Highest risk of death in the southeastern United States termed the "stroke belt."
- Etiology:
  ○ 80% ischemic, 20% hemorrhagic.
  ○ Mechanisms.
    - Thrombosis: Obstruction of artery due to arteriosclerosis, dissection, fibromuscular dysplasia with or without superimposed thrombosis.
    - Embolism: Debris translocating from one area to another causing obstruction; occurs from cardiac, arterial, or unknown sources.
    - Hypoperfusion: Low circulatory flow for necessary tissue metabolism resulting in tissue injury.

○ Definitions:
  – Transient ischemic attack: Change in neurological symptoms lasting less than 24 hours.
  – Large vessel occlusion: Obstruction of the extracranial (common and internal carotid) and intracranial (circle of Willis, proximal branches) arteries.
  – Small vessel disease: Disease of distal vessels from the vertebral, basilar, or middle cerebral artery; results in lipohyalinosis and atheroma.
  – Lacunar infarct: Injury to vessels of the basal ganglia, internal capsule, thalamus, or pons.
  – Cryptogenic stroke: Cerebral ischemia due to unknown origin after workup.
○ High-risk cardiac features for stroke include atrial fibrillation, valvular disease, or arrhythmia.
○ Hypercoagulopathy risk factors include blood disorders (e.g., sickle cell anemia) or coagulation disorders (e.g., factor V Leiden).
○ Trial of Org 10172 in Acute Stroke Treatment (TOAST) classification of ischemic stroke divides stroke into five categories: large artery atherosclerosis, cardioembolism, small vessel occlusion, stroke of other determined etiology, and stroke of undetermined etiology.
• Diagnosis:
○ See Chapter 16.2 Intubation, ACLS/PALS, Cardiac Arrest, and Stroke Reference.
○ History, physical, and neurological exam performed; time of stroke onset noted from patient, family, and/or emergency medical services; evaluation of current patient anticoagulation performed; standard labs evaluated (complete blood count, complete metabolic panel, coagulation factors, type and screen, troponin); EKG used to evaluate cardiac arrhythmia as potential cause and rule out concomitant myocardial infarction; other select tests performed in select patients (liver function test, toxicology, blood alcohol, pregnancy tests, arterial blood gas, chest X-ray).
○ Rapid assessment of stroke includes evaluation of deficits in face, drift/weakness, and abnormal speech.
○ National Institutes of Health Stroke scale (see ▶ Table 16.21): Obtained with almost all protocolized brain attacks or stroke evaluations; scored 0–42 with 42 being highest possible score; scores of 5–15 indicate moderate stroke and scores > 22–25 suggest a higher risk of hemorrhage with use of tissue plasminogen activator (TPA).
○ Noncontrast CT of the head prerequisite for any medical management to identify stroke burden and rule out hemorrhagic stroke.
○ Vascular imaging involving CT angiography and CT perfusion most commonly used to rapidly assess areas of core stroke (i.e., nonsalvageable tissue) and penumbra (i.e., potentially salvageable tissue with hypoperfusion).
○ Further workup of stroke etiology may include lipid panels, A_{1c} levels, transthoracic or transesophageal echocardiography, MRI of the brain, diagnostic cerebral angiography, laboratory evaluation of coagulopathy or vasculitis, as well as telemetry and Holter monitoring.
• Medical management:
○ Stabilization of airway, circulation, and blood pressure performed; hypoglycemia corrected to goal of 140–180 mg/dL; use of isotonic fluids (i.e., normal saline) used to avoid cerebral vasogenic edema.
○ Blood pressure stabilized ≤ 185 mm Hg systolic and ≤ 110 mm Hg diastolic for at least 24 hours after thrombolytic treatment utilizing labetalol, nicardipine, and clevidipine as the first-line therapy and IV nitroprusside as the second-line therapy.
○ Patient management in a stroke critical care unit has been associated with improved patient outcomes and reduced complications.
○ Tissue plasminogen activator (TPA) indicates for stroke < 4.5 hours' duration with newer studies suggesting that CT perfusion and the presence of penumbra can potentially further this time window; checklist utilized to evaluate eligible patients (see ▶ Table 16.2); door-to-needle time of < 60 minutes recommended.
○ Aspirin initiated within 48 hours of ischemic stroke.
○ Control of blood sugar and administration of statin performed.
○ Inpatient or outpatient rehabilitation commonly recommended after acute stabilization.
• Surgical management:
○ Clot retrieval occurs via use of an stent retriever device and suction catheter; postoperatively patients closely monitored for reperfusion hemorrhage; intravascular stenting or carotid stenting with angioplasty (i.e., balloon dilation of stenotic blood vessels) can be utilized for maintaining vessel patency.

- Several key studies (MR CLEAN,[46] SWIFT-PRIME,[47] EXTEND IA,[48] ESCAPE,[49] and REVASCAT[50]) suggested improved outcomes for mechanical thrombectomy in the presence of large vessel occlusion with penumbra on advanced vascular imaging.
- Newer studies (DAWN[51]) have extended the window for thrombectomy up to 24 hours based on vascular imaging.
- Complications:
  - Prophylactic treatment of deep vein thrombosis and pulmonary embolism initiated as soon as safe; later evaluation of dysphagia and aspiration risk performed in all stroke patients.
  - Patients with large hemispheric or cerebellar strokes are closely monitored for the potential need of decompressive craniectomy in the setting of worsened edema, hemorrhage, and/or mass effect; early decompression shown to improve outcome but does result in a higher number of patients who would have otherwise died to remain severely disabled or vegetative.
  - Medical complications are most common after stroke: Falls (25%), urinary tract infection (24%), pneumonia (22%), pressure sores (21%), depression (16%), shoulder pain (9%), deep vein thrombosis (2%), pulmonary embolism (1%), cardiac arrhythmia or myocardial infarction (1%), aspiration, gastrointestinal bleeding, and nutritional deficiencies.

14.3.5 Other Topics

- Unruptured cerebral aneurysms:
  - Five-year rupture rate of 1,692 patients was studied in the International Study of Unruptured Intracranial Aneurysms (ISUIA).[52]
  - Increasing size of aneurysm, > 7 mm in maximal dimension, and location in the posterior circulation conferred increased risk of rupture.[52]
  - Endovascular intervention and surgical clipping remain the two methods for aneurysm treatment. The best technique depends on both aneurysm and patient characteristics.
- Arteriovenous malformations (AVM)[53]:
  - Anomalous connection of arteries to veins without intermediary brain parenchyma or a capillary network. Predisposes patients to intracerebral and/or intraventricular hemorrhages.
  - Annual risk of hemorrhage is approximately 3%.
  - Deep venous drainage, deep seated lesions, and previous hemorrhage represent increased risk factors of hemorrhage.
  - Best identified with vessel imaging, such as CTA or DSA.
  - Spetzler–Martin grading scale, a five-point scale, helps determine whether or not to offer treatment of an AVM. Treatment is often recommended in Grades 1 and 2 patients, while conservative management is recommended for Grades 4 and 5 patients (► Table 14.16).

Table 14.16 Spetzler–Martin grading of arteriovenous malformations

Characteristic	Number of points
Size of arteriovenous malformation	
Small (<3 cm)	1
Medium (3–6 cm)	2
Large (>6 cm)	3
Location	
Noneloquent	0
Eloquent[a]	1
Pattern of venous drainage	
Superficial only	0
Deep component	1

[a] Eloquent cortex: sensorimotor, language, visual cortex, hypothalamus, thalamus, internal capsule, brainstem, cerebellar peduncles, or cerebellar nuclei.

- Stereotactic radiosurgery (e.g., Gamma knife) has been shown to have good results with smaller lesions with obliteration rates between 2 and 4 years.
- Endovascular intervention for embolization of feeding vessels for complete or partial occlusion of the AVM. Generally used as an adjunct for surgical resection in difficult cases.
- Craniotomy for resection of Spetzler–Martin Grade 1 and 2 lesions have low morbidity and mortality compared with Grade 3 or higher.[54]
- Dural arteriovenous malformations (dAVF)[55]:
  - An acquired pathologic connection between meningeal vessels and dural venous sinuses or cortical veins.
  - Rare, accounts for 10–15% of all intracranial vascular malformations.
  - Usually presents in the fifth and sixth decades of life with annual rates of hemorrhage reported between 7.4 and 19% for dAVF with cortical venous drainage and 1.4–1.5% without.
  - Classified most commonly by the Borden or Cognard classifications.[56]
  - Can be managed conservatively in low-risk cases. Endovascular embolization is considered the first-line treatment for dAVFs requiring treatment. Stereotactic radiosurgery and surgical ligation remain options in select cases.
- Cerebral cavernous malformations[57]:
  - Also known as cavernomas or cavernous angiomas. Low-flow clusters of sinusoidal channels that can rupture and cause ICH.
  - Angiographically occult aside from visualization of developmental venous anomalies (DVAs) which are associated with 33% of cavernoma patients.
  - Multiple small hemorrhagic events lead to characteristic "popcorn" appearance of cavernomas on imaging studies.
  - Familial forms may represent up to 20% of all cases and exhibit an autosomal dominant inheritance pattern. Can be associated with loss of function mutations in CCM 1, 2, or 3. Hemorrhage rate varies from 0.5 to 10% annually from initial presentation. Patients generally present in the third or fourth decade of life.
  - Annual risk of hemorrhage tends to decrease 2.5 years after initial hemorrhage.[58]
  - Surgical resection remains the treatment of choice for cavernomas in surgically accessible locations with multiple hemorrhages, neurological deficits, and/or progressive seizures.
  - Stereotactic radiosurgery for cavernomas remains controversial.

14.4 Neurosurgical Neoplasms

Michael Karsy and Randy L. Jensen

14.4.1 Epidemiology

- World Health Organization has classified tumors into four grades which correlate with survival, seven categories of nervous system tumors identified (e.g., neuroepithelial, cranial and paraspinal nerves, meninges, lymphomas and hematopoietic cells, germ cell tumors, sellar region, metastatic tumors).[59,60]
- Adult tumors:
  - Annual adult incidence: 40.82 per 100,000 persons (> 40 years) and 10.94 per 100,000 persons (18–40 years).
  - Mostly metastatic lesions.
  - Among primary tumors, meningiomas are the most common tumor followed by gliomas.
- Pediatric tumors:
  - Annual pediatric incidence: 2–5 cases per 100,000; second to leukemia for most common type of tumor; high mortality relative to other types of tumors.
  - Most commonly posterior fossa (60% of cases).
  - Most commonly cerebellar astrocytomas (15%), medulloblastoma (14%), brain stem gliomas (12%), ependymomas (9%).
  - Tumors in infants < 1 year of life are rare, primarily of neuroectodermal origin, and more likely to be aggressive.

14.4.2 Diagnosis

- Presentation: Progressive neurological deficits (two-thirds of cases), motor weakness (50% for cases), headaches (50% of cases), seizure (25% of cases).
- Neurological changes can localize to tumor location:
  - Frontal lobe: Personality changes, language dysfunction, apraxia.
  - Temporal lobe: Memory impairment, contralateral superior quadrantanopsia.
  - Parietal lobe: Contralateral motor or sensory impairment, homonymous hemianopsia.
  - Occipital lobe: Visual field deficits.
  - Posterior fossa: Obstructive hydrocephalus, nausea, vomiting, ataxia, vertigo, diplopia, seizures are rare.
- Molecular markers commonly used for diagnosis and prognosis, genomic classification applied to tumors to improve prognostication, and identification of targeted treatments.
- Metastatic lesions:
  - 10–30% of patients with cancer will develop metastatic brain lesions owing to improved radiochemotherapy treatment improving life-span and improved imaging of metastatic lesions.
  - Annual incidence of 200,000–300,000 cases in the United States.
  - Most commonly in older adults.
  - Most common primary lesions involve lung, breast, colorectal, renal cell, and melanoma, although other types are possible.
  - Metastatic lesions spread from primary tumors by blood stream.
  - Metastatic lesions to the brain can be solitary in two-thirds of cases, requires workup of other lesions in the body to identify other tumors.
- Meningiomas:
  - Most common primary brain tumor.
  - Most are WHO grade I (90%) followed by WHO grades II and III.
  - Arise from arachnoid cap cells.
  - Occur in cerebral convexity, sphenoid wing, along the skull base, within the cerebellopontine angle, and posterior fossa.
  - Primary lesions > 3 cm amenable to surgery, while smaller lesions can undergo stereotactic radiotherapy using imaging diagnosis alone; small lesions treated with radiotherapy show > 90% local control rates at 5 years.
  - Efficacy of tumor resection assessed by Simpson grading where Simpson grade I resections (e.g., all tumor, involved dura and bone) result in > 90% 5-year disease-free rates.
- Gliomas:
  - Second most common tumor, most common malignant primary brain tumor.
  - Encompass a broad group of tumors, heavily involves molecular testing for diagnosis.
  - Arise from glial or stem-like progenitor cells.
  - Isocitrate dehydrogenase 1/2 (IDH1/2): Enzyme of the Kreb cycle, when mutated promotes formation of 2-hydroxyglutarate and correlates with improved prognosis of gliomas.
  - O-6-methylguanine-DNA methyltransferase (MGMT): A DNA repair enzyme with reduced gene translation when MGMT promoter is methylation in gliomas, thus improving the efficacy of alkylating agents.
  - Chromosome 1p/19q codeletion: Pathognomonic for oligodendroglioma, unknown mechanism for influence on tumors.
  - P53: Most common mutation in tumors and in gliomas.
  - Epidermal growth factor (EGFR): tyrosine kinase growth factor receptor, EGFRvIII mutation results in constitutive activity and growth signaling pathway, increased copy number of EGFR confers worse prognosis.
  - Spectrum of disease including pilocytic astrocytoma (WHO grade I), diffuse astrocytoma IDH mutant (grade II), oligodendroglioma 1p/19q co-deleted (grade II), anaplastic astrocytoma (grade III), anaplastic oligodendroglioma (grade III), and glioblastoma (grade IV).
  - Maximal tumor resection improves mortality and reduces recurrence in all grades of tumors; treatment followed with chemoradiotherapy for higher grade lesions.
- Midline gliomas:
  - Midline high-grade glioma (WHO grade IV), median age of diagnosis 5–11 years.

- ○ Associated with K27 M mutation in histone H3F3A.
- ○ Uniformly poor prognosis.
- Ependymal tumors:
  - ○ Ependymomas (WHO grade II) and subependymomas (WHO grade I) arise from the lining of the ventricles.
  - ○ Commonly intracranial in pediatric patients and spinal in adults.
  - ○ Myxopapillary ependymomas are found in the spinal lesions of young adults.
- Choroid plexus tumors:
  - ○ Choroid plexus papillomas: WHO grade I tumors arising within the ventricles; benign and can produce cerebrospinal fluid and result in obstructive hydrocephalus.
  - ○ Choroid plexus carcinomas: WHO grade III tumors arising within the ventricles, malignant.
- Mixed neuronal-glial tumors: Range of tumors with mixed cell populations; includes ganglioglioma, gangliocytoma, dysembryoplastic neuroepithelial tumor, central neurocytoma.
- Pineal tumors:
  - ○ Pineocytoma: Slow growing WHO grade I primary tumor of the pineal gland.
  - ○ Pineoblastoma: WHO grade IV tumor, rare, common in young children.
- Medulloblastoma:
  - ○ WHO grade IV tumor commonly in children.
  - ○ Arises from cerebellar progenitor cells in the posterior fossa.
  - ○ Four histological types including sonic hedgehog, WNT type, group 3 and 4 types with variation in patient age, prognosis, and treatment options.
- Nerve sheath tumors:
  - ○ Schwannoma: Grade I lesion, extraneural tumor arising from well-differentiated Schwann cells, associated with NF2 mutation; arises from trigeminal, facial, and vestibular nerves.
  - ○ Neurofibroma: Grade I lesion, intraneural or extraneural tumor consisting of Schwann cells and nonneoplastic cells, associated with NF1 mutation.
- Mesenchymal tumors:
  - ○ Chordoma: Mesenchymal tumor arising in the midline, one-half arising in the sacrum, one-third arising in the occiput and the rest throughout the spine, arises from notochord cells, most common in adults, benign but usually surrounding neurovascular structures.
  - ○ Chondrosarcoma: aggressive paramidline tumors commonly in adults.
- Pituitary adenomas:
  - ○ Commonly benign tumors but can be invasive (35%) and carcinomas (0.1–0.2%).
  - ○ More common in adults.
  - ○ Termed microadenomas (< 10 mm) or macroadenomas (> 10 mm).
  - ○ Most commonly are nonsecreting tumors; most common secreting tumors in order are prolactinomas, growth-hormone secreting tumors, and adrenocorticotropic secreting tumors (Cushing disease).
  - ○ Can be associated with bitemporal hemianopsia or other visual field defects due to pressure placed on the optic nerves and chiasm.
- Craniopharyngioma:
  - ○ Benign tumor of the sellar lesion, commonly seen in children.
  - ○ Associated with tumor calcifications.
  - ○ High rate of pituitary dysfunction with resection due to adherent nature of the tumor to the pituitary gland.
- Germ cell and non–germ cell tumors:
  - ○ Heterogenous collection of tumors similar to gonadal or other extraneuraxial germ cell neoplasms.
  - ○ Main types: Germinoma, teratoma, yolk sac tumor, embryonal carcinoma, choriocarcinoma.
  - ○ Can be mixed types of germ cell or non–germ cell tumors.
  - ○ Teratoma: Heterogeneous tumor population with cells from all three germ layers (e.g., endoderm, mesoderm, ectoderm).
  - ○ Seen more commonly in the pineal region and parasellar areas.
  - ○ Tumor markers including alpha-fetoprotein, beta–human chorionic gonadotropin, and placental alkaline phosphatase can be sent from serum and CSF for diagnosis.

- Germ cell tumors can be radiosensitive, mixed types, and teratomas show reduced sensitivity to chemotherapy and radiation.
- Hemangioblastoma:
  - Posterior fossa tumor involving disorganized vascular formation with tumor cells, seen more commonly in adults.
  - Associated with von Hippel–Lindau gene mutations.
  - Can present with tumor hemorrhage.

14.4.3 Imaging

- MRI with contrast is the primary method of evaluating tumors.
- CT imaging can be helpful in identifying calcifications in certain tumors (e.g., meningiomas, oligodendrogliomas, choroid plexus papillomas, and craniopharyngiomas among others).
- Tumor location (▶ Table 14.17) and patient age can help with an initial differential diagnosis.
- Evaluation of intra- versus extra-axial compartment, contrast enhancement, vasogenic edema in surrounding areas, and single versus multiple lesions, midline crossing, displacement of neurovascular structures, evaluation of dural base, and bone reaction.
- Functional MRI can be utilized to identify eloquent regions of brain for surgical treatment.
- Other lesions that must be ruled out on imaging include abscess or infections, demyelinating or inflammatory lesions, aneurysms, and other vascular lesions.
- Stereotactic MRI scans involve thin-cut sequences utilized intraoperatively with neuronavigation to improve resection efficacy and safety.

14.4.4 Medical Management

- Patient observation with close follow-up imaging can be a useful strategy in patients with small tumors who are asymptomatic.
- Patient treatment often discussed in multidisciplinary tumor board to delineate treatment and clinical trial options; neurosurgeons with or without specialization in oncology are primarily involved in managing brain tumors; otolaryngologists can be involved in managing tumors of the face and neck.
- Steroids (dexamethasone 10 mg IV once followed by 4–6 mg every 6 hours with a proton pump inhibitor or H2 blocker; pediatric patients 0.5–1 mg/kg IV once followed by 0.25–0.5 mg/kg every 6 hours) can be used to reduce vasogenic edema, should be avoided in patients with suspected leukemia or lymphomas until definitive diagnosis obtained.
- Prophylactic anticonvulsants controversial, 20–40% of patients will have seizure by the time of tumor diagnosis, level II recommendations to use prophylactic anticonvulsants with taper 1 week postoperatively.

Table 14.17 Differential diagnosis of brain tumors and lesions by location

Location	Differential diagnosis
Supratentorial	Gliomas, meningiomas, metastatic tumors
Skull base	Chordoma, chondrosarcoma, esthesioneuroblastoma, sinonasal carcinoma, lymphoma, metastasis, myeloma, paraganglioma
Sellar region	Pituitary adenoma, craniopharyngioma, meningioma, Rathke cyst, dermoid, epidermoid, germinoma, schwannoma, metastasis
Pineal region	Pineocytoma, pineoblastoma, germ cell tumor, tectal glioma, meningioma, dermoid
Intraventricular	Ependymoma, subependymoma, choroid plexus papilloma, central neurocytoma, colloid cyst, meningioma, subependymal giant cell astrocytoma
Posterior fossa	Pilocytic astrocytoma, medulloblastoma, ependymoma, hemangioblastoma
Cerebellopontine angle	Vestibular schwannoma, meningioma, epidermoid

- Chemotherapy agents with good blood–brain barrier penetration utilized.
  - Alkylating agents: temozolomide, procarbazine.
  - Nitrosourea: carmustine, lomustine, nimustine.
  - Carboplatin/cisplatin.
  - Nitrogen mustards: cyclophosphamide.
  - Vinca alkaloids: vincristine, vinblastine, paclitaxel.
  - Topoisomerase inhibitors: topotecan, irinotecan.
  - Anti-monoclonal antibodies: bevacizumab.
- Radiotherapy:
  - Whole brain radiotherapy (WBRT) utilized to provide radiation to the whole brain, fractionated treatment to improve overall dosing and reduce toxicity.
  - Stereotactic radiation therapy (e.g., Gamma Knife, Cyberknife) involve single, conformed doses of treatment to specific tumor areas.

14.4.5 Surgical Management

- Maximal safe resection with preservation of neurovascular structures is generally performed, boundaries of resection are determined on preoperative imaging (e.g., contrast-enhanced portions or T2 hyperintense areas).
- Postoperative monitoring of neurosurgical complications (e.g., hemorrhage, seizures, hyponatremia, vasogenic edema, and stroke).
- Postoperative MRI with and without contrast utilized for certain tumors (e.g., gliomas) to identify extent-of-resection, evaluate for complications, evaluate for ischemia/stroke, and serve as a baseline for further follow-up.

14.5 Peripheral Nerve Injury

Erin McCormack, Mansour Mathkour, Hussam Abou-Al-Shaar, Michael Karsy, and Mark A. Mahan

14.5.1 Introduction

- The incidence of peripheral nerve injury (PNI) is approximately 2–3% of emergency room or trauma admissions; the most common mechanisms of PNIs are typically due to laceration, blunt or penetrating injury, or acute limb compression[61-64].
- The frequency of PNIs in the upper extremity relates to the depth and location of the nerve, with greater incidence in the hand (e.g., digital nerves), followed by superficial locations in the forearm (e.g., median, ulnar, and radial nerves). Proximal PNIs (e.g., brachial plexus), while less frequent, tend to have worst neurological outcomes, whereas digital nerves have the best prognosis.
- Similar patterns of PNIs exist in the lower extremity, with injury to the common peroneal nerve being most common, due to the superficial location at the fibular head. Proximal injuries have worse outcomes, but injuries in the foot are not as common as in the hand.
- PNIs fit into three basic grades of injury[65-70]:
  - Apraxia: Mild mechanism of injury leading to a conduction block, with variable degree of loss of sensation and motor function. Typically a transient injury with excellent recovery over a few hours to a few months.
  - Axonotmesis: More severe mechanism of PNI that causes to axonal damage and leads to muscle atrophy over time. Variable recovery, with some patients experiencing improvement over months while others do not demonstrate any signs of recovery.
  - Neurotmesis: Most severe PNI leading to complete nerve transection. Recovery is not possible without surgical repair.

14.5.2 Injury Types

- Injury types:
  - Stretch/traction, with special types:
    - Avulsion (preganglionic) from the spinal cord.
    - Rupture (postganglionic) of the nerve distal to the spinal cord.
  - Laceration.
  - Direct compression/crush.
  - Concussive, e.g., gunshot injuries.
  - Iatrogenic.
  - Ischemic, especially compartment syndrome.
  - Combined.
  - Less common injuries:
    - Chronic injuries (e.g., entrapment, which may appear acute sometimes).
    - Immunologic (see below).
    - Burn, skin loss, electrocution, iatrogenic, etc.
- PNI can result in three basic grades of injury. Injury classification can aid in predicting the degree of nerve recovery (► Table 14.18). Injury classification can be hard to distinguish in the acute period after injury. The type of injury is usually determined by the success of natural peripheral nerve recovery/regeneration, unless the injury can be observed (visible laceration or radiologic demonstration of injury).
  - Apraxia: conduction block, with loss of sensation and motor function.
    - Usually low-energy mechanism (e.g., compression).
    - Transient injury with excellent recovery over a few hours to a few months.
  - Axonotmesis: axonal loss, which leads to muscle atrophy over time.
    - Moderate mechanisms, e.g., joint dislocation.
    - Usually proven on electrodiagnostic studies, including nerve conduction and electromyographic studies (EMG, see below).
    - Variable recovery, with some patients experiencing improvement over months, while others do not demonstrate any signs of recovery.
  - Neurotmesis: Complete nerve transection.
    - High-energy mechanisms (e.g., fractures, non-closed vehicle collisions)or transection injuries.
    - Recovery is not possible without surgical repair.
- Workup[71,72]:
  - Radiographs:
    - Limited sensitivity for nerve injuries. Helpful for the identification of fractures or dislocations associated with PNIs.
    - Can be suggestive of phrenic nerve injury by detection of a hemidiaphragm.
  - Ultrasound: Excellent for evaluation of nerve transection or nerve swelling, especially when magnetic resonance imaging (MRI)is contraindicated (e.g., metallic foreign bodies or pacemakers). Practitioner variability.
  - MRI: Excellent for direct visualization of nerve injury as well as denervation changes within muscles in chronic injuries. Less practitioner variability than ultrasound, but requires skill of interpretation, which can vary substantially.

Table 14.18 Nerve structures injured withSunderland and Seddon classification

Sunderland	Seddon	Myelin	Axon	Endoneurium	Perineurium	Epineurium	Recovery
I	Neuropraxia	X					Complete recovery within days to weeks
II	Axonotmesis	X	X				Regeneration within weeks to months
III			X	X	X		Partial recovery
IV			X	X	X	X	Permanent deficits
V	Neurotmesis	X	X	X	X	X	Permanent deficits

○ CT myelogram: Can be used to identify nerve root avulsion from the spinal cord.Used when MRI is equivocal or cannot be obtained especially when an avulsion is still suspected.
○ Nerve conduction studies and EMG:
  – Rarely indicated in the acute setting, as distal denervation requires 2–3 weeks to develop characteristic signals. Nerve conduction studies can be normal for the first 1–2 days after complete nerve laceration, as Wallerian degeneration has not commenced.
  – Evaluation of nerve conduction studies (nerve conduction velocity, amplitude, and latency) as well as EMG (acute changes: muscle reactivity to needle insertion, and chronic changes: recruitment patterns) serves to evaluate the severity and acuity of injury. May provide information on the degree of nerve recovery.

14.5.3 Specific Injury Patterns

• Significant cross-innervation of muscles is seen in both the upper and lower limbs with variation in deficits depending on injured nerve (▶ Table 14.19).
  ○ Dermatome patterns are distinct from peripheral nerve distributions (i.e., PNIs can usually be readily distinguished from spinal level injuries).
  ○ Plexus level injuries typically involve multiple nerves and fit patterns (e.g., lateral cord injury is distinguished by the involvement of the musculocutaneous and median sensory and possible proximal median motor innervation—such that elbow flexion, pronation, and wrist flexion are weak, along with loss of sensation in the lateral forearm and radial side of the hand).

Table 14.19 Nerves and muscles associated with thebrachial plexus

Peripheral nerve	Nerve root components	Motor/ sensory	Function
Dorsal scapular	C3, C4, C5	Motor	Levator scapulae
	C4, C5	Motor	Rhomboids
Suprascapular	C5, C6	Motor	Supraspinatus
	C5, C6	Motor	Infraspinatus
Long thoracic	C5, C6, C7	Motor	Serratus anterior
Nerve to subclavius	C5, C6	Motor	Subclavius
Subscapular	C5, C6	Motor	Teres major
	C5, C6	Motor	Subscapularis
Lateral pectoral	C5, C6, C7	Motor	Clavicular pectoralis major
Medial pectoral	C6, C7, C8, T1	Motor	Sternal pectoralis major
	C6, C7, C8, T1	Motor	Pectoralis minor
Thoracodorsal	C7, C8	Motor	Latissimus dorsi
Musculocutaneous	C5, C6	Motor	Biceps
	C5, C6	Motor	Brachialis
	C5, C6, C7	Motor	Coracobrachialis
Axillary	C5, C6	Motor	Deltoid
	C5, C6	Motor	Teres minor
Median	C6, C7, C8, T1	Motor	Flexors of the wrist
Radial	C5, C6	Motor	Brachioradialis
	C5, C6	Motor	Supinator
	C6, C7, C8	Motor	Triceps
	C6, C7, C8	Motor	Extensors of the wrist
	C7, C8	Motor	Extensors of the fingers
Ulnar	C7, C8, T1	Motor	Flexors of the wrist
	C7, C8, T1	Motor	Flexors of the fingers

(Continued)

Table 14.19 (*Continued*) Nerves and muscles associated with thebrachial plexus

Peripheral nerve		Nerve root components	Motor/ sensory	Function
Iliohypogastric	Anterior	T12, L1, L2	Sensory	Anterior abdominal wall above the pubis
	Posterior		Sensory	Skin over the outer buttock and hip
Ilioinguinal		L1	Sensory	Medial thigh below the inguinal ligament; skin of thesymphysis pubis; skin of external genitalia
Genitofemoral	Genital	L1–L2	Sensory	Scrotum
	Femoral		Sensory	Femoral triangle
			Motor	Cremaster muscle
Lateral femoral cutaneous		L2, L3	Sensory	Anterior thigh; upper half of the lateral aspect ofthe thigh
Femoral	Anterior	L2, L3, L4	Motor	Sartorius muscle
			Sensory	Anterior/medial thigh
	Posterior		Motor	Quadriceps femoris
			Sensory	Medial leg/foot
Obturator		L2, L3, L4	Motor	Adductor magnus/longus/brevis
			Sensory	Medial thigh
Superior gluteal		L4, L5, S1	Motor	Gluteus medius, gluteus minimus, tensor fasciaelatae
Inferior gluteal		L5, S1, S2	Motor	Gluteus maximus
Sciatic	Common peroneal	L4, L5, S1, S2, S3	Motor	Tibialis anterior, muscles of foot eversion
	Tibial		Sensory	Sensation posterior thigh, dorsolateralleg/foot
Posterior femoral cutaneous		S1, S2, S3	Sensory	Sensation to posterior thigh/popliteal fossa
Pudendal		S2, S3, S4	Motor	Perineal muscles, external anal sphincter
			Sensory	Perineum, penis/clitoris, scrotum/labia majora,anus

Upper Limb

- Axillary nerve:
  - Acute injury most commonly occurs from humeral neck fracture or dislocation, due to the nerve's course through the quadrangular space.
  - Patients areunable to abduct shoulder greater than 20 degreeswith atrophy to the deltoid muscle.
- Radial nerve:
  - Acute injury most commonly occur after midshaft humeral fracture or injury to the antecubital fossa. May also occur after compression injuries (e.g., the so-called Saturday night palsy), where deep sleep may compress the nerve against the humerus.
  - Loss of elbow extension is rare (branches to the triceps originate in the axilla), with wrist and finger drop being more commonly observed.
  - Posterior interosseous nerve (PIN) injury results in a unique pattern of isolated wrist extension weakness with radial deviation (as innervation of extensor carpi radialis longus is not from the PIN) and weakness of finger extension. Acute forms of an isolated PIN injury may be viral or immunological in etiology other than direct nerve injury. Chronic forms may occur from entrapment.
- Median nerve:
  - Acute injury most commonly results from acute carpal tunnel syndrome (e.g., pyogenic finger flexor tenosynovitis), nerve laceration, or forearm injury.

- Distal (wrist level) injury of the median nerve results in reduced palmar sensation of the radial 3½ digits, loss of lumbrical to digits 2 and 3 (inability to extend the finger with flexion at the metacarpophalangeal joint), and weakness of the thenar muscles (inability to elevate the thumb away from the palm or oppose it towards the fifth digit). Dual innervation of the thenar muscles by the ulnar nerve can mask some elements of median nerve injury.
  - Proximal injury of the median nerve results in the same deficits as proximal injury, *plus* loss of sensation of the palm, loss of long finger and thumb flexors (flexor digitorum superficialis, flexor digitorum profundus, and flexor pollicis longus muscles), and, if very proximal, loss of pronation and wrist flexion.
  - Injury to anterior interosseous nerve (AIN) results in weakness of the flexor digitorum profundus, flexor pollicis longus, and pronator quadratus muscles with inability to make "ok" sign. Similar to the PIN syndrome, acute, isolated AIN weakness may be viral or immunological in etiology, other than direct nerve injury.
- Ulnar nerve:
  - Acute injury is commonly secondary to supracondylar humeral fractures or direct elbow injury. Acute injury at the wrist can also occur. Chronic ulnar neuropathy is commonly due to entrapment at the elbow. Rare chronic injures can occur at the Guyon canal in the wrist(e.g., bicycle riding).
  - Distal (wrist level) injury leads to loss of hand intrinsic strength, specifically finger and thumb adduction and abduction. Loss of lumbrical innervation may lead to clawing of the fourth and fifth digits. Palmar finger sensation to the ulnar one and a half digits is diminished.
  - Proximal (elbow and above) injury leads to the same pattern as distal injury, plus loss of sensation on the ulnar side of the palm and dorsal hand, and weakness of flexion of the distal phalanx of fourth and fifth digits (ulnar side of flexor digitorum profundus muscle) and ulnar wrist flexion (flexor carpi ulnaris muscle).
- Musculocutaneous nerve:
  - Acute injury is commonly encountered from proximal arm injuries or lateral chest injuries (e.g., clavicle fractures or shoulder dislocation).
  - Patients typically present with weakness in elbow flexion, supination (biceps is a powerful forearm supinator), and loss of lateral forearm sensation (as the lateral antebrachial cutaneous nerve arises from the musculocutaneous nerve).
- Brachial plexus:
  - Not uncommonly confused with cervical nerve root injuries, e.g., acute radiculopathy. However, brachial plexus injuries disrupt the innervation from multiple nerve roots. Thus, if a patient's symptoms can only be explained by injury to multiple cervical roots, one should consider a brachial plexus injury in the differential diagnosis.
  - Pan-plexus injury (C5–T1 contributions to the brachial plexus):
    - Most common form of brachial plexus injury, typically caused by high-energy collisions. Injury leads to a flail arm with no motor or sensory function below the acromioclavicular joint Sensation to the top of the shoulder (C4 distribution) is spared. Shoulder shrug (trapezius) is commonly intact. Variable preservation of proximal brachial plexus nerves, such as dorsal scapular nerve (rhomboid muscle, leading to scapular retraction) and long thoracic nerve (serratus anterior, leading to shoulder forward rotation). Horner syndrome (pupil small in a dark room) is suggestive of spinal nerve/root avulsion.
  - Upper trunk (C5–C6 contributions to the brachial plexus):
    - Acute injury is most commonly due tostretch injury from head/neck combined with shoulder stretch (e.g., unrestrained motor vehicle collisions). Penetrating neck trauma is another common cause. May occur during birth, typically from infant shoulder dystocia during vaginal delivery.
    - Injury leads to loss of shoulder abduction, elbow flexion, and loss of sensation from the shoulder to the thumb. Elbow extension, wrist, forearm, and hand strength are typically spared.
  - Extending upper trunk (C5-7 contributions to the brachial plexus):
    - Same causes as upper trunk injuries.
    - Loss of function similar to upper trunk injury *plus* loss of elbow extension and some loss of wrist and forearm strength. Sensory deficits will include the middle finger. Hand movement, particularly

finger flexion, is the only movement preserved in the upper extremity, making this type of lesion very classic for diagnosis.

- Isolated lower trunk (C8–T1 contributions to the brachial plexus):
  - Most commonly due to proximal humeral shaft fracture with an upward displacement.
  - Injury results in loss of hand intrinsic muscles (finger and thumb adduction and abduction) and claw position of all four fingers—unlike ulnar nerve injuries that lead to clawing of only fourth and fifth digits.
- Lateral cord:
  - Occurs commonly with clavicle fracture or humeral dislocation.
  - Results in weakness to the biceps and coracobrachialis muscles (musculocutaneous nerve), forearm, and wrist flexors; reduced sensation in the lateral surface of the forearm and midprone forearm.
- Medial cord:
  - Most commonly seen with penetrating injuries, e.g., gunshot wounds. Compression can also occur with thoracic outlet syndrome.
  - Results in weakness in ulnar innervated muscles of the forearm/hand (flexor carpi ulnaris, flexor digitorum profundus, lumbrical muscles, opponens digiti minimi, flexor digiti minimi, abductor digiti minimi, interossei, adductor pollicis), reduced sensation to the ulnar side of the forearm and hand as well as weakness in hand muscles innervated by the median nerve, which will give rise to a claw hand.
- Posterior cord:
  - Most commonly occurs in shoulder dislocations, due to tethering of the posterior cord by the axillary and radial nerves to the posterior arm.
  - Results in weakens of elbow, wrist, and metacarpophalangeal joint extension (radial nerve; resulting in wrist and finger drop), as well as weakness of shoulder abduction (axillary nerve) and reduced sensation on the dorsal aspect of forearm and hand.
- Neuralgic amyotrophy (brachial neuritis/Parsonage-Turner syndrome):
  - Monophasic inflammatory disorder of the brachial plexus. Classically presents with acute, severe pain in the shoulder with 2-week delayed onset of weakness of the muscles of the upper extremity. Usually a complex and patchy pattern of muscle atrophy with minimal to no sensory loss.
  - Painless, sensory dominant, and other forms exist in a spectrum of disease. When occurs in a diabetic patient, often referred to as diabetic radiculoplexoneuropathy.
  - Idiopathic form is often unilateral and does not recur. Hereditary form is inherited in an autosomal dominant pattern and is often bilateral and recurrent.
  - A similar form may occur in the lower extremity.

Lower Limb

- Iliohypogastric nerve:
  - Injury is most commonly iatrogenicduring abdominal surgery (e.g., herniorrhaphy).
  - Results in sensory deficit in lower abdomen superior to pubis symphysis. Proximal injury can also lead to a flank bulge (i.e., pseudohernia).
- Ilioinguinal nerve:
  - Most commonly an iatrogenic injury during abdominal or inguinal surgery.
  - Results in sensory deficit in pubis symphysis, genitals, and medial thigh, which is typically painful.
- Genitofemoral nerve:
  - Most commonly an iatrogenic injury from femoral artery surgery or angiography. The genitofemoral nerve is medial to the femoral artery, whereas the femoral nerve is lateral to the femoral artery.
  - Results in numbness in scrotum/labia and proximal anteromedial thigh.
- Femoral and saphenous nerve:
  - Most commonly due to penetrating trauma (e.g., laceration or an iatrogenic injury from femoral artery surgery), angiography, or psoas lesions, such as psoas hematomas and as a consequence of lateral access lumbar spine surgery.
  - Results in quadriceps femoris weakness and numbness in the anterior thigh and anteromedial shin (saphenous nerve territory).

- Isolated saphenous (exclusively sensory nerve) can occur from medial knee injury.
- Lateral femoral cutaneous nerve:
  - Injury occurs secondary to chronic overuse, blunt trauma, or entrapment, especially in obese individuals.
  - Results in numbness and paresthesias at the lateral thigh.
  - Management of lateral femoral cutaneous nerve injuries includes tricyclic antidepressants, gabapentin, and topical steroids. Spinal cord stimulator trial could be considered. For distal lesions, decompression of the nerve can be considered.
- Sciatic nerve:
  - Injury most commonly occurs due to an acute compression of the nerve against the hip capsule, femur fracture, laceration, or iatrogenic (e.g., intramuscular injection).
  - Injury results in hamstring, gastrocnemius, and soleus weakness, ankle dorsiflexion weakness, loss of inversion and eversion and toe flexion and extension, reduced sensation of the foot, and pain radiating down the posterolateral surface.
  - Piriformis syndrome is a controversial diagnosis, with vague sciatic pain aggravated by sitting without observable neurologic signs. More likely due to musculoskeletal injuries, imbalances, or tendonopathies.
- Common fibular nerve:
  - Acute injury arises from direct lateral knee injury or during varus trauma (e.g., rupture of the lateral collateral ligament).
  - Results in loss of deep peroneal nerve and superficial peroneal nerve function. The deep peroneal nerve provides ankle and toe dorsiflexion as well as sensation to the webspace between the first and second digits. The superficial peroneal nerve provides ankle eversion strength and sensation to the dorsum of the foot.
  - The treatment of peroneal nerve injury is focused on prevention with appropriate limb positioning during surgery. Simple (i.e. in situ) decompression can provide excellent outcomes in cases of partial injury.
- Tibial nerve:
  - Commonly occurs from compression of the tibial nerve at the tarsal tunnel (e.g., swelling, abnormal bony growth, flat feet), or direct trauma to the nerve.
  - Patients typically present with weakness of plantar and toe flexion as well as weakness in foot inversion and reduced sensation in the bottom of the foot.
- Obturator nerve:
  - Rare isolated injury—more commonly associated with plexus level injury. May be iatrogenic injury during hip surgery. Isolated obturator nerve palsy may be viral or immunologic in nature.
  - Results in thigh adductor weakness and numbness on the distal medial thigh.
- Superior gluteal nerve:
  - Rare isolated injury—More commonly associated with plexus level injury. Acute injury is most commonly from penetrating trauma.
  - Results in weakness in gluteus medius; demonstrates Trendelenburg sign with waddling gait.
- Inferior gluteal nerve:
  - Rare isolated injury—More commonly associated with plexus level injury. Acute injury most commonly from penetrating trauma or from iatrogenic injury from hip surgeries.
  - Results in weakness in gluteus maximus in the form of weakness of thigh extension.
- Pudendal nerve:
  - May occur from iatrogenic injury during urogenital procedures. Pudendal nerve acute entrapment (e.g., long distance bicycle ride) may occur, but is controversial.
  - Results in loss of sensation to the scrotum/labia. May cause denervation of the levator ani muscle and laxity of sphincters leading to incontinence.

Treatment of Nerve Injuries

- Optimal treatment depends on the severity and mechanism of injury[71,84]:
  - Initial diagnosis of the severity of the PNI is based on physical examination and imaging.

- Mechanism is based on the clinical history—higher energy injuries should raise suspicion for severe nerve injuries.
- Surgical indications:
  - Immediate surgical intervention should be offered for patients with vascular injuries, penetrating trauma, compartment syndrome, and progressive neurologic deterioration.
  - Expectant management can be considered for up to 3 months to monitor recovery of neuropraxiaand axonotmesis (e.g., stretch and low-velocity gunshot wounds). Surgical repair or reanimation procedures (nerve or tendon transfers) can be performed for failure of natural nerve recovery or regeneration.
  - Avulsion injuries may benefit from surgical reanimation procedures with in the first month of injury.
- Treatment algorithm:
  - Sharp laceration: Primary nerve repair/coaptation within 3 days.
    - Nerves have intrinsic tension and will retract away when cut.
    - If left longer than a few days, severed nerve ends will scar in place, away from the other cut end, making primary suture repair challenging, if not impossible.
  - Contused laceration: Explore, tack to fascial tissues, and repair within 3 weeks.
    - Blunt nerve lacerations (e.g., propellers and chainsaws) often have more proximal injury to the nerve due to stretching during the transection.
    - Allowing time for the contused end to die back proves the limit of the healthy nerve.
    - Suturing to fascia at the index exploration allows for a short repair distance. However, an intervening nerve graft or synthetic conduit may be necessary.
  - Closed injuries: Surgical decision making within 3 months:
    - Closed injuries present a diagnostic challenge of determining whether the injury is predominantly low severity with failure to conduct (and hence no function) or severe injury that will fail to have natural nerve recovery/regeneration.
    - Many practitioners place emphasis on expectant management, with serial electrodiagnostic studies. Others may recommend exploration and intraoperative measurement of nerve-to-nerve action potentials, as an estimate for likelihood of nerve recovery/regeneration.
  - Avulsion injuries:
    - Distal nerve transfer should be considered within the first 4 weeks of injury.
- Surgical treatments include:
  - Primary nerve coaptation/suture repair:
    - Cutting back to healthy nerve generally should be done as soon as feasibly possible to achieve success.
    - Suture repair of two clean nerve ends with as little tension as possible.
    - May need to release/transpose nerve to facilitate primary repair.
  - Exploration and neurolysis:
    - Release of nerve from incarcerating scar can immediately improve neurophysiologic function.
    - Intraoperative electrophysiology, such as nerve-to-nerve action potentials, can be performed to assess for likelihood of nerve recovery/regeneration.
  - Nerve grafting:
    - Graft repair utilizes a donor nerve as a conduit to place between cut nerve ends that cannot be repaired primarily. This is often the case when a neuroma-in-continuity needs to be resected—in order to repair a healthy proximal nerve to a denervated distal nerve.
    - Autograft is commonly used for vital nerves (e.g., median nerve). One of the most common sites for nerve graft harvest is the sural nerve. Small caliber grafts are preferred for a decreased risk of central necrosis.
    - Allograft repairs are becoming more common, especially with lower extremity vital nerves (e.g., digital sensory nerves) where the consequence of allograft harvest is nearly as severe as achieving repair of the injured nerve. Processed, detergent-washed fresh-frozen cadaveric nerves are immunogenically nonreactive and commercially available.
    - Nerve conduits, typically hollow tubes of either processed xenograft or purified protein or polymers, can be used for nerve gaps of up to 1–2 cm.
    - Similarly, nerve grafting should be done within 3–6 months to achieve success.

- Nerve, tendon, and muscle transfers for patients who fail to improve:
  - Nerve transfer: A functionally redundant (or potentially less valuable) nerve is transferred to a more clinically valuable nerve, close to the injured nerve's entry into the enervated muscle. The classic example is transfer of a fascicle of the median or ulnar nerve at the upper arm, typically a fascicle innervating wrist flexion, to the biceps or brachialis branch of the musculocutaneous nerve. The procedure is performed distally, creating shorter time to reinnervation, less axon loss, and motor-to-motor transfer. Nerve transfers typically have excellent recovery in comparison to proximal grafting procedures and involve less complex surgery; many practitioners prefer nerve transfers to nerve grafting procedures. Nerve transfers can be considered after the 3–6-month window for primary or graft repairs, but success after 1 year is considered to have lower odds.
  - Tendon transfer: The insertion of the tendon is released and re-routed to be sutured to a tendon of a denervated muscle. These procedures have good historical success rates, but the functional result is very technique-driven and the degree of success is not uniform. Tendon procedures can be performed at any time after nerve injury but can be limited in success if joint ankylosis has formed.
  - Free-functioning or pedicled muscle transfer: The entire muscle, typically the gracilis, rectus abdominis, or latissimus dorsi, is transferred to a new site and repaired with a new vascular supply and innervation. Essentially a nerve transfer performed with a fresh nerve injury. Good success rates, but technically challenging procedure with numerous pitfalls and should be limited to major centers with expertise.
- Pain should be managed optimally with appropriate pain medications (i.e., anticonvulsants, selective serotonin and norepinephrine reuptake inhibitors, tricyclic antidepressants, lidocaine patches, tramadol, and opioids).

14.6 Hydrocephalus

Michael Karsy and John R. Kestle

14.6.1 Epidemiology

- 0.6% of all annual pediatric admissions in the United States; 1–5:1000 live births; most common cause for neurosurgery in children; varies by region of the world.[85]
- Less common in adults (3.4–17 per 100,000 adults).[86]
- Broad types:
  - Communicating: Flow of CSF is blocked after exiting ventricles, CSF can flow between ventricles, can result from CSF overproduction or poor absorption; postmeningitis, subarachnoid hemorrhage, disseminated tumors, postsurgical, posttraumatic hemorrhage.
  - Noncommunicating: Obstructive hydrocephalus, flow of CSF is blocked within the ventricles, commonly at narrowed portions of the ventricles (e.g., Foramen of Monro, aqueductal of Sylvius) but can occur anywhere; aqueductal stenosis, obstructive tumor.
- Specific pathologies:
  - Congenital hydrocephalus: Hydrocephalus at birth due to structural issues (e.g., aqueductal stenosis, Dandy–Walker syndrome, holoprosencephaly).
  - Hydrocephalus associated with myelomeningocele: up to 80% of patients with open myelomeningocele may require a shunt; the 2011 Management of Myelomeningocele Study (MOMS) multicenter trial of in-utero repair of myelomeningocele showed a reduction in shunt placement from 82 to 40% in patients undergoing repair compared to expectedly managed babies, higher risk of preterm delivery, and uterine dehiscence.
  - Posthemorrhagic hydrocephalus: secondary hydrocephalus due to intraventricular hemorrhage, incidence of 40–70% after hemorrhage.
  - Hydrocephalus ex vacuo: brain tissue loss from injury resulting in appearance of enlarged ventricles.
  - Normal pressure hydrocephalus (NPH): pathologically enlarged ventricles with normal opening pressure on lumbar puncture seen in older adults; presents with Hakim triad of dementia, magnetic

gait, and urinary incontinence; probably underdiagnosed and undertreated; 5% of diagnosed dementia may be actually undiagnosed NPH; a potentially reversible cause of dementia.

○ Pseudotumor cerebri or idiopathic intracranial hypertension: increase intracranial pressure without dilatation of the ventricles necessarily, arises commonly in overweight women due to increased abdominal venous pressure or venous stenosis causing obstructing venous return and reducing CSF absorption, can result in optic neuropathy leading to blindness.

○ Benign external hydrocephalus: common cause of macrocephaly seen in children; associated with elevated subarachnoid fluid collections; evaluated by monitoring head growth curves, ensuring milestone functional development, and assessing the presence of macrocephaly in parents.

• Mechanism:

○ CSF produced in choroid plexus (60–80% of total production) and by brain parenchyma, CSF flows from the lateral ventricles through the foramen of Monro to the third ventricle then through the aqueduct of Sylvius to the fourth ventricle and finally out the foramen of Magendie and Lushka, CSF absorbed by arachnoid granulations at the superior sagittal sinus into the venous system, CSF also absorbed by ependymal lining of the ventricles, the choroid plexus, and spinal subarachnoid space.

○ Brain contains 125–150 mL of CSF at one time, 500 mL produced per day which is similar between children and adults, CSF allows buoyancy of the brain acting as a shock absorber and aids in clearance of waste.

○ Overproduction or under absorption of CSF results in hydrocephalus.

• Long-term outcomes for patients treated for hydrocephalus showed 54% had an average of four or more revisions, 45% require treatment of depression, 75% showed education beyond high school, 50% were employed and living independently, and chronic headache remains a common problem.[87]

14.6.2 Diagnosis

• Clinical signs of acute pediatric or adult hydrocephalus include lethargy, nausea, vomiting, poor memory, and cognition; focal neurological deficits are rare and suggest a specific lesion and headache[88]; rare symptoms include seizures; mothers of pediatric patients can especially assess for subtle behavioral changes which are highly predictive of shunt failure; shunt failures present similarly from event to event.

• Shunt infection presents with fever, rarely causes signs of meningitis or signs of bacterial peritonitis; can be evaluated with labs including complete blood count, C-reactive protein and erythrocyte sedimentation rate, as well as shunt tap to evaluate CSF analysis and culture.

• Symptoms of patients with shunts can fluctuate due to intermittent shunt obstruction but usually progressively worsening as hydrocephalus worsens.

• Ruling out of other masking medical issues often required (e.g., acute viral illnesses, urinary tract infections [UTIs]); UTIs can present identically to shunt malfunction in myelomeningocele patients.

• Evaluating reason for prior shunt placement, prior revisions, and prior symptoms of failure can aid in evaluating new changes; "mother's intuition" that something is wrong with their child should not be dismissed and can be predictive of shunt failure.

• Clinical diagnosis supported with imaging studies; symptoms from hydrocephalus vary depending on age, etiology, and acuity.

• Causes vary for children and adults, but it is important for understanding the need and acuity of treatment with shunt failure (▶ Table 14.20).

• Hydrocephalus in premature newborns evaluated by presence of bradycardic events (HR < 50), fullness and bulging of the fontanelle with splaying of the suture, and ultrasound measurements showing dilated ventricles; bradycardia and apnea can result from hydrocephalus or many other causes related to prematurity in newborns.

• Head growth curves utilized for children measuring head circumference for adjusted gestational age; increased head size crossing over multiple growth lines or poor functional development suggests a need for surgical treatment; patients with achondroplasia utilize a different head growth curve chart.

• Open fontanelles in children can be palpated when a child is flat or slightly inclined to evaluate for hydrocephalus; splaying of sutures by more than 1 finger breadth can be abnormal.

Table 14.20 Common causes of hydrocephalus for children and adults

Children	Adults
Premature intraventricular hemorrhage	Subarachnoid hemorrhage (e.g., aneurysms)
Neural tube defects (e.g., myelomeningoceles)	Meningitis
X-linked aqueductal stenosis	Traumatic brain injury
Dandy–Walker malformation	Choroid plexus papilloma, carcinoma, or other tumors
Congenital/syndromic	Postsurgical
CNS malformations	
Congenital syndromes	
Intrauterine or postnatal meningitis	
Choroid plexus papilloma, carcinoma, or other tumors	
Postsurgical	

14.6.3 Imaging

- Ventricle obstruction can cause dilation of proximal areas and helps localize the focus of the obstruction.
- CT imaging of the head with comparison to prior films is the most objective method of assessing for ventricular dilatation in hydrocephalus and widely available; rapid MR protocols are becoming first-line imaging choice especially in pediatric patients to reduce radiation exposure.
- Shunt X-ray series involves a combination of AP and lateral X-rays covering the shunt tubing to evaluate shunt valve settings, valve type, catheter disconnection, and catheter malposition.
- CT or rapid MRI head and shunt X-ray series are the minimum imaging needed to begin evaluating shunt failures or infections.
- Ultrasound imaging of the head utilized in children with open fontanelles to evaluate ventricular size and progression; evaluation of the frontal-occipital horn ratio (FOR) can be performed. FOR = (lateral ventricle width + occipital horn width)/(2 × biparietal width), where an FOR > 0.35 is considered abnormal, but a threshold FOR > 0.55 is often used to initiate treatment.
- CT of the abdomen may be necessary in patients with abdominal pain/distension to rule out other causes of acute abdomen, and evaluate for pseudocysts which suggest shunt infection.
- MRI studies play a limited role in acute hydrocephalus; rapid MR can be performed without sedation for assessing ventricles; detailed MRI can be useful in evaluating for transependymal flow on T2 imaging suggesting CSF accumulation; FIESTA imaging can evaluate blockages or stenosis (e.g., aqueductal stenosis) causing obstructive hydrocephalus, loculated cystic fluid pockets possibly requiring multiple shunt procedures, and anatomy for potential interventions (e.g., endoscopic third ventriculostomy).

14.6.4 Medical Management

- Symptomatic management is important for patient comfort and ruling out other mimicking diseases; one-third of patients with hydrocephalus can present with migraine-like, hydrocephalus-related headaches; fluid hydration with migraine cocktails (diphenhydramine, ketorolac, and prochlorperazine; diphenhydramine, ketorolac, and ondansetron).
- Dexamethasone (2–4 mg every 6 hours) can alleviate temporize edema causing obstruction in the setting of tumors.

14.6.5 Surgical Management

- External ventricular drain (EVD) placement for acute hydrocephalus can temporize patients until definitive treatment especially in the setting of infection delaying shunt placement, risk of upward herniation in patients with posterior fossa lesions; EVD height depends on pathology and goals of treatment (see Chapter 2.2 Neurological Monitoring).

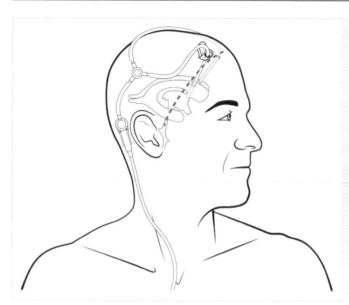

Fig. 14.8 Schematic of ventriculoperitoneal shunt placement.

- Shunts:
  - Diversion of cerebrospinal fluid to cavities of the body where fluid absorption can be performed.
  - Most common types include ventriculoperitoneal, ventriculopleural, ventriculoatrial, and lumboperitoneal.
  - Proximal catheter placed in the frontal or occipital horn of the lateral ventricles, tunneled to a valve and distal catheter using a shunt passer.
  - Ventriculoperitoneal shunt shows the longest lifespan and lowest complication rate; overall failure rates of 30% within first year and 50% within second year with decreasing risk thereafter, 5–10% risk of shunt obstruction, 5–10% risk of infection, 1–4.5% risk of abdominal pseudocyst, 0.1–0.7% risk of bowel perforation, 20% of subdural hematoma formation from overdrainage mostly in NPH population (▶ Fig. 14.8).
  - Occult shunt disconnection/fracture can be possible in some patients with long-term treatment for hydrocephalus by allowing drainage of fluid down a fistulous tract.
  - Valves can be programmable/adjustable (e.g., Codman, Strata, Sophysa) or nonadjustable (e.g., PS Medical, Delta, Orbis-Sigma), fixed differential pressure, or flow regulated, with or without anti-siphon devices.
  - No difference in shunt malfunction rate or patient outcomes by valve type; valve adjustments to treat patient symptoms of over- or underdrainage can be performed in an outpatient setting to allow for several days of follow-up in assessing symptom changes; settings must be checked by skull X-ray after MRI scans which may later alter settings; however, newer valves (e.g., Codman Certas Plus) are MRI compatible.[89]
  - Valve aspiration utilized to assess infection of shunt system; valve aspiration has potential risk of introducing skin flora and causing meningitis.
  - Slit ventricle syndrome: Small lateral ventricles seen in patients treated with chronic shunted hydrocephalus, suggests brain and ventricles lack compliance to dilate with shunt failures.
  - After shunting, patients are followed up at 2–3 months to ensure ventricular size is decreasing, then followed up yearly thereafter to help with detecting early problems; signs/symptoms of shunt failure are taught to patients and caregivers.
  - Fever in the setting of shunts: Most infections occur within 3–6 months after an intervention, otherwise rare unless caused by bowel perforation or abdominal pseudocyst.
- Endoscopic third ventriculostomy (ETV):
  - Utilized in patients with aqueductal stenosis due to congenital reasons or tumor obstruction and who have adequate anatomy (e.g., space in the floor of the third ventricle without proximity of the basilar artery).

Table 14.21 Endoscopic ventriculostomy (ETV) success score

ETV success score = probability of shunt freedom at 6 mo of age + etiology + previous shunt score			
Score	Age	Etiology	Previous shunt
0	<1 mo	Postinfectious	Previous shunt
10	1–6 mo		No previous shunt
20		Myelomeningocele, intraventricular hemorrhage, nontectal brain tumor	
30	6–12 mo	Aqueductal stenosis, tectal tumor, other etiology	
40	1–10 y		
50	≥10 y		

- Utilized an endoscopic lateral approach from the lateral ventricle to the third ventricle, generate a perforation in the membrane anterior to the mammillary bodies, can be used in conjunction with biopsy of tectal or intraventricular lesions, can be utilized with choroid plexus cauterization to potentially improve the outcome of hydrocephalus treatment in infants.
- ETV success score generates the probability of ETV success and shunt freedom at 6 months (▶ Table 14.21).[90]

References

[1] Echemendia RJ, Meeuwisse W, McCrory P, et al. The Sport Concussion Assessment Tool 5th Edition (SCAT5): background and rationale. Br J Sports Med. 2017; 51(11):848–850

[2] Ravindra VM, Bollo RJ, Sivakumar W, et al. Predicting blunt cerebrovascular injury in pediatric trauma: validation of the "Utah Score". J Neurotrauma. 2017; 34(2):391–399

[3] The CRASH Trial Management Group, The CRASH Trial Collaborators. The CRASH trial protocol (Corticosteroid randomisation after significant head injury) [ISRCTN74459797]. BMC Emerg Med. 2001; 1(1):1

[4] Hutchinson PJ, Kolias AG, Timofeev IS, et al. RESCUEicp Trial Collaborators. Trial of decompressive craniectomy for traumatic intracranial hypertension. N Engl J Med. 2016; 375(12):1119–1130

[5] Cooper DJ, Rosenfeld JV, Murray L, et al. DECRA Trial Investigators, Australian and New Zealand Intensive Care Society Clinical Trials Group. Decompressive craniectomy in diffuse traumatic brain injury. N Engl J Med. 2011; 364(16):1493–1502

[6] Morgenstern LB, Frankowski RF, Shedden P, Pasteur W, Grotta JC. Surgical treatment for intracerebral hemorrhage (STICH): a single-center, randomized clinical trial. Neurology. 1998; 51(5):1359–1363

[7] Carney N, Totten AM, O'Reilly C, et al. Guidelines for the management of severe traumatic brain injury, fourth edition. Neurosurgery. 2017; 80(1):6–15

[8] Brain Trauma Foundation (BTF). 2018. Available at: https://www.braintrauma.org/. Accessed January 5, 2020

[9] Wijdicks EF, Varelas PN, Gronseth GS, Greer DM, American Academy of Neurology. Evidence-based guideline update: determining brain death in adults: report of the Quality Standards Subcommittee of the American Academy of Neurology. Neurology. 2010; 74 (23):1911–1918

[10] Ontario Neurotrauma Foundation (ONF), Institut national d'excellence en santé et en services sociaux (INESSS). 2018. Available at: https://braininjuryguidelines.org/. Accessed January 5, 2020

[11] Brain Injury Association of America (BIAA). 2018. Available at: https://www.biausa.org/. Accessed January 5, 2020

[12] Steyerberg EW, Mushkudiani N, Perel P, et al. Predicting outcome after traumatic brain injury: development and international validation of prognostic scores based on admission characteristics. PLoS Med. 2008; 5(8):e165–, discussion e165

[13] National Spinal Cord Injury Statistical Center. National Spinal Cord Injury Statistical Center, Facts and Figures at a Glance. 2016; Available at: https://www.nscisc.uab.edu/. Accessed January 15, 2020

[14] Karsy M, Hawryluk G. Pharmacologic management of acute spinal cord injury. Neurosurg Clin N Am. 2017; 28(1):49–62

[15] Biffl WL, Moore EE, Offner PJ, Brega KE, Franciose RJ, Burch JM. Blunt carotid arterial injuries: implications of a new grading scale. J Trauma. 1999; 47(5):845–853

[16] Markus HS, Hayter E, Levi C, Feldman A, Venables G, Norris J, CADISS Trial Investigators. Antiplatelet treatment compared with anticoagulation treatment for cervical artery dissection (CADISS): a randomised trial. Lancet Neurol. 2015; 14(4):361–367

[17] Bracken MB, Shepard MJ, Collins WF, et al. A randomized, controlled trial of methylprednisolone or naloxone in the treatment of acute spinal-cord injury. Results of the Second National Acute Spinal Cord Injury Study. N Engl J Med. 1990; 322(20):1405–1411

[18] Bracken MB, Shepard MJ, Hellenbrand KG, et al. Methylprednisolone and neurological function 1 year after spinal cord injury. Results of the National Acute Spinal Cord Injury Study. J Neurosurg. 1985; 63(5):704–713

[19] Bracken MB, Shepard MJ, Holford TR, et al. Administration of methylprednisolone for 24 or 48 hours or tirilazad mesylate for 48 hours in the treatment of acute spinal cord injury. Results of the Third National Acute Spinal Cord Injury Randomized Controlled Trial. National Acute Spinal Cord Injury Study. JAMA. 1997; 277(20):1597–1604

[20] Hadley MN, Walters BC. Introduction to the guidelines for the management of acute cervical spine and spinal cord injuries. Neurosurgery. 2013; 72 Suppl 2:5–16

[21] Fehlings MG, Vaccaro A, Wilson JR, et al. Early versus delayed decompression for traumatic cervical spinal cord injury: results of the Surgical Timing in Acute Spinal Cord Injury Study (STASCIS). PLoS One. 2012; 7(2):e32037

[22] France JC, Karsy M, Harrop JS, Dailey AT. Return to play after cervical spine injuries: a consensus of opinion. Global Spine J. 2016; 6(8):792–797

[23] Patchell RA, Tibbs PA, Regine WF, et al. Direct decompressive surgical resection in the treatment of spinal cord compression caused by metastatic cancer: a randomised trial. Lancet. 2005; 366(9486):643–648

[24] Chew BG, Swartz C, Quigley MR, Altman DT, Daffner RH, Wilberger JE. Cervical spine clearance in the traumatically injured patient: is multidetector CT scanning sufficient alone? Clinical article. J Neurosurg Spine. 2013; 19(5):576–581

[25] Tomycz ND, Chew BG, Chang YF, et al. MRI is unnecessary to clear the cervical spine in obtunded/comatose trauma patients: the four-year experience of a level I trauma center. J Trauma. 2008; 64(5):1258–1263

[26] Maddox S. Paralysis Resource Guide. 2017. Available at: https://www.christopherreeve.org/about-us. Accessed January 5, 2018

[27] Suarez JI, Tarr RW, Selman WR. Aneurysmal subarachnoid hemorrhage. N Engl J Med. 2006; 354(4):387–396

[28] de Rooij NK, Linn FH, van der Plas JA, Algra A, Rinkel GJ. Incidence of subarachnoid haemorrhage: a systematic review with emphasis on region, age, gender and time trends. J Neurol Neurosurg Psychiatry. 2007; 78(12):1365–1372

[29] Feigin VL, Rinkel GJ, Lawes CM, et al. Risk factors for subarachnoid hemorrhage: an updated systematic review of epidemiological studies. Stroke. 2005; 36(12):2773–2780

[30] Greenberg MS. Handbook of Neurosurgery. New York, NY: Thieme; 2019

[31] Hunt WE, Hess RM. Surgical risk as related to time of intervention in the repair of intracranial aneurysms. J Neurosurg. 1968; 28(1):14–20

[32] Teasdale GM, Drake CG, Hunt W, et al. A universal subarachnoid hemorrhage scale: report of a committee of the World Federation of Neurosurgical Societies. J Neurol Neurosurg Psychiatry. 1988; 51(11):1457

[33] Fisher CM, Kistler JP, Davis JM. Relation of cerebral vasospasm to subarachnoid hemorrhage visualized by computerized tomographic scanning. Neurosurgery. 1980; 6(1):1–9

[34] Frontera JA, Claassen J, Schmidt JM, et al. Prediction of symptomatic vasospasm after subarachnoid hemorrhage: the modified fisher scale. Neurosurgery. 2006; 59(1):21–27, discussion 21–27

[35] Dorsch NW, King MT. A review of cerebral vasospasm in aneurysmal subarachnoid haemorrhage Part I: Incidence and effects. J Clin Neurosci. 1994; 1(1):19–26

[36] Dorai Z, Hynan LS, Kopitnik TA, Samson D. Factors related to hydrocephalus after aneurysmal subarachnoid hemorrhage. Neurosurgery. 2003; 52(4):763–769, discussion 769–771

[37] Fewel ME, Thompson BG, Jr, Hoff JT. Spontaneous intracerebral hemorrhage: a review. Neurosurg Focus. 2003; 15(4):E1

[38] Qureshi AI, Tuhrim S, Broderick JP, Batjer HH, Hondo H, Hanley DF. Spontaneous intracerebral hemorrhage. N Engl J Med. 2001; 344(19):1450–1460

[39] Juvela S, Hillbom M, Palomäki H. Risk factors for spontaneous intracerebral hemorrhage. Stroke. 1995; 26(9):1558–1564

[40] Hart RG, Boop BS, Anderson DC. Oral anticoagulants and intracranial hemorrhage. Facts and hypotheses. Stroke. 1995; 26(8):1471–1477

[41] Hemphill JC, III, Bonovich DC, Besmertis L, Manley GT, Johnston SC. The ICH score: a simple, reliable grading scale for intracerebral hemorrhage. Stroke. 2001; 32(4):891–897

[42] Passero S, Rocchi R, Rossi S, Ulivelli M, Vatti G. Seizures after spontaneous supratentorial intracerebral hemorrhage. Epilepsia. 2002; 43(10):1175–1180

[43] Hanley DF, Thompson RE, Rosenblum M, et al. MISTIE III Investigators. Efficacy and safety of minimally invasive surgery with thrombolysis in intracerebral haemorrhage evacuation (MISTIE III): a randomised, controlled, open-label, blinded endpoint phase 3 trial. Lancet. 2019; 393(10175):1021–1032

[44] Mendelow AD, Gregson BA, Rowan EN, Murray GD, Gholkar A, Mitchell PM, STICH II Investigators. Early surgery versus initial conservative treatment in patients with spontaneous supratentorial lobar intracerebral haematomas (STICH II): a randomised trial. Lancet. 2013; 382(9890):397–408

[45] Mendelow AD, Gregson BA, Fernandes HM, et al. STICH Investigators. Early surgery versus initial conservative treatment in patients with spontaneous supratentorial intracerebral haematomas in the International Surgical Trial in Intracerebral Haemorrhage (STICH): a randomised trial. Lancet. 2005; 365(9457):387–397

[46] Berkhemer OA, Fransen PS, Beumer D, et al. MR CLEAN Investigators. A randomized trial of intraarterial treatment for acute ischemic stroke. N Engl J Med. 2015; 372(1):11–20

[47] Saver JL, Goyal M, Bonafe A, et al. SWIFT PRIME Investigators. Stent-retriever thrombectomy after intravenous t-PA vs. t-PA alone in stroke. N Engl J Med. 2015; 372(24):2285–2295

[48] Campbell BC, Mitchell PJ, Kleinig TJ, et al. EXTEND-IA Investigators. Endovascular therapy for ischemic stroke with perfusion-imaging selection. N Engl J Med. 2015; 372(11):1009–1018

[49] Goyal M, Demchuk AM, Menon BK, et al. ESCAPE Trial Investigators. Randomized assessment of rapid endovascular treatment of ischemic stroke. N Engl J Med. 2015; 372(11):1019–1030

[50] Jovin TG, Chamorro A, Cobo E, et al. REVASCAT Trial Investigators. Thrombectomy within 8 hours after symptom onset in ischemic stroke. N Engl J Med. 2015; 372(24):2296–2306

[51] Nogueira RG, Jadhav AP, Haussen DC, et al. DAWN Trial Investigators. Thrombectomy 6 to 24 hours after stroke with a mismatch between deficit and infarct. N Engl J Med. 2018; 378(1):11–21

[52] Wiebers DO, Whisnant JP, Huston J, III, et al. International Study of Unruptured Intracranial Aneurysms Investigators. Unruptured intracranial aneurysms: natural history, clinical outcome, and risks of surgical and endovascular treatment. Lancet. 2003; 362(9378):103–110

[53] Solomon RA, Connolly ES, Jr. Arteriovenous malformations of the brain. N Engl J Med. 2017; 377(5):498

[54] Bervini D, Morgan MK, Ritson EA, Heller G. Surgery for unruptured arteriovenous malformations of the brain is better than conservative management for selected cases: a prospective cohort study. J Neurosurg. 2014; 121(4):878–890

[55] Reynolds MR, Lanzino G, Zipfel GJ. Intracranial dural arteriovenous fistulae. Stroke. 2017; 48(5):1424–1431

[56] Borden JA, Wu JK, Shucart WA. A proposed classification for spinal and cranial dural arteriovenous fistulous malformations and implications for treatment. J Neurosurg. 1995; 82(2):166–179

[57] Stapleton CJ, Barker FG, II. Cranial cavernous malformations: natural history and treatment. Stroke. 2018; 49(4):1029–1035

[58] Barker FG, II, Amin-Hanjani S, Butler WE, et al. Temporal clustering of hemorrhages from untreated cavernous malformations of the central nervous system. Neurosurgery. 2001; 49(1):15–24, discussion 24–25

[59] Ostrom QT, Gittleman H, Fulop J, et al. CBTRUS Statistical Report: primary brain and central nervous system tumors diagnosed in the United States in 2008–2012. Neuro-oncol. 2015; 17 Suppl 4:iv1–iv62

[60] Louis DN, Perry A, Reifenberger G, et al. The 2016 World Health Organization Classification of Tumors of the Central Nervous System: a summary. Acta Neuropathol. 2016; 131(6):803–820

[61] Belzberg A, Malessy MJ. Early management of brachial plexus injuries. In: Winn HR, ed. Youmans Neurological Surgery. 6th ed. Philadelphia: Saunders; 2011

[62] Colbert SH, Mackinnon SE. Nerve transfers for brachial plexus reconstruction. Hand Clin. 2008; 24(4):341–361, v

[63] Kim DH, Hudson AR, Kline DG. External and internal neurolysis. In: Atlas of Peripheral Nerve Surgery, 2nd ed. Philadelphia: Elsevier; 2014: chapter 21

[64] Ducker TB. Pathophysiology of peripheral nerve trauma. In: Omer GE, Spinner M, eds. Management of Peripheral Nerve Problems. Philadelphia: WB Saunders; 1980

[65] Ferrante MA, Wilbourn AJ. The utility of various sensory nerve conduction responses in assessing brachial plexopathies. Muscle Nerve. 1995; 18(8):879–889

[66] Ferrante MA. Brachial plexopathies: classification, causes, and consequences. Muscle Nerve. 2004; 30(5):547–568

[67] Foad SL, Mehlman CT, Ying J. The epidemiology of neonatal brachial plexus palsy in the United States. J Bone Joint Surg Am. 2008; 90 (6):1258–1264

[68] Gentili F, Hudson AR, Midha R. Peripheral nerve injuries: types, causes, and grading. In: Wilkins RH, Rengachary SS, eds. Neurosurgery. New York: McGraw-Hill Company; 1996:3105–3114

[69] Highet WB, Sanders FK. The effects of stretching nerves after suture. BJ Soc 1943; 30(120):355–369

[70] Kline DG, Hudson AR. Acute injuries of peripheral nerves. In: Winn HR, ed. Youmans Neurological Surgery. Philadelphia: WB Saunders; 1990

[71] Kim D, Hudson A, Kline D. Atlas of Peripheral Nerve Surgery. 2nd ed. Philadelphia, PA: Elsevier/Saunders; 2013

[72] Kretschmer T, Birch R. Management of acute peripheral nerve injuries. In: Winn HR, ed.Youmans Neurological Surgery. 6th ed. Philadelphia: Saunders; 2011

[73] Liang C, Malessy M. Techniques in nerve reconstruction and repair. In: Winn H, ed. Youmans and Winn Neurological Surgery. 7th ed. Philadelphia: WB Saunders 2017:2051–2058

[74] Alberstone C, Benzel E, Najm I, et al. Lumbosacral plexus. In: Anatomic Basis of Neurologic Diagnosis. 1st ed. Thieme; 2009

[75] Midha R, Zager E. Surgery of Peripheral Nerves. A Case-Based Approach. 1st ed. Thieme; 2008

[76] Nadi M, Midha R. Management of peripheral nerve injuries. In: Principles of Neurological Surgery. 4th ed. Elsevier; 2018:832–841

[77] Principles and indications for nerve transfers. In: Mackinnon S, ed. Nerve Surgery. 1st Edition. Thieme; 2015

[78] Sulaiman W. Management of acute peripheral nerve injuries. In: Winn H, ed. Youmans and Winn Neurological Surgery. 7th ed. Philadelphia: WB Saunders 2017:2064–2071

[79] Sulaiman OAR, Midha R, Gordon T. Pathophysiology of surgical nerve disorders. In: Winn HR, ed. Youmans Neurological Surgery. 6th ed. Philadelphia: Saunders; 2011

[80] Sulaiman O, Kline D. Outcomes of treatment for adult brachial plexus injuries. In: Chung K, Yang L, McGillicudy J, eds. Practical Management of Pediatric and Adult Brachial Plexus Palsies. Edinburgh: Churchill Livingston; 2012

[81] Sunderland S. A classification of peripheral nerve injuries producing loss of function. Brain. 1951; 74(4):491–516

[82] Sunderland S. Nerve and Nerve Injuries. Edinburgh: Livingstone; 1978

[83] Tharin BD, Kini JA, York GE, Ritter JL. Brachial plexopathy: a review of traumatic and nontraumatic causes. AJR Am J Roentgenol. 2014; 202(1):W67–75

[84] Surgical techniques for peripheral nerve repair. In: Wolfa C, Resnick F, eds. Neurosurgical Operative Atlas: Spine and Peripheral Nerves. 3rd ed. Thieme; 2016

[85] Vinchon M, Rekate H, Kulkarni AV. Pediatric hydrocephalus outcomes: a review. Fluids Barriers CNS. 2012; 9(1):18

[86] Dewan MC, Rattani A, Mekary R, et al. Global hydrocephalus epidemiology and incidence: systematic review and meta-analysis. J Neurosurg. 2018:1–15–. [Epub ahead of print]

[87] Gupta N, Park J, Solomon C, Kranz DA, Wrensch M, Wu YW. Long-term outcomes in patients with treated childhood hydrocephalus. J Neurosurg. 2007; 106(5) Suppl:334–339

[88] Riva-Cambrin J, Kestle JR, Holubkov R, et al. Hydrocephalus Clinical Research Network. Risk factors for shunt malfunction in pediatric hydrocephalus: a multicenter prospective cohort study. J Neurosurg Pediatr. 2016; 17(4):382–390

[89] Lollis SS, Mamourian AC, Vaccaro TJ, Duhaime AC. Programmable CSF shunt valves: radiographic identification and interpretation. AJNR Am J Neuroradiol. 2010; 31(7):1343–1346

[90] Kulkarni AV, Drake JM, Kestle JR, Mallucci CL, Sgouros S, Constantini S, Canadian Pediatric Neurosurgery Study Group. Predicting who will benefit from endoscopic third ventriculostomy compared with shunt insertion in childhood hydrocephalus using the ETV Success Score. J Neurosurg Pediatr. 2010; 6(4):310–315

15 Orthopaedics

Edited by Jim Lai and Mohit Gilotra

15.1 Fracture Basics and Compartment Syndrome

Jim Lai and Mohit Gilotra

15.1.1 Acute Fracture Management

- Fractures occur when bone fails due to loads exceeding the load-bearing capacity.[1]
- Fractures undergo specific radiographic imaging views for evaluation (▶ Table 15.1).
- Fracture description: Specific position on specific bone, extension into joints (e.g., intra-articular), involvement of the growth plate (Salter–Harris classification, ▶ Table 15.2), fracture line pattern (transverse, oblique, spiral), amount of displacement and angulation, comminuted (> 2 fragments) versus segmental (> 3 fragments), compression (e.g., vertebral endplates), impaction (e.g., telescoping of fractures in long bone), open versus closed.
- Bone stress and fracture patterns:
  - Tension → transverse fracture.
  - Compression → oblique fracture.
  - Bending → butterfly fracture.
  - Torsion → spiral fracture.
- Periosteum promotes callus formation and healing, periosteum is thicker and stronger in children who resist fracture displacement and open fracture formation compared to adults.
- Pathologic fractures involve injuries due to bone weakened by an underlying abnormality that requires treatment (e.g., cancer, rickets, McCune–Albright syndrome, juvenile osteoporosis, renal disease, osteogenesis imperfect).
- Pediatric fractures:
  - Buckle/torus fracture: Compression between metaphysis and diaphysis with or without disrupted periosteum; commonly in distal radius; managed by splitting.

Table 15.1 Common radiographic views for fractures[a]

Location	X-ray
Wrist	AP, lateral, oblique, scaphoid
Elbow	AP, lateral, oblique
Shoulder	AP, scapular Y, axillary
Knee	AP, lateral, oblique (internal or external rotation), sunrise (axial, tangential)
Foot	AP, lateral, oblique
Tibia, femur, forearm	AP, lateral
Ankle	AP, lateral, mortise (10–20-degree internal rotation)

Abbreviation: AP, anteroposterior.

[a] Views depend on practice patterns, and suspicion of fracture type based on clinical history.

Table 15.2 Salter–Harris fracture classification

Mnemonic description		Fracture type	Description
S	"Straight across"	I	Fracture across growth plate
A	"Above"	II	Fracture through physis and metaphysis
L	"Lower"	III	Fracture through physis and epiphysis
T	"Two"	IV	Fracture through physis and both metaphysis and epiphysis
ER	"ERasure of growth plate"	V	Compression of growth plate

- ○ Plastic deformation/bowing fracture: Tension force resulting in accentuation of bone curve; commonly in ulna and radius; deformation < 20 degrees or in children < 4 years often self-corrects.
- ○ Greenstick fracture: Incomplete fracture with plastic deformation; high risk for repeat fracture; treated with casting.
- ○ Physeal/growth plate fracture: Various injury levels of growth plates; higher degree of deformity with higher grades; occurs in 20–30% of long bone fractures; 30% of physeal fractures interrupt growth.
- ○ Apophyseal avulsion: Injury to fibrocartilage from overuse traction and inflammation; commonly in tibial tuberosity, calcaneus, pelvis, patella; more common in adolescents and athletes; can be subtle and identified more on clinical exam.
- ○ Child abuse red flags: Long bone fractures in nonambulatory children, metaphyseal corner (bucket handle) fractures, rib fractures, sternal fractures, multiple fractures with various stages of healing, bilateral acute long-bone fracture, fractures without high level of force, digital fractures in children < 36 months, displaced physeal fractures, complex skull fractures, vertebral body fractures.

15.1.2 Open Fractures

- Open fracture refers to osseous disruption in which a break in the skin and underlying soft-tissue communicates directly with the fracture and hematoma.
- One-third of patient with open fractures are polytraumas. Any wound in the same limb segment as a fracture are open until proven otherwise.
- Soft-tissue injuries in an open fracture may be contaminated with exposure to the external environment. Crushing, stripping, and devascularization of the soft tissue increase risk of infection and result in loss of function of musculature, nerve, vascular, or skin damage.
- Open fractures are the result of high-energy injury. The amount of bony displacement and comminution along with soft-tissue injury is proportional to the amount of applied force.
- Classification:
  - ○ Gustilo–Anderson classification (▶ Table 15.3): Originally designed to classify open tibia fractures and was later extended to include all open fractures except hand fractures. Subcutaneous soft-tissue injury is potentially more important than skin wound; so, definitive classification is reserved until observation in the operating room.
- Treatment:
  - ○ Open fractures constitute orthopaedic emergencies. Surgical intervention is almost always needed for formal wound exploration, irrigation, and debridement.
  - ○ Do not irrigate, debride, or probe the wound in the emergency room, as it may further contaminate the wound. Bone fragments should not be removed in the emergency room.
  - ○ Antibiotic coverage for open fractures is dependent on classification type (▶ Table 15.3).

Table 15.3 Gustilo–Anderson classification

Type	Description	Antibiotics use[a]
I	Clean skin wound < 1 cm	First-generation cephalosporin
II	Wound > 1 cm but < 10 cm with extensive soft-tissue damage	
III	Wound > 10 cm with extensive soft-tissue damage	First-generation cephalosporin plus aminoglycoside
IIIA	Extensive soft-tissue laceration with adequate tissue for bone coverage. Includes segmental fractures, gunshot wounds, and minimal periosteal stripping	
IIIB	Extensive soft-tissue injury with periosteal stripping and bone exposure requiring soft-tissue flap coverage. Usually with massive contamination	
IIIC	Vascular injury requiring repair	

[a]Farm injuries: first-generation cephalosporin, aminoglycoside, and penicillin.

- Operative treatment:
  - Adequate irrigation and debridement are the most important parts of open fracture treatment.
  - Careful debridement needs to be performed to evaluate the zone of injury and all surrounding tissue including bone fragments, tendons, and muscle.
  - Extension into joints necessitates additional exploration.
  - Foreign bodies/debris must be removed.
  - Fracture stabilization helps provide protection against additional soft-tissue injury.
- Complications:
  - Cellulitis and osteomyelitis are the most common infections.
  - Gross contamination, soft-tissue compromise, nutritional status, and polytrauma are all risk factors for infection.

15.1.3 Fracture Healing

- Complex and sequential set of events involved in restoring bone injury to stable conditions.
- Strain below 2% induces primary bone healing (i.e., intramembranous healing), occurs in highly stable constructs (e.g., compression plating).
- Strain between 2 and 10% induces secondary bone healing (i.e., endochondral healing), occurs with nonrigid fixation (e.g., braces, external fixation, bridge plating, intramedullary nailing).
- Stages of healing:
  - Inflammation: Induces infiltration of immune cells and fibroblasts, release of cytokines, proliferation of osteoblasts and fibroblasts.
  - Repair: Callus formation within 2 weeks if bone ends not touching, callus formation depends on amount of immobilization, formed cartilage replaced by bone, endochondral ossification converts soft callus to hard callus.
  - Remodeling: Begins in repair phase and continues after union, chondrocytes undergo terminal differentiation, extra-articular matrix undergoes calcification, and matrix is proteolyzed, cartilaginous calcification occurs.
- Bone remodeling proceeds according to Wolff's law (mechanical stress) and piezoelectric charges (electric signals from stress).
- Factors influencing healing: Blood supply, soft-tissue attachments, mechanical stability, injury location, degree of bone loss, fracture pattern, bone stimulators, cyclooxygenase-2 (COX-2) inhibitors, nutrition (e.g., vitamin D, calcium), nicotine, radiation exposure, infection, diabetes.
- Nonunion types: Septic (inadequate healing in the setting of infection), pseudoarthrosis (nonbony union and instead fibrous union), hypertrophic (inadequate stability, adequate blood supply), atrophic (inadequate stability and blood supply), oligotrophic (inadequate reduction with fragment displacement).
- Bone grafts:
  - Osteoconductive: Material acts as structure for bone growth (e.g., demineralized bone matrix).
  - Osteoinductive: Material promotes bone growth, induces stem cells (e.g., bone morphogenic protein).
  - Osteogenic: Material provides cells producing bone (e.g., cancellous bone, autologous bone).

15.1.4 Compartment Syndrome

- Definition: Clinical diagnosis where osseofascial compartment pressure increases to a level decreasing perfusion leading to irreversible muscle and nerve damage.
- Epidemiology:
  - Compartment syndrome may occur anywhere in the body where muscle is surrounded by fascia. Most common areas are leg, forearm, hand, foot, thigh, and buttocks.
- Mechanism of injury:
  - High-energy trauma with resulting fracture is the most common cause.
  - Other causes include crush injuries, extravasation of IV fluids, burns, tight casts/wrappings, or arterial injury.

- Clinical evaluation[2]:
  - Severe pain out of proportion to situation, decreased sensation, and tense extremity are all signs of possible compartment syndrome.
  - May be difficult to assess in polytrauma patient or in sedated patient.
  - Pain with passive stretch is the most sensitive finding. Paresthesias may indicate nerve ischemia.
  - Paralysis and pulselessness are late findings that suggest ischemia and necrosis already occurred.
- Compartment pressure measuring[3]:
  - May be necessary to diagnose compartment syndrome especially in polytrauma patients who are unreliable with inconclusive exam findings and altered mentation.
  - Compartment pressures with a reading > 30 mm Hg should raise concern.
  - Compartment pressures within 30 mm Hg of the diastolic blood pressure indicates compartment syndrome.
- Treatment: Emergent fasciotomies of all involved compartments.

15.2 Upper Extremity Fractures

Jim Lai and Mohit Gilotra

15.2.1 Clavicle Fractures

- Epidemiology:
  - Common injuries in young active individuals who participate in sports or activities where high-speed falls or collisions are frequent.
  - Account for 2.6% of all fractures: 29 per 100,000 population per year.
  - Highest incidence among young males under 20 and decreases with subsequent decade of life until elderly age.
  - 80% of fractures occur in the middle third, 15% lateral, and 5% medial.
- Anatomy:
  - S-shaped bone with medial side convex forward and lateral side concave forward, widest medially and thins out laterally.
  - Functions as a strut to brace the shoulder away from the trunk to allow the shoulder to function optimally.
  - The medial third of the clavicle articulates with the sternum forming the sternoclavicular joint (SC joint) and protects the brachial plexus, subclavian vessels, and superior lung.
  - The distal clavicle articulates with the acromion of the scapula to form the acromio-clavicular joint (AC joint) and is attached by the acromio-clavicular ligament. Additional ligaments attach the distal clavicle to the coracoid via the coracoclavicular ligaments (CC ligaments). CC ligaments include the conoid and trapezoid ligaments that provide vertical stability to the AC joint.
- Mechanism of injury:
  - Falls onto the affected shoulder are the most common mechanism for clavicle fractures (87%). Direct impact accounts for 7% and falls onto outstretched hand account for 6%.
  - Direct blows applied to the shoulder along with the small cross-sectional area in the midshaft lead to bony failure. Motor vehicle/motorcycle crashes, bicycle crashes, skiing/snowboarding falls, sports collisions, and falls are the most common mechanisms.[4]
  - Lack of soft-tissue structures in the midshaft of the clavicle (which may help dissipate force) results in highest incidence of clavicle fractures to the middle third.
  - Compressive forces applied laterally leads to failure in three ways: (1) failure of the AC joint, (2) fracture of the clavicle, (3) dislocation of the SC joint.
  - Simple falls from standing height are unlikely to produce clavicle fractures in healthy young adults but can be possible cause in elderly osteoporotic individuals.
  - Failure of the bone can also occur in traction injuries to upper extremity and is more associated with proximal third clavicle fractures.

- Clinical evaluation:
  - History and mechanism of injury are important aspects that determine the patient's care.
  - Careful neurovascular exam of the affected shoulder is necessary to assess for injuries to the brachial plexus and axillary artery. Examination of the overlying skin integrity for tenting, bruising, deformity, and swelling should also be noted.
  - High-energy mechanisms require careful evaluation for other associated injuries such as rib fractures, pneumothorax, or head injuries.
- Radiographic evaluation:
  - Simple AP radiographs are usually sufficient to visualize a clavicle fracture and the amount of displacement.
  - AP chest X-ray can also be used to visualize the clavicle for side-to-side comparison along with additional nearby structures such as ribs and scapula.
  - The best visualization of the clavicle employs a 20–30-degree superior tilt to eliminate the thoracic cage overlap.
  - CT scans may be used to visualize the SC joint which can be difficult to view on plain films if an injury is suspected.
- Classification: Multiple classification systems based on anatomic location, fracture pattern, and fracture prevalence; Allman classification (▶ Table 15.4) and Orthopedic Trauma Association (OTA) classification[5] are the most common.
- Nonoperative treatment:
  - The majority of clavicle fractures can be managed nonoperatively with immobilization.
  - Numerous studies have demonstrated good outcomes with a variety of immobilization techniques including slings, figure-of-eight bandaging, braces, and swathes.[6]
  - Goals of immobilization include supporting the shoulder girdle by elevating the distal fragment superiorly and posteriorly and depressing the medial fragment.
  - No one technique of immobilization has been shown to be superior to any other.[7,8]
  - Nonunion is the most common complication and has been reported to be about 15% for midshaft fractures.[9]
  - It is widely accepted that simple sling immobilization is sufficient as nonoperative treatment.
- Operative treatment:
  - Operative indications for clavicle fractures are controversial and their indications have been changing; recent studies suggest patients with clavicle fractures may benefit from primary surgical fixation; fixation is preferred for patients who are active and can benefit from anatomy restoration.[6]
  - Relative indications of midshaft clavicle fractures: (1) displacement > 2 cm, (2) shortening > 2 cm, (3) increased comminution > 3 fragments, (4) open fracture, (5) impending soft-tissue compromise (skin tenting), (6) vascular compromise requiring repair, (7) neurologic deficit, (8) ipsilateral upper extremity/rib fractures, (9) "floating shoulder" (ipsilateral clavicle and glenoid neck fracture), (10) bilateral clavicle fractures, (11) patient motivation for rapid return to function.
  - Surgical fixation is obtained using either plate fixation (more common, biomechanically superior to intramedullary fixation,[7,10] anteroinferior placement, reduced hardware irritation but greater surgical

Table 15.4 Allman classification system for clavicular fractures

Group	Description
Group I	Fracture of the middle third, most common type
Group II	Fracture of the distal third
• Type I	Minimally displaced, ligaments all intact
• Type II	Displaced secondary to fracture medial to coracoclavicular ligaments
• Type IIA	Conoid and trapezoid ligament attached to distal segment
• Type IIB	Conoid torn, trapezoid attached to distal segment
• Type III	Fracture extending into the AC joint with no ligament involvement
Group III	Fracture of the proximal third

exposure) or intramedullary (less common, smaller incision but more difficult to control axial length and prevent rotation) fixation.

- Complications:
  - Deep infections (2.2%) and superficial infections (4.4%),[7] nonunion (15–20%),[6]
  - Nonunion risk factors include age, female gender, fracture displacement, and comminution.[11]
  - Distal third clavicle fractures have higher nonunion rates when treated nonoperatively, as much as 40% for completely displaced fractures.
  - Malunion: Common cause of patient complaints and symptoms after midshaft clavicle fractures; typically diagnosed in young active patients with significant degree of shortening resulting in abnormal biomechanics of the shoulder joint; results in weakness, loss of endurance, and upper back pain.
  - ≥ 2 cm of shortening was associated with poor function outcome and patient dissatisfaction.[12]

15.2.2 Scapula Fractures

- Epidemiology:
  - Uncommon injury that represents 0.5–1% of all fractures and 3–5% of shoulder fractures.
  - Mean age of patients is 35–45 years of age.
- Anatomy:
  - Flat triangular bone that connects the upper extremity to the axial skeleton.
  - Protected from impact due to large amount of surrounding muscle mass as well as mobility of the scapula on the chest wall.
- Mechanism of injury:
  - Significant high-energy trauma is usually required including motor vehicle accidents (50% injuries) and motorcycle accidents (11–25%).
  - Direct trauma occurs from blows or fall to the acromion or coracoids. Indirect injury occurs from axial loading on an outstretched arm.
  - Shoulder dislocations may cause glenoid fracture. Muscles/ligaments can cause avulsion fracture.
- Clinical evaluation:
  - Affected upper extremity is in an adducted and immobile position supported by the contralateral hand; range of motion is painful; neurovascular and trauma exam warranted.
  - Associated injuries warrant full trauma evaluation[13]: High association with comorbid injuries; fractured ribs, clavicle, sternum, or shoulder trauma; pneumothorax; pulmonary contusion; brachial plexus injuries; spine injuries.
- Radiographic evaluation:
  - Initial X-rays of the shoulder include true AP, axillary, and scapular Y view. These should be able to demonstrate glenoid, scapular neck, body, and acromion fractures.
  - Stryker notch view (45-degree cephalic tilt) is for coracoid fractures.
  - CT scan is used for intra-articular glenoid fractures.
- Classification: Multiple strategies (▶ Table 15.4) and OTA classification.[5]
- Nonoperative treatment:
  - Most extra-articular scapular fractures are managed with nonoperative treatment consisting of sling and early range of motion; wide range of shoulder joint motion allows functional compensation.
  - Scapula body fractures: Surgical fixation is rarely indicated.
- Open reduction internal fixation (ORIF):
  - Surgical indications controversial but include (1) displaced intra-articular glenoid fractures involving > 25% of articular surface with/without subluxation, (2) scapular neck fractures with > 40-degree angulation or 1-cm medial translation, (3) scapular neck fractures with associated displaced clavicle fracture. Fixation of clavicle fracture generally results in adequate stabilization, (4) acromion fractures that impinge on subacromial space, (5) fractures of coracoids that result in AC separation. Complete third degree AC separation with a displaced coracoid fracture, (6) comminuted fractures of scapula spine.
  - Complications:
    - Increased mortality with concomitant first rib fracture.

Table 15.5 Various classifications for scapular fractures

Anatomic classification	
Type I	Scapular body
Type II	Apophyseal fractures including acromion and coracoids
Type III	Fractures of the superolateral angle including scapular neck and glenoid
Ideberg classification of intra-articular glenoid fractures	
Type I	Avulsion fracture of the anterior margin
Type IIA	Transverse fracture through glenoid fossa exiting inferiorly
Type IIB	Oblique fracture through glenoid fossa exiting inferiorly
Type III	Oblique fracture exiting superiorly and associated with acromioclavicular joint injury
Type IV	Transverse fracture through the medial border of scapula
Type V	Combination of II and IV
Type VI	Comminuted glenoid fracture
Acromion fracture	
Type I	Minimally displaced
Type II	Displaced but maintains subacromial space
Type III	Displaced with narrowing of subacromial space
Coracoid fractures	
Type I	Proximal to coracoclavicular ligament
Type II	Distal to coracoclavicular ligament
Scapulothoracic dissociation	
Type I	Musculoskeletal injury
Type IIA	Musculoskeletal injury with vascular disruption
Type IIB	Musculoskeletal injury with neurologic disruption
Type III	Musculoskeletal injury with neurologic and vascular disruption

- Malunion: Generally well tolerated but may result in scapulothoracic crepitus.
- Suprascapular nerve injury: May occur with fractures that involve the suprascapular notch.
- Scapulothoracic dissociation: Rare, life-threatening injury involving traumatic disruption of scapula from posterior chest wall; essentially a traumatic four-quarter amputation; caused by violent traction and rotational force; associated with complete (80%) or partial (15%) brachial plexopathy, subclavian or axillary artery injury (88%); may or may not have bony injury; scapula laterally displaced on chest X-ray; presents with pulseless arm, neurologic deficit, and massive shoulder swelling; increased grades of injury (▶ Table 15.5); evaluation includes angiography with urgent vascular repair, EMG, or MRI with early brachial plexus exploration, bone stabilization; limb may require amputation.

15.2.3 Proximal Humerus Fractures

- Epidemiology:
  - 4–5% of all fractures, most common humerus fracture (45%).
  - Increased incidence in older population but most (85%) are nondisplaced.
  - 2:1 female:male ratio.
- Anatomy:
  - Shoulder has the greatest range of motion of any joint in the body due to the shallow glenoid fossa that is only 25% of humeral head.
  - Major contributors to stability are not bony constraints but ligaments, muscle, and capsule.
  - Proximal humerus is 30 degrees relative to epicondylar axis.

○ The proximal humerus consists of four osseous segments (Neer classification) with associated deforming muscular forces: Humeral head, greater tuberosity (displaces superiorly and posteriorly by supraspinatus and infraspinatus), lesser tuberosity (displaces medially by subscapularis), humeral shaft (displaces medially by pectoralis major and abducts by deltoid).

○ Vascular supply: Primary blood supply is the anterior and posterior humeral circumflex arteries.

• Mechanism of injury:

○ Fall onto outstretched upper extremity is the most common cause in elderly population.

○ High-energy trauma or direct blow is most common in younger patients.

○ Pathologic fractures can also occur but are less common.

• Clinical evaluation:

○ Upper extremity is held close to the chest by contralateral extremity with pain, swelling, tenderness, limited painful range of motion, and crepitus.

○ Careful neurovascular exam with focus on axillary nerve function.

○ Standard shoulder views are sufficient on X-rays.

• Classification:

○ Neer classification: Proximal humerus divided into four parts, each part is defined as > 1 cm of displacement or 45-degree angulation (► Table 15.6).

• Nonoperative treatment:

○ Most proximal humerus fractures can be treated nonoperatively (sling immobilization for comfort followed by early shoulder motion) as they are minimally displaced or nondisplaced (85%).[14]

• Operative treatment:

○ ORIF, arthroplasty, and percutaneous pinning are the main methods for surgical fixation of proximal humerus fractures depending on the fracture pattern.

○ Two-part fracture:

– Anatomic neck: ORIF or hemiarthroplasty.

– Surgical neck: Percutaneous pinning if reducible, ORIF if irreducible.

– Greater tuberosity: ORIF with or without rotator cuff repair.

– Lesser tuberosity: Nonoperative management unless internal rotation is blocked.

– Two-part fracture dislocations can be treated nonoperatively after shoulder reduction unless the fragments are displaced.

○ Three-part fracture:

– Often requires ORIF due to unstable muscle forces making closed reduction difficult.

○ Four-part fracture:

– Highest incidence of osteonecrosis.

– Hemiarthroplasty can also be considered, especially in elderly.

– Four-part fracture dislocations should be treated operatively with ORIF in younger patients or hemiarthroplasty in the elderly.

○ Complications:

– Vascular injury: Rare, axillary artery is most commonly injured, higher rate in elderly due to atherosclerosis.

– Neural injury: Axillary nerve most common as it courses along the inferior capsule.

– Myositis ossificans: Associated with repeated attempts of closed reduction in chronic dislocations.

– Osteonecrosis[15]: 14% of three-part and 34% of four-part fractures.

– Nonunion/malunion: Soft-tissue interposition, inadequate closed reduction, or failed surgical repair.

Table 15.6 Neer classification of humeral fractures

Number of fragments	Description
One part	No displaced fragments
Two parts	Any fragment from anatomical neck, surgical neck, greater tuberosity, or lesser tuberosity
Three parts	Fragment from surgical neck plus either a greater tuberosity or lesser tuberosity fragment
Four parts	All four fragments are displaced/angulated

15.2.4 Humeral Shaft Fractures

- Epidemiology:
  - Represents 3–5% of all fractures; 2–10% are open fractures.
  - 60% involve the middle third of the diaphysis, 30% at proximal third of diaphysis, and 10% at distal third of diaphysis.
  - Peak age distribution is young males and elderly females.
- Anatomy:
  - Humeral shaft: From the pectoralis major insertion to the supracondylar ridge, tapers distally.
- Mechanism of injury:
  - Direct trauma is the most common mechanism, usually from motor vehicle crash that results in transverse or comminuted fracture patterns.
  - Indirect trauma such as fall onto outstretched arm or rotational injury results in spiral or oblique fracture patterns.
  - Fracture patterns are dependent on type of force applied.
- Clinical evaluation:
  - Pain, swelling, deformity, and shortening of the injured arm.
  - Careful neurovascular exam with attention to radial nerve function.
  - Abrasions and superficial lacerations must be distinguished from open fractures.
- Radiographic evaluation:
  - AP and lateral views including shoulder and elbow joints are obtained.
  - The patient not the arm should be rotated to obtain orthogonal views as rotating the arm will only move the distal fragment.
- Classification:
  - Classification based on position (open vs. closed; proximal third, middle third, distal third) and fracture pattern (transverse, oblique, spiral, segmental, comminuted) or OTA classification.[2]
- Nonoperative treatment[16,17]:
  - Multiple factors: Age, functional level, associated injuries, and fracture pattern.
  - Most isolated humeral shaft fractures can be treated nonoperatively.
  - Requires compliant, mobile, upright position of patient, and close follow-up and maintains reduction.
  - Significant amount of deformity can be tolerated (< 20 degrees of anterior angulation, < 30 degrees of varus/valgus angulation, and < 3 cm of shortening).
  - Reduction with gravity:
    - Hanging arm cast: Weight of arm and cast produce dependent traction to maintain reduction.
    - Coaptation splint: Utilizes hydrostatic pressure and dependent traction to maintain reduction, less distraction than hanging arm cast with more stability.
    - Thoracobrachial immobilization: Used for minimally displaced or nondisplaced fractures in elderly and children.
    - Functional bracing: Utilizes hydrostatic soft-tissue compression for alignment but allows for motion of adjacent joints.
- Operative treatment:
  - Indications: Polytrauma, inadequate closed reduction, pathologic fracture, associated neurovascular injury, floating elbow, segmental fracture, intra-articular extension, bilateral humerus fracture, or open fracture.
  - ORIF: Best functional results due to direct reduction and stable fixation.
  - Intramedullary nail: Can use flexible or interlocked nails.
  - Interlocked nails provide rotational and axial stability but have high incidence of shoulder pain due to penetration of rotator cuff.
  - External fixation: Used in cases of infections, burn patients, or extensive soft-tissue loss.
- Complications[18]:
  - Potential injury to axillary nerve during screw insertion.
  - Radial nerve injury (18% cases), most common with middle to distal third fractures as it travels along spiral groove, can also be result of attempted fracture reduction where the nerve becomes entrapped during manipulation.

- Vascular injury is uncommon but can occur with the humeral shaft lacerating the brachial artery, greatest risk in the proximal and distal third of the arm.
- Nonunion (15% cases).

15.2.5 Distal Humerus Fractures

- Epidemiology:
  - Relatively uncommon, 2% all fractures, 30% of humerus fractures.
  - Bimodal age distribution with high incidence in young males and older females.
  - Intercondylar fractures are most common; most are caused from falls landing directly on the elbow or from motor vehicle accidents.
- Anatomy:
  - Medial and lateral columns composed of nonarticulating epicondyle and articulating condyle.
  - Capitellum and trochlea projects anteriorly at about 40–45 degrees; trochlea axis (carrying angle) is approximately 3-8 degrees of valgus in relation to the longitudinal axis.
- Clinical evaluation:
  - Swelling, gross instability, and displacement are most obvious; crepitus may be present.
  - Careful neurovascular exam is needed, as the sharp bony fragments may injury the brachial artery, median nerve, or radial nerve.
- Radiographic evaluation:
  - Standard AP and lateral views of the elbow are sufficient; fat pad sign (displacement of adipose), effusions, or hemarthrosis may be present on lateral radiograph of nondisplaced fractures as indirect markers of fracture.
  - CT scans may be utilized to further visualize fracture pattern.
- Classification:
  - Descriptive on region and pattern: Supracondylar, transcondylar, intercondylar, condylar, capitellum, trochlea, lateral epicondyle, and medial epicondyle or OTA classification.[2]
- Nonoperative treatment:
  - Indicated for either nondisplaced or minimally displaced fractures or for severely comminuted fractures in elderly patients with limited functional abilities.[19]
  - Posterior splint immobilization for 1–2 weeks followed by early range-of-motion exercises in a hinged brace.
  - Frequent radiographic follow-up is needed to monitor maintenance of reduction and healing.
- Operative treatment[20]:
  - General treatment principles: anatomic articular reduction, stable internal fixation of articular surface, restoration of articular axial alignment, stable internal fixation of articular segment to metaphysis, early elbow range of motion.
  - Significantly displaced fractures, open fracture, vascular injury, or failure of nonoperative management/inability to maintain reduction.
  - ORIF with plate and screws fixation is the preferred treatment method.
  - Total elbow arthroplasty may also be considered but only if the distal humerus is deemed non-reconstructible and the patient had good preinjury functional abilities.
- Complications:
  - Volkmann contractures are the result of unrecognized compartment syndrome of the volar compartment.
  - Loss of elbow range of motion is a common complication from fractures around the elbow, as stiffness results from prolonged immobilization, callus formation in the olecranon fossa limits extension, capsular contraction restricts flexion; range-of-motion exercises should begin as soon as possible to prevent loss of motion[21].
  - Heterotopic bone formation may occur.
  - Posttraumatic arthritis results from injury to articular surface and failure to restore articular congruity[22].
  - Neurologic injury: Ulnar nerve is most commonly injured (15 of cases).

15.2.6 Olecranon Fractures

- Epidemiology:
  - 8–10% of elbow fractures.
  - Bimodal distribution, younger patients (high-energy trauma) versus elderly (falls).
- Anatomy:
  - Articulation with the trochlea allows for only flexion–extension motion but provides the intrinsic stability of the elbow joint.
  - Triceps tendon envelops the articular capsule before inserting into the olecranon; displacement results in loss of elbow extension.
  - Subcutaneous position makes the olecranon susceptible to direct trauma.
- Mechanism of injury:
  - Direct trauma: Comminuted olecranon fracture.
  - Indirect trauma: Strong eccentric contraction of triceps on flexed elbow produces transverse or oblique fracture.
- Clinical evaluation:
  - Injured extremity typically supported by contralateral hand in flexed position.
  - Palpable defect at the olecranon with inability to extend elbow.
  - Careful neurovascular exam is needed due to likelihood of ulnar nerve injury.
- Radiographic evaluation:
  - Standard AP and lateral views of the elbow need to be obtained and are usually enough to demonstrate the extent of fracture, comminution, and displacement.
  - Schatzker or Mayo classification used (▶ Table 15.7).
- Treatment goals:
  - Restoration of articular surface.
  - Restoration and preservation of elbow extensor mechanism.
  - Restoration of elbow motion and prevention of stiffness.
- Nonoperative treatment:
  - Nondisplaced fractures and displaced fractures in low-functioning individuals.
  - Immobilization in long arm splint in 45–90 degrees of flexion. Protected range of motion can begin in 3 weeks avoiding active flexion and extension past 90 degrees.
- Operative treatment:
  - Indications include disruption of extensor mechanism or articular incongruity.
  - Tension band wiring is the treatment of choice. Converts tensile forces to compressive forces.
  - Intramedullary fixation.
  - ORIF.

Table 15.7 Schatzker and Mayo classifications of olecranon fractures

Schatzker classification	
Type A	Simple transverse
Type B	Transverse impacted
Type C	Oblique
Type D	Comminuted
Type E	More distal fracture, extra-articular
Type F	Fracture dislocation
Mayo classification	
Type I	Undisplaced
Type II	Displaced, stable
	A: noncomminuted, B: comminuted
Type III	Unstable
	A: noncomminuted, B: comminuted

○ Excision of fragment with repair of triceps tendon.
- Complications[23]:
  ○ Symptomatic hardware (80% of patients) is the most common complication, up to 66% of patients may require removal.
  ○ Infection, pin migration, ulnar nerve injury, heterotopic ossification, and decreased range of motion (50%) are all possible.

15.2.7 Radial Head Fractures

- Epidemiology:
  ○ Up to 5.4% of all fractures and 30% of all elbow fractures.
  ○ 30% with associated injuries to shoulder, humerus, forearm, or wrist.
- Anatomy:
  ○ Capitellum and radial head are reciprocally curved; force transmission across the radiocapitellar articulation occurs at all angles of elbow flexion and is greatest in extension.
  ○ Radial head contributes to valgus stability of the elbow as a secondary restraint especially if there are injuries to ligamentous and muscle-tendon restraints.
- Mechanism of injury:
  ○ Most injuries are from fall onto outstretched hand, from height or sports related.
  ○ Radial head fracture occurs from impact onto the capitellum from axial load, rotational force, or from posterior dislocation of the radial head.
  ○ Ligamentous injuries are frequent.
- Clinical evaluation:
  ○ Pain with elbow motion and forearm rotation.
  ○ Tenderness directly over the radial head may be present with an effusion.
  ○ Examination of the ipsilateral distal forearm and wrist should be performed to evaluate for an Essex-Lopresti lesion (see below).
- Radiographic evaluation:
  ○ Standard AP and lateral views of the elbow.
  ○ Oblique views (Greenspan view): Further visualizes the radiocapitellar articulation, performed with the forearm in neutral rotation with the beam directed 45 degrees inferiorly.
  ○ Associated forearm and wrist pain imaged appropriately.
- Classification:
  ○ Mason classification (▶ Table 15.8) used.
- Nonoperative treatment:
  ○ Most radial head fractures can be treated nonoperatively.
  ○ Sling and early range of motion are advocated.
  ○ Injection of local anesthesia into the joint may provide pain relief.
- Operative treatment:
  ○ Correct forearm rotation, maintain range of motion in elbow and forearm, stabilization of elbow and forearm.
  ○ Surgical indications depend on the fracture pattern.
  ○ ORIF is indicated for simple fracture patterns with a rotational block and adequate bone stock, optimal fracture patterns typically have three or fewer bony fragments without deformity that can accept screw fixation[24].

Table 15.8 Mason classification of radial fractures

Type	Description
I	Nondisplaced fractures
II	Marginal fractures of the radial head with displacement
III	Comminuted fractures involving the entire radial head
IV	Associated elbow dislocation

- ○ Prosthetic replacement of the radial head is indicated in comminuted fractures involving the entire radial head in unstable injuries, act as spacers to prevent proximal migration of the radius[25].
- ○ Radial head excision is a last resort option in certain cases.
- ○ Essex-Lopresti lesion:
  - – Longitudinal disruption of forearm interosseous ligament with radial head fracture/dislocation and distal radial ulnar joint injury, easy to miss, and difficulty to diagnose.
  - – Treatment involves stabilizing the elbow and distal radioulnar joint.
- • Complications:
  - ○ Contractures from immobilization, pain, or inflammation may represent a osteochondral lesion of the capitellum.
  - ○ Chronic wrist pain from unrecognized interosseus ligament, DRUJ, or triangular fibrocartilage complex.
  - ○ Posttraumatic radiocapitellar arthritis.

15.2.8 Radius and Ulna Shaft Fractures

- • Epidemiology:
  - ○ More common in men than in women due to higher incidence of motor vehicle accidents, athletic competition, altercations, and falls from height.
  - ○ Second highest ratio of open fractures after tibia.
- • Anatomy:
  - ○ Forearm resembles a ring; fracture on either bone will result in either a fracture or dislocation of the other forearm bone proximally or distally.
  - ○ Ulna acts as the axis for the radius to rotate around in supination and pronation; lateral curvature of the radius allows for rotation to occur (radial bow).
  - ○ Interosseous membrane occupies the space between the radius and ulna.
  - ○ Deforming muscle forces are determined by fracture location.
- • Fractures of both radius and ulna shaft:
  - ○ Most commonly caused by high-energy injuries or direct trauma such as protecting one's head, sporting events, or gunshot wounds.
  - ○ Clinical evaluation:
    - – Gross deformity of the forearm with swelling, pain, and loss of hand/forearm function.
    - – Careful neurovascular exam of radial and ulnar pulses and radial, median, and ulnar nerves.
    - – Ulna border is subcutaneous and open wounds easily connect to fracture site creating open fracture.
    - – Excruciating, unremitting pain with swollen compartments may indicate pending compartment syndrome.
  - ○ Radiographic evaluation:
    - – AP and lateral views should include the entire length of the forearm.
    - – Ipsilateral wrist and elbow films should also be obtained to rule out associated fracture or dislocation.
  - ○ Classification: Descriptive patterns include open versus closed, location, comminution, displacement, angulation, and rotational alignment.
  - ○ Nonoperative treatment: Rarely nonoperative as very difficult to maintain the reduction.
  - ○ Operative treatment[26,27]:
    - – ORIF with plate and screw fixation is the treatment of choice for radius and ulna shaft fractures.
    - – Goals of ORIF include restoring length, restoring alignment, and restoring the radial bow which is essential for rotational function.
    - – External fixation may be used in cases with severe bone or soft-tissue loss, gross contamination, or infected settings.
- • Fractures of the ulna shaft:
  - ○ Nightstick fracture: Direct trauma to the ulna while attempting to protect one's head.
  - ○ Monteggia fractures: Proximal ulna fractures with radial head dislocation.

○ Clinical evaluation:
– Pain, swelling, tenderness, deformity, and painful range of motion can be present.
○ Radiographic evaluation:
– AP and lateral views of forearm along with complete views of elbow and wrist obtained.
○ Classification:
– Descriptive patterns include open versus closed, location, comminution, displacement, angulation, and rotational alignment.
– The Bado classification is used for Monteggia fractures (▶ Table 15.9).
○ Nonoperative treatment:
– Nondisplaced or minimally displaced nightstick fracture may be treated with splint immobilization for 7–10 days followed by functional bracing for range-of-motion exercises. Close follow-up is needed to assess maintenance of reduction.
○ Operative treatment:
– Displacement of more than 10-degree angulation in any direction or > 50% displacement of the shaft requires ORIF.
– All Monteggia fractures require ORIF with plate fixation, closed reduction of the radial head is done first followed by fixation of the ulna shaft.
○ Complications:
– Radial and/or median nerve injury along with their terminal branches; the anterior/posterior interosseous nerve may be injured during initial injury or as a result of surgery.
– Radial head instability may occur if the ulna is poorly reduced[28].
• Fractures of radial shaft:
○ Proximal fractures of the radial shaft may be isolated.
○ Distal third radial shaft fractures are assumed to be associated with a distal radioulnar joint injury unless proven otherwise.
○ Galeazzi fracture: Fracture of the distal third of radius with distal radioulnar joint disruption.
○ Reverse Galeazzi fracture: Distal third ulna fracture with associated distal radioulnar joint disruption.
○ Mechanism of injury:
– Direct trauma to the forearm or indirect trauma such as fall onto outstretched hand.
– Proximal radial shaft has more soft-tissue musculature surrounding it; so, most injuries that fracture the proximal radius also fracture the ulna.
– Galeazzi fractures may result from direct trauma to the wrist, typically on the dorsolateral aspect or fall onto outstretched hand with forearm pronation.
– Reverse Galeazzi fractures can result from fall onto outstretched hand with forearm supination.
○ Clinical evaluation:
– Pain, swelling, point tenderness at the fracture site are typically present.
– Elbow range of motion, supination, and pronation should be assessed.
○ Radiographic evaluation:
– AP and lateral views of the forearm, elbow, and wrist should all be obtained.
– Radiographic signs of distal radioulnar joint injury include fracture at base of ulnar styloid, widened distal radioulnar joint, subluxed ulna, or radial shortening.
○ Treatment:
– Nondisplaced proximal radius fractures can be treated in a cast, close follow-up is required, and loss of reduction or radial bow is indication for ORIF.
– All Galeazzi fractures require ORIF as nonoperative management is associated with a high rate of failure.

Table 15.9 Bado classification for Monteggia fractures

Type	Description
I	Anterior dislocation of the radial head with anterior angulation of ulna shaft fracture
II	Posterior dislocation of the radial head with posterior angulation of the ulna shaft fracture
III	Lateral dislocation of the radial head with ulna fracture
IV	Anterior dislocation of the radial head with both radius and ulna fractured at the same level

– Kirschner wire fixation may be used to maintain reduction of the distal radioulnar joint.
○ Complications[29]:
– Malunion results from nonanatomic reduction of the radius and loss of radial bow needed for supination/pronation.
– Compartment syndrome.
– Nerve injury is usually iatrogenic from surgical repair.
– Recurrent radial head dislocation may occur from poor radial reduction.

15.2.9 Distal Radius

- Epidemiology:
  ○ Among the most common fractures of upper extremity, represent approximately 1/6 of all fractures treated in emergency departments.
  ○ Incidence increases in elderly patients due to osteopenia similar to hip fractures.
  ○ Risk factors include decreased bone mineral density, female, white ethnicity, family history, and early menopause.
- Anatomy:
  ○ 80% of axial load is supported by distal radius versus 20% by ulna and triangular fibrocartilage complex.
  ○ Numerous ligamentous attach to distal radius and often remain intact facilitating reduction.
- Mechanism of injury:
  ○ Fall onto outstretched hand is the most common mechanism with wrist extended.
  ○ High-energy injuries may result in significantly displaced or highly comminuted unstable fractures to the distal radius.
- Clinical evaluation:
  ○ Wrist deformity, hand displacement, swelling, ecchymosis, tenderness, and painful range of motion noted.
  ○ Ipsilateral elbow and shoulder should be examined for associated injuries.
  ○ Careful neurovascular exam with particular attention to median nerve function.
- Radiographic evaluation:
  ○ AP and lateral views of the wrist obtained, oblique views may also be used.
- Classification:
  ○ Multiple classification schemes for the distal radius exist based on intra-articular involvement, mechanism based, or descriptive.
  ○ Multiple eponyms for distal radius fracture:
    – Colles fracture: Dorsal angulation or dorsal displacement of the distal fragment, 90% of distal radius fractures are pattern, fall onto extended hand, radially deviated wrist with forearm pronation.
    – Smith fracture: Aka reverse Colles fracture, palmar angulation, or displacement of the distal fragment, fall onto flexed wrist with forearm supination.
    – Barton fracture: Shearing mechanism resulting in fracture/dislocation of the wrist where the rim of the distal radius is displaced, fall onto extended wrist with forearm fixed in pronation.
    – Chauffeur's fracture, backfire fracture, Hutchinson fracture: Avulsion fracture of radial styloid, compression of scaphoid against the radius with the wrist extended and ulnar deviated.
- Nonoperative treatment:
  ○ Radiologic parameters for acceptable closed reduction depending on radial length (within 2–3 mm of normal), palmar tilt (0–10 degrees of dorsal angulation), intra-articular step-off (< 2 mm), radial inclination (< 5-degree loss).
  ○ Loss of reduction is associated with initial displacement of the fracture, age, and comminution.
  ○ All displaced fractures should undergo initial closed reduction even if surgical treatment is needed in the future to limit swelling, provide pain relief, and minimize median nerve compression.
  ○ Splinting is done initially due to swelling followed by casting once swelling subsides.
  ○ Extreme flexion of wrist is to be avoided, as it increases pressure inside the carpal tunnel.
  ○ Immobilization is needed for 6 weeks or until radiologic evidence of healing.

- Operative:
  - Indications for surgical intervention include high-energy injury mechanism, loss of initial reduction, articular comminution, bone loss, distal radioulnar joint incongruity, and open fractures.
  - Percutaneous pinning: Used for extra-articular or two-part intra-articular fractures, used to supplement casting or external fixation.
  - External fixation[30]: Spanning external fixation using ligamentotaxis can restore radial length and radial inclination but not palmar tilt, usually not sufficient to prevent collapse and is supplemented by percutaneous pinning; nonspanning external fixation stabilizes the distal radius fragment alone but requires a large distal radius fragment.
  - ORIF: Dorsal plating versus palmar plating of the distal radius fragment.
  - Complications:
    – Median nerve injury may occur from the initial injury or after closed reduction and manipulation[31].
    – Malunion/nonunion from poor reduction or fixation.
    – Arthritis.
    – Finger, wrist, elbow stiffness from prolonged immobilization.
    – Tendon rupture[32]: Specifically extensor pollicis longus has been associated with distal radius fractures as an early or late complication due to disruption of the tendon sheath or from irritation from healing callus.

15.2.10 Carpal Bone Fractures

- Epidemiology:
  - Approximate incidence: Scaphoid (68.2%), triquetrum (18.3%), trapezium (4.3%), lunate (3.9%), capitate (1.9%), hamate (1.7%), pisiform (1.3%), trapezoid (0.4%).
  - 70% are fractures to scaphoid/proximal row.
- Anatomy:
  - Proximal row: Scaphoid, lunate, triquetrum, pisiform.
  - Distal row: Trapezium, trapezoid, capitates, hamate; connected by strong ligaments to the metacarpals and less mobile.
  - Lunate is key to carpal stability.
  - Zero-degree capitolunate angle is a straight line down the third metacarpal shaft, capitates, lunate, and radial shaft.
  - Extrinsic ligaments connect the radius to carpal bones and carpal bones to the metacarpals, intrinsic ligaments connect the carpal bones to each other, and palmar ligaments are stronger than dorsal ligaments.
  - Triangular fibrocartilage complex: Major stabilizer of the ulnar carpal bones and distal radioulnar joint, "meniscus of the wrist," absorbs 20% of axial load across the wrist joint.
  - Transverse arterial arches are formed by radial, ulna, and anterior interosseous arteries.
  - Blood supply to the scaphoid comes primarily from radial artery, palmar scaphoid branches supply the distal 20–30% of the scaphoid, and dorsal braches supply proximal 70–80% forming a watershed area at the scaphoid waist and makes it susceptible to nonunions.[33]
  - Normal motion: 70-degree flexion, 70-degree extension, 20-degree radial deviation, 40-degree ulnar deviation.
- Mechanism of injury: Most common mechanism is fall onto outstretched hand resulting in axial compressive force and the wrist hyperextended.
- Clinical evaluation: Well-localized tenderness is the most consistent sign, gross deformity may be present, and provocative tests may indicate individual carpal bone injury.
- Radiographic evaluation:
  - AP and lateral films of the wrist are taken in neutral position. The Gilula lines are three smooth radiographic curves along the proximal carpal row and the distal carpal row seen on AP view. Disruption of these arcs suggests ligamentous instability.
  - Special views of the carpal bones include the scaphoid view, oblique view, and clenched fist view.
  - CT scans are useful to evaluate carpal fractures, malunion, nonunion, and bone loss.
  - MRIs are sensitive to occult fractures and osteonecrosis along with soft-tissue disruptions.

- Specific fractures:
  - Scaphoid:
    - Most common carpal bone fracture, divided into proximal pole, tubercle, waist, and distal pole.
    - Fractures of the waist or proximal one-third depend on fracture union for revascularization.
    - Presents with tenderness to palpation over the anatomic snuffbox; special tests include scaphoid shift test and Watson test.
    - Initial X-rays may be nondiagnostic 25% of the time; if clinical suspicion of fracture, then trial of immobilization followed by repeat films in 1–2 weeks may demonstrate fracture.[34]
    - Classified based on fracture pattern, displacement, or location.
    - Nonoperative treatment: Indicated for nondisplaced distal one-third or tuberosity fractures; immobilization in thumb spica cast until fracture is performed.
    - Expected time to union is 6–8 weeks for distal 1/3, 8–12 weeks for middle 1/3, and 12–24 weeks for proximal 1/3.
    - Operative treatment: Indications include displacement > 1 mm, increased radiolunate or scapholunate angles, or nonunion, treated with placement of screws across fracture line percutaneously or ORIF.
    - Complications: Delayed union, nonunion, or malunion with delays in treatment; osteonecrosis is most common with fractures to proximal pole due to blood supply.
  - Lunate:
    - Fourth most fractured carpal bone, referred to as carpal keystone as it is well protected and anchored by interosseous ligaments.
    - Presents with tenderness to palpation on the dorsal wrist overlying distal radius.
    - AP and lateral X-rays usually not sufficient to visualize lunate fractures due to overlap of other carpal bones; CT scans are the best at demonstrating fractures.
    - Nonoperative treatment used for nondisplaced fractures via splint/cast immobilization with close follow-up to evaluate healing; operative treatment used for displaced or angulated fractures.
    - Complications: Osteonecrosis of the lunate may result in collapse and radiocarpal degeneration requiring further surgical intervention.
  - Triquetrum:
    - Second most commonly fractured carpal bone after scaphoid.
    - Most are avulsion or impaction injuries.
    - Presents with tenderness on the dorsoulnar aspect of the wrist.
    - AP, lateral, and oblique views may all be needed to fully visualize triquetral fractures.
    - Treatment is with short arm splint/cast for nondisplaced or chip fractures; displaced fractures require surgical fixation.
  - Pisiform:
    - Rare fracture type.
    - Presents with tenderness to volar aspect of wrist.
    - Poorly visualized on standard AP and lateral views; special views are needed to properly visualize the pisiform.
    - Treatment is similar to other carpal bone fractures.
  - Trapezium:
    - High likelihood of poor outcomes due to degenerative changes.
    - Caused by forceful adduction of the thumb driving the first metacarpal into the trapezium.
    - Tenderness to the radial aspect of wrist with painful motion of the first metacarpal joint.
    - Standard AP and lateral views are usually sufficient to identify the fractures.
    - Treatment is similar to other carpal bone fractures; immobilization for nondisplaced fractures in thumb spica cast; surgical treatment for displaced, comminuted, or carpometacarpal joint involvement.
  - Trapezoid:
    - Rare fractures due to position of trapezoid at the base of second metacarpal.
    - Tenderness at the base of second metacarpal and painful range of motion may be present.
    - AP view may be sufficient enough to visualize trapezoid fractures. Oblique view or CT scan may be needed if details are obscured by overlap.
    - Treatment is the same principle as other carpal bones.

○ Capitate:
  – Rare fracture.
  – May be more likely fractured in perilunate dislocation.
  – Fractures can be seen on scaphoid view X-rays.
  – Requires closed reduction to reduce risk of osteonecrosis, otherwise surgical fixation is needed to restore normal anatomy.
○ Hamate:
  – Multiple potential articular fracture sites; fracture of the hook is a frequent athletic injury when the palm is struck by an object; distal hamate fractures may occur with fifth metacarpal injuries.
  – Can usually be visualized on AP view of the wrist; carpal tunnel view may be needed to visualize the hook of hamate fracture; CT scan may be best modality.
  – Treatment is similar to other carpal bone fractures, immobilization for nondisplaced fractures; displaced fractures may be fixed with pinning or screws; hook of the hamate fractures may also be excised.
  – Complications: Nonunion, ulnar/median neuropathy, or flexor tendon ruptures of the small finger.
○ Perilunate dislocations and fracture dislocations.
  – Load is applied to the thenar eminence and transmitted from radial to ulnar direction.
  – Lunate can dislocate palmarly out of the lunate fossa of the distal radius creating a lunate dislocation.
  – Presents with tenderness distal to Lister tubercle and generalized swelling.
  – AP and lateral X-rays are usually sufficient; CT scan may be useful for details; lateral X-ray most important and shows spilled tea cup sign with palmar dislocation of lunate.
  – Described by Mayfield classification (▶ Table 15.10), sequence of progressive perilunate instability as the injury spreads.
  – Close reduction with or without pinning requires adequate sedation for manipulation, early surgical reconstruction is performed if swelling permits, and immediate surgery is needed if there is median nerve compromise.
  – Complications include median neuropathy from compression, posttraumatic arthritis, chronic perilunate injury with instability, pain, and deformity.
○ Carpal dislocation:
  – Continuum of perilunate dislocations with lunate dislocation as the final stage due to fall onto outstretched hand or direct trauma.
  – Present with painful, limited range of motion and possible median neuropathy; specific maneuvers for carpal instability may be done.
  – Most carpal dislocations can be diagnosed with AP and lateral X-rays.
  – Carpal dislocations need to be reduced and immobilized; irreducible dislocations or unstable injuries can be treated with ORIF.
  – Complications include arthritis or recurrent instability.
○ Scapholunate dissociation:
  – Ligamentous analog of scaphoid fracture.
  – Most common and significant ligamentous disruption of the wrist due to loading of extended carpus in ulnar deviation.
  – Presents with tenderness of the wrist, pain with hand grip, decreased grip strength, painful range of motion.
  – AP, lateral, clenched fist, supinated AP, and radial/ulnar deviated films are obtained. A "Terry Thomas" sign is widening of the scapholunate space.
  – Treatment is with closed or open reduction with percutaneous pinning.

Table 15.10 Mayfield classification of scapholunate joint

Stage	Description
I	Disruption of scapholunate joint
II	Disruption of midcarpal joint
III	Disruption of lunotriquetral joint
IV	Disruption of radiolunate joint

15.2.11 Hand Fractures

- Epidemiology:
  - Metacarpal and phalange fractures are very common, comprising 10% of all fractures.
  - Fracture incidence: Distal phalanx (45%) followed by metacarpals (30%), proximal phalanx (15%), and middle phalanx (10%).
  - Sports injuries and work-related injuries are most common causes.
- Mechanism of injury:
  - A variety of mechanisms account for the injury to the hand.
  - Axial loading is frequently sustained during sports or reaching for objects such as catching a falling object.
  - Diaphyseal fractures and dislocations usually require a bending component in the mechanism of injury.
  - Individual digits can easily be caught in workplace equipment, clothes, furniture causing spiral fractures or dislocations.
  - Industrial settings with heavy equipment lead to crush injuries.
- Clinical examination:
  - Important aspects of hand examination include digit viability, neurologic status including sensation and motor function, deformity, range of motion, and soft-tissue disruption.
  - AP, lateral, and oblique of the hand should be obtained; individual films of injured digits should be maintained to reduce overlap.
- Classification[35]:
  - Descriptive: Open versus closed injury, bone involvement and location, fracture pattern (comminuted, transverse, spiral), displacement and deformity, extra-articular versus intra-articular, stable versus unstable.
  - Open fractures in the hand are classified differently than other parts of the body:
    - Type I: Clean wound without significant contamination or delay in treatment; treated with primary wound closure.
    - Type II: Contamination with gross dirt/debris, bite injury, water injury, or barnyard injury; treated with delayed wound closure.
- General treatment principles:
  - Fight bite injuries: Any laceration overlying a joint in the hand must be assumed to be from a tooth and contaminated with oral flora, broad-spectrum antibiotics including anaerobic coverage and irrigation and debridement.
  - Animal bites: Requires coverage for Pasteurella and Eikenella.
  - Five treatment methods for hand injuries: Immediate motion, temporary splinting, closed reduction and pinning, ORIF, immediate reconstruction.
  - General indications for surgery include open fracture, unstable fracture, irreducible fracture, bone loss, and tendon lacerations.
  - Treatment of stable fractures is with buddy taping or splinting.
  - Unstable fractures or irreducible fractures require pinning or internal fixation.
- Specific fracture patterns:
  - Metacarpals:
    - Fractures of the metacarpals can be at the head, neck, shaft, or base.
    - Fourth and fifth metacarpals can usually tolerate greater deformity than the second and third metacarpals.
    - Most metacarpal fractures can be treated with splinting and immobilization.
    - Metacarpal head fractures require anatomic reduction to reestablish joint congruity.
    - Rotational deformity is the least tolerated deformity; > 10-degree malrotation is the upper limit of normal for metacarpal shaft fractures.
    - Surgical fixation includes closed reduction/pinning, ORIF with screws, nails, or plates.
  - Metacarpal base:
    - Fractures of the metacarpal base for digits 2–5 usually involve carpal–metacarpal fracture dislocations.

- Special attention is needed to the thumb metacarpal base fractures.
- Extra-articular fractures can usually be treated with closed reduction and immobilization.
- Intra-articular fractures are usually unstable and require surgery.
- Bennett fracture: Oblique fracture line through first metacarpal base.
- Rolando fracture: Comminuted fracture pattern in the shape of "T" or "Y."
○ Proximal and distal phalanges:
  - Intra-articular condylar fractures of the base of the phalanx require surgical fixation for anatomic reduction of the joint space and are difficult to maintain the reduction in splint.
  - Shaft fractures are treated with pinning or ORIF if displaced or unstable; closed reduction should be attempted first but may be difficult to maintain due to pull of the flexor digitorum superficialis muscle.
○ Distal phalanx:
  - Mallet finger is avulsion fracture of the extensor tendon off distal phalanx, may be purely ligamentous, treatment is controversial.
  - Jersey finger: Avulsion of flexor digitorum profundus, most commonly involving ring finger, treatment is primary repair.
  - Extra-articular fractures are transverse, longitudinal, or comminuted, treated with splinting with aluminum finger splints.

15.3 Lower Extremity Fractures

Jim Lai and Mohit Gilotra

15.3.1 Pelvic Fracture

- Epidemiology[36,37]:
  ○ Under age of 35, more common in males. Over age of 35, more common in females.
- Anatomy:
  ○ Pelvic ring consists of sacrum and two innominate bones joined anteriorly at symphysis and posteriorly at sacroiliac joints
  ○ Stability maintained by ligamentous structures from sacrum to ilium, the sacroiliac ligamentous complex (anterior and posterior), sacrotuberous ligament, and sacrospinous ligaments
- Mechanism of injury:
  ○ High-energy blunt force trauma, crush injuries. 1–15% mortality for closed fractures, 50% mortality for open fractures.
  ○ High-energy mechanisms in younger people versus low energy in elderly.
- Subtypes:
  ○ Anterior inferior iliac spine avulsion injury: Forceful avulsion from rectus femoris muscle during hip extension, most common in ages 14–17 from sports with kicking, managed conservatively.
  ○ Anterior superior iliac spine avulsion injury.
  ○ Duverney fracture: Isolated iliac wing fracture from direct blow.
  ○ Malgaigne fracture: Vertical sheer injury with two ipsilateral pelvic rings, fracture anterior and posterior to acetabulum, associated with disruption of the ipsilateral pubic rami and sacroiliac joint or public symphysis diastasis, unstable lateral fragment containing acetabulum.
  ○ Wind-swept pelvis fracture: Unilateral anteroposterior compression and contralateral compression injury.
  ○ Pelvic bucket handle fracture: Ipsilateral superior and inferior pubic rami fracture with contralateral sacroiliac joint disruption.
  ○ Pelvic insufficiency fracture: Osteoporotic fracture commonly in sacrum, medial ileum, supra-acetabular region, iliac wing, pubic rami, or parasymphyseal.
  ○ Open book fracture: High-energy anteroposterior compression fracture to both anterior (public diastasis, sacrotuberous or sacrospinous ligamentous disruption, pubic rami fracture) and posterior (sacroiliac joint widening or diastasis, ilium fracture, sacral ala fracture) injuries, associated with vascular and urethral injuries, significant morbidity, and mortality.

- ○ Pubic rami fracture.
- • Sacroiliac (SI) joint:
  - ○ Incomplete (posterior ligaments intact, vertically stable, rotationally unstable), complete (vertically and rotationally unstable), fracture-dislocation/crescent fracture (iliac wing injury into SI joint).
  - ○ Ligaments: Sacrospinous, sacrotuberous, anterior sacroiliac, posterior sacroiliac.
  - ○ No clear classification system.
  - ○ Treatment: Skeletal traction (vertical translation of hemipelvis), ORIF (anterior and/or posterior ring, ilium).
  - ○ Complications: DVT, neurovascular injury, nonunion/malunion.
- • Clinical evaluation:
  - ○ Full trauma evaluation due to likely high energy injury mechanism.
  - ○ Associated with polytrauma (head/abdominal injury, spine fracture, long bone injury, chest injury).
  - ○ Abnormal lower limb positioning (rotation or length), ecchymosis or hematoma, vaginal and rectal exam to evaluate sphincter and perirectal sensation, urogenital exam.
  - ○ Pelvic instability test should only be done once so as to not disrupt the clot.
- • Radiographic evaluation:
  - ○ AP, inlet, outlet views of the pelvis.
  - ○ CT scan to evaluate posterior pelvis.
- • Sacral fractures:
  - ○ Forceful axial loading of spine and pelvis fractures the sacrum through the neural foramina.
  - ○ Classification of sacral fractures is the Denis Classification
    - – Denis I: Lateral to foramen.
    - – Denis II: Through foramen.
    - – Denis III: Medial to foramen.
  - ○ Additional injury to SI joint and SI ligaments are incorporated into Young–Burgess Classification I joint).
- • Classification: Tile (▶ Table 15.11) and Young–Burgess (▶ Table 15.12) used.
- • Treatment:

Table 15.11 Tile classification of pelvic fractures

A: Stable	
A1	Fracture not involving the ring
A2	Stable or minimally displaced fracture of the ring
A3	Transverse sacral fracture (Denis zone III sacral fracture)
B: Rotationally unstable, vertically stable	
B1	Open book injury (external rotation)
B2	Lateral compression injury (internal rotation)
• B2–1	With anterior ring rotation/displacement through ipsilateral rami
• B2–2	With anterior ring rotation/displacement through contralateral rami
B3	Bilateral
C: Rotationally and vertically unstable	
C1	Unilateral
• C1–1	Iliac fracture
• C1–2	Sacroiliac fracture dislocation
• C1–3	Sacral fracture
C2	Bilateral with one side type B and one side type C
C3	Bilateral with both sides type C

Table 15.12 Young–Burgess classification of pelvic fractures

Anterior posterior compression (APC)	
APC I	Symphysis widened < 2.5 cm
APC II	Symphysis widened > 2.5 cm, anterior sacroiliac (SI) joint diastasis, posterior SI ligament intact, disruption of sacrospinous and sacrotuberous ligaments, rotationally unstable
APC III	Disruption of anterior SI, posterior SI, sacrospinous and sacrotuberous ligaments; associated with vascular injury, vertically and rotationally unstable
Lateral compression (LC)	
LC I	Oblique or transverse ramus fracture, ipsilateral anterior sacral ala compression fracture
LC II	Rami fracture, ipsilateral posterior ilium fracture dislocation (crescent fracture)
LC III	Ipsilateral lateral compression and contralateral APC (windswept pelvis)
Vertical shear (VS)	
VS	Vertical pelvis or hemipelvis displacement, associated with high risk of vascular injury

- ○ Management of hemorrhage (80% venous, 10–20% arterial, most common arteries: Superior gluteal, internal pudendal, obturator), resuscitation, pelvic binder/sheet, external fixation, angiography with embolization.
- ○ External fixation: Used for pelvic ring injuries with external rotation or unstable ring resulting in ongoing blood loss.
- ○ Indications for ORIF (symphysis diastasis > 2.5 cm, sacroiliac joint displacement > 1 cm, sacral fracture with
  displacement > 1 cm, malalignment of hemipelvis, open fracture, fracture diastasis > 4–6 cm).
- ○ Diverting colostomy (used in perineal injury or rectal involvement).
- • Surgical stabilization goals: Anterior ring, cposterior ring, acetabular and pelvis.
- • Associated injuries[38,39,40]: L5 nerve root, DVT (60% pelvic fractures), PE (25% pelvic fractures), infection, urogenital injury (12–20% of pelvic fractures), bladder rupture.

15.3.2 Acetabular Fracture

- • Anatomy:
  - ○ Described as a two column construct forming an inverted Y.
  - ○ Anterior column: Extends from iliac crest to the pubic symphysis containing the anterior wall of the acetabulum.
  - ○ Posterior column: Extends from superior gluteal notch to the ischial tuberosity and includes posterior wall of acetabulum.
- • Mechanism of injury:
  - ○ Usually due to high energy trauma.
  - ○ Fracture pattern depends on position of the femoral head in the acetabulum at time of injury, force, and age of patient.
- • Clinical evaluation:
  - ○ Trauma evaluation is usually necessary.
  - ○ Careful assessment of neurovascular status as sciatic nerve injury is common, especially with posterior dislocations.
  - ○ Ipsilateral extremity injuries in the knee must be ruled out.
- • Radiographic evaluation:
  - ○ AP and Judet views (oblique) of the pelvis are obtained.
  - ○ Evaluation of iliopectineal line (anterior column), ilioischial line (posterior column), anterior wall, posterior wall, and dome of acetabulum.
  - ○ CT scans can better help identify fracture pattern.

Table 15.13 Judet and Letournel classification of acetabular fractures

Elemental acetabular fractures	Associated acetabular fractures
Anterior wall	T-shaped[a]
Posterior wall[a]	Transverse with posterior wall[a]
Anterior column	Posterior column and posterior wall
Posterior column	Both columns[a]
Transverse[a]	Anterior column/wall with posterior hemitransverse

[a] Account for 80% of fractures.

- Judet and Letournel classification commonly used (▶ Table 15.13)[41]: Divided into five elemental (posterior column, posterior wall, anterior column, anterior wall, transverse) and five associated fracture patterns.
- Diagnosis: X-rays (AP, Judet/oblique, inlet/outlet; evaluation of iliopectineal line/anterior column, ilioischial line/posterior column, anterior wall, posterior wall, superior weight bearing roof, angulation of femoral head) and CT scan with 3D reconstruction can be helpful in identifying fracture type.
- Treatment:
  - Nonoperative: Displacement less than 3 mm, maintenance of roof arcs greater than 45 degrees, and smaller fragments < 20% are generally nonoperative; quality of reduction correlates most with clinical outcome.[42]
  - ORIF (< 3 weeks from injury, roof displacement > 2 mm, unstable fracture pattern, impaction, intra-articular loose body, irreducible fracture dislocation; column vs. wall fixation strategies, anterior vs. posterior approaches).[43]
- Total hip arthroplasty for fractures: Used in elderly, osteopenia, significant fracture comminution; anterior versus posterior approaches.[44]
- Complications: Posttraumatic degenerative joint disease, heterotopic ossification, osteonecrosis (6–7%), DVT/PE, infection, bleeding, neurovascular injury, hardware malposition.

15.3.3 Femoral Fracture

- Femoral neck fractures:
  - Epidemiology:
    - One of the most common fractures that occurs especially in the elderly.
    - Over 250,000 hip fractures annually with 50% involving the femoral neck.
    - Younger patients tend to sustain femoral neck fractures through high-energy trauma.
  - Anatomy:
    - Neck–shaft angle is approximately 130 degrees.
    - Femoral anteversion is approximately 10 degrees.
    - Hip joint capsule attachment extends to intertrochanteric line with three ligaments, iliofemoral, pubofemoral, and ischiofemoral.
  - Mechanism of injury:
    - Low-energy trauma from falls is most common in older patients.
    - High-energy trauma in the setting of motor vehicle crashes in younger patients.
    - Repetitive overuse may also be a cause of stress fractures in the femoral neck.
  - Clinical evaluation:
    - Shortening, external rotation of affected extremity, pain with ROM and palpation of groin.
    - AP of the pelvis and cross table lateral of the hip are indicated.
    - CT scans can be useful in trauma setting.
    - MRIs can be used to evaluate occult femoral neck fractures not seen on plain films.
  - Classification:
    - Classification can be based on anatomic location (subcapital, transcervical, basicervical).
    - Pauwels or Gardner classification used (▶ Table 15.14).

Table 15.14 Femoral fracture classification

Pauwels classification (femoral neck fracture; angle of fracture line from horizontal)	
Type I	< 30 degrees
Type II	30–70 degrees
Type III	> 70 degrees
Garden classification (femoral neck fractures; based on valgus displacement)	
Type I	Valgus impacted/incomplete
Type II	Complete but nondisplaced
Type III	Complete with partial displacement
Type IV	Completely displaced
Winquist and Hansen classification (proximal femoral shaft fractures)	
0	No comminution
I	Minimal comminution
II	>50% cortical contact
III	<0% cortical contact
IV	Segmental fracture, no contact between Segmental fracture, no contact between

OTA classification (proximal fractures)

Simple (A1—spiral; A2—oblique; A3—transverse)

Wedge (B1—spiral; B2—bending; B3—fragmented)

Complex (C1—spiral; C2—segmental; C3—irregular)

OTA classification (distal femoral shaft fractures)

Extra-articular

Partial articular

Complete articular

Abbreviation: OTA, Orthopaedic Trauma Association.

- ○ Treatment[45,46]:
  - – Goals of treatment are to minimize pain, restore hip function, and allow early return to ambulatory function.
  - – Nonoperative treatment is reserved only for patients with extreme surgical risk or nonambulators with dementia and minimal pain.
  - – Operative treatment depends on age and functional abilities of patient. Young patients with displaced femoral neck fractures require urgent internal fixation to preserve blood supply to the femoral head. Fixation can be obtained with percutaneous screws or other implants.
  - – Treatment for elderly patients is controversial depending on patient's abilities.
  - – Highly functional patients may benefit from internal screw fixation but also results in higher rate of revisions and future surgeries.
  - – Lower demand patients are often treated with hemiarthroplasty to allow earlier weight-bearing and remove risk of nonunion/osteonecrosis.
  - – Total hip arthroplasty has also been used as primary treatment option for displaced femoral neck fractures with better long-term results. Disadvantages include more extensive surgery, blood loss, and higher dislocation rate.
- • Intertrochanteric:
  - ○ Epidemiology:
    - – Account for approximately other 50% of hip fractures with femoral neck being the other 50% as previously described.

- Anatomy:
  - The region between the greater and less trochanters in the proximal femur sometimes extending to the subtrochanteric region.
  - Extracapsular fractures with abundant blood supply. Osteonecrosis and nonunion are less likely.
- Evaluation: Same modalities as femoral neck fractures as described previously.
- Classification:
  - Evans classification: Stable or unstable based on the posteromedial cortex of the femur.
- Treatment:
  - Nonoperative treatment is rare and reserved for those with extreme surgical risk or nonambulators with dementia and minimal pain.
  - Operative treatment is to allow early mobilization and weight bearing. Variety of implants can be used including sliding hip screw, intramedullary hip screw nail, and arthroplasty for patients who fail initial fixation.
- Complications:
  - Loss of fixation and malrotation deformity are the most common.
  - Osteonecrosis and nonunion are less common with intertrochanteric fractures.
- Subtrochanteric:
  - Anatomy:
    - Subtrochanteric femur fracture is a fracture between the lesser trochanter to 5 cm distal.
    - It is subject to high biomechanical forces and less vascularity.
    - Strong deforming forces proximally from glutes and psoas muscles.
  - Mechanism of injury:
    - Low-energy mechanisms in elderly patients. Also a frequent site for pathologic fractures.
    - High-energy mechanisms in young adults.
  - Radiologic evaluation:
    - AP and lateral of the pelvis and affected hip.
    - AP and lateral of the full femur should also be done.
  - Classification[47]:
    - Descriptive methods based on location relative to lesser trochanter, bone fragments, and comminution.
    - OTA classifications.
  - Atypical subtrochanteric fractures due to prolonged bisphosphonate uses:
    - Minimal to no trauma, fall from standing.
    - Fracture originates at lateral cortex.
    - Noncomminuted.
    - Complete fracture through both cortices with medial spike
    - Incomplete fracture only through lateral cortex, local periosteal/endosteal thickening.
  - Treatment:
    - Nonoperative treatment is now only for historical purposes when skeletal traction was used.
    - Operative treatment is indicated in nearly all subtrochanteric fractures with intramedullary nails or 95 degree fixed angle device.
  - Complications:
    - Neurovascular injury, heterotopic ossification, infection, malunion with rotational malalignment or shortening.
  - Complications:
    - Loss of fixation, nonunion, malunion.
- Femoral shaft fractures:
  - Epidemiology:
    - Bimodal distribution in ages 25 and 65.
    - Occurs in high-energy trauma or as a result of falls.
  - Anatomy:
    - Largest tubular bone in the body.
    - Femur is surrounded by large mass of muscle, separated into three compartments—anterior, medial, and posterior.

- 10 degrees of anterior bow in the femoral shaft is an important feature.
- Good blood supply to the femur is provided by the profunda femoral artery.
○ Mechanism of injury:
  - Almost always due to high-energy trauma in adults.
  - Pathologic fractures may occur from low-energy falls in the elderly.
○ Evaluation:
  - Full trauma evaluation is often necessary due to high-energy trauma.
  - Obvious deformity but evaluation of the entire extremity must be done to evaluate for more additional injuries at the knee and hip.
○ Radiographs:
  - Full length femur, hip, knee, and pelvis films must be obtained to look for associated fractures especially in the femoral neck.
  - CT scan of the pelvis can also be obtained to evaluate femoral neck.
○ Classification:
  - Winquist and Hansen or OTA classifications for femoral shaft fractures (► Table 15.14).
○ Treatment[48]:
  - Nonoperative treatment: Skeletal traction is reserved only for adult patients with severe surgical risk.
  - Skeletal traction can restore length, limit rotation, and reduce pain but results in prolonged bedrest, respiratory/skin complications, malunion, and thromboembolism risks.
  - Operative: Surgical fixation is standard of care usually within 24 hours. Treatment options include intramedullary nailing (antegrade or retrograde), external fixation, or plate fixation.
  Intramedullary nailing is the standard of care. Benefits of IM nailing include earlier ambulation, high union, and less extensive dissection of tissue.
○ Complications:
  - Neurovascular injury, heterotopic ossification, infection, malunion with rotational malalignment or shortening.
• Distal femur:
○ Epidemiology:
  - Much less common than hip fractures. Account for about 7% of all femur fractures.
  - Similar bimodal age distribution as other lower extremity fractures. High-energy trauma in young adults, and falls in the elderly.
○ Anatomy:
  - Distal femur consists of the distal 15 cm of the femur.
  - Forms two curved condyles medially and laterally that account for the physiologic 9-degree valgus of the femur.
  - Deforming muscular forces from the gastrocnemius, hamstrings, and quadriceps characterize displacement patterns.
○ Evaluation:
  - Close assessment of initial neurovascular status is needed. Full assessment of entire extremity to look for additional fractures.
  - AP and lateral of the entire femur and knee should be obtained. CT scan of the knee assists with evaluating intra-articular fragments.
○ Classification:
  - Mostly descriptive based on location, fracture pattern, articular involvement, and displacement.
  - OTA classification.
○ Treatment:
  - Nonoperative: Nondisplaced, stable fractures can be treated with mobilization in a hinged knee brace with limited weight bearing.
  - Operative: Most displaced femur fractures are best treated with ORIF. Anatomic reduction is necessary in articular fractures. Other surgical techniques that can be used include intramedullary nails, fixed angle plates, or external fixation.
  - Complications: Fixation failure, malunion, posttraumatic arthritis, knee stiffness.

15.3.4 Patella, Tibial, and Ankle Fractures

- Patella fractures:
  - Epidemiology:
    - Uncommon injury. Represents only 1% of all skeletal injuries.
    - Most common in younger age group, 20–50.
  - Anatomy:
    - Largest sesamoid bone.
    - Quadriceps tendon inserts superiorly, patella tendon originates inferiorly.Functions to increase mechanical advantage and lever arm of the quadriceps tendon.
  - Mechanism of injury:
    - Direct injury: Direct trauma to the patella.
    - Indirect injury: More common. Caused by forcible eccentric contraction of the quadriceps exceeding the strength of the patella.
  - Evaluation:
    - Limited ambulatory function with pain and swelling of the knee.
    - Active knee extension needs to be evaluated along with associated lower extremity injuries.
    - AP, lateral, and sunrise view of the patella should be obtained.
  - Classification:
    - Open vs. closed.
    - Displaced vs. nondisplaced.
    - Fracture patterns: Stellate, comminuted, transverse, vertical, polar, osteochondral.
  - Treatment[49,50]:
    - Nonoperative: Nondisplaced or minimally displaced (<3 mm) with minimal articular disruption (<2 mm). Place leg in knee immobilizer or long leg cylinder cast with weight bearing.
    - Operative: Indications for ORIF include loss of extension, >3 mm of displacement, >2 mm articular disruption, or open fracture. Fixation techniques include tension banding, cerclage wiring, or screw fixation.
    - Partial vs. total patellectomy is another possibility but less frequently done.
  - Complications:
    - Infection, loss of fixation, hardware irritation, posttraumatic arthritis, loss of knee motion, or nonunion.
- Tibia plateau fractures[51]:
  - Epidemiology:
    - Constitute 1% of all fractures.
    - Lateral tibia plateau more commonly injured than medial plateau.
  - Anatomy:
    - Consists of medial and lateral tibia plateaus with articular cartilage and meniscus.
    - Intercondylar eminence separates the two sides and serves as attachment for cruciate ligaments.
    - Medial plateau is stronger than lateral side and less likely to be injured. Medial plateau injuries are more likely to be high energy.
  - Mechanism of injury:
    - Varus or valgus forces with axial loading.
    - High-energy mechanisms in young adults. Falls in elderly patients.
  - Evaluation:
    - Complete neurovascular exam to evaluate for compartment syndrome.
    - Examination of skin and soft tissues to evaluate for open fractures or intra-articular involvement. Intra-articular injection of saline may be required to definitively rule out communication with knee joint.
    - AP, lateral, oblique, and plateau view plain films of the knee are initially obtained. CT scan for delineating extend of fragmentation.
    - Associated injuries include meniscus tears, cruciate/collateral ligamentous injuries, neurovascular injury.

- Classification:
  - Schatzker classification (▶ Table 15.15): Types I–III are low-energy injuries. Types IV–VI are high energy. Medial plateau fractures are clinical equivalent of knee dislocations.
  - OTA classification.
- Treatment[52,53]:
  - Nonoperative: Indicated for nondisplaced or minimally displaced. Protected weight bearing with hinged knee brace with progression to full weight bearing.
  - Operative: Surgical indications include articular depression (2–10 mm), instability (>10 degrees), open fractures, associated compartment syndrome, or neurovascular injury.
  - Goals of treatment are to reconstruct the articular surface and realignment of the tibia.
  - ORIF, percutaneous fixation, and external fixation are common options.
- Complications:
  - Arthrofibrosis, infections, compartment syndrome, malunion/nonunion, and posttraumatic arthritis are all common.
- Tibial shaft:
  - Epidemiology:
    - Most common long bone fracture.
    - Highest among young males and elderly females.
  - Anatomy:
    - Long tubular bone with triangular cross-section.

Table 15.15 Tibial fracture classification

Gustilo–Anderson classification of open tibial fractures	
I	Periosteal stripping, clean wound
II	Mild-moderate periosteal stripping, wound > 1 cm
IIIA	Soft-tissue injury, periosteal stripping, wound > 5 cm
IIIB	Soft-tissue injury, flap required from gastrocnemius, soleus, or free flap
IIIC	Soft tissue, vascular injury, comminuted fracture
Schatzker classification of tibial plateau	
I	Lateral split (low energy)
II	Lateral split depression (low energy)
III	Lateral pure depression (low energy)
IV	Medial plateau (high energy; knee dislocation)
V	Bicondylar (high energy)
VI	Metaphyseal–diaphyseal (high energy)
OTA classification (proximal tibial third)	
Simple	
Wedge	
Comminuted	
OTA classification (tibial plafond/pilon)	
Extra-articular	
Partial articular	
Complete articular	
Lauge–Hansen classification (ankle fractures)	
Supination–adduction	
Supination–external rotation (most common)	
Pronation–abduction	
Pronation–externalrotation (Maisonneuve fracture is a variant of this mechanism with associated proximal fibula fracture)	

- – Anteromedial section is directly subcutaneous. Four fascial compartments surround the tibia: anterior, lateral, posterior, deep posterior.
- – Intramedullary blood supply can be disrupted when injured.
- o Mechanism of injury:
  - – Direct mechanisms include high energy, penetrating, or bending.
  - – Indirect mechanisms includestress fractures, torsion with a fixed foot.
- o Clinical evaluation:
  - – Complete neurovascular exam is critical. Highest rate of compartment syndrome in the body.
  - – Soft-tissue exam as the tibia is directly subcutaneous.
- o Radiographic evaluation:
  - – AP and lateral films must include the entire tibia with visualization of knee and ankle.
  - – Evaluate for comminution, displacement, and bone quality on X-rays.
  - – CT scans are usually not needed for tibia shaft fractures.
- o Classification:
  - – Descriptive based on location, fragments, fracture pattern, angulation, rotation, and shortening.
  - – Associated with soft-tissue injuries; used Oestern and Tscherne classification for grading soft-tissue injury.
  - – Gustilo–Anderson open tibia fracture classification (▶ Table 15.15).
- o Treatment[54,55]:
  - – Nonoperative: Long leg cast with progressive weight bearing for isolated, closed, low-energy fractures with minimal displacement. Acceptable reduction is <5 degrees of varus/valgus angulation, < 10 degrees of AP angulation, <10 degrees of rotation, < 1 cm shortening, and 50% cortical contact.
  - – Operative: Treatment options include intramedullary nail, ORIF, external fixation, or percutaneous plating.
  - – Proximal third tibia fractures are known to be difficult to nail leading to malalignment.
- o Complications:
  - – Highest rate of nonunion in any long bone.
  - – Soft-tissue loss, knee pain, symptomatic hardware, compartment syndrome, neurovascular injury.
- • Proximal tibial third:
  - o 5–11% of tibial shaft fractures, low-energy torsional injury or high-energy trauma.
  - o AO classification (▶ Table 15.15).
  - o Diagnosis: X-rays (AP, lateral, ipsilateral knee, tibia, ankle), CT rarely.
  - o Treatment: Closed reduction and immobilization, external fixation, IM nailing, percutaneous locking plate.
- • Tibial plafond/pilon:
  - o Epidemiology:
    - – Pilon fractures refer specifically to fractures extending from the distal tibia into the articular surface.
    - – 7–10% of tibia fractures. Most common in men 30–40. High association with fibula fractures.
  - o Mechanism of injury:
    - – High-energy mechanism: Axial compression from talus directly into the plafond.
    - – Rotational: Torsion combined with varus or valgus stress.
  - o Clinical evaluation:
    - – Careful assessment of neurovascular status and soft tissues for swelling and skin breakdown.
    - – Usually high-energy mechanism;therefore, associated injuries to the entire extremity must be evaluated.
    - – AP, lateral, and mortise views of the ankle should be obtained. Full-length tibia should also be obtained. CT scans of the ankle to evaluate fracture pattern in articular involvement.
  - o Classification:
    - – OTA classification (▶ Table 15.15).
    - – Ruedi and Allgower classification: nondisplaced, simple displacement with incongruous joint, comminuted articular surface.
  - o Treatment:
    - – Nonoperative: Long leg casting used primarily for nondisplaced fracture patterns or severely debilitated patients.

– Operative: Most pilon fractures are treated operatively with ORIF.
– Timing of definitive fixation is usually delayed to allow soft-tissue swelling to subside.
– External fixation may be done initially to provide stabilization and maintain length.
– Goals of surgical fixation are to maintain length as well as stability and to restore tibia articular surface and graft defects.
  ○ Complications[58]:
– Wound dehiscence and infection are the most devastating complications but can be kept at around 10% with modern techniques.
– Varus malunion, nonunion, posttraumatic arthritis, and chondrolysis.
- Ankle fractures:
  ○ Epidemiology:
– Highest incidence of ankle fractures occurs in elderly women.
– Most are isolated malleolar fractures.
  ○ Anatomy:
– Complex hinge joint composed of articulations of fibula, tibia, and talus and complex ligamentous system.
– Distal tibia surface is called the plafond and along with medial and lateral malleoli forms the ankle mortise.
– Syndesmotic ligament exists between distal tibia and fibula resisting axial, rotational, and translational forces to maintain the mortise. Deltoid ligament medially and fibula collateral ligaments provide additional support.
  ○ Clinical evaluation:
– Careful neurovascular exam with comparison to contralateral extremity.
– Evaluate soft tissues for wounds and skin tenting.
– Entire fibula should be palpated so that proximal fibula fractures are not missed. Syndesmosis injury should be assessed.
– AP, lateral, and mortise views of the ankle should be obtained. Full-length tibia film to assess proximal fibula is suspicious for fracture proximally. Stress views can be used to identify medial side injuries.
  ○ Classification:
– Lauge–Hansen (injury mechanism), Danis–Weber (level of fibula fracture relative to tibia plafond), or OTA classification (▶ Table 15.15).
  ○ Treatment[56,57]:
– Closed reduction and splinting should be performed immediately to reduce swelling, pressure on articular cartilage, skin breakdown risk, and pressure on neurovascular structures.
– Nonoperative: Nondisplaced stable ankle fracture patterns as well as displaced fractures with stable anatomic reduction can be treated with short leg cast or removable boot.
– Operative: ORIF is indicated for failure to obtain or maintain closed reduction, widened ankle mortise, or syndesmotic injury.
  ○ Complications:
– Wound breakdown, infection, posttraumatic arthritis, loss of reduction.

15.3.5 Foot Fractures

- Talus fractures[59,60]:
  ○ Epidemiology:
– Frequency ranges from 0.1 to 0.85% of all fractures.
– Second most common tarsal bone fracture.
  ○ Anatomy:
– Talus body is covered with articular cartilage through which the entire body weight is transmitted. 60% of talus is covered with articular cartilage; so, there is less surface area for vascular perforation making it susceptible to osteonecrosis.
– Articulates with medial, lateral malleoli and tibia plafond.

Table 15.16 Hawkins classification of talar neck fracture

I	Nondisplaced
II	Subtalar dislocation
III	Subtalar and tibiotalar dislocation
IV	Subtalar, tibiotalar, and talonavicular dislocation

    – Talar neck is most vulnerable to fracture.
  ○ Mechanism of injury:
    – Commonly associated with high-energy mechanisms with a component of ankle hyperdorsiflexion.
    – Talus fractures are a common snow-boarding injury, specifically the lateral process.
  ○ Clinical evaluation:
    – Pain, swelling, and crepitus are common.
    – Associated foot and ankle fractures are also commonly seen.
    – AP, lateral, and mortise views of the ankle. AP, lateral, and oblique views of the foot. Canale view is a specific view for the talar neck but difficult to obtain in acute setting.
    – CT scans may be used to characterize fracture fragments and displacement.
  ○ Classification (▶ Table 15.16):
    – Anatomic based on location: Lateral process, posterior process, talar head, neck, or body.
    – Hawkins classification for talar neck fractures.
  ○ Treatment:
    – Nondisplaced fractures can be treated with short leg cast or boot and non-weight-bearing.
    – Displaced fractures are treated with immediate reduction and immobilization followed by urgent surgical fixation with screws or wires. ORIF is the standard of treatment.
    – Fragment excision can also be done for posterior process fractures.
  ○ Complications:
    – Osteonecrosis is directly related to initial fracture displacement.
    – Infection, nonunion, malunion, skin breakdown, or foot compartment syndrome can all occur.
• Calcaneus fractures:
  ○ Epidemiology:
    – Most frequently fractured tarsal bone.
    – Account for about 2% of all fractures. Most are young men aged 21–45.
  ○ Anatomy:
    – Three facets on the superior surface that articulates with the talus. Posterior facet is the largest and is the major weight-bearing surface.
    – Middle and anterior facets are contiguous.
    – Sustentaculum tali is medial and supports the talus with the middle facet.
    – Flexor hallucis longus and peroneal tendon pass medially and laterally, respectively, around the calcaneus. The Achilles tendon attaches posteriorly.
  ○ Mechanism of injury:
    – Axial loading from falls is the most common mechanism. The talus is driven down into the calcaneus.
    – Twisting forces may cause extra-articular fractures or avulsions.
  ○ Clinical evaluation:
    – Heel pain with swelling about the heel. Ecchymosis is highly suggestive of calcaneus fractures.
    – Soft tissue and skin evaluation is essential.
    – High association with lumbar spine or other lower extremity fractures.
    – AP and lateral of the foot with a Harris axial view of the calcaneus. CT scan is often obtained to evaluate the articular surface.
  ○ Classification:
    – Extra-articular fractures: Do not involve the posterior facet; classified by anatomic location.
    – Intra-articular fractures: Essex-Lopresti classification (based on primary and secondary fracture lines produced by the amount of axial loading during injury); Sander classification (▶ Table 15.17;

Table 15.17 Sanders classification of calcaneus fractures

I	Nondisplaced
II	One fracture line in posterior facet, two fragments
III	Two fracture lines in posterior facet, three fragments
IV	Comminuted

  based on CT scans in the coronal plane counting the number of articular fragments); OTA classification.

- ○ Treatment:
  - – Severely disabling injuries with variable degrees of functional debility.
  - – Nonoperative: nondisplaced fractures, patients with severe PVD, severe blistering, or soft-tissue edema may be treated nonoperatively. Splinting followed by fracture boot with non-weight-bearing.
  - – Operative: Displaced fractures, fracture dislocations, and fractures involving > 25% of the anterior process all require surgical treatment but not be attempted until swelling subsides.
  - – Surgical techniques include percutaneous pinning and ORIF.
  - – Goals are to restore subtalar articulation, restore normal height and width, correct varus malalignment, and maintain calcaneocuboid articulation.
  - – Primary arthrodesis can also be performed.
- ○ Complications:
  - – Wound dehiscence up to 25% is the most common complication due to minimal soft-tissue coverage.
  - – Posttraumatic arthritis, loss of subtalar motion, sural nerve injury, and chronic pain.
- • Fracture of midfoot and forefoot:
  - ○ Anatomy:
    - – Midfoot consists of five tarsal bones: navicular, cuboid, and the three cuneiforms (medial, middle, lateral).
    - – Midtarsal joints work with subtalar joint to invert and evert the foot.
  - ○ Mechanism of injury:
    - – High-energy trauma due to direct impact of combination of axial load and torsion.
    - – Low-energy injuries from athletic injuries resulting in sprains.
  - ○ Clinical evaluation:
    - – Variable presentation from simple limp to significant swelling, pain, and deformity.
    - – AP, lateral, and oblique views of the foot should be obtained. Stress views or weight-bearing films can also help distinguish subtle injuries.
- • Navicular fractures:
  - ○ Anatomy:
    - – Navicular is the keystone to the medial longitudinal arch of the foot.
    - – Posterior tibialis attaches to the medial prominence, navicular tuberosity.
    - – The talonavicular joint where the subtalar joint motion transmits to the forefoot and where forefoot inversion and eversion are initiated.
    - – Thick ligaments including the spring ligament and deltoid provide strong support.
  - ○ Mechanism of injury:
    - – Often indirect forces of axial loading injure the navicular.
    - – Stress fractures may occur due to overuse in running and jumping.
  - ○ Clinical evaluation:
    - – Foot pain localized to the dorsomedial aspect.
    - – Evaluate all bony prominences of the foot to rule out associated injuries.
    - – AP, lateral, and oblique views of the foot should be obtained. Weight-bearing films help detect ligamentous injuries.
    - – MRI may be used to evaluate for stress fracture if suspected and not visualized on plain films.

- Classification:
  - Based on location: avulsion, tuberosity, or body fractures; avulsion is most common.
- Treatment[61]:
  - Nonoperative: Nondisplaced fractures can be treated with short leg cast or fracture brace with restricted weight bearing. Repeat radiographs to evaluate for any instability that may require surgical treatment.
  - Operative: Goal is to restore medial column length and articular congruity of the talonavicular joint. Indications are any loss of articular congruity of more than 2 mm or significant involvement of dorsal surface from avulsions. Surgical techniques include K-wire or screw fixation. Primary fusion can also be considered if more than 40% of the articular surface cannot be restored.
- Complications:
  - Osteonecrosis, posttraumatic arthritis, nonunion, loss of foot alignment, or collapse can occur.
- Tarsometatarsal injuries (Lisfranc injury):
  - Anatomy:
    - Second metatarsal is recessed between medial and lateral cuneiforms, limiting movement in the frontal plane.
    - Second metatarsal base is the keystone in the transverse arch of the foot.
    - Limited motion exists between the tarsometatarsal joints.
    - Strong ligaments connect the base of the second to fifth metatarsals; the most important is the Lisfranc ligament that connects the base of the second metatarsal to the medial cuneiform.
  - Mechanism of injury:
    - Twisting: Forceful abduction of the forefoot.
    - Axial loading on a fixed foot.
    - Crush injuries.
  - Clinical evaluation:
    - Foot deformity, pain, swelling over the dorsum of the foot. Plantar ecchymosis is pathognomonic for Lisfranc injury.
    - Requires high degree of clinical suspicion as they are frequently missed injuries.
    - Dorsalis pedis artery may be injured; so care neurovascular exam is needed.
    - Stressing the midfoot with passive abduction while hindfoot stabilized can suggest diagnosis.
    - AP, lateral, oblique views of the foot are sufficient for diagnosis. Medial border of second metatarsal should be collinear with medial border of middle cuneiform. Widening of joint space suggests Lisfranc injury.
    - Weight-bearing films provide stress view of the complex.
  - Classification:
    - Ouene and Kuss: Homolateral, isolated, divergent.
    - Myerson classification: total incongruity, partial incongruity, divergent.
  - Treatment[62]:
    - Nonoperative: Nondisplaced ligamentous injuries with or without avulsions should be placed in short leg cast or boot and be made non-weight-bearing.
    - Operative: Displacement of the tarsometatarsal joint is greater than 2 mm. Anatomic reduction and stable fixation are required with screw or Kirschner wire fixation.
  - Complications:
    - Posttraumatic arthritis, compartment syndrome, infection, symptomatic hardware, or hardware failure.
- Metatarsal fracture:
  - Anatomy:
    - Metatarsals are major weight-bearing complex of the forefoot. Fractures disrupt the normal distribution of weight in the forefoot.
    - Mobile in the sagittal plane to accommodate for uneven ground.
  - Mechanism of injury:
    - Direct: Heavy object lands on the forefoot.
    - Twisting: Body torque when the toes are fixed in place.

- Avulsions.
- Stress fractures.
  - Clinical evaluation:
    - Evaluation of pain, swelling, and tenderness; soft tissues and ambulatory function.
    - Weight-bearing AP and lateral films should be obtained.
- First metatarsal fracture:
  - More mobile and stronger than other metatarsals, so less frequently injured.
  - Injuries due to direct trauma.
  - Stress radiographs are best way to determine displacement.
  - Displacement requires surgical fixation.
  - Nondisplaced injuries without evidence of instability can be treated with short leg cast or boot and be weight bearing as tolerated.
  - Malunion, nonunion, and arthritic changes are possible complications.
- Second, third, fourth metatarsal fracture:
  - More frequently injured than first metatarsal due to ligamentous connections.
  - Twisting mechanisms cause a spiral fracture pattern.
  - Most central metatarsal fractures can be treated with hard-sole show and weight bearing as tolerated.
  - Surgical treatment criterion is 10 degrees of dorsal angulation or 3–4 mm of translation.
- Fifth metatarsal fracture (Jones fracture):
  - Result of direct trauma.
  - Classification:
    - Separated into proximal base and distal spiral fractures.
    - Proximal base fracture separated into three zones.[63,64]
    - Zone 1: Cancellous tuberosity involves the metatarsocuboid joint. Pseudo-Jones fracture usually from avulsions. Treatment is hard sole shoe.
    - Zone 2: Distal to tuberosity. True Jones fracture from adduction or inversion of forefoot. Treatment is controversial regarding operative vs. nonoperative due to risk of nonunion.
    - Zone 3: Distal to proximal ligaments and extends to diaphysis for 1.5 cm. Less common. Often seen in athletes. Highest risk of nonunion. Treatment is short leg cast with non-weight-bearing unless concern for nonunion at which time surgical fixation can be done. More aggressive treatment may be required.
- Phalanges fracture:
  - More common fracture in the forefoot.
  - First and fifth digits are most vulnerable.
  - Usually caused by dropping a heavy object or stubbing the injury with axial load.
  - Pain, swelling, and variable deformities.
  - AP, lateral, and oblique views of the foot are sufficient.
  - Classified based on proximal, middle, or distal phalanx and description of fracture pattern.
  - Treatment is usually nonoperative with hard-sole shoe and protected weight bearing.
  - Buddy taping of adjacent toes helps provide pain relief. Closed reduction can be performed if needed.
- Other:
  - Ottawa ankle X-ray rules: Suggest ankle X-rays with pain in malleolar zone or pain in midfoot and/or inability to walk.
  - Ottawa foot X-ray rules: Suggest foot X-ray with pain at base of fifth metatarsal/navicular bone *or* navicular bone *or* inability to walk.
- Ankle sprain:
  - Epidemiology:
    - Ankle sprains are among the most common musculoskeletal injuries.
    - Intermittent pain can occur in 40% of patients 1 year after injury.
  - Anatomy:
    - Lateral collateral ligament is made up of three ligaments that provide lateral support to the ankle laterally. Anterior talofibular ligament, calcaneofibular ligament, posterior talofibular ligament.
    - Deltoid ligament (superficial and deep portions) provides medial support to the ankle. It is composed of superficial and deep portion.

Table 15.18 Classification of low ankle sprains

Grade	Description
I	No ligamentous disruption, minimal ecchymosis, no pain with weight bearing
II	Ligament stretch without tear, moderate ecchymosis, mild pain with weight bearing
III	Complete tear, severe ecchymosis, and pain with weight bearing

- Syndesmotic ligament connects the distal tibia and fibula. Consists of anterior inferior tibiofibular ligament, posterior tibiofibular ligament, transverse tibiofibular ligament, interosseous ligament.
  ○ Mechanism of injury:
    - Twisting or turning event to the ankle, either internal or external rotation.
    - Ligaments injured depend on position of the foot and direction of stress. Plantar-flexion inversion injuries first strain the anterior talofibular ligament followed by calcaneofibular ligament.
    - Dorsiflexion and inversion injure the calcaneofibular ligament.
    - Dorsiflexion and external rotation will injure syndesmotic ligaments.
  ○ Classification (▶ Table 15.18):
    - Mild: Minimal loss of function, no limp or swelling. Pain with palpation.
    - Moderate: Limp with walking, inability to stand on the injured ankle, local swelling, and tenderness.
    - Severe: Diffuse swelling and preference for non-weight-bearing.
  ○ Clinical evaluation:
    - Popping or tearing sensation around the ankle followed by immediate pain. Swelling, ecchymosis, tenderness, instability, crepitus, and deformity may all be present.
    - Location of tenderness helps identify the involved ligaments.
    - Ottawa ankle X-ray rules: Suggest ankle X-rays with pain in malleolar zone or pain in midfoot and/ or inability to walk.
    - Ottawa foot X-ray rules: Suggest foot X-ray with pain at base of fifth metatarsal/navicular bone or navicular bone or inability to walk.
    - Most patients should undergo plain films to rule out fractures to the fifth metatarsal, navicular, lateral malleolus, calcaneus, or talus.
    - MRI used for pain > 6–8 weeks to evaluate peroneal tendon injury, osteochondral injury, or syndesmotic injury.
  ○ Treatment:
    - Nonoperative treatment: Rest, cold compression, elevation, and limited weight bearing. Immobilization of moderate or severe sprains may be necessary in a boot or with crutches; outpatient therapy for range of motion exercises, strengthening, proprioception, and protective bracing; 30% of patients can have persistent pain after injury.
    - Arthroscopy used to reconstruct intra-articular pathology or ATFL impingement.
    - Repaired via Gould modification of Brostrom anatomic reconstruction (reinsertion of ATFL and CFL) or tendon transfer/tenodesis.
- Syndesmosis sprains (high ankle sprain):
  ○ Account for only 1% of ankle sprains.
  ○ Often go undiagnosed and cause chronic pain and greater impairment than lateral ankle sprains.
  ○ Classification:
    - Diastasis of the distal tibiofibular syndesmosis classified by Edwards and DeLee.
    - Type I: Lateral subluxation without fracture.
    - Type II: Lateral subluxation with plastic deformation of the fibula.
    - Type III: Posterior subluxation/dislocation of fibula.
    - Type IV: Superior subluxation/dislocation of the talus within the mortise.
  ○ Clinical evaluation:
    - Patients usually present later after the injury with difficulty weight bearing, ecchymosis, and swelling extending up to the leg.
    - Vague ankle pain with push-off.

– Squeeze test: Squeezing the fibula and tibia at the midcalf reproduces distal tibiofibular pain.
– External rotation stress test: Externally rotate the foot with leg stabilized.
– Standard AP, lateral, and mortise views of the ankle along with stress views should be obtained. Widening of the space between medial malleolus and medial border of talus suggests injury.
○ Treatment:
– Slower to recover than other ankle injuries. Initially non-weight-bearing for 2–3 weeks followed by protective boot limiting motion.
– Operative treatment for patients with irreducible diastasis by screw fixation.

15.4 Joint Injuries

Jim Lai

15.4.1 Glenohumeral Dislocations

- Epidemiology:
  ○ Most commonly dislocated joint (45% dislocations) in the body.
  ○ Most are anterior dislocations (90%).
  ○ Peaks at young men aged 21–30 and elderly women aged 61–80.
- Anatomy:
  ○ Stability: joint conformity and vacuum effect of synovial fluid, joint capsule, and ligamentous restraints (e.g., superior glenohumeral ligament, middle glenohumeral ligament, inferior glenohumeral ligament), glenoid labrum, bony restraints (acromion, coracoids, and glenoid fossa), rotator cuff tendons, and biceps tendon provide active stability.
  ○ Mechanism of shoulder dislocation: stretching/tearing of capsule usually off glenoid, labral damage (e.g., Bankart lesion—avulsion of anteroinferior labrum from glenoid rim), associated fracture of glenoid (e.g., bony Bankart).
  ○ Hill–Sachs lesion: Defect on the posterolateral humeral head caused by impression fracture on the glenoid rim.
- Anterior glenohumeral dislocation:
  ○ Most common (90% dislocations) type.
  ○ Causes: Indirect trauma to the upper extremity with the shoulder in abduction, extension, and external rotation; direct impaction to posterior shoulder or recurrent instability.
  ○ Clinical evaluation:
    – Clinical history including nature of trauma, chronicity, history of laxity/instability, and inciting events is helpful to know.
    – Injured shoulder typically held in abduction and external rotation.
    – Exam typically shows prominence anteriorly and hollow space beneath the acromion.
    – Careful neurovascular exam is needed paying particular attention to the axillary nerve function.
  ○ Radiographic examination: Standard AP, scapular Y, and axillary views sufficient; multiple special views can also be done to fully assess the humeral head and glenoid (e.g., Velpeau axillary view, West Point axillary view, Hill–Sachs view, Stryker Notch view).
  ○ Nonoperative treatment:
    – Closed reduction with adequate sedation and analgesics can be done using multiple techniques, followed by immobilization.
    – Traction–countertraction: Requires two people to perform. Wrap a sheet under the axilla of the injured side. One person pulls the two ends of the sheet while another pulls the injured arm gently at 30-degree abduction. It is important that both people maintain the same line of force when pulling.
    – Hippocratic technique: Effective if only one person is performing the reduction. Place one foot on the axillary fold and gentle internal/external rotation and gentle traction of the injured extremity.
    – Stimson technique: The patient is prone on a stretcher with the injured arm dangling off the edge. Hang 5–10 lb of weight off the wrist to obtain reduction after 15–20 minutes.

- – Milch technique: Patient is supine with upper extremity abducted and externally rotated; direct pressure is applied to the humeral head to push it back into place.
  - ○ Operative treatment:
    - – Indications: Soft-tissue interposition, displaced greater tuberosity fracture > 5 mm, glenoid rim fracture > 5 mm.
    - – Stabilization methods include labral repair, capsular shift, muscle/tendon transfers, and bony transfers.
  - ○ Complications[65]:
    - – Recurrent dislocation: Most common, prognosis worse with dislocation at early age.
    - – Osseous lesions: Hill Sachs lesion, bony Bankart lesion, greater tuberosity fracture, and acromion/coracoid fracture.
    - – Soft-tissue injuries: Rotator cuff, capsular, or subscapularis tendon tears.
    - – Vascular injuries: More common in elderly patients and involve axillary artery, may be a result of closed reduction attempt.
    - – Nerve injuries: Most commonly involve musculoskeletal and axillary nerves; more common in elderly.
- • Posterior glenohumeral dislocations:
  - ○ Represent 10% of shoulder dislocations, easily missed injury.
  - ○ Caused by indirect trauma to shoulder in adduction, flexion, and internal rotation; electric shock or seizures may cause posterior dislocations due to greater musculature of internal rotators compared to external rotators.
  - ○ Clinical evaluation:
    - – Does not present with obvious deformity. Typically held in the sling position of internal rotation and adduction.
    - – Limited external rotation and forward elevation are noted.
    - – Palpable posterior mass and flattening of anterior shoulder.
  - ○ Radiographic evaluation:
    - – Standard AP, scapula Y, and axillary views of the shoulder may be obtained.
    - – Signs suggestive of posterior glenohumeral dislocation on AP view include absence of normal overlap of humeral head on glenoid, humerus in full internal rotation, and impaction fracture of the anterior humeral head (reverse Hill–Sachs lesion).
    - – Axillary view most easily visualizes glenohumeral dislocations.
  - ○ Nonoperative treatment:
    - – Closed reduction techniques similar to reduction for anterior dislocations, followed by immobilization with sling o shoulder spica.
    - – Traction applied in line to the adducted arm with gentle lifting of the humeral head into the glenoid fossa.
  - ○ Operative treatment:
    - – Surgical indications: Displacement of lesser tuberosity fracture, posterior glenoid fragment, irreducible dislocation or impaction fracture, > 20% humeral head involvement.
    - – Open reduction, infraspinatus/long head of biceps tendon transfers, osteotomies, or capsulorrhaphy.
  - ○ Complications:
    - – Recurrent dislocation is likely in atraumatic posterior dislocations.
    - – Neurovascular injuries are less common in posterior dislocations than in anterior ones.
    - – Anterior subluxation may occur from overtightening posterior structures forcing the humeral head anteriorly.

15.4.2 Elbow Dislocation

- • Epidemiology:
  - ○ 11–28% of injuries to the elbow.
  - ○ Posterior dislocations are most common (80–90% of dislocations).
  - ○ Simple dislocations are purely ligamentous; complex dislocations occur with an associated fracture (nearly 50% of dislocations).

- Highest incidence is within the 10–20-year age group related to sports injuries.
- Anatomy:
  - Hinged joint with high degree of stability due to joint congruity, opposing muscle tension, and ligamentous constraints.
  - Three articulations of the elbow joint are the ulnotrochlear joint, radiocapitellar joint, and proximal radioulnar joint that provide combination of hinge and rotation.
  - Anteroposterior stability is provided by the trochlea-olecranon fossa, coronoid fossa, radiocapitellar joint, and biceps/triceps/brachialis muscles.
  - Valgus stability is provided by the medial collateral ligament complex; anterior bundle is the primary stabilizer.
  - Varus stability is provided by lateral ulnar collateral ligament and anconeus muscle.
  - Normal range of motion is 0–150-degree flexion, 85-degree supination, 80-degree pronation; functional range of motion is 100-degree arc of 30–130-degree flexion and 50-degree supination to 50-degree pronation.
- Mechanism of injury:
  - Most commonly caused by fall onto outstretched hand or elbow with a levering force that dislodges the olecranon from the trochlea and translation of the articular surfaces.
  - Posterior dislocation is the result of hyperextension, valgus stress, arm abduction, and forearm supination.
  - Anterior dislocations occur when a direct force hits the posterior forearm with the elbow flexed.
  - Capsuloligamentous stabilizers of the elbow get injured from medial to lateral.
- Clinical evaluation:
  - Variable instability and swelling are noted.
  - Careful neurovascular exam must be done prior to imaging or manipulation and after any manipulation has been performed.
  - Serial exams should be performed if there is massive swelling or suspicion for compartment syndrome.
  - Angiography may be needed to evaluate vascular injury such as brachial artery.
- Radiographic evaluation:
  - Standard AP and lateral of the elbow should be obtained.
  - Careful evaluation of the films for associated fractures around the elbow.
  - CT scans may be used to identify bony fragments not seen on X-rays.
- Classification:
  - Simple versus complex, association of fracture.
  - Based on direction of ulna displacement relative to the humerus (anterior, posterior, medial, lateral, posterolateral, posteromedial, divergent).
- Treatment principles[66]:
  - Restoration of bony stability includes the trochlear notch, coronoid process, and radiocapitellar contact.
  - Lateral collateral ligament is more important than MCL; MCL rarely needs to be repaired and will heal with active motion.
- Fracture dislocations:
  - Associated fractures include the radial head, medial/lateral epicondyle, coronoid process.
  - Intra-articular fractures are associated with greatest risk of chronic instability.
  - Distinct injury patterns:
    - Posterior dislocation with fracture of radial head.
    - Posterior dislocation with fracture of radial head and coronoid process known as terrible triad.
    - Varus posteromedial rotational instability with coronoid fracture.
    - Anterior olecranon fracture dislocation.
    - Posterior olecranon fracture dislocation.
  - Elbow instability patterns:
    - Posterolateral rotator instability: Fall onto outstretched arm creating valgus, axial, and posterolateral rotatory force. Injures the radial head or coronoid.

- Varus posteromedial rotational instability: Fall onto outstretched arm with varus, axial, and posteromedial rotational force. Results in fracture of coronoid process along with lateral collateral ligament, olecranon fracture, or additional fracture of coronoid process at the base.
- Nonoperative treatment:
  - Simple dislocations:
    - Closed reduction under adequate sedation and analgesia.
    - Longitudinal traction and flexion along with correction of medial/lateral displacement is usually sufficient for posterior dislocation.
    - Reassessment of neurovascular status and postreduction imaging is needed.
    - Splint immobilization initially followed by transition to hinged elbow brace for range of motion.
  - Fracture dislocations:
    - Only acceptable in patients with non or minimally displaced fracture of the radial head.
    - Reasonable to begin active motion within 1 week after injury.
- Operative treatment[67]:
  - Simple dislocations:
    - Indicated for unstable dislocations that cannot be held in a concentrically reduced position.
    - ORIF, repair of soft tissues to distal humerus or external fixation.
  - Fracture dislocations:
    - Repair or replacement of radial and lateral collateral ligaments.
    - Addition of coronoid fracture to dislocated elbow with radial head fracture dramatically increases instability and likelihood of problems.
    - Repair of coronoid along with repair/replacement of radial head and lateral collateral ligament repair are all necessary for best outcome.
- Complications:
  - Loss of motion: Immobilization after elbow dislocation should not go beyond 2 weeks.
  - Neurologic injury: Ulnar neuropathy.
  - Vascular injury: Brachial artery is most commonly disrupted.
  - Compartment syndrome.
  - Persistent instability/dislocation.
  - Arthrosis.
  - Heterotopic bone formation: Increases with multiple reduction attempts due to soft-tissue trauma.

15.4.3 Hand Joint Dislocations

- Metacarpophalangeal joint dislocations[68,69]:
  - Dorsal dislocations are the most common and are usually reducible.
  - Irreducible dislocations are usually the result of volar plate interposition.
  - Dorsal dislocations are usually stable and do not require surgical intervention.
- Thumb metacarpophalangeal joint dislocations[70]:
  - Involves one-sided collateral ligament injury.
  - Stener lesions: Torn ulnar collateral ligament stump lies on top of the adductor pollicis aponeurosis preventing it from healing to the correct location.
  - Nonoperative treatment with thumb spica cast is for partial thumb MCP joint collateral ligaments.
  - If the metacarpophalangeal joint opens up > 30 or > 15 degrees compared to the contralateral side, surgical repair is warranted as it is a complete ligament injury.
- Proximal interphalangeal joint dislocations:
  - Often missed and diagnosed as sprains due to spontaneous reduction, very common sports-related injury.
  - Dislocations can be dorsal, palmar, and rotator; injured structures include the volar plate, collateral ligament, and central slip.
  - Once reduced, range of motion can usually begin with buddy taping to adjacent digits.
  - Surgical repair is rarely needed.
- Distal interphalangeal and thumb interphalangeal dislocations:

○ Dislocations are usually the result of ball-catching sports in the dorsal direction and associated with PIP joint dislocations.
○ Often present late and not at the time of injury.
○ Reduced dislocations can begin immediate range of motion.
○ Delayed presentation > 3 weeks may require surgical treatment to resect scar tissue to obtain reduction.
○ Pinning is usually sufficient to provide enough stability.
• Complications:
○ Malunion: Poor angulation can result in pain with functional use of the hands and cosmetic disturbances especially in the second and third metacarpals.
○ Nonunion: May result from soft-tissue injury or bone loss.
○ Infection: Grossly contaminated wounds require meticulous debridement and antibiotics.
○ Contracture, loss of motion, and arthritis can also occur.

15.4.4 Hip Dislocation

• Anatomy:
○ Ball and socket joint with stability from bony and ligamentous restraints.
○ 40% of femoral head is covered by bony acetabulum at any position. Labrum deepens the acetabulum to increase stability.
○ Hip joint capsule formed by thick ligamentous fibers of the iliofemoral, pubofemoral, and ischiofemoral ligaments.
○ Femoral head blood supply is from the medial and lateral circumflex arteries. Extracapsular arteries from at the base of the femoral neck and enter the hip joint.
○ Sciatic nerve exits at the greater sciatic notch and is susceptible to impingement.
• Mechanism of injury (almost always the result of high energy trauma):
○ Posterior dislocation: 90% of cases, dashboard injury with knee flexed and adducted, associated with osteonecrosis, posterior wall acetabular fracture, femoral head fracture, sciatic nerve injury, ipsilateral knee injury.
○ Anterior dislocation: 10% of cases, femoral head impaction with hip in abduction and external rotation.
• Classification by Thompson and Epstein method or OTA (▶ Table 15.19).
• Clinical evaluation:
○ Full trauma evaluation is usually warranted due to nature of injury mechanism.
○ Classic position of posterior hip dislocation is flexed, internally rotated and adducted. Anterior hip dislocation is mild flexion, external rotation, and abduction.
○ Careful neurovascular exam is needed due to likelihood of injury to sciatic nerve or femoral vessels.
○ Associated fractures to the pelvis, knee, femur, and patella are common.
○ AP pelvis and cross table lateral are essential. Dislocation direction can be determined based on size of femoral head appearance on X ray. Smaller on posterior dislocations vs larger on anterior dislocations.
○ CT scan is also useful to check for intra-articular bone fragments.
○ Femoral neck fracture must be ruled out before any treatment manipulation.
• Treatment:
○ Closed reduction within 6 hours using inline traction, Allis method involves standing on stretcher and pulling below knee in line with femur, assistant places downward pressure on both anterior superior iliac spines, and gentle adduction and rotation of the pelvis can be helpful; repeat x-rays evaluates adequate reduction; repeat CT evaluates intra-articular bone fragment migration.
○ ORIF indications: Inability to obtained closed reduction, nonconcentric reduction needed, fracture of acetabulum or femoral head requiring fragment removal or ORIF, ipsilateral femoral neck fracture.
• Complications[71]: Posttraumatic arthritis (20%), femoral head necrosis (5–40%), sciatic nerve injury (8–20%), recurrent dislocation (< 2%), femoral head fractures (10% risk with posterior dislocations, 25–75% risk with anterior dislocations), recurrent dislocation (2%), heterotopic ossification (2%), DVT/PE.
• Outcomes are generally good with simple dislocations and worsen with associated fractures.

Table 15.19 Classification of hip dislocation

Thompson–Epstein classification (posterior dislocation)	
Type I	Simple dislocation with or without small posterior wall fragment
Type II	Dislocation with a single large posterior wall fragment
Type III	Dislocation with comminuted posterior wall fragment
Type IV	Dislocation with fracture of the acetabular floor
Type V	Dislocation with fracture of the femoral head
Epstein classification (anterior dislocation)	
Type I	Superior dislocation
A	No associated fractures
B	Fracture or impaction of femoral head
C	Fracture of acetabulum
Type II	Inferior dislocation
A	No associated fractures
B	Fracture or impaction of femoral head
C	Fracture of acetabulum
OTA classification	
1	Anterior
2	Posterior
3	Medial or central (fracture through acetabulum)
4	Obturator
5	Other

15.4.5 Knee Dislocation

- Epidemiology[72]:
  - 0.02% of orthopaedic injuries.
  - 50% of dislocations self-reduce and are misdiagnosed.
- Anatomy and injury mechanisms:
  - Dislocation at the tibiofemoral articulation/knee joint.
  - High-energy mechanisms: Motor vehicle collision, crush, fall, dashboard injury.
  - Low-energy mechanisms: Athletic injury, routine walking, low-energy impact in setting of morbid obesity.
  - Hyperextension leads to anterior dislocation.
  - Posterior force (dashboard injury) leads to posterior dislocation.
  - Posterior cruciate ligament (PCL), anterior cruciate ligament (ACL), lateral collateral ligament (LCL), medial collateral ligament (MCL), and posterolateral corner of knee (PLC) all at risk of injury; 3 out of 4 ligaments are usually ruptured for a knee dislocation[73].
  - Associated with high risk of vascular injuries, common peroneal injuries, fractures, and soft-tissue disruption.
- Classification:
  - Organized by Kennedy or Schenck classifications (▶ Table 15.20).
- Clinical evaluation:
  - Gross knee deformity unless it spontaneously reduces in the field. Immediate reduction should be performed without waiting for plain films. Careful evaluation of neurovascular status is paramount.
  - Spontaneously reduced knee dislocation may appear normal with only subtle signs of injury such as abrasions or effusion.
  - Evaluation of major knee ligaments including ACL, PCL, LCL, and MCL.
  - Careful neurovascular exam before and after reduction of the dorsalis pedis and posterior tibialis arteries with palpation or Doppler.

Table 15.20 Kennedy and Schenck classification of knee dislocation

Kennedy classification	
Anterior	30–50% of injuries, due to hyperextension, results in tear of PCL
Posterior	30–40% of injuries, due to axial loading of flexed knee (dashboard injury), highest rate of vascular injury with popliteal artery tear (25%)
Lateral	13% of injuries, due to varus or valgus force, associated with ACL and PCL tears, highest rate of peroneal nerve injury
Medial	3% of injuries, due to varus or valgus force, associated with PLC and PCL disruption
Rotational	4% of injuries, usually irreducible, knee usually rotates posterolaterally
Schenck classification	
KD I	Multiligamentous injury involving ACL or PCL
KD II	Injury to ACL and PCL
KD IIIM	Injury to ACL, PCL, and PMC
KD IIIL	Injury to ACL, PCL, and PLC
KD IV	Injury to ACL, PCL, PMC, and PCL
KD V	Multiligamentous injury with periarticular fracture

Abbreviations: ACL, anterior cruciate ligament; KD, knee dislocation; LCL, lateral collateral ligament; MCL, medial collateral ligament; MLC, mediolateral corner of knee; PCL, posterior cruciate ligament; PLC, posterolateral corner of knee.

- ○ Peroneal nerve injury occurs 10–35% of the time.[74]
- ○ Plain films of the knee to evaluate for fracture and associated injuries.
- ○ MRI of the knee is also obtained to evaluate all soft tissues.
- ○ Dimple sign: Button holing of medial femoral condyle, indicates irreducible rotational dislocation and contraindication to closed reduction.
- • Treatment[75,76]:
  - ○ Immediate reduction if obvious deformity or absent pulses except in cases of rotational deformity which may require operative reduction.
  - ○ Serial vascular exams of the dorsalis pedis and posterior tibial pulses are required.
  - ○ Serial ankle-brachial index (ABI) measurements performed in all patients, ABI > 0.9 warrants serial examination, ABI < 0.9 warrants arterial duplex ultrasound or CT angiograms.
  - ○ Ischemia time > 8 hours has an amputation rate of > 90%; fasciotomy should be performed for ischemia times greater than 6 hours when indicated.
  - ○ Imaging withheld if it will delay surgical revascularization.
  - ○ Serial neurologic exams of peroneal and tibial nerve performed.
  - ○ Imaging: Pre-reduction AP and lateral X-rays of knee along with postreduction AP and lateral X-rays of knee performed; 45-degree oblique views are optional; CT may be performed postreduction to identify fracture patterns; RI may be performed postreduction to identify soft-tissue injuries.
  - ○ Immobilization used rarely for fractures without vascular injury, but most cases require surgical stabilization.
  - ○ Open reduction used for irreducible knees, posterolateral dislocation, open fracture dislocation.
  - ○ Early ligamentous reconstruction performed < 3 weeks from injury, can be done arthroscopically to re-build ACL or PCL, open repair more common with PLC and MC repair due to proximity of neurovascular structures, intra-articular injuries addressed (e.g., menisci, cartilage defects, capsular injury).
- • Complications:
  - ○ Vascular compromise (5–15% of dislocations), stiffness/arthrofibrosis (40%) of complications, laxity/instability (40%), peroneal injury (25%).
- • Patella dislocation:
  - ○ Anatomy:
    - – Patella dislocations are more common in women due to physiologic laxity.
    - – Q angle is the line from the ASIS to the center of the patella intersecting with the line from the center of patella to tibia tubercle. Higher Q angles predisposes to patella dislocation.

- Mechanism of injury:
  - Lateral dislocation: Most common dislocation. Forced internal rotation of the femur on an externally rotated tibia with knee in flexion.
  - Medial dislocation is rare and usually iatrogenic, congenital, or associated with atrophy of quadriceps muscles.
  - Superior dislocation: Occurs in elderly patients with forced hyperextension in which the patella gets locked onto an anterior femoral osteophyte.
- Clinical evaluation:
  - Knee pain, swelling, and displaced patella noted on palpation.
  - AP, lateral, and sunrise views of the patella should be obtained.
  - Assessment of patella alta or baja based on the lateral.
  - Insall–Salvati ratio: Ratio of length of patella tendon (numerator) to patella length (denominator). Should be 1.0. Ratio of 1.2 is patella alta, 0.8 is patella baja.
- Classification: Based on location, acute vs chronic, congenital vs acquired.
- Treatment:
  - Nonoperative: Reduction of patella followed by immobilization of knee locked in extension for 3 weeks. Afterwards, physical therapy for quad strengthening exercises.
  - Operative treatment: Primarily used for recurrent dislocations. May be done for acute dislocations to repair medial patellofemoral ligament in highly active patients; other methods include lateral release or patella realignment.
- Complications:
  - Recurrent dislocation: higher in patients younger than 20 at time of initial dislocation.
  - Loss of motion and patellofemoral pain.

15.4.6 Subtalar Dislocation

- Epidemiology:
  - Rare, 1% of all dislocations.
  - 25% may be open.
  - Due to high-energy mechanisms.
- Anatomy:
  - Associated with talonavicular dislocation and fractures.
  - Medial dislocation: Associated with fracture of dorsomedial talar head, posterior process of talus, navicular bone.
  - Lateral dislocation: Associated fracture of cuboid, anterior calcaneus, lateral process of talus or fibula.
- Classification:
  - Classified by dislocation direction:
    - Medial: Most common (65–80% cases), results from inversion on plantarflexed foot.
    - Lateral: More likely to be open, results from eversion on plantarflexed foot.
    - Anterior: Rare.
    - Posterior: Rare.
    - Total dislocation/extruded talus: Usually open, talus dislocated from ankle, subtalar joint, and talonavicular joints.
- Presentation:
  - Foot locked in supination or pronation.
  - AP and lateral X-rays used, CT used after reduction to look for additional injuries.
- Treatment:
  - Closed reduction and non–weight bearing cast for 4–6 weeks used as first-line treatment for most patients (60–70% of cases).
  - Open reduction used after failure of closed reduction due to blocking from medial or lateral structures.
- Complications[77]:
  - Posttraumatic arthritis most common in subtalar joint (89% of cases).

15.4.7 Joint Replacement

- Shoulder arthroplasty:
  - Total shoulder arthroplasty (TSA):
    - Replacement of humeral head and glenoid resurfacing, requires functional and intact rotator cuff.
    - Good 10-year implant survival (93%) and range of motion.
    - Indications: Shoulder pain, inability to utilize arm, posterior humeral head subluxation, glenoid chondral wear to bone.
    - Contraindications: Poor bone quality, rotator cuff arthropathy, deltoid dysfunction, irreparable rotator cuff, infection, brachial plexus injury.
    - Preoperative imaging includes X-rays, CT, and MRI.
    - Significant technical nuances to place properly.
    - Complications: Axillary nerve and posterior humeral circumflex artery damage within quadrilateral space, glenoid loosening (2.9% reoperation rate), humeral stem loosening, component malposition, subscapularis repair failure, iatrogenic rotator cuff injury, stiffness, infection, insufficient soft tissue, periprosthetic fractures.
  - Reverse shoulder arthroplasty (RSA):
    - Convex glenoid (ball) and concave humerus (articulating cup), reverses components from normal anatomy or TSA, requires functional deltoid.
    - Good 10-year survival (90%) with variability due to indication.
    - Indications: Inability to elevate arm due to irreparable rotator cuff tear and glenohumeral arthritis, incomplete coracoacromial arch, proximal humeral fractures in elderly with poor bone quality, prior arthroplasty nonunion or malunion, failed arthroplasty, rheumatoid arthritis, low functional demands on shoulder, age > 70.
    - Contraindications: Deltoid palsy, acromion deficiency, glenoid osteoporosis, infection.
    - Lower center of rotation allows deltoid to have improved mechanical advantage in the setting of deficient rotator cuff muscles, can be combined with latissimus dorsi transfer.
    - Significant technical nuances to place properly.
    - Complications: Scapular notching (injury to scapula from humeral cup), dislocation (2–3.4%), glenoid loosening, infection, acromion and scapular fractures, neurovascular injury.
  - Shoulder hemiarthroplasty:
    - Humeral articular surface replaced with attached/stemmed humeral component.
    - Outcomes depend on rotator cuff status, good pain control for humeral fractures.
    - Indications: Deficient rotator cuff, osteoporosis, high risk of glenoid loosening due to activity (e.g., young patients), rotator cuff arthropathy with inability to flex > 90 degrees, proximal humeral fracture (three-part with poor bone quality or four-part fracture, head-splitting fracture, fracture with disruption of the joint).
    - Contraindications: Infection, neuropathic joint, poor tolerance for postoperative therapy, coracoacromial ligament deficiency.
    - X-rays, CT, and MRI used for preoperative workup.
    - Significant technical nuances to place properly.
    - Complications: Glenoid arthritis, tuberosity displacement/malunion, joint overstuffing with stiffness or worsened glenoid arthritis, subcutaneous hardware dislodgement.
- Knee arthroplasty:
  - Indicated for joint cartilage destruction from osteoarthritis (95% of cases), inflammatory arthritis (e.g., rheumatoid, psoriatic, spondylitic), trauma, tumor, or osteonecrosis.
  - Used after failure of conservative therapy including physical therapy, nonsteroidal anti-inflammatory drugs (NSAIDs), steroid injections, and/or arthroscopic surgery.
  - Absolutely contraindicated during active infection in the knee or elsewhere and in skeletal immaturity.
  - Relatively contraindicated in patients with neurologic deficits in the muscles of the leg, chronic lower extremity ischemia, and patients who cannot participate in postoperative rehabilitation.
  - Total knee arthroplasty: involves replacement of entire knee structure; consists of femoral, tibial, and/or patellar components with polyethylene spacers; variation in removal of posterior cruciate ligament

seen, but all result in sacrifice of anterior cruciate ligament; cement used to fix implants or bone grows into implants.

- Alternatives:
  - Unicompartmental or partial knee arthroplasty: Improved recovery with reduced surgical reconstruction; ideally in medial compartment disease, age < 60 years, low level of activity, low body weight, angular deformity < 15 degrees, intact cruciate ligaments, preoperative flexion of 90 degrees, minimal flexion contracture or pain at rest, no chondrocalcinosis, or patellofemoral osteoarthritis.
  - Knee osteotomy: Used for unicompartmental disease with varus or valgus knees especially in younger patients.
- Important to rule out pathology of the hip and back as a potential cause of knee pain.
- Patients with antalgic gait suggest knee arthritis; abnormal knee thrusting in a varus or vagus direction indicates deformity; Trendelenburg gait suggests pain when loading hip which can be from back, hip, or knee.
- Important to assess pulses in the leg.
- Imaging includes X-rays (standing AP, lateral, tangential patellar views, and other views), MRI, and CT imaging not routinely required but can be used to plan instrumentation and individualized cutting guides.
- Complications overall 0.5–1% including venous thromboembolism and surgical-site infection, neurovascular injury, and implant failure.
- Surgical treatment is via anterior, parapatellar approach.
- Risk of surgical revision increases with age, obesity, and time.
- Risk of DVT following knee replacement ranges from 40 to 88%, risk of asymptomatic pulmonary embolism (PE) is 10–20%, risk of symptomatic PE is 0.5–3%, risk of death is 2%; variability in postoperative anticoagulation types and duration.

- Total hip arthroplasty (THA):
  - Indicated for osteoarthritis, inflammatory arthritis (e.g., rheumatoid, psoriatic, spondylitic), femoroacetabular impingement syndrome, developmental hip dysplasia, childhood hip disorders (e.g., Legg–Calve–Perthes disease, slipped capital femoral epiphysis), trauma, tumors, osteonecrosis.
  - Hip replacement involves a femoral component, acetabular component, and bearing surface; most systems are modular; fixation with cement or bony ingrowth performed; usually acetabular liner usually highly crosslinked polyethylene and articulates with ceramic or cobalt-chrome femoral head.
  - Used after failure of conservative therapy including physical therapy, NSAIDs, and/or steroid injections, arthroscopic surgery.
  - Absolutely contraindicated with active infection, significant medical comorbidities, skeletal immaturity, quadriplegia, neuromuscular weakness.
  - Relatively contraindicated in paraplegia, difficulty with ambulation, neuropathic/Charcot joint, obesity.
  - Leg length discrepancy must be carefully evaluated.
  - Evaluation of gait, posture, and other potential causes of pain (e.g., back, knees) must be evaluated.
  - Surgical treatment is via a posterolateral/Kocher–Langenbeck, direct lateral/Hardinge, anterior/Smith–Petersen–Hueter approaches.
  - Heterotopic ossification reduced in patients with high risk using NSAIDs or external beam radiation; high risk in males, bilateral hypertrophic osteoarthritis, ankylosing spondylitis, diffuse idiopathic skeletal hyperostosis, older age, or lateral approach.
  - Complications: hardware fracture (0.1–1% for cemented components; 3–18% for uncemented components), nerve injury (0–3%), vascular injury (0.2–0.3%), cement-related hypotension, thromboembolic disease, infection, dislocation (0–2%), osteolysis and bone resorption, metal-on-metal wear debris, hardware wear and loosening, periprosthetic fracture (< 1%), limb leg discrepancy, heterotopic ossification.

15.4.8 Periprosthetic Fractures

- Total hip arthroplasty/femoral shaft periprosthetic fractures:
  - Can occur intraoperatively or postoperatively. More likely to happen intraoperatively with noncemented components.

- Risk factors: Osteopenia, rheumatoid arthritis, revision surgery, inadequate implant site preparation, loose components.
- Classification:
- Multiple classifications exist including Johansson, Cooke and Newman, AAOS, and Vancouver.
- Vancouver classification most commonly used[78]:
  - Type A: Fracture around trochanteric region, either greater or lesser troch.
  - Type B: Fracture around or just distal to the stem. Further classified as stable, unstable, or unstable with poor bone stock.
  - Type C: Distal to the stem.
- Treatment[79]:
  - Treatment depends on location, stability, bone stock, and patient's medical condition.
  - Nonoperative treatment for stable/minimally displaced fractures can be limited weight bearing and immobilization.
  - Operative treatment falls into two categories: ORIF using cables/plates and screw fixation.
  - Revision of the prosthesis and cortical allograft.
- Acetabulum periprosthetic fractures:
  - Nondisplaced fractures can be treated with limited weight bearing but monitored closely for late loosening.
  - Displaced fractures should be treated with ORIF.
  - Associated with underreaming of acetabular cup intraoperatively.
- Total knee arthroplasty/supracondylar femur periprosthetic fractures[80]:
  - Usually occurs in the setting of minor trauma.
  - Risk factors include osteoporosis, knee stiffness, notching of the anterior cortex during primary TKA.
  - Lewis and Rorabeck classification:
    - Type I: Nondisplaced fracture with bone–prosthesis interface intact.
    - Type II: Displaced fracture with interface intact.
    - Type III: Displaced or nondisplaced fracture with loosening.
  - Treatment:
    - Nonoperative: Long leg cast with non-weight-bearing for minimally displaced fractures.
    - Operative: Similar principle applies to all periprosthetic fractures.
    - Displaced fractures are almost always managed with ORIF including intramedullary nailing, screw/plate fixation for revision of the femoral component.
    - Cortical strut grafts for autologous grafting may be done in case of poor bone stock.
    - Acceptable alignment includes< 10-degree angulation, < 5-mm translation, < 10-degree rotation, and< 1-cm shortening.
- Tibia periprosthetic fractures:
  - Risk factors include trauma, tibia component malalignment, component loosening.
  - Classification: Based on location, type of fracture, stability of implant, and intraoperative or postoperative occurrence.
  - Treatment:
    - Nonoperative: Closed reduction and casting if alignment is maintained.
    - Operative: ORIF if tibia plateau is not involved. If the plateau is involved, the revision is needed as it involves the bone–prosthesis interface.
- Patella periprosthetic fracture:
  - Risk factors: Large central peg, excessive resection of patella, malalignment, and lateral release.
  - Classification: Goldberg[81]:
    - Type I: Fractures not involving implant–bone interface and extensor mechanism intact.
    - Type II: Implant–bone interface or extensor mechanism disrupted.
    - Type III: Inferior pole of patella with or without patella tendon disruption.
    - Type IV: Fracture/dislocation.
  - Treatment:
    - Nonoperative treatment for any fracture without disruption of the patella/quad tendons or bone–implant interface involvement can be treated with knee immobilizer and partial weight bearing.

- – Operative for any disruption of the extensor mechanism, dislocation, or loosening. Can be done with ORIF with revision, excision of fragments, or patellectomy.[82]
- Total shoulder arthroplasty:
  - ○ Risk factors: Excessive reaming, over-impaction of humerus, excessive torque during implantation.
  - ○ Classification: Multiple classification systems exist. All are based on fracture line location relative to prosthesis.
  - ○ Wright and Cofield classification[83]:
    - – Type A: Fractures at the tip extending proximally.
    - – Type B: Fractures at the tip with minimal proximal extension and extends distally.
    - – Type C: Fractures distal to the tip.
  - ○ Treatment[84,85]:
    - – Nonoperative treatment with bracing, isometric exercises, and early-range of motion.
    - – Operative treatment includes ORIF with cerclage wiring and bone grafting. Revision of the prosthesis may be needed if loose.
- Controversial regarding which fracture types can be successfully managed nonoperatively vs. more aggressively.
- Total elbow arthroplasty:
  - ○ Risk factors: Osteoporosis, abnormal humeral bow, excessive reaming, revision elbow surgery.
  - ○ Classification[86]: Based on the location of the fracture at the metaphysic (type I), stemmed shaft (type II), or beyond the stem (type III) with assessment of stable or loose prosthesis.
  - ○ Treatment:
    - – Nondisplaced fractures with implant stability may be split at 90 degrees and allowed for isometric exercise.
    - – Surgical treatment of types II and III is similar to that of the periprosthetic hip with ORIF techniques. Type I fractures may require revision of implants.

15.4.9 Septic Joints

- Epidemiology:
  - ○ Incidence of 6:100,000 patients annually; incidence 30–60:100,000 patients with joint disease or prosthetic joints annually.
- Etiology:
  - ○ Risk factors: age, joint disease, recent joint surgery, skin or soft-tissue infection, IV drug abuse, catheters or sepsis, immunosuppression, diabetes.
  - ○ Arises from hematogenous spread most often.
  - ○ Most commonly due to *Staphylococcus aureus*; other causes from *Streptococcus pneumoniae*, *Pseudomonas*.
- Presentation:
  - ○ Presents with single, swollen, painful joint; restricted joint movement, warm joint.
  - ○ Most commonly occurs in knees (50%) followed by wrists, ankles, and hips; less commonly in axial joints.
  - ○ Polyarticular infection (> 2 joints) occurs in 20% of cases; more common in rheumatoid arthritis, connective tissue disorder, or sepsis.
  - ○ Highly associated with infective endocarditis especially in IV drug abuse.
- Diagnosis:
  - ○ Physical exam, laboratory studies, blood culture, and joint aspiration used for diagnosis; inflammatory labs (C-reactive protein, erythrocyte sedimentation rate, procalcitonin) can be used as ancillary
    testing but have limited sensitivity; joint X-rays, ultrasound, or other imaging used for evaluation; echocardiography used to evaluate endocarditis; synovial biopsy rare but used to evaluate osteomyelitis, slow growing infections, or coinfection with *Mycobacterium tuberculosis*.
  - ○ Blood cultures positive in 50% of cases.
  - ○ Synovial fluid analysis demonstrates positive Gram stain organism, leukocyte count ($50–150,000$ cells/mm^3; mostly neutrophils).

- ○ Differential diagnosis: Septic bursitis, gonococcal arthritis, Lyme disease, tuberculous arthritis, viral arthritis, fungal arthritis, traumatic arthritis, crystal-induced arthritis (i.e., gout or pseudogout), spondyloarthritis, rheumatoid arthritis.
- Treatment:
  - ○ Joint drainage or surgical washout used to clear infectious burden and obtain diagnosis.
  - ○ Empiric antibiotics administered (vancomycin and third/fourth-generation cephalosporin) before narrowing; antibiotic duration ranges between 14 and 21 days depending on clinical factures.

15.5 Orthopaedic Neoplasms

Jim Lai

15.5.1 General Approach to Orthopaedic Neoplasms

- Epidemiology:
  - ○ Overall rare, 0.2% of malignancies, incidence 0.9:100,000 people annually; 5% of all cancers in children.
  - ○ 5-year overall survival is 68%.
  - ○ Bimodal age distribution: First peak in second decade and second peak in sixth decade.
- Presentation:
  - ○ Patients can present with localized pain or swelling; presentation is often asymptomatic.
  - ○ Assessment of fracture risk and need for prophylactic fixation suggested by functional pain, > 50% destruction of cortical bone, Harington criteria or Mirels criteria (▶ Table 15.21).
- Diagnosis:
  - ○ Bone with sharp, well-defined zones of transition from normal bone suggest slow lesion growth.
  - ○ Bone with sclerotic zone of transition suggests rapid growth and an aggressive lesion.
  - ○ Wide zones of transition suggest aggressive lesions; mimickers include infection and eosinophilic granuloma.
  - ○ Limited periosteal thickening, lamellated periosteum, speculated periosteum, and erosive periosteal reaction (i.e., Codman triangle) suggest increasing degrees of aggressiveness.
  - ○ Cortical bone destruction common in malignant lesions; mimickers include infection and eosinophilic granuloma.
  - ○ Differential depends on age (▶ Table 15.22), tumor characteristics (▶ Table 15.23), and location (▶ Table 15.24).
  - ○ Other features used to differentiate tumor include lesion origin on bone site (i.e., epiphysis, metaphysis, and diaphysis), centric versus eccentric lesion center on bone cortex, formation of tumor matrix, presence of multiple lesions in separate bones.
  - ○ Consideration of soft tissue, muscle, and vascular tumors should be considered due to proximity and similarity to some bone neoplasm.

Table 15.21 Harington and Mirels criteria for impending fracture from bone tumors

Harington criteria

- > 50% destruction of diaphyseal cortices
- > 50–75% destruction of metaphysis (> 2.5 cm)
- Permeative destruction of subtrochanteric femoral region
- Persistent pain following irradiation

Mirels criteria (score ≥ 8 suggests prophylactic fixation)

Score	1	2	3
Site	Upper limb	Lower limb	Peritrochanteric
Pain	Mild	Moderate	Functional
Lesion	Blastic	Mixed	Lytic
Lesion size compared to bone	< 1/3	1/3–2/3	> 2/3

Table 15.22 Differential diagnosis of orthopaedic neoplasms by age

Age group	Benign tumors	Malignant tumors
Children (0–5 y)	Osteofibrous dysplasia	Metastatic rhabdomyosarcoma
	Osteomyelitis	Metastatic neuroblastoma
		Leukemia
Teenagers, young adults (10–40 y)	Fibrous dysplasia	Osteosarcoma
	Osteoid osteoma	Ewing sarcoma
	Giant cell tumors	Desmoplastic fibroma
	Aneurysmal bone cyst	Leukemia/lymphoma
	Nonossifying fibroma	
	Unicameral bone cyst	
	Osteochondroma	
	Chondroblastoma	
	Osteomyelitis	
	Eosinophilic granuloma	
	Endochondroma	
Older adult (40–80 y)	Endochondroma	Metastatic bone disease
	Bone infarct	Multiple myeloma
	Paget disease	Leukemia/lymphoma
	Hyperparathyroid disease	Chondrosarcoma
		Malignant fibrous histioma
		Secondary sarcoma (Paget irradiation)

Table 15.23 Differential diagnosis of orthopaedic neoplasms by X-ray characteristics

Age	Well-defined	Ill-defined	Sclerotic
0–10	Eosinophilic granuloma	Ewing sarcoma	Osteosarcoma
	Unicameral bone cyst	Osteosarcoma	
		Leukemia	
10–20	Nonossifying fibroma	Ewing sarcoma	Osteosarcoma
	Fibrous dysplasia	Eosinophilic granuloma	Fibrous dysplasia
	Unicameral bone cyst	Osteosarcoma	Eosinophilic granuloma
	Aneurysmal bone cyst		Osteoid osteoma
	Chondroblastoma		Osteoblastoma
	Chondromyxoid fibroma		
20–40	Giant cell tumor	Giant cell tumor	Endochondroma
	Endochondroma		Osteoma
	Chondrosarcoma		Bone island
	Hyperthyroidism		Periosteal osteosarcoma
	Osteoblastoma		Healed lesions
>40	Metastasis	Metastasis	Metastasis
	Multiple myeloma	Multiple myeloma	Bone island
	Geode	Chondrosarcoma	

Note: Consider infective osteomyelitis in all age groups and appearance categories.

Table 15.24 Differential diagnosis of orthopaedic neoplasms by location

Location	Differential
Skull	Eosinophilic granuloma, metastasis, multiple myeloma, fibrous dysplasia, osteosarcoma
Mandible	Adamantinoma, odontogenic cyst
Humerus	All tumors, unicameral bone cyst
Distal radius	Giant cell tumor, eosinophilic granuloma
Hands	Endochondroma
Ribs	Metastasis, endochondroma, chondrosarcoma, Ewing sarcoma
Spine	Metastasis, multiple myeloma, osteoblastoma, chordoma, hemangioma, aneurysmal bone system, osteoid osteoma, lymphoma, eosinophilic granuloma, plasmacytoma
Pelvis	Osteosarcoma, chondrosarcoma, unicameral bone cyst, lymphoma, Ewing sarcoma, eosinophilic granuloma, chordoma
Proximal femur	Unicameral bone cyst, fibrous dysplasia, eosinophilic granuloma
Knee	All tumors, osteosarcoma, Ewing sarcoma
Tibia	Nonossifying fibroma, fibrous dysplasia, adamantinoma, osteoid osteoma
Calcaneus	Unicameral bone cyst, Ewing sarcoma, osteoblastoma, chondroblastoma

- ○ Imaging commonly includes plain films; imaging can include CT or MRI for improving characterization of a lesion; PET imaging recommended for evaluating primary bone tumors; skeletal survey X-rays utilized for multiple myeloma to evaluate lesions.
- • Treatment:
  - ○ Primary bone sarcomas staged by Musculoskeletal Tumor Society (MSTS)/Enneking staging (▶ Table 15.25); American Joint Committee on Cancer TNM staging (▶ Table 15.25) not widely utilized for bone tumors.
  - ○ Bone biopsy used for diagnosis of benign or malignant lesion, when histology could alter treatment, or in identifying diagnosis with potentially high-risk lesions; planned to allow potential resection of biopsy tract.
  - ○ Bone biopsy results range from 90 to 95% for metastatic lesions and 70–80% for primary bone tumors or infections.
  - ○ Resection can involve localized removal with reconstruction or wide-spread en bloc resection depending on pathology.
  - ○ Radiation can be used for fractures with low risk of fracture or deformity.
  - ○ Stabilization of bone required for impending fracture (▶ Table 15.21) or after resection.

15.5.2 Specific Benign Orthopaedic Lesions

- • Unicameral bone cyst[87,88]:
  - ○ Nonneoplastic bone lesion, occurs near the physis in patients < 20 years.
  - ○ Commonly on proximal humerus.
  - ○ Decreases in size with skeletal maturity but requires monitoring due to fracture risk.
  - ○ Presents asymptomatically (50%) or with pain from pathologic fracture (50%).
  - ○ Diagnosed with radiographs.
  - ○ Treated with immobilization, aspiration, and injection of methylprednisolone; curettage with bone grafting and internal fixation; most heal spontaneously.
- • Aneurysmal bone cyst[88,89]:
  - ○ Nonneoplastic bone lesion with bone filled by blood-filled cavities, can be large and destructive.
  - ○ Most commonly in spine (25%) and long bones (20%); most common in metaphysis, metatarsal bone, or pelvis.
  - ○ Associated with other tumors in 30% of cases.
  - ○ Presents with pain or pathologic fracture.

Table 15.25 Staging of primary bone sarcomas

Grade	Description
Musculoskeletal Tumor Society (MSTS)/Enneking staging[a]	
1	Latent lesion
2	Active lesion
3	Aggressive lesion
I	Low grade
• A	Intracompartmental
• B	Extracompartmental
II	High grade
• A	Intracompartmental
• B	Extracompartmental
III	High grade with regional node or metastatic spread
American Joint Committee on Cancer TNM staging	
T (appendicular skeleton, trunk, skull, facial bones)[b]	
T1	Tumor ≤ 8 cm
T2	Tumor > 8 cm
T3	Discontinuous tumors in primary bone site
T (spine)[b]	
T1	Tumor confined to ≤ 2 adjacent vertebra
T2	Tumor confined to 3 adjacent vertebrae
T3	Tumor confined to ≥ 4 adjacent vertebrae or any nonadjacent vertebrae
T4	Extension into spinal canal or great vessels
T (pelvis)[b]	
T1	Tumor confined to 1 pelvic segment without extraosseous extension (T1a: ≤ 8 cm, T1b: > 8 cm)
T2	Tumor confined to 1 pelvic segment with extraosseous extension or 2 segments without extraosseous extension (T2a: ≤ 8 cm, T2b: > 8 cm)
T3	Tumor spanning 2 pelvic segments with extraosseous extension (T3a: ≤ 8 cm, T3b: > 8 cm)
T4	Tumor spanning 3 pelvic segments or crossing sacroiliac joint (T4a: tumor involving sacroiliac joint and medial to foramen; T4b: tumor encasing external iliac vessels or thrombus in pelvic vessels)
N	
• N0	No regional lymph node metastasis
• N1	Regional lymph node metastasis
M	
• M1	Distant metastasis
G	
• G1	Well differentiated, low grade
• G2	Moderately differentiated, high grade
• G3	Poorly differentiated, high grade

[a] Intracompartmental tumors are confined to the cortex of the bone, while extracompartmental tumors extend beyond the bone cortex.

[b] TX: primary tumor cannot be assessed; T0: no evidence of primary tumor.

- Diagnose with radiographs; MRI or CT may show fluid-fluid levels from blood.
- Treated nonoperatively in setting of some fractures which can heal the cyst, curettage with bone grafting.
- 25% risk of recurrence.

- Fibrous dysplasia[88]:
  - Developmental abnormality resulting in poor mineralization of normal bone.
  - Most common proximal femur but can occur in any bone.
  - Most common in adolescents/young adults.
  - Monostotic (one bone involved, 80% of cases) or polyostotic (multiple bones involved, 20% of cases).
  - Associated with McCune–Albright syndrome (skin abnormalities, precocious puberty, mono-ostotic fibrous dysplasia), Mazabraud syndrome (polyostotic fibrous dysplasia), osteofibrous dysplasia.
  - Can result in cranial nerve compression, most commonly the optic nerve.
  - 1% risk of malignant transformation.
  - Diagnosed with radiographs or bone scans.
  - Treated with observation, bisphosphonate therapy, fixation and bone grafting, osteotomies.
- Paget disease[90]:
  - Abnormal bone remodeling due to increased osteoclastic resorption possibly caused by a subacute viral infection.
  - Most common in fifth decade.
  - Monostotic or polyostotic; can be hereditary.
  - Rare risk of progression to Paget sarcoma (1% of cases).
  - Presents with pain, swelling, stress fractures, cardiac symptoms from high-output cardiac failure.
  - Diagnosed with radiographs; bone scan can identify disease; MRI and CT can better evaluate some lesions.
  - Treated with observation, nonsteroidal anti-inflammatory drugs (NSAIDs), bisphosphonates, calcitonin, surgical resection, and stabilization.
- Eosinophilic granuloma/histiocytosis X/Langerhans cell histiocytosis[88,91]:
  - Three types of presentations:
    - Eosinophilic granuloma: Single lesion in younger patients.
    - Hand–Schuller–Christian disease: Chronic, disseminated disease with bone and visceral lesions.
    - Letterer–Siwe disease: Fatal disease in younger patients.
  - Most common in skull, ribs, clavicle, scapula, and mandible; can have isolated lesions in the spine or diaphysis of long bones and pelvis.
  - Diagnosed with radiographs but can mimic other tumors.
  - Treated with observation, bracing, low-dose radiation, chemotherapy, corticosteroid injections, curettage and bone grafting, or spine fixation.
- Nonossifying fibroma[88,92]:
  - Most common benign tumor of childhood, occurs in 30–40% of skeletally immature children mostly in the metaphysis of the lower extremity.
  - Usually asymptomatic but can present with pathologic fracture.
  - Diagnosed by radiographs, most found incidentally when taking X-rays for different reason.
  - Most need no treatment unless risk for pathologic fracture, greater than ⅔ diameter of bone. The older, bigger, or active the patient, the high likelihood of needing surgical treatment. Curettage and bone grafting can be used for symptomatic and large lesions.
- Giant cell tumor[94,93]:
  - Benign tumor of metaphysis of long bones.
  - Most common in femur around knee (50%), tibia, radius, and sacral ala/vertebra (10%).
  - Progresses to malignant tumor in 2–5% of cases.
  - Presents with pain localized to the adjacent joint
  - Radiolucent and well defined on plain films. 2% present with clinically indolent lung metastasis
  - Diagnosed with radiographs, chest X-rays, or CT used to evaluate pulmonary metastasis.
  - Treated with radiation, bisphosphonates, denosumab, curettage, and reconstruction; 15–25% risk of recurrence.

15.5.3 Specific Benign Orthopaedic Neoplasms

- Osteoid ostema and osteoblastoma[88,93,95]:
  - Small, painful lesion

- Size distinguishes types: Osteoid osteoma (< 2 cm) vs. osteoblastoma (> 2 cm).
- Most common in patients aged 5–25 years.
- Most common in lower extremity (> 50%), spine (10–15%), hand (5–10%), and foot (< 5%).
- Pain highly responsive to NSAIDs, worse at night and with alcohol.
- Distinction between lesion nidus and reactive perilesional bone.
- Osteoid osteoma represents 10% of benign tumors, while osteoblastoma demonstrates 3% of benign tumors.
- Treatment can be observation, NSAIDs, percutaneous radiofrequency ablation, surgical resection with curettage.
- 10–15% recurrence rate with percutaneous radiofrequency ablation.
- Enchondroma[88,93,96]:
  - Benign tumor of hyaline cartilage located in medullary cavity.
  - Most common in 20–50-year-olds in the hands (60%), distal femur (20%), proximal humerus (10%), and tibia.
  - Associated with Ollier disease (multiple enchondromatosis) and Maffucci syndrome (multiple enchondromas and soft-tissue angiomas).
  - Undergo skeletal surveys if polyostotic disease suspected; CT can be useful to distinguish chondrosarcomas.
  - Treated with observation, intralesional curettage with bone grafting, or immobilization followed by curettage and bone grafting.
  - Rare risk of malignant transformation to chondrosarcoma (1%), higher risk in genetic conditions (25–30%).
- Periosteal chondroma:
  - Rare lesion of surface of long bones in 10–20 years, most common on proximal humerus.
  - Treated with marginal excision of bone and underlying cortex.
- Osteochondroma[88,93]:
  - Most common benign bone tumor overall.
  - Presents in adolescents/young adults.
  - Located at sites of tendon insertion in knee, proximal femur, or proximal humerus.
  - Rare malignant transformation (< 1%) to secondary chondrosarcoma.
  - Multiple hereditary exostosis: Multiple osteochondromas, 5–10% risk of transformation to chondrosarcoma.
  - Can occur after Salter–Harris fractures, trauma, or radiation therapy.
  - Present with painless mass and deformity.
  - Diagnosed by radiographs; CT and MRI used to better characterize lesion.
  - Treated with observation, or marginal resection.
- Chondroblastoma[88,93]:
  - Rare lesion in the epiphyseal region of young patients.
  - Most common in distal femur and proximal tibia.
  - Presents with pain and deformity.
  - Diagnosed by radiographs; CT and MRI not routinely used.
  - Treated with surgical resection with or without bone grafting.
- Chondromyxoid fibroma[88,93]:
  - Rare benign lesion with chondroid and myxoid elements.
- Nonossifying fibroma[88,93]:
  - Most common benign tumor of childhood, occurs in 30–40% of skeletally immature children mostly in the metaphysis of the lower extremity.
  - Usually asymptomatic but can present with pathologic fracture.
  - Diagnosed by radiographs.
  - Treated nonoperatively as most lesions self-resolve, casting can be used for pathologic fractures, curettage and bone grafting can be used for symptomatic and large lesions.
- Desmoplastic fibroma[88,93]:
  - Low-grade malignant tumor of the bone in adolescents and young adults, commonly in the mandible and metaphysis of long bones.

- Presents with pain.
- Treated with wide surgical resection to reduce recurrence rate.
- Giant cell tumor[88,93]:
  - Benign tumor of metaphysis of long bones.
  - Most common in femur around knee (50%), tibia, radius, and sacral ala/vertebra (10%).
  - Progresses to malignant tumor in 2–5% of cases.
  - Presents with pain and palpable mass.
  - Diagnosed with radiographs, chest X-rays, or CT used to evaluate pulmonary metastasis.
  - Treated with radiation, bisphosphonates, denosumab, curettage, and reconstruction.
  - 15–25% risk of recurrence.

15.5.4 Specific Malignant Orthopaedic Neoplasms

- Most common malignant tumors are:
  - 36%: Osteosarcomas of the leg bones in children/young adults.
  - 30%: Chondrosarcomas of patients > 40.
  - 16%: Ewing sarcoma of thigh, upper arm, shin, or pelvis in children/teenagers.
- Osteosarcoma[88,97,98]:
  - Intramedullary osteosarcoma is the most common primary sarcoma; 76% long-term survival currently; 2nd most common sarcoma is liposarcoma and 3rd most common sarcoma is synovial sarcoma.
  - Other subtypes:
    - Parosteal osteosarcoma is a low-grade variant on the metaphysis surface of long bones, 95% survival.
    - Periosteal osteosarcoma: Rare, occurs on the diaphysis of long bones; most common in femur and tibia; intermediate prognosis between parosteal and intramedullary osteosarcoma.
    - Telangiectatic osteosarcoma: Rare, similar to survival as intramedullary osteosarcoma.
  - Occurs primarily in the second decade and elderly with Paget disease.
  - Most commonly at distal femur and proximal tibia.
  - Most commonly stage IIB, 10–20% present with pulmonary metastasis requiring chest CT for workup.
  - Predisposing mutations include retinoblastoma (Rb) and RECQL4 (Rothmund–Thomson syndrome).
  - Patients present with significant pain, fever, swelling, and can feel a mass; alkaline phosphatase may be elevated.
  - Significant blastic changes are seen on radiographs; MRI used to evaluate soft-tissue involvement; bone scans used to evaluate local disease and presence of bone metastasis.
  - Treatment with preoperative chemotherapy and maintenance chemotherapy after surgical resection.
  - Wide surgical excision is performed with attempts to salvage limbs.
- Chondrosarcoma[88,98]:
  - Malignant primary tumor of chondrocytes.
  - Primary versus secondary from osteochondroma, multiple hereditary exostosis, enchondroma, Ollier disease, or Maffucci syndrome.
  - More common in older patients (40–75 years).
  - Most common in pelvis, proximal femur, distal femur, and scapula.
  - Grade 1 has 90% 5-year survival, while grade III has 30–50% 5-year survival; most lesions present as grade 1 or 2 (85%).
  - Presents with pain and bowel/bladder obstruction from mass effect in the pelvis.
  - Diagnosed with radiographs; MRI useful to evaluate soft-tissue involvement; CT used to evaluate cortical involvement.
  - Treated with chemotherapy and radiation alone but resistant to treatment; intralesional curettage for low-grade lesions, wide surgical excision for high-grade lesions, resection with chemotherapy.
  - 5–15% rate of recurrence for grade I lesions versus 25% rate of recurrence for grade III lesions; recurrence dependent on resection margins.
- Multiple myeloma:
  - Proliferation of plasma cells and skeletal lesions.
  - Types include multiple myeloma, solitary plasmacytoma, osteosclerotic myeloma.

- ○ Most common in patients > 40 years.
- ○ 5-year survival of 30% but variable pending on clinical features and tumor mutations.
- ○ Presents with pain, anemia, hypercalcemia, renal insufficiency.
- ○ Radiographs show punched-out lytic lesions; skeletal surveys can be useful to identify secondary lesions as PET scanning cannot identify 30% of lesions; MRI can be useful for pelvis and spine imaging.
- ○ Treatment with multiagent chemotherapy combined with steroids (e.g., lenalidomide and dexamethasone), autologous and allogenic stem cell transplantation, and/or surgical stabilization and irradiation.
- Histiocytoma[88,99]:
  - ○ Benign fibrous histiocytoma: Rare, benign lesion of the bone.
  - ○ Malignant fibrous histiocytoma/fibrosarcoma.
    - – Rare, lesion presenting similarly with osteosarcoma.
    - – Affects patients aged 20–80 years, most common in metaphysis of long bones.
    - – 50–60% 5-year survival, presents with pulmonary metastasis in 30% of cases.
    - – Treated with neoadjuvant chemotherapy, wide surgical resection, and multiagent maintenance chemotherapy.
- Ewing sarcoma[88,98]:
  - ○ Small round cell tumor, common in patients 5–25 years of age.
  - ○ 50% found in diaphysis of long bones.
  - ○ t(11:22) translocation resulting in EWS–FLI1 fusion protein found in 95% of cases and can be used to distinguish Ewing sarcoma from other small blue cell tumors (e.g., neuroblastoma, leukemia, eosinophilic granuloma, lymphoma, myeloma).
  - ○ 65–80% 5-year survival for localized disease, 25–50% 5-year survival for metastatic disease.
  - ○ Poor risk factors: Larger tumors, older age, male sex, elevated lactate dehydrogenase, p53 and t(11;22) mutation, elevated Ki-67, elevated HER-2/neu, metastasis, < 90% necrosis with chemotherapy.
  - ○ Presents with pain and fever.
  - ○ Diagnosed with radiographs, bone scans, MRI to evaluate soft tissue, and CT chest to evaluate pulmonary metastasis.
  - ○ Treated with chemotherapy and radiation alone for nonresectable tumors, limb salvage resection where able.
- Metastatic disease:
  - ○ Most common cause of bone destruction in adults.
  - ○ Tumors commonly spreading to the bone: breast, lung, thyroid, renal, prostate.
  - ○ Presents in older adults with pain, pathologic fracture, or during staging.
  - ○ Most common in spine (see Chapter 14.2 Spine Injury), proximal femur, and humerus.
  - ○ Tumors spread hematogenously to the bone and secrete cytokines to activate osteoclastic bone lysis.
  - ○ Diagnosed with radiographs, CT imaging, or MRI depending on location; biopsy can be used to identify primary pathology.
  - ○ Treated with bracing, bisphosphonate therapy, radiotherapy alone, stabilization with postoperative radiation, or preoperative embolization.

References

[1] Egol K, Koval KJ, Zuckerman JD. Handbook of Fractures. 6th ed. Philadelphia, PA: Lippincott,Williams &Wilkins;2019

[2] Ulmer T. The clinical diagnosis of compartment syndrome of the lower leg: are clinical findings predictive of the disorder? J Orthop Trauma. 2002; 16(8):572–577

[3] McQueen MM, Court-Brown CM. Compartment monitoring in tibial fractures. The pressure threshold for decompression. J Bone Joint Surg Br. 1996; 78(1):99–104

[4] Canadian Orthopaedic Trauma Society. Nonoperative treatment compared with plate fixation of displaced midshaft clavicular fractures. A multicenter, randomized clinical trial. J Bone Joint Surg Am. 2007; 89(1):1–10

[5] Meinberg EG, Agel J, Roberts CS, Karam MD, Kellam JF. Fracture and dislocation classification compendium-2008. J Orthop Trauma. 2018; 32 Suppl 1:S1–S170

[6] Donnelly TD, Macfarlane RJ, Nagy MT, Ralte P, Waseem M. Fractures of the clavicle: an overview. Open Orthop J. 2013; 7:329–333

[7] Stanley D, Norris SH. Recovery following fractures of the clavicle treated conservatively. Injury. 1988; 19(3):162–164

[8]   Andersen K, Jensen PO, Lauritzen J. Treatment of clavicular fractures. Figure-of-eight bandage versus a simple sling. Acta Orthop Scand. 1987; 58(1):71–74

[9]   Zlowodzki M, Zelle BA, Cole PA, Jeray K, McKee MD, Evidence-Based Orthopaedic Trauma Working Group. Treatment of acute midshaft clavicle fractures: systematic review of 2144 fractures: on behalf of the Evidence-Based Orthopaedic Trauma Working Group. J Orthop Trauma. 2005; 19(7):504–507

[10] Golish SR, Oliviero JA, Francke EI, Miller MD. A biomechanical study of plate versus intramedullary devices for midshaft clavicle fixation. J Orthop Surg Res. 2008; 3:28

[11] Robinson CM, Court-Brown CM, McQueen MM, Wakefield AE. Estimating the risk of nonunion following nonoperative treatment of a clavicular fracture. J Bone Joint Surg Am. 2004; 86(7):1359–1365

[12] Hill JM, McGuire MH, Crosby LA. Closed treatment of displaced middle-third fractures of the clavicle gives poor results. J Bone Joint Surg Br. 1997; 79(4):537–539

[13] Fischer RP, Flynn TC, Miller PW, et al. Scapular fractures and associated major ipsilateral upper-torso injuries. Curr Concepts Trauma Care.. 1985; 1:14–16

[14] Koval KJ, Gallagher MA, Marsicano JG, Cuomo F, McShinawy A, Zuckerman JD. Functional outcome after minimally displaced fractures of the proximal part of the humerus. J Bone Joint Surg Am. 1997; 79(2):203–207

[15] Gerber C, Hersche O, Berberat C. The clinical relevance of posttraumatic avascular necrosis of the humeral head. J Shoulder Elbow Surg. 1998; 7(6):586–590

[16] Sarmiento A, Zagorski JB, Zych GA, Latta LL, Capps CA. Functional bracing for the treatment of fractures of the humeral diaphysis. J Bone Joint Surg Am. 2000; 82(4):478–486

[17] Sarmiento A, Kinman PB, Galvin EG, Schmitt RH, Phillips JG. Functional bracing of fractures of the shaft of the humerus. J Bone Joint Surg Am. 1977; 59(5):596–601

[18] Farragos AF, Schemitsch EH, McKee MD. Complications of intramedullary nailing for fractures of the humeral shaft: a review. J Orthop Trauma. 1999; 13(4):258–267

[19] Brown RF, Morgan RG. Intercondylar T-shaped fractures of the humerus. Results in ten cases treated by early mobilisation. J Bone Joint Surg Br. 1971; 53(3):425–428

[20] Cobb TK, Morrey BF. Total elbow arthroplasty as primary treatment for distal humeral fractures in elderly patients. J Bone Joint Surg Am. 1997; 79(6):826–832

[21] Kundel K, Braun W, Wieberneit J, Rüter A. Intraarticular distal humerus fractures. Factors affecting functional outcome. Clin Orthop Relat Res. 1996(332):200–208

[22] Ring D, Jupiter JB, Gulotta L. Articular fractures of the distal part of the humerus. J Bone Joint Surg Am. 2003; 85(2):232–238

[23] Jobe FW, Stark H, Lombardo SJ. Reconstruction of the ulnar collateral ligament in athletes. J Bone Joint Surg Am. 1986; 68(8):1158–1163

[24] Herbertsson P, Josefsson PO, Hasserius R, Karlsson C, Besjakov J, Karlsson M, Long-Term Follow-Up Study. Uncomplicated Mason type-II and III fractures of the radial head and neck in adults. A long-term follow-up study. J Bone Joint Surg Am. 2004; 86(3):569–574

[25] Moro JK, Werier J, MacDermid JC, Patterson SD, King GJ. Arthroplasty with a metal radial head for unreconstructible fractures of the radial head. J Bone Joint Surg Am. 2001; 83(8):1201–1211

[26] Anderson LD, Sisk D, Tooms RE, Park WI, III. Compression-plate fixation in acute diaphyseal fractures of the radius and ulna. J Bone Joint Surg Am. 1975; 57(3):287–297

[27] Matthews LS, Kaufer H, Garver DF, Sonstegard DA. The effect on supination-pronation of angular malalignment of fractures of both bones of the forearm. J Bone Joint Surg Am. 1982; 64(1):14–17

[28] Ring D, Jupiter JB, Waters PM. Monteggia fractures in children and adults. J Am Acad Orthop Surg. 1998; 6(4):215–224

[29] Schemitsch EH, Richards RR. The effect of malunion on functional outcome after plate fixation of fractures of both bones of the forearm in adults. J Bone Joint Surg Am. 1992; 74(7):1068–1078

[30] Edwards GS, Jr. Intra-articular fractures of the distal part of the radius treated with the small AO external fixator. J Bone Joint Surg Am. 1991; 73(8):1241–1250

[31] Bourrel P, Ferro RM. Nerve complications in closed fractures of the lower end of the radius. Ann Chir Main. 1982; 1(2):119–126

[32] Hove LM. Delayed rupture of the thumb extensor tendon. A 5-year study of 18 consecutive cases. Acta Orthop Scand. 1994; 65(2):199–203

[33] Gelberman RH, Gross MS. The vascularity of the wrist. Identification of arterial patterns at risk. Clin Orthop Relat Res. 1986(202):40–49

[34] Gäbler C, Kukla C, Breitenseher MJ, Trattnig S, Vécsei V. Diagnosis of occult scaphoid fractures and other wrist injuries. Are repeated clinical examinations and plain radiographs still state of the art? Langenbecks Arch Surg. 2001; 386(2):150–154

[35] Swanson TV, Szabo RM, Anderson DD. Open hand fractures: prognosis and classification. J Hand Surg Am. 1991; 16(1):101–107

[36] Halawi MJ. Pelvic ring injuries: emergency assessment and management. J Clin Orthop Trauma. 2015; 6(4):252–258

[37] Durkin A, Sagi HC, Durham R, Flint L. Contemporary management of pelvic fractures. Am J Surg. 2006; 192(2):211–223

[38] Montgomery KD, Geerts WH, Potter HG, Helfet DL. Thromboembolic complications in patients with pelvic trauma. Clin Orthop Relat Res. 1996(329):68–87

[39] Flancbaum L, Morgan AS, Fleisher M, Cox EF. Blunt bladder trauma: manifestation of severe injury. Urology. 1988; 31(3):220–222

[40] Majeed SA. Neurologic deficits in major pelvic injuries. Clin Orthop Relat Res. 1992(282):222–228

[41] Judet R, Judet J, Letournel E. Fractures of the acetabulum: classification and surgical approaches for open reduction. Preliminary report. J Bone Joint Surg Am. 1964; 46:1615–1646

[42] Matta JM, Anderson LM, Epstein HC, Hendricks P. Fractures of the acetabulum. A retrospective analysis. Clin Orthop Relat Res. 1986 (205):230–240

[43] Matta JM. Fractures of the acetabulum: accuracy of reduction and clinical results in patients managed operatively within three weeks after the injury. J Bone Joint Surg Am. 1996; 78(11):1632–1645

[44] Mears DC, Velyvis JH. Acute total hip arthroplasty for selected displaced acetabular fractures: two to twelve-year results. J Bone Joint Surg Am. 2002; 84(1):1–9

[45] Skinner P, Riley D, Ellery J, Beaumont A, Coumine R, Shafighian B. Displaced subcapital fractures of the femur: a prospective randomized comparison of internal fixation, hemiarthroplasty and total hip replacement. Injury. 1989; 20(5):291–293

[46] Tidermark J, Ponzer S, Svensson O, Söderqvist A, Törnkvist H. Internal fixation compared with total hip replacement for displaced femoral neck fractures in the elderly. A randomised, controlled trial. J Bone Joint Surg Br. 2003; 85(3):380–388

[47] Balach T, Baldwin PC, Intravia J. Atypical femur fractures associated with diphosphonate use. J Am Acad Orthop Surg. 2015; 23(9):550–557

[48] Winquist RA, Hansen ST, Jr, Clawson DK. Closed intramedullary nailing of femoral fractures. A report of five hundred and twenty cases. J Bone Joint Surg Am. 1984; 66(4):529–539

[49] Leung PC, Mak KH, Lee SY. Percutaneous tension band wiring: a new method of internal fixation for mildly displaced patella fracture. J Trauma. 1983; 23(1):62–64

[50] Tang SC, Goulet JA, McClellan RT, et al. Results of treatment of displaced patellar fractures by partial patellectomy. J Bone Joint Surg Am. 1991; 73(8):1273–1274

[51] Prat-Fabregat S, Camacho-Carrasco P. Treatment strategy for tibial plateau fractures: an update. EFORT Open Rev. 2017; 1(5):225–232

[52] Schatzker J, McBroom R, Bruce D. The tibial plateau fracture. The Toronto experience 1968–1975. Clin Orthop Relat Res. 1979(138):94–104

[53] Rasmussen PS. Tibial condylar fractures. Impairment of knee joint stability as an indication for surgical treatment. J Bone Joint Surg Am. 1973; 55(7):1331–1350

[54] Sarmiento A, Sharpe FE, Ebramzadeh E, Normand P, Shankwiler J. Factors influencing the outcome of closed tibial fractures treated with functional bracing. Clin Orthop Relat Res. 1995(315):8–24

[55] Freedman EL, Johnson EE. Radiographic analysis of tibial fracture malalignment following intramedullary nailing. Clin Orthop Relat Res. 1995(315):25–33

[56] Bauer M, Jonsson K, Nilsson B. Thirty-year follow-up of ankle fractures. Acta Orthop Scand. 1985; 56(2):103–106

[57] Lindsjö U. Operative treatment of ankle fracture-dislocations. A follow-up study of 306/321 consecutive cases. Clin Orthop Relat Res. 1985(199):28–38

[58] Sands A, Grujic L, Byck DC, Agel J, Benirschke S, Swiontkowski MF. Clinical and functional outcomes of internal fixation of displaced pilon fractures. Clin Orthop Relat Res. 1998(347):131–137

[59] Mayer SW, Joyner PW, Almekinders LC, Parekh SG. Stress fractures of the foot and ankle in athletes. Sports Health. 2014; 6(6):481–491

[60] Bica D, Sprouse RA, Armen J. Diagnosis and management of common foot fractures. Am Fam Physician. 2016; 93(3):183–191

[61] Miller CM, Winter WG, Bucknell AL, Jonassen EA. Injuries to the midtarsal joint and lesser tarsal bones. J Am Acad Orthop Surg. 1998; 6(4):249–258

[62] Kuo RS, Tejwani NC, Digiovanni CW, et al. Outcome after open reduction and internal fixation of Lisfranc joint injuries. J Bone Joint Surg Am. 2000; 82(11):1609–1618

[63] Johnson JT, Labib SA, Fowler R. Intramedullary screw fixation of the fifth metatarsal: an anatomic study and improved technique. Foot Ankle Int. 2004; 25(4):274–277

[64] Nielsen TR, Lindblad BE, Faun P. Long-term results after fracture of the fifth metatarsal. Foot Ankle Surg. 1998; 4:227–232

[65] teSlaa RL, Wijffels MP, Brand R, Marti RK. The prognosis following acute primary glenohumeral dislocation. J Bone Joint Surg Br. 2004; 86(1):58–64

[66] Pugh DM, Wild LM, Schemitsch EH, King GJ, McKee MD. Standard surgical protocol to treat elbow dislocations with radial head and coronoid fractures. J Bone Joint Surg Am. 2004; 86(6):1122–1130

[67] Broberg MA, Morrey BF. Results of treatment of fracture-dislocations of the elbow. Clin Orthop Relat Res. 1987(216):109–119

[68] al-Qattan MM, Murray KA. An isolated complex dorsal dislocation of the MP joint of the ring finger. J Hand Surg [Br]. 1994; 19(2):171–173

[69] Moneim MS. Volar dislocation of the metacarpophalangeal joint. Pathologic anatomy and report of two cases. Clin Orthop Relat Res. 1983(176):186–189

[70] Sollerman C, Abrahamsson SO, Lundborg G, Adalbert K. Functional splinting versus plaster cast for ruptures of the ulnar collateral ligament of the thumb. A prospective randomized study of 63 cases. Acta Orthop Scand. 1991; 62(6):524–526

[71] Brav EA. Traumatic dislocation of the hip. J Bone Joint Surg Am. 1962; 44:1115–1134

[72] Wascher DC, Dvirnak PC, DeCoster TA. Knee dislocation: initial assessment and implications for treatment. J Orthop Trauma. 1997; 11(7):525–529

[73] Sisto DJ, Warren RF. Complete knee dislocation. A follow-up study of operative treatment. Clin Orthop Relat Res. 1985(198):94–101

[74] Hill JA, Rana NA. Complications of posterolateral dislocation of the knee: case report and literature review. Clin Orthop Relat Res. 1981(154):212–215

[75] Stannard JP, Sheils TM, Lopez-Ben RR, McGwin G, Jr, Robinson JT, Volgas DA. Vascular injuries in knee dislocations following blunt trauma: evaluating the role of physical examination to determine the need for arteriography. J Bone Joint Surg Am. 2004; 86(5):910–915

[76] Green NE, Allen BL. Vascular injuries associated with dislocation of the knee. J Bone Joint Surg Am. 1977; 59(2):236–239

[77] Bibbo C, Anderson RB, Davis WH. Injury characteristics and the clinical outcome of subtalar dislocations: a clinical and radiographic analysis of 25 cases. Foot Ankle Int. 2003; 24(2):158–163

[78] Duncan CP, Masri BA. Fractures of the femur after hip replacement. In: Jackson D, ed. Instructional Course Lectures 44. Rosemont, IL: American Academy of Orthopaedic Surgeons;1995:293–304

[79] Masri BA, Meek RM, Duncan CP. Periprosthetic fractures evaluation and treatment. Clin Orthop Relat Res. 2004(420):80–95

[80] Lesh ML, Schneider DJ, Deol G, Davis B, Jacobs CR, Pellegrini VD, Jr. The consequences of anterior femoral notching in total knee arthroplasty. A biomechanical study. J Bone Joint Surg Am. 2000; 82(8):1096–1101

[81] Goldberg VM, Figgie HE, III, Inglis AE, et al. Patellar fracture type and prognosis in condylar total knee arthroplasty. Clin Orthop Relat Res. 1988(236):115–122

[82] Ortiguera CJ, Berry DJ. Patellar fracture after total knee arthroplasty. J Bone Joint Surg Am. 2002; 84(4):532–540

[83] Wright TW, Cofield RH. Humeral fractures after shoulder arthroplasty. J Bone Joint Surg Am. 1995; 77(9):1340–1346

[84] Campbell JT, Moore RS, Iannotti JP, Norris TR, Williams GR. Periprosthetic humeral fractures: mechanisms of fracture and treatment options. J Shoulder Elbow Surg. 1998; 7(4):406–413

[85] Kumar S, Sperling JW, Haidukewych GH, Cofield RH. Periprosthetic humeral fractures after shoulder arthroplasty. J Bone Joint Surg Am. 2004; 86(4):680–689

[86] O'Driscoll SW, Morrey BF. Periprosthetic fractures about the elbow. Orthop Clin North Am. 1999; 30(2):319–325

[87] Campanacci M, Capanna R, Picci P. Unicameral and aneurysmal bone cysts. Clin Orthop Relat Res. 1986(204):25–36

[88] Fletcher CDM, Bridge JA, Hogendoorn PCS, Mertens F, eds. World Health Organization Classification of tumors of Soft tissue and Bone. 4th ed. Lyon, France: IARC Press;2013

[89] Lichtenstein L. Aneurysmal bone cyst; observations on fifty cases. J Bone Joint Surg Am. 1957; 39-A(4):873–882

[90] Siris ES. Paget's disease of bone. J Bone Miner Res. 1998; 13(7):1061–1065

[91] Velez-Yanguas MC, Warrier RP. Langerhans' cell histiocytosis. Orthop Clin North Am. 1996; 27(3):615–623

[92] Arata MA, Peterson HA, Dahlin DC. Pathological fractures through non-ossifying fibromas. Review of the Mayo Clinic experience. J Bone Joint Surg Am. 1981; 63(6):980–988

[93] Garcia RA, Inwards CY, Unni KK. Benign bone tumors–recent developments. Semin Diagn Pathol. 2011; 28(1):73–85

[94] Goldenberg RR, Campbell CJ, Bonfiglio M. Giant-cell tumor of bone. An analysis of two hundred and eighteen cases. J Bone Joint Surg Am. 1970; 52(4):619–664

[95] Kneisl JS, Simon MA. Medical management compared with operative treatment for osteoid-osteoma. J Bone Joint Surg Am. 1992; 74 (2):179–185

[96] Schwartz HS, Zimmerman NB, Simon MA, Wroble RR, Millar EA, Bonfiglio M. The malignant potential of enchondromatosis. J Bone Joint Surg Am. 1987; 69(2):269–274

[97] Klein MJ, Kenan S, Lewis MM. Osteosarcoma. Clinical and pathological considerations. Orthop Clin North Am. 1989; 20(3):327–345

[98] Hameed M, Dorfman H. Primary malignant bone tumors–recent developments. Semin Diagn Pathol. 2011; 28(1):86–101

[99] Pritchard DJ, Reiman HM, Turcotte RE, Ilstrup DM. Malignant fibrous histiocytoma of the soft tissues of the trunk and extremities. Clin Orthop Relat Res. 1993(289):58–65

16 Medications and Rapid Access Information

16.1 Medications

Chad Condie, Logan Kelly, Wayne Shipley, and Ryan McTish

16.1.1 Analgesia

- See ▸ Table 16.1 and ▸ Table 16.2.[1,2,3]
- Self-reported pain should be assessed in all surgical patients using a validated assessment tool: visual analog, numeric rating, verbal rating, or faces pain scales.
- Pain assessment in critically ill patients who are unable to self-report pain: Behavioral Pain Score (BPS) and the Critical-Care Pain Observation Tool (CPOT).
- Nonopioid analgesics:
  - Acetaminophen and nonsteroidal anti-inflammatory drugs (NSAIDs) should be administered first to minimize opioid analgesic requirements and their resulting side effects.
  - NSAIDs inhibit platelet activating pathways and must be used cautiously in surgical patients, renal dysfunction, and gastrointestinal bleeding/ulceration.
  - Low-quality evidence links NSAID use and nonunion rates in orthopaedic procedures.
  - Patients with neuropathic pain: Gabapentin or pregabalin can improve pain control and minimize opioid analgesic requirements.
  - Ketamine: Consider for postoperative pain control after major surgeries, opioid intolerance, or high opioid tolerance.
- Opioid analgesia:
  - Oral administration of opioids is preferred to intravenous (IV) administration.

Table 16.1 Comparison of nonopioid analgesic medications

Drug	Route	Doses	Onset (min)	Duration (h)	Half-life (h)
Acetaminophen	IV	325–1,000 mg q6h	5–10	4–6	2–3
	PO	325–975 mg q6h	30–60	4–6	2–3
Ibuprofen	PO	200–800 mg q6–8h	30	6–8	2–2.5
Ketorolac	IV	15–30 mg q6h	10–30	4–6	2.5–8.5
Ketamine	IV	Bolus 0.25–0.5 mg/kg	0.5–1	1–2	2–3
		Continuous 0.05–0.5 mg/kg/h			

Abbreviations: IV, intravenous; PO, oral.

Table 16.2 Comparison of opioid analgesic medications

Drug	Route	Equianalgesic doses (mg)	Onset (min)	Duration (h)	Half-life (h)
Fentanyl	IV	0.1	1–2	0.5–1	2–4
Hydromorphone	IV	1.5	5–15	3–4	2–3
	PO	7.5	15–30	3–4	2–3
Morphine	IV	10	5–10	3–5	2–4
	PO	30	30–60	3–5	2–4
Oxycodone	PO	20	10–15	3–6	3–4
Hydrocodone	PO	30	10–20	3–6	4
Tramadol	PO	120	30–60	5–6	6

Abbreviations: IV, intravenous; PO, oral.

- When parenteral pain control is required postoperatively, consider utilizing patient controlled analgesia (PCA) in those who maintain adequate cognitive function and require analgesia for at least several hours; evidence supports PCA use to improve efficacy and patient satisfaction.
- Monitor patients who receive opioid analgesia for respiratory depression, excessive sedation, opioid-induced constipation, and postoperative nausea and vomiting.

16.1.2 Anesthetics (Local)

- See ▶ Table 16.3.[3,4,5,6]
- All local anesthetics share the same mechanism of action—reversibly binding to sodium channels to inhibit sodium ion flow across nerve cell membranes, preventing signal conduction.
- Adverse effects to local anesthetics typically manifest with higher doses and relate to systemic sodium channel blockade; they are shared across all medications in the class.
- Common adverse effects: Injection-site reaction, paralysis, hypotension, heart block, central nervous system depression.
- True allergies to local anesthetics are uncommon; consider preservative-free, epinephrine-free agent or switch between amide and ester types.
- Simplified formula for approximating maximum doses:

Table 16.3 Local anesthetics

	Medication	Dose	PK/Considerations
Amide type	Lidocaine[a] 0.5, 1, 2, or 4%	Infiltration (+ /− Epi): 1–60 mL 0.5% 1–30 mL 1% Nerve block: 3–20 mL 1–1.5%	Onset: 1–3 min Duration: 1–2 h Max dose = 4.5 mg/kg/dose; max: 300 mg (if Epi: 7 mg/kg/dose; max: 500 mg) per 2-h interval
	Bupivacaine[a] 0.25, 0.5, or 0.75%	Infiltration (+ /− Epi): 1–70 mL 0.25% 1–35 mL 0.5% Nerve block: 5–80 mL 0.25–0.5% PF	Onset: 5–15 min Duration: 3–6 h Max dose = 2.5 mg/kg; max: 400 mg per 24-h interval
	Mepivacaine[b] 1, 1.5, or 2%	Infiltration (+ /− Epi): 1–60 mL 0.5% 1–30 mL 1% Nerve block: 3–20 mL 1–1.5% PF	Onset: 3–20 min Duration: 2–3 h Max dose = 7 mg/kg; max: 1,000 mg per 24-h interval; 400 mg per dose
	Ropivacaine[c] 0.2, 0.5, 0.75, or 1%	Infiltration (+ /− Epi): 1–60 mL 0.5% 1–30 mL 1% Nerve block: 10–50 mL 0.5–0.75%	Onset: 3–15 min Duration: 3–15 h Max dose = 3 mg/kg; incremental dosing recommended
Ester type	Chloroprocaine[b] 1, 2, or 3%	Infiltration: 1–80 mL 1% 1–40 mL 2% Nerve block: 1–25 mL 1–3%	Onset: 6–12 min Duration: ~ 1 h Max dose = 11 mg/kg or 800 mg, whichever is less

[a] ± Epinephrine, ± preservative.

[b] ± Preservative.

[c] Preservative free.

   ○ Maximal allowable dose (mg/kg) × (weight in kg/10) × 1/concentration of local anesthetic = mL anesthetic. Thus, for 1% lidocaine with epinephrine (7 mg/kg) in a 60-kg male, 7 × (60/10) × 1 = 42 mL of lidocaine.

16.1.3 Anesthetics (Rapid Sequence Intubation Medications)

- See ▶ Table 16.4 and Chapter 1.3 Anesthesia.[3,5,7]
- Ensure induction agent is given before paralytic agent.
- Etomidate and ketamine are commonly used as induction agents due to low incidence of adverse effects (AEs) and minimal effect on cardiovascular function.
- Ensure postintubation analgesia is available once induction agents wears off; nondepolarizing agents may mask need for analgesia due to their prolonged duration of activity.

16.1.4 Antiarrhythmic Medications

- See ▶ Table 16.5.[3,8,9,10]
- Four main classes based on how they affect certain ion channels and receptors located on the myocardial cell membrane.
- Despite the common classification of antiarrhythmic medications into four classes, each drug is unique with a specific pharmacological profile, and antiarrhythmic medications are not considered interchangeable with other members of drug in the same class.
- Most antiarrhythmic medications are potent and have a relatively narrow therapeutic index; inappropriate dosing or monitoring can result in toxicity.
- Antiarrhythmic therapies should be custom matched to each patient based on pharmacological properties of the medication as well as patient factors (i.e., age, coexisting disease, other patient medication therapies, and the presence of an implantable cardioverter defibrillator).

Table 16.4 Rapid sequence intubation

	Medication	Dose	Pharmacokinetics	Considerations/AEs
Anesthetics (induction agents)	Etomidate	0.3 mg/kg IVP Use TBW	Onset: < 60 s Duration: 3–5 min	May cause adrenal suppression No effect on BP, HR
	Ketamine	1–2 mg/kg IVP 3–5 mg/kg IM Use IBW	Onset: 30 s IV 3–5 min IM Duration: 10 min IV; 15–20 min IM	Can increase BP, HR No evidence to suggest it increases ICP
	Propofol	1–2 mg/kg IVP Use ABW	Onset: 15–30 s Duration: 5 min	Can cause hypotension
	Midazolam	0.2–0.3 mg/kg IVP/IM	Onset: ~ 90 s Duration: 30–80 min	Delayed onset Prolonged duration
Paralytics	Succinylcholine (depolarizing)	1–1.5 mg/kg IVP 3–4 mg/kg IM Use TBW	Onset: < 60 s Duration: 5–7 min	Can cause hyperkalemia Repeat dose associated with bradycardia
	Rocuronium (nondepolarizing)	1–1.2 mg/kg IVP Use IBW	Onset: 1–2 min Duration: 30–40 min	Use if contraindications to succinylcholine Prolonged duration
	Vecuronium (nondepolarizing)	0.1–0.2 mg/kg IVP Use IBW	Onset: 2–3 min Duration: ~45 min	Longest duration

Abbreviations: ABW, adjusted body weight; AE, adverse effects; IBW, ideal body weight; IM, intramuscular; IVP, intravenous push; TBW, total body weight.

Table 16.5 Antiarrhythmic medications (Van William's classification)

Class	Mechanism	Medication	Indication	Dosing range	Side effects and cautions
Ia	Moderately blocks Na$^+$ channels, prolongs APD	Quinidine	AFib, AFlutter, VT	PO: 300 mg q8–12h	SE: QT prolongation, hypotension, diarrhea, vertigo, vision changes Caution: heart block, pregnancy risk C
		Procainamide	VT, AFib	Load: 100 mg q5 min until arrhythmia is controlled up to a maximum of 17 mg/kg Maintenance: 1–6 mg/min	SE: hypotension, widened QRS, rash, agranulocytosis, drug-induced lupus Caution: complete heart block, torsades de pointes. Monitor NAPA levels. Pregnancy risk: C
		Disopyramide	VT, AFib	150 mg q6h or 300 mg q12h	SE: hypotension, HF, widened QRS, QT prolongation, anticholinergic effects Caution: 1st/2nd degree HB Pregnancy risk: C
Ib	Weakly blocks Na$^+$ channels with rapid dissociation	Lidocaine	VF, VT	Load: 1–1.5 mg/kg IV/IO × 1; 0.5–0.75 mg/kg IV repeat q 3–5 min (max: 3 mg/kg) Maintenance: 30–50 µg/kg/min	SE: hypotension, dizziness, drowsiness, and seizures at high levels Caution: reduce dose in liver disease or left ventricular dysfunction Pregnancy risk: B
		Mexiletine	VT	200 mg PO q8h (max dose: 1,200 mg/d)	SE: acute liver injury, leukopenia, agranulocytosis, tremor, blurry vision, lethargy, and nausea Caution: sick sinus syndrome, heart block, hypotension, HF Pregnancy risk: C
Ic	Strongly blocks Na$^+$ channels with slow dissociation	Propafenone	PSVT and PAF without structural heart disease, VT	IR formulation: 150 mg q8h with dose increased q3–4d up to a max of 900 mg/d SR formulation: 225 mg bid (up to 425 mg bid)	SE: arrhythmias, worsen HF, dose-related increase in QRS and QT intervals, heart block Caution: bradycardia, shock, CAD, prolonged QT interval Pregnancy risk: C
		Flecainide	PSVT and PAF without structural heart disease, VT	50–100 mg q12h (max: 400 mg/d)	SE: arrhythmias, worsen HF, dose-related increase in QRS and QT intervals, heart block Warnings: bradycardia, shock, prolonged QT interval, CAD Pregnancy risk: C

(Continued)

Table 16.5 (*Continued*) Antiarrhythmic medications (Van William's classification)

Class	Mechanism	Medication	Indication	Dosing range	Side effects and cautions
II	β-Adrenergic blocker	Esmolol and other β-adrenergic antagonists	VT, AFib, AFlutter, ST	Doses vary based on specific drug and indication	SE: bradycardia, hypotension, exacerbation of HF, bronchospasm Caution: asthma, decompensated HF Pregnancy risk: C
III	Inhibits K$^+$ channel conduction prolongs APD	Amiodarone	VT, VF, AFib, AFlutter, PSVT	Inj: pulseless VT/VF: 300 mg IV/IO push VT/VF: 150 mg IV over 10 min Afib: 1.2–1.8 g/d until 10 g total, then lowest effect dose (100–400 mg/d)	SE: hypo and hyperthyroidism, pulmonary fibrosis, liver toxicity, blue skin discoloration, optic neuropathy Caution: heart block Pregnancy risk: D
		Sotalol	VT, AFib, AFlutter	80 mg bid, then up to 120 bid	SE: increase in QT interval, Torsade de pointes Caution: bradycardia, HF, hypokalemia Pregnancy risk: B
		Ibutilide	Conversion of AFib, AFlutter	<60 kg: 0.01 mg/kg over 10 min >60 kg: 1 mg IV over 10 min (a second dose may be given × 1 after initial dose complete)	SE: Increase in QT interval, Torsade de pointes Caution: bradycardia Pregnancy risk: C
		Dofetilide	Conversion of AFib, AFlutter	Dosing ranges: 0.125–0.5 mg bid based on CrCl and QTc	SE: increase QT interval, Torsade de pointes Caution: bradycardia Pregnancy risk: C Prescriber and pharmacy must be registered
IV	Ca$^+$ channel blocker (nondihydropyridine)	Verapamil	Angina, AFib, AFlutter with RVR	2.5–5 mg IV over 2 min then 5–10 mg PRN q15–30 min (max dose of 20 mg)	SE: bradycardia, HB, worsening HF, decrease BP Caution: sick sinus syndrome, HB Pregnancy risk: C
		Diltiazem	AFib, AFlutter with RVR	15–20 mg IV over 2 min may repeat in 15 min at 20–25 mg	SE: bradycardia, HB, worsening HF, decrease BP Caution: sick sinus syndrome, HB Pregnancy risk: C

Table 16.5 *(Continued)* Antiarrhythmic medications (Van William's classification)

Class	Mechanism	Medication	Indication	Dosing range	Side effects and cautions
Misc	Adenosine receptor agonist	Adenosine	AFib, AFlutter	6 mg IV rapid bolus over 1–3 s (flush with 20 mL of NS), may repeat with 12 mg in 1–2 min	SE: AV block, flushing, bronchospasm, brief period of asystole on monitor Caution: HB, wide-complex VT Pregnancy risk: C
	Na+ and K+ ATPase inhibitor	Digoxin	AFib, AFlutter with RVR, HF	0.4–0.6 mg IV over 5–10 min, may repeat 0.1–0.3 mg IV over 5–10 min	SE: arrhythmias, nausea Caution: bradycardia, HB, renal failure, hypokalemia Pregnancy risk: C
	Structurally related to amiodarone, exhibits properties of all 4 antiarrhythmic classes	Dronedarone	AFib, AFlutter	400 mg bid	SE: HF, HB, bradycardia, QT prolongation Caution: use with 3A4 inhibitors, Class IV HF, liver disease Pregnancy risk: X Stop class I or III agents before initiating

Abbreviations: AFi, atrial fibrillation; AFlutter, atrial flutter; APD, action potential duration; HB, heart block; HF, heart failure; Inj, injection; IR, immediate release; IV, intravenous; NAPA, N-acetylprocainamide; PAF, paroxysmal atrial fibrillation; PSVT, paroxysmal supraventricular tachycardia; RVR, rapid ventricular rate; SE, side effects; SR, sustained release; VF, ventricular fibrillation; VT, ventricular tachycardia.

16.1.5 Anticoagulant Agents and Anticoagulant Reversal Agents

- See ▶ Table 16.6 and ▶ Table 16.7.[3,11,12]
- Anticoagulants are used by a large number of patients with varying disease states; indications and treatment options have rapidly shifted; utilize expert consultation for anticoagulation and reversal when able.
- Anticoagulant use has increased over the last decade and should continue to rise into the next decade.

Table 16.6 Anticoagulants

Agent	Dose range	Mode of action	Half-life (h)	Reversal (preferred agent is listed first)
Apixaban (Eliquis)	PX: 2.5 mg BID	Xa inhibitor	8–15	• Andexanet alfa
	T: 5–10 mg BID			• PCC
Argatroban	T: 0.5–2 µg/kg/min	Reversible IIa inhibitor	0.75	• PCC
Betrixaban (Bevyxxa)	PX: 160 mg × 1 then 80 mg QD	Xa inhibitor	19–27	• PCC
Bivalirudin (Angiomax)	T: 0.5–2.5 mg/kg/h	DTI	0.5	• aPCC
				• PCC
Dabigatran (Pradaxa)	PX: 220 mg QD	DTI	12–17	• Idarucizumab
	T: 150 mg BID			• PCC
Dalteparin (Fragmin)	PX: 5,000 unit QD	Xa inhibitor	3–5	• Protamine
	T: IV 10–15 µg/kg/h			• rFVIIa
	T: SQ 100 µg/kg			
Edoxaban (Lixiana)	T: 30–60 mg QD	Xa inhibitor	10–14	• Andexanet alfa
				• PCC
Enoxaparin (Lovenox)	PX:30 mg BID	Xa inhibitor	4.5–7	• Protamine
	40 mg QD			
	T: 1 mg/kg BID			
	1.5 mg/kg QD			
Fondaparinux (Arixtra)	PX: 2.5 mg QD	Binds AT III to inhibit Xa	17–21	• aPCC[a]
	T: 5–10 mg QD			• rFVIIa[a]
Rivaroxaban (Xarelto)	PX: 10 mg QD	Xa inhibitor	5–10	• Andexanet alfa
	T: 15 mg BID × 21 d then 20 mg QD			
Tinzaparin (Innohep)	PX: 75 anti-Xa u/kg	Binds AT III	1.5	• Protamine
	T: 175 anti-Xa u/kg			• rFVIIa
Unfractionated heparin	PX: 5,000 u TID	Inhibits thrombin, factors IX, X, XI, XII	1–2	• Protamine
	T: variable dosed in u/kg/h			
Warfarin (Coumadin)	T: 1–20 mg QD, based on INR	VKA	20–60	• PCC
				• FFP
				Vitamin K 10 mg should be given along with either of the above agents

Abbreviations: aPCC, activated prothrombin complex concentrate (anti-inhibitor coagulant complex); AT, antithrombin; BID, twice daily; DTI, direct thrombin inhibitor; PCC, prothrombin complex concentrate; PX, prophylactic dose; QD, daily; rFVIIa, recombinant factor VIIa; T, therapeutic dose; TID, three times daily; u, units; VKA, vitamin K antagonist.

[a] No reversal for fondaparinux exists, low-quality evidence in animals or healthy adults indicate that aPCC (20 IU/kg) or rFVIIa (90 µg/kg) may have benefit in severe bleeds.

Table 16.7 Anticoagulant reversal agents

Agent	Dose	Onset (min)	Adverse reactions	Anticoagulants reversed
Anti-inhibitor coagulant complex (**aPCC, Feiba**)	• 50 units/kg for DOACs • 20 units/kg for fondaparinux • 500–1,000 units for warfarin	15–30	• Embolic events • Urticaria • Chills	• Apixaban • Betrixaban • Dabigatran • Edoxaban • Fondaparinux • Rivaroxaban • Warfarin
Andexanet alfa (**Andexxa**)[a]	**High dose** • Bolus 800 mg over 27 min followed by • Infusion 8 mg/min for 120 min **Low dose** • Bolus 400 mg over 14 min followed by • Infusion 4 mg/min for 120 min	2–5	• Embolic events • Flushing • Urticaria	• Apixaban • Rivaroxaban
4-Factor **PCC** (**Kcentra**)	• 50 units/kg for DOAC **Warfarin reversal** • 25 units/kg for INR 2 to <4 • 35 units/kg for INR 4–6 • 50 units/kg for INR >6	<10 (INR reversal)	• Hypotension • Headache • Embolic events	• Apixaban • Dabigatran • Edoxaban • Rivaroxaban • Warfarin
FFP	• 10–20 mL/kg for warfarin • 1 unit FFP = 200–250 mL	Delayed	• Transfusion reactions	• Warfarin
Idarucizumab (**Praxbind**)	• 5 g IV × 1 • May repeat 5 g dose × 1 for refractory bleeding	<10	• Headache • Constipation • Embolic events	• Dabigatran
Protamine	**Heparin** • 1 mg per ~ 100 units given over previous 2–3 h • Max dose 50 mg • Infuse over 10 min **Enoxaparin** • 1 mg for each 1 mg given over last 8 h • Max dose 50 mg • Infuse over 10 min **Dalteparin, nadroparin, tinzaparin** • 1 mg for every 100 anti-Xa units given • Max dose 50 mg • Infuse over 10 min	~5	• Bradycardia • Flushing • Hypotension • Dyspnea	• Dalteparin • Enoxaparin • Heparin • Nadroparin • Tinzaparin

Abbreviations: DOACs, direct oral anticoagulants; FFP, fresh frozen plasma; PCC, prothrombin complex concentrate.

[a] Andexanet alfa is FDA approved only for apixaban and rivaroxaban; further studies are ongoing to investigate role in reversing edoxaban, enoxaparin, and betrixaban.

• Bleeding is the most significant side effect of these medications; prompt reversal is needed to minimize patient morbidity and mortality; reversal strategies vary by bleeding risk, last dose of patient anticoagulation use, and institutional guidelines.
• Recent FDA approval of Andexanet alfa and Idarucizumab has helped in the management of life-threatening bleeds caused by direct oral anticoagulants.

16.1.6 Antihypertensive Medications

• See ▶ Table 16.8.[3,13,14,15]
• Hypertensive urgency: Higher than 180 mm Hg systolic blood pressure (SBP) and/or 110 mm Hg diastolic blood pressure (DBP) or greater without evidence of acute organ damage.

Table 16.8 Hypertension urgencies and emergencies (IV administration)

Agent	Class	Dosing	Onset	Duration	Hemodynamic effects			Special considerations
					PL	AL	CO	
Nitroglycerin	NOD	5–200 µg/m T:5–20 µg/m q5–10 min	I	5 min	↓	↓↔	↔↑	• V > A vasodilator • Potential rapid TP
Nitroprusside	NOD	0.25–10 µg/k/m T:0.25 µg/k/m q5 m	I	5 min	↓	↓	↑	• Increase ICP • TCN tox in RF • CYN tox in LF • Avoid Inf>72 h or rate>3 µg/k/m • Monitor serum CYN TCN levels
Hydralazine	DAV	5–20 mg q30 m PRN	10 min	2–6 h	↕	↓	↑	• Risk of reflex TC
Nicardipine	CCB	5–15 mg/h T: 2.5 mg/h q5–10 m	10 min	2–6 h	↕	↓	↑	• Risk of reflex TC • Monitor fluid status
Clevidipine	CCB	1–6 mg/h T: Double dose q90s (Max = 32 mg/h)	4 min	15 min	↕	↓	↑	• CI with soy or egg allergies • 2 kcal/mL of lipids
Esmolol	BB	25–300 µg/k/m T: 25 µg/k/m q3–5 m	10 min	20 min	↕	↕	↓	• CI in acute DHF • Useful for TA • Monitor fluid status
Metoprolol	BB	Bolus 5–15 mg q5–15 m PRN	20 min	2–6 h	↕	↕	↓	• CI in acute DHF • Useful for TA
Labetalol	BB	10–20 mg, may redose 20–80 mg q10m Inf: 0.5–2 mg/m T:1–2 mg/m q2h	5 min	2–18 h	↓	↓	↓	• Possible monotherapy in AAD • CI in acute DHF
Enalaprilat	ACEi	1.25–5 mg IV q6h	15–30 min	12–24 h	↓	↓	↑	• CI in pregnancy
Fenoldopam	DA	0.01–1.6 µg/k/m T:0.05–0.1 µg/k/m q15 m	5–15 min	30–60 min	↕	↓	↑	• Reflex TC • Increase ICP

Abbreviations: A, arterial; AAD, acute aortic dissection; ACEi, angiotensin-converting enzyme inhibitor; AL, after load; BB, β-adrenergic blocker; CI, contraindicated; CO, cardiac output; CYN, cyanide; DA, dopamine agonist; DHF, decompensated heart failure; I, immediate; ICP, intracranial pressure; LF, liver failure; NOD, nitric oxide dilator; PL, pre load; PRN, as needed; Q, every; RF, renal failure; T, titrate; TA, tachyarrhythmias; TC, tachycardia; TCN, thiocyanate; Tox, toxicity; TP, tachyphylaxis; V, venous.

Table 16.9 Guidelines for BP reduction during hypertensive emergencies

Goal time	BP target
First hour	Reduce MAP by 25% (while maintaining goal DBP > 100 mm Hg)
Hours 2–6	SBP 160 mm Hg and/or DBP 100–100 mm Hg
Hours 6–24	Maintain goal for hours 2–6 during first 24 h
Hours 24–48	Outpatient BP goal

Abbreviations: BP, blood pressure; DBP, diastolic blood pressure; MAP, mean arterial pressure; SBP, systolic blood pressure.

Table 16.10 Acute nebulized medications

Medication/Formulation	Mechanism	Common dosing	Adverse effects
Albuterol 0.63 mg/3 mL 1.25 mg/3 mL 2.5 mg/3 mL	Selective β2 agonist	**Asthma exacerbation:** 2.5–5 mg nebulized every 1–4 h **Severe asthma:** 10–15 mg/h as continuous nebulization	Nervousness Tremor Tachycardia
Hypertonic saline 3%, 7%, 10%	Mucolytic and expectorant	**Increased secretions:** 4 mL nebulized every 6–12 h	Cough Mucosal irritation
Ipratropium 0.5 mg/3 mL	Anticholinergic	**COPD:** 0.5 mg nebulized every 6–8 h **Severe asthma:** 0.5 mg nebulized every 20 min × 3 doses	Xerostomia Mydriasis Urinary retention
Lev-albuterol 0.63 mg/3 mL 1.25 mg/3 mL	Selective β2 agonist	**Asthma exacerbation:** 1.25–2.5 mg nebulized every 1–4 h	Theoretically less tachycardia compared to albuterol
Racemic epinephrine 2.25%	Mixed α, β1, and β2 agonist	**Airway edema:** 0.5 mL of 2.25% solution nebulized every 20 min	Nervousness Tachycardia Hypertension

- Hypertensive emergency: Abrupt and significantly elevated blood pressure (SBP > 200 mm Hg and/or DBP > 120 mm Hg) with target-organ dysfunction.
  - Target-organ dysfunction: Eclampsia/preeclampsia, acute kidney injury, acute aortic dissection, unstable angina, seizures, retinopathy, flash pulmonary edema, acute intracranial bleeding (nontraumatic), acute myocardial ischemia/infarction, acute left ventricular failure with pulmonary edema.
  - Common causes of hypertensive emergency include intoxications (e.g., cocaine, amphetamines, and stimulant diet supplements), nonadherence to antihypertensive regimens, withdrawal syndromes (e.g., clonidine or β-antagonist), drug–drug interactions, spinal cord disorders, collagen vascular diseases, and pregnancy.
- BP management considerations:
  - Hypertensive urgency—lowers BP slowly over 24–48 hours using oral medications (consider starting and/ or titrating home regimens), avoid overaggressive BP correction in patients with chronic hypertension.
  - Hypertensive emergency—requires intravenous medications and intensive care unit admission for monitoring, gradual blood pressure reduction (▶ Table 16.9).
  - Compelling conditions that require exceptions to general BP targets include patient with aortic dissections, acute stroke (ischemic and hemorrhagic), and pregnancy-associated hypotension emergency.
  - Drug of choice for hypertensive emergency is IV nitroprusside except in neurosurgical patients due to accumulation and intracranial pressure concerns.

16.1.7 Asthma/COPD Nebulized Medications

- See ▶ Table 16.10.[3,16]
- Use of a tiered approach to asthma treatment with escalation of care depending on patient symptoms is recommended.

- Ipratropium nebulization can cause mydriasis, including unilateral pupil dilation.
- In patients with asthma, use of ipratropium is reserved for severe exacerbations as there is no benefit in mild, moderate exacerbations.
- For asthma exacerbations refractory to maximum albuterol therapy, systemic corticosteroids are indicated.

16.1.8 Bowel Regimen Medications

- See ▶ Table 16.11.[3,17,18]
- Perioperative constipation affects a large number of surgical patients (2–20%).
- Risk factors for constipation: Decreased mobility postoperatively, opioid pain medications, dehydration.
- Tiered approach:
  - First: Can be used daily during the perioperative period.
  - Second: Options used when no bowel movement was produced with first-tier therapies.
  - Third: Therapies are reserved for patients with refractory constipation not relieved with first or second-tier therapies; intestinal or other blockage must be ruled out prior to use.

16.1.9 Muscle Relaxants

- See ▶ Table 16.12.[2,3,19]
- Skeletal muscle relaxants include a mix of agents that are generally classified as antispasticity or antispasmodic agents.
- Antispasticity agents have activity in upper motor neuron diseases, whereas antispasmodics are utilized for peripheral muscle pain.
- Antispasmodics should be reserved for second-line treatment of muscle pain after failure of first-line treatment.
- These agents should be used cautiously in elderly patients due to high prevalence of anticholinergic side effects.
- The minimum tolerated effective dose should be used in all patients due to the high rate of intolerability.

16.1.10 Sedation

- See ▶ Table 16.13.[3,20]
- Sedation is used for comfort, anxiolysis, or amnesia during surgical procedures and management of post-op agitation and anxiety in critically ill patients.
- Frequent monitoring of the patient's consciousness, hemodynamics, oxygenation, and ventilation should be performed.
- When sedation is required for critically ill surgical patients, sedation should be initiated using a nonbenzodiazepine sedative and titrated to the lightest depth of sedation.
- Light rather than deep sedation is associated with shorter duration of mechanical ventilation and intensive care unit (ICU) length of stay.
- Benzodiazepines:
  - Gamma-aminobutyric acid (GABA) receptor mediating agents.
  - Demonstrates sedating, anxiolytic, amnestic, hypnotic, and anticonvulsant effects.
  - Descending potency: Lorazepam, midazolam, and diazepam.
  - Delayed emergence from sedation can occur after long-term administration, old age, and hepatic/renal impairment.
  - Monitor patients for respiratory depression and systemic hypotension in addition to the development of tolerance after long-term administration.
- Propofol:
  - Gamma-aminobutyric acid (GABA) receptor mediating agent.
  - Displays sedative, anxiolytic, amnestic, antiemetic, and anticonvulsant properties.
  - Highly lipophilic with rapid onset of action.
  - Due to rapid hepatic and extrahepatic clearance, propofol demonstrates a short duration of action after short-term administration.
  - Monitor patients for respiratory depression, hypotension, hypertriglyceridemia, pancreatitis, and propofol-related infusion syndrome (PRIS).

Table 16.11 Bowel regimen medications

Medication	Dose	Onset	MOA	Side effects
First tier therapies				
Bisacodyl	PO: 5–15 mg daily PR: 10 mg daily	PO: 6–12 h PR: 15–60 min (suppository), 5–20 min (enema)	Stimulates peristalsis by irritating smooth muscle of intestine	• Abdominal cramps • Nausea • Rectal irritation • Vomiting
Docusate	PO: 50–360 mg daily in divided doses PR: 283 mg QD to TID	PO: 12–72 h PR: 5–15 min	Enhanced incorporation of water and fat into stool	• Cramps • Nausea
Polycarbophil	PO: 1,250 mg calcium polycarbophil QD to QID	PO: 12–72 h	Provides intestinal bulk	• GI fullness
Polyethylene glycol	PO: 17 g QD to BID	PO: 24–96 h	Osmotic agent causing water retention in stool	• Abdominal pain • Diarrhea • Flatulence • Nausea
Psyllium	PO: 2.5–30 g per day in divided doses	PO: 12–72 h	Soluble fiber that absorbs water to promote peristalsis	• Abdominal cramps • Esophageal or intestinal obstruction • Diarrhea
Senna/Sennosides	PO: 8.6–34.4 mg QD to BID	PO: 6–24 h	Stimulates intestinal mucosa resulting in increased peristalsis	• Abdominal cramps • Diarrhea • Nausea • Vomiting
Second tier therapies				
Glycerin	PR: Enema 5.4 g PR: Suppository 1–2 g	PR: 15–30 min	Draws fluid into colon to stimulate evacuation	• Rectal discomfort • Anal burning • Abdominal cramps
Lactulose	PO: 10–20 g QD to QID	PO: 24–48 h	Osmotic effect that causes distention promoting peristalsis	• Dehydration • Abdominal distention • Hypernatremia • Hypokalemia • Flatulence

Table 16.11 *(Continued)* Bowel regimen medications

Medication	Dose	Onset	MOA	Side effects
Magnesium citrate	PO: 150–300 mL QD	PO: 0.5–6 h	Osmotic retention, colonic distension leading to increased peristalsis	• Avoid in RF • Avoid in MG • Flatulence • Diarrhea
Magnesium hydroxide	PO: 1,200–2,400 mg 1–3 times daily Tablet: 311 mg/tab LQ: 400 mg/5 mL, 800 mg/5 mL, 1,200 mg/5 mL	PO: 0.5–6 h	Osmotic retention, colonic distension leading to increased peristalsis	• Avoid in RF • Avoid in MG • Flatulence • Diarrhea
Methylnaltrexone	PO: 450 mg once daily SQ: <38 kg = 0.15 mg/kg; 38 to <62 kg = 8 mg; 62–114 kg = 12 mg; >114 kg = 0.15 mg/kg	SQ: Tmax 30 min PO: Tmax 1.5 h	Mu-opioid receptor antagonist which blocks opioid binding at the mu-receptors of the GI tract	• Abdominal pain • Flatulence • Nausea • Dizziness • Headache
Mineral oil	PO: Plain: 15–45 mL/24 h Emulsion: 30–90 mL/24 h Rectal: 118 mL as a single dose	PO: 6–8 h PR: 2–15 min	Decreased colonic absorption of water, intestinal lubricate	• Abdominal cramps • Nausea • Diarrhea • Oily rectal leakage
Naloxegol	PO: 12.5–25 mg daily	PO: Tmax <2 h	Mu opioid receptor antagonist within the GI tract	• Abdominal pain • Flatulence • Headache • Nausea
Sodium phosphate	PO: 15–45 mL once PR: 135 mL once	PO: 3–6 h PR: 2–5 min	Osmotic effect on the small intestine, producing distention and promoting peristalsis	• Bloating • Nausea • Abdominal pain • Hyperphosphatemia • Hypocalcemia

Table 16.11 (*Continued*) Bowel regimen medications

Medication	Dose	Onset	MOA	Side effects
Sorbitol	PO: 30–45 mL (70% solution) once PR: 120 mL (25–30% solution) once	PR: 0.25–1 h	Osmotic cathartic	• Edema • Electrolyte depletion • Lactic acidosis • Abdominal pain
Third tier therapies				
Linaclotide	PO: 145 µg QD	N/A	A guanylate cyclase C agonist	• Abdominal pain • Diarrhea • Headache
Lubiprostone	PO: 24 µg BID	PO: Tmax 1.1 h	Intestinal type-2 chloride channel activator, increases fluid secretion and improves small intestinal transit	• Abdominal pain • Diarrhea • Edema • Headache • Nausea
Neostigmine	IV: 0.5–2 mg × 1	IV: 10–30 min	Acetylcholinesterase inhibitor which facilitates impulse transmission across myoneural junction	• **Advanced monitoring required due to bradycardia, need atropine at bedside**
SMOG (sorbitol, mineral oil, glycerin) enema	PR: sorbitol 70% 473 mL, mineral oil 473 mL, glycerin 120 mL combined in enema bag given once	PR: rapid (see individual ingredients)	(See individual ingredients)	• (See individual ingredients)

Abbreviations: BID, twice daily; GI, gastrointestinal; IV, intravenous; LQ, liquid; MG, myasthenia gravis; MOA, mechanism of action; PO, oral; PR, per rectum; QD, daily; QID, four times daily; SQ, subcutaneous; TID, three times daily; Tmax, time to peak plasma concentration.

Table 16.12 Comparison of muscle relaxant medications

Drug	Dosage range	Onset/duration (h)	Half-life (h)	Side effects
Baclofen	5–25 mg TID Max: 80 mg/d	O: 72–96 D: unknown	2.5–4	Confusion, HA, insomnia, urinary frequency, WD
Carisoprodol	250–350 mg TID	O: 0.5 D: 4–6	2	D/D, HA
Chlorzoxazone	250–750 mg TID/QID	O: 1 D: 3–4	1.1	D/D, GI bleeding, allergic-type skin reactions
Cyclobenzaprine	5–10 mg TID	O: < 1 D: 8–12	8–37	D/D, xerostomia, asthenia urinary retention, constipation
Dantrolene	Start: 25 mg QD Taper q7d Max: 400 mg/d	O: Up to 1 wk D: Unknown	8.7	Hepatotoxicity, HF, AV block, TC, somnolence, N, diarrhea, flushing
Metaxalone	400–800 mg TID–QID	O: 1 D: 4–6	2–4	D/D, irritability, N, V, leukopenia, hemolytic anemia
Methocarbamol	1,000–2,000 mg QID	O: 0.5 D: 8	1–2	Bradycardia, syncope, hypotension, diplopia, D/D, dyspepsia, jaundice
Orphenadrine	100 mg BID	O: < 1 D: 8	14	TC, agitation, drowsiness, tremor, xerostomia, N, V, muscle weakness
Tizanidine	2–12 mg TID Max: 36 mg/d	O: 1–2 D: 3–6	2.5	Asthenia, D/D, xerostomia, hypotension, syncope, WD

Abbreviations: AV, arteriovenous; BID, twice daily; D, duration; D/D, drowsiness/dizziness; HA, headache; HF, heart failure; N, nausea; O, onset; Q, every; QD, daily; TC, tachycardia; TID, three times daily; WD, withdrawal.

Table 16.13 Comparison of sedation medications

Drug (IV)	Onset (min)	Half-life (h)	Duration (h)	Usual dosing
Midazolam	2–5	2–6	0.5–4	Bolus: 0.01–0.2 mg/kg Continuous: 0.02–0.1 mg/kg/h
Lorazepam	2–3	8–15	6–10	Bolus: 0.02–0.04 mg/kg Continuous: 0.01–0.1 mg/kg/h
Diazepam	2–5	33–45	0.5–2	Bolus: 0.01–0.1 mg/kg Continuous: N/A
Propofol	1–2	0.5–7	5–15 min	Bolus: 0.5–1.5 mg/kg Continuous: 5–50 µg/kg/min
Dexmedetomidine	5–10	1.8–3	1–2	Bolus: 0.5–0.1 µg/kg Continuous: 0.2–1.5 µg/kg/h
Ketamine	0.5	2–3	1–2	Bolus: 0.5–2 mg/kg Continuous: 0.05–2.5 mg/kg/h

- Dexmedetomidine:
  - α_2-Adrenoreceptor agonist.
  - Demonstrates sedative, analgesic, and sympatholytic properties; retains arousability and respiratory drive.
  - Demonstrates analgesic effects and evidence supports its opioid-sparing benefit.
  - Monitor patients for hypotension and bradycardia.

- Ketamine:
  - Unclear mechanism but modulates N-methyl-D-aspartate (NMDA) receptors and other targets.
  - Demonstrates dissociative sedation, analgesic, and amnestic properties.
  - Preserves airway reflexes, respiratory effort, and cardiovascular stability.
  - Monitor patients for emergence reactions which manifest as hallucinations, vivid dreams, and delirium.
  - Avoid ketamine in patients with a history of schizophrenia.

16.1.11 Seizure and Initial Status Epilepticus Management

- See ▶ Table 16.14.[3,21]
- Status epilepticus (SE) requires emergent action to prevent morbidity and mortality.
- Status epilepticus occurs when a seizure lasts longer than 5 minutes or a patient has several seizures and does not return to baseline mental status between seizures.

Table 16.14 Initial status epilepticus/seizure management medications

Medication	Dose	Administration issues	Side effects
Benzodiazepines			
• Diazepam[a]	• 0.15 mg/kg, max 10 mg per dose • May repeat in 5 min	• IV or IM or PR • Dose based on IV route	• Hypotension • Respiratory depression • Sedation
• Lorazepam[a]	• 0.1 mg/kg, max 4 mg per dose • May repeat in 5–10 min	• IV or IM • Dose based on IV route	
• Midazolam[a,b]	• 0.2 mg/kg, max 10 mg per dose	• IV or IM or intranasal • Dose based on IV route	
Fosphenytoin[c] Or Phenytoin	• LD 20 mg/kg • MD 100–150 mg q8h	Fosphenytoin: • Max infusion rate is 150 mg/min • IV only • If available, is preferred due to faster infusion rates Phenytoin: • Max infusion rate is 50 mg/min • Available IV or PO	Infusion-related cardiac effects (hypotension, arrhythmias)
Lacosamide	• LD 200–400 mg • MD 100–200 mg BID	• Give 200 mg IV over 5 min • Available IV or PO	• ECG PR interval prolongation • Hypotension
Levetiracetam[c]	• LD 40–60 mg/kg • Max dose: 4,500 mg • MD 1,000–2,000 mg q12h • Peds LD 20–60 mg/kg • Peds MD 500–1,000 mg q12h	• Infuse time < 10 min • Available IV or PO	• Agitation • Sedation • Leukopenia • Thrombocytopenia
Phenobarbital[b]	• LD 20 mg/kg • MD 2 mg/kg/d in divided doses	• Infusion rate 50–100 mg/min • Available IV or PO	• Hypotension • Respiratory depression
Topiramate[c]	• LD 200–400 mg • MD 200–1,600 mg/d in divided doses (2–4 times)	• Oral route only • No IV formulation	• Metabolic acidosis
Valproic acid[c]	• LD 20–40 mg/kg • MD 10–15 mg/kg/d IV or PO	• Infuse at 3–6 mg/kg/min • Available IV or PO	• Hyperammonemia • Pancreatitis • Thrombocytopenia • Hepatotoxicity

Abbreviations: IV, intravenous; IM, intramuscular; LD, loading dose; MD, maintenance dose; PO, oral route; PR, per rectal.

[a] First-line agents.

[b] Third-line agents.

[c] Second-line agents.

- SE can be convulsive (clinical demonstration of tonic–clonic movements), nonconvulsive status epilepticus (electrographic seizure) or refractory status epilepticus (clinical or electrographic seizures despite initial doses of a benzodiazepine and another appropriately dosed anticonvulsant medication).
- Initial treatment should be a benzodiazepine followed by fosphenytoin/phenytoin, levetiracetam, phenobarbital, or valproic acid.
- Monitoring of patient vitals and oxygenation should be performed early.
- For seizures related to delirium tremens, intravenous benzodiazepines are first line but can also consider oral chlordiazepoxide 25–100 mg.
- Hypoglycemia-induced seizures in children: consider using dextrose as first line.
- Lacosamide or topiramate can be used if the initial treatments do not stop the seizures.
- If seizures continue, patient will likely need ICU level care, continuous monitoring, and expert consultation.
- Tertiary therapies include continuous infusions of benzodiazepines, propofol, and pentobarbital.

16.1.12 Steroid Medications

- See ▶ Table 16.15.[3,5]
- For steroids with intravenous and oral formulations, doses are considered equivalent.

Table 16.15 Comparison of oral and injectable steroids

Medication/Dosing routes	Equipotent dose (mg)	Duration of activity (h)	GC potency	MC potency
Betamethasone	0.75	36–54	30	0
IM, IA, ID				
Cortisone	25	8–12	0.8	0.8
PO only				
Dexamethasone	0.75	36–54	30	0
IV, IM, IA, ID, PO				
Fludrocortisone	N/A	24–36	N/A	150
PO only				
Hydrocortisone	20	8–12	1	1
IV, IM, PO				
Methylprednisolone	4	12–36	5	0.5
IV, IM, IA, ID, PO				
Prednisone	5	12–36	4	0.8
PO only				
Prednisolone	5	12–36	4	0.8
PO only				
Triamcinolone	4	12–36	5	0
IM, IA, ID				

Common steroid dosing regimens

Asthma exacerbation: IV methylprednisolone 40 mg every 12 h; PO prednisone 40–60 mg divided once or twice daily

Chronic immunosuppression: PO prednisone 5–20 mg daily

COPD exacerbation: IV methylprednisolone 60–125 mg every 24 h; PO prednisone 40 mg daily for 5–7 daily

Cerebral edema: IV dexamethasone 10 mg × 1 dose followed by 4 mg IV every 6 h

High-dose immunosuppression:

IV methylprednisolone 500–1,000 mg IV daily for 3–5 d followed by PO prednisone taper as appropriate

Septic shock:

IV hydrocortisone 200–300 mg/d divided every 6–8 h for at least 3 d

Stress dosing for patients already on glucocorticoids:

IV hydrocortisone 50–150 mg/d divided every 8–12 h for 1–2 d

Abbreviations: GC, glucocorticoid; IA, intra-articular; ID, intradermal; IM, intramuscular; IV, intravenous; MC, mineralocorticoid; PO, oral.

- Glucocorticoid and mineralocorticoid potencies are in comparison to hydrocortisone activity.
- For prolonged steroid courses (> 1 month), consider *Pneumocystis jirovecii* prophylaxis as well as gastric ulcer prophylaxis.

16.1.13 Thrombolytic Bleeding Management

- See ▶ Table 16.16.[3,11]
- Thrombolytic agents which work as plasminogen activators converting entrapped plasminogen to plasmin which degrade fibrinogen and fibrin causing thrombolysis.
- Thrombolytic agents are used for a wide variety of indications including ischemic stroke, pulmonary embolism, and myocardial infarction.
- Thrombolytic agents include Alteplase, Defibrotide, Reteplase, and Tenecteplase.
- No reversal agent currently exists for thrombolytic agents.
- If a serious bleed occurs during thrombolytic infusion or shortly after (< 24 hours) its infusion, do the following:
  - Stop infusion.
  - Check fibrinogen level.
  - Administer cryoprecipitate *and/or* either tranexamic acid *or* aminocaproic acid.

16.1.14 Vasopressors and Inotropes

- See ▶ Table 16.17.[3]
- Definitions:
  - Vasopressor: A drug causing the constriction of blood vessels.
  - Inotropy: Ability to contract in relation to a given preload, afterload, and HR.
  - Chronotropy: Ability to generate an electrical impulse at an intrinsic rate.
- Considerations:
  - Adrenergic medications should not be administered with alkaline solutions or sodium bicarbonate because they are inactivated, and line compatibility and distance from patient are critical with use of vasopressors.
  - Central line is recommended for administration particularly with any agent with α-agonist properties because of extravasation and tissue necrosis concerns.
  - High doses of epinephrine or norepinephrine are associated with increasing α_1 activity.
  - Dopamine—demonstrates dose-related receptor activity and does not provide exclusive receptor activity across dosing ranges; use cautiously in patients with history of heart disease or arrhythmias.
  - Epinephrine—mixed α and β activity, drug of choice for hemodynamically unstable anaphylactic reactions.
  - Norepinephrine—currently first line for septic shock and should be used in volume-resuscitated patients.

Table 16.16 Thrombolytic bleeding management dosing

Agent	Dose	Mechanism	Side effects
Aminocaproic acid (Amicar)	4–5 g IV over 1 h	Binds plasminogen to prevent fibrinolysis	• Bradycardia • Hypotension • Thrombosis
Cryoprecipitate	10 units IV infuse over 10–30 min Redose if repeat fibrinogen is < 150 mg/dL	Cryoprecipitate contains fibrinogen (200 mg/unit), FVIII, fibronectin, FXIII, and vWF	• Infusion reactions
Tranexamic acid (Cyklokapron)	1g 10–15 mg/kg IV over 20 min	Displaces plasminogen inhibiting fibrinolysis	• Headache • Hypotension • Sedation • Thrombosis

Abbreviations: IV, intravenous; FVIII/FXIII, factor VIII or XIII, respectively.

Table 16.17 Vasopressors and inotropes to support end-organ perfusion

	Medication	Dosing range	Site of action	Hemodynamic effects	Adverse effects
Vasopressors	Dopamine	1–3 µg/kg/min	D++++, β_1+	INT++, CHT+	Tachycardia, arrhythmias, mesenteric hypoperfusion, GI motility inhibition
		3–10 µg/kg/min	D++++, β_1++++, β_2+	INT++++, CHT++, HR↑, CI↑, SVR↑	
		>10–20 µg/kg/min	α_1+++, β_1++++, β_2+	INT+++, CHT+++, HR↑↑, CI↑, SVR↑↑	
	Epinephrine	0.01–0.3 µg/kg/min	α_1++, β_1++++, β_2+++	INT++++, CHT++, HR↑↑, CI↑↑ SVR (low dose) ↓, SVR (high dose) ↑	Tachycardia, arrhythmias, increased lactate, hyperglycemia, mesenteric hypoperfusion
	Norepinephrine	0.01–0.3 µg/kg/min	α_1++++, β_1+++, β_2+	INT+, CHT++, HR↑, CI↑↑, SVR ↑↑	Mesenteric hypoperfusion, peripheral ischemia, tachycardia
	Phenylephrine	0.1–3 µg/kg/min	α_1+++++	INT(0), CHT (0), CI↓ or ↑, SVR ↑	Peripheral ischemia, reflex bradycardia
	Vasopressin	0.01–0.04 units/min	V_1+V_2 agonism	INT(0), CHT (0), CI↔ or ↑, SVR ↑	Arrhythmias, peripheral ischemia
Inotropes	Dobutamine	2–20 µg/kg/min	α_1+, β_1++++, β_2++	INT++++, CHT++, HR↑, CI↑	Tachycardia, arrhythmias
	Isoproterenol	2–10 µg/kg/min	β_1+++++, β_2+++++	INT+++, CHT++++, HR↑↑, CI↑	Arrhythmias, cardiac ischemia, hypertension, hypotension
	Milrinone	0.3–0.75 µg/kg/min	PDE_3 inhibition	INT+++, CHT+++, HR↑↑, CI↑, SVR ↓	Arrhythmias, hypotension, cardiac ischemia

Abbreviations: CHT, chronotropy; D, dopamine receptor; HR, heart rate; INT, inotropy; PDE_3, phosphodiesterase type 3; V, arginine vasopressin receptor.

○ Phenylephrine—pure α agonist, ideal agent when a vasopressor is needed in tachycardic patients, should be used in volume-resuscitated patients.
○ Dobutamine—used to treat low cardiac index (CI), α_1-agonist and β_2-agonist counterbalance, leading to little change in systemic vascular resistance (SVR), use with caution in patients with a history of heart disease or arrhythmias.
○ Milrinone—used to treat low CI, longer duration of action than dobutamine, more pulmonary and systemic vasodilation than dobutamine, less tachycardia than dobutamine, accumulates in renal dysfunction.

16.2 Intubation, ACLS/PALS, Cardiac Arrest, and Stroke Reference

Michael Karsy

16.2.1 Intubation Checklist

- Introduction:
  - Formulation of a preintubation strategy and checklist has been shown to improve first-pass intubation and reduce complications.
  - Customization of a checklist should be performed for each institution (▶ Table 16.18).
  - Regarding selection of patients requiring intubation, see Section 2.3—Ventilator Management.
  - Regarding selection of medications for intubation, see Section 1.3—Anesthesia and 16.1—Key Medications.
  - Regarding postintubation patient management, see Section 1.3—Anesthesia.
- Rapid sequence intubation:
  - Simultaneous administration of induction agent and neuromuscular blocking agent.
  - Highly dependent on preoxygenation and reduced use of bag-mask ventilation to minimize risk of aspiration.
  - Increased risk of hypotension with induction especially in critical patients.
  - 14% of first-pass intubation show complication compared to 50% with second attempts.
  - Steps: Preparation, preoxygenation, paralysis with induction, intubation, postintubation management (▶ Table 16.18).
    - Preparation: Development of airway management plan, acquisition of personnel, medications and equipment, anticipation of airway difficulties, preparation for possible hypoxia and hypotension, establishment of IV access, patient positioning (20–30 degrees of elevated head of bed).
    - Preoxygenation: Increased functional reserve, utilization of 3 minutes of oxygen at highest flow rates; after preoxygenation healthy 70-kg adult can maintain saturation > 90% for 6–8 minutes of apnea; after preoxygenation children can maintain saturation > 90% for 4 minutes; highly dependent on patient physiology and pulmonary status; continuous passive oxygenation by nasal cannula can be used during intubation and can extend apnea time; jaw thrust and gentle ventilation assistive ventilation can be performed.
    - Postintubation management: Confirmation of endotracheal intubation is key and most accurate by waveform capnography; secondary methods include colorimetric capnography, visualization of the cords, misting of the tube, and auscultation of breath sounds and are not reliable for confirming placement; chest X-ray can only confirm depth of placement and securement of tube; and postintubation medications are used.
  - Postintubation hypotension:
    - Can be due to cardiogenic (e.g., poor cardiac function), distributive (e.g., sepsis, hemorrhagic shock, anaphylaxis), or obstructive shock (e.g., cardiac tamponade, pulmonary embolism) requiring specific recognition and treatment.

Table 16.18 Mnemonic for preparation of endotracheal intubation (STOPMAID)

Mnemonic	Description
S	Suction
T	Tools for intubation (laryngoscope blades, handles, video laryngoscope, Bougie, advance airway equipment)
O	Oxygen source: preoxygenation and ventilation
P	Positioning
M	Monitors: ECG, pulse oximetry, blood pressure, wave form capnography, colorimetric capnography, stethoscope
A	Assistant, Ambu bag with face mask, airway devices: endotracheal tube, syringes
I	Intravenous access
D	Drugs: induction agent, neuromuscular blocking agent, adjuncts

- Poor physiological reserve requiring IV fluids and pressors.
- High thoracic pressure from overventilation.
- Airway obstruction from mucous plug, fluids, or clots.
- Pediatric tube sizing:
  - ET tube size:
    - Uncuffed tube size = (age/4) + 4.
    - Cuffed tube size = (age/4) + 3.
  - ET tube depth:
    - Children > 1 year = age/2 + 13.
    - Children < 1 year = weight/2 + 8.

16.2.2 Advanced Cardiac Life Support (ACLS) Protocols

- Specific set of algorithms and knowledge used to improve patient outcomes after events; similar protocol between adult and pediatric patients but with differences in duration and vitals for pediatric patients (▶ Table 16.19).[22]
- For recognition of cardiac arrhythmias, see Chapter 2.5 Cardiac Arrhythmia and Chapter 16.1 Key Medications.
- For management of stroke, see Chapter 14.3 Vascular Diseases.[23]
- Management of bradycardia (▶ Fig. 16.1), tachycardia (▶ Fig. 16.2), cardiac arrest (▶ Fig. 16.3 and ▶ Fig. 16.4, ▶ Table 16.20), and stroke (▶ Table 16.21 and ▶ Table 16.22, ▶ Fig. 16.5).

Table 16.19 Pediatric vitals reference

Age	Heart rate (beats/min)	Systolic/diastolic blood pressure (mm Hg)[a]	Respiratory rate (breaths/min)
Premature	110–170	55–75/35–45	40–70
0–3 mo	110–160	65–85/45–55	35–55
3–6 mo	110–160	70–90/50–65	30–45
6–12 mo	90–160	80–100/55–65	22–38
1–3 y	80–150	90–105/55–70	22–30
3–6 y	70–120	95–110/60–75	20–24
6–12 y	60–110	100–120/60–75	16–22
> 12 y	60–100	110–135/65–85	12–20

[a] PALS guidelines for hypotension:

Neonate (0–28 d): SBP < 60 mm Hg.

Infant (1–12 mo): SBP < 70 mm Hg.

Young children (1–10 y): SBP < 70 + (2 × age in years) mm Hg.

Older children (> 10 y): SBP < 90 mm Hg.

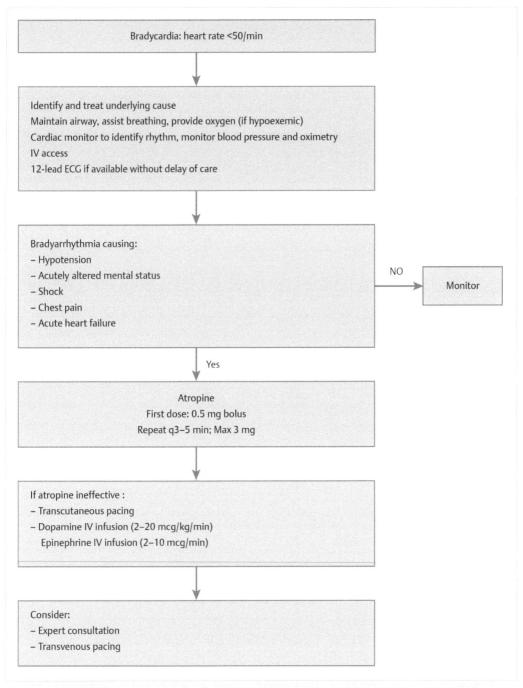

Fig. 16.1 Bradycardia protocol for adult and pediatric patients. PALS doses: atropine (0.02 mg/kg, repeat once, min: 0.1 mg, max: 0.5 mg), epinephrine (0.01 mg/kg 1:10,000 concentration q3–5 min IV/IO; 0.1 mg/kg 1:1,000 ET tube).

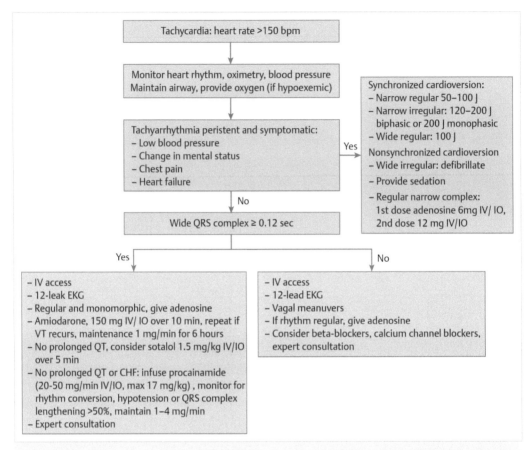

Fig. 16.2 Tachycardia protocol. PALS doses: adenosine (first dose 0.1 mg/kg, IV/IO, max: 6 mg; second dose: 0.2 mg/kg, IV/IO, max 12 mg), amiodarone (5 mg/kg IV/IO, over 20–60 min), procainamide (15 mg/kg, IV/IO, over 30–60 min). Cardioversion shock energy: monophasic or biphasic, 0.5–1.0 J/kg. Defibrillation shock energy: monophasic or biphasic, 2 J/kg for first attempt, 4 J/kg for second attempt, ≥4 J/kg for subsequent attempts. bpm, beats per minute; CHF, congestive heart failure.

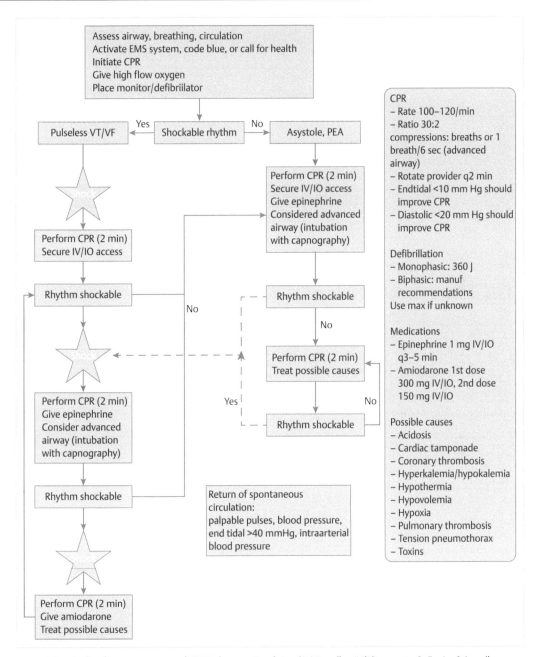

Fig. 16.3 ACLS/cardiac arrest protocol. PALS doses: epinephrine (0.01 mg/kg, IV/IO, repeat q3–5 min; 0.1 mg/kg through endotracheal tube); amiodarone (5 mg/kg, IV/IO, may repeat up to two times) *or* lidocaine (1 mg/kg load, IV/IO, maintenance 20–50 µg/kg/min, repeat bolus if infusion initiated > 15 min after initial bolus). Cardioversion shock energy: monophasic or biphasic, 0.5–1.0 J/kg. Defibrillation shock energy: monophasic or biphasic, 2 J/kg for first attempt, 4 J/kg for second attempt, ≥ 4 J/kg for subsequent attempts. CPR, cardiopulmonary resuscitation; EMS, emergency medical system.

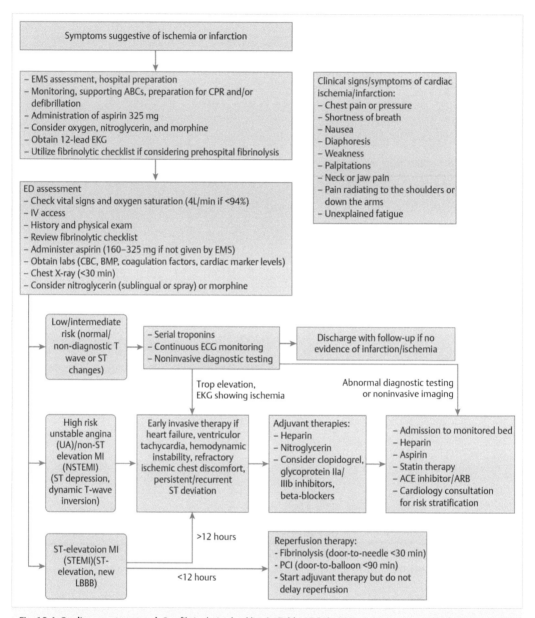

Fig. 16.4 Cardiac arrest protocol. See fibrinolytic checklist (► Table 16.21). ACE, angiotensin-converting enzyme; ARB, angiotensin II receptor blocker; BMP, basic metabolic panel; CBC, complete blood count; ED, emergency department; EMS, emergency medical service; LBBB, left bundle branch block.

Table 16.20 Tissue plasminogen activator checklist for myocardial infarction

Inclusion	• Chest discomfort for > 15 min and < 12 h • EKG showing STEMI or new LBBB
Contraindications	• Systolic BP > 180–200 mm Hg, diastolic BP > 100–100 mm Hg • Right vs. left systolic BP difference > 15 mm Hg • History of structural central nervous system disease • Significant closed head/facial trauma within previous 3 mo • Stroke > 3 h or < 3 mo • Major trauma, surgery (including laser eye surgery), gastrointestinal/genitourinary bleeding within previous 2–4 wk • Any history of intracranial hemorrhage • Bleeding or clotting disorders; blood thinners • Pregnancy • Serious systemic disease (advanced cancer, liver disease, or kidney disease)
High-risk criteria, consider transfer to PCI facility	• Contraindications to fibrinolytic therapy • Heart rate ≥ 100/min and systolic BP < 100 mm Hg • Pulmonary edema • Signs of shock • Required CPR

Table 16.21 National Institutes of Health stroke scale

1a. Level of consciousness	0: alert
	1: drowsy
	2: stuporous
	3: coma
1b. Level of consciousness questions (month, age)	0: answers both correctly
	1: answers one correctly
	2: incorrect
1c. Level of consciousness commands (open/close eyes, make fist/let go)	0: obeys both correctly
	1: obeys one correctly
	2: incorrect
2. Best gaze (eyes open, patient follows examiner's finger or face)	0: normal
	1: partial gaze palsy
	2: forced deviation
3. Visual fields (introduce visual stimulus/threat to patient visual field quadrants)	0: no visual loss
	1: partial hemianopia
	2: complete hemianopia
	3: bilateral hemianopia/blindness
4. Facial paresis (shows tech, raise eyebrows, squeeze eye shut)	0: normal
	1: minor
	2: partial
	3: complete
5a. Motor left arm	0: no drift
5b. Motor right arm	1: drift
(elevate arm to 90 degrees if patient is sitting, 45 degrees if supine)	2: cannot resist gravity
	3: no effort against gravity
	4: no movement
	x: untestable (joint fusion or limb amp)
6a. Motor left leg	0: no drift

(Continued)

Table 16.21 *(Continued)* National Institutes of Health stroke scale

6b. Motor right leg	1: drift
	2: cannot resist gravity
	3: no effort against gravity
	4: no movement
	X: untestable (joint fusion or limb amp)
7. Limb ataxia (finger-nose, heel-to-shin)	0: no ataxia
	1: present in 1 limb
	2: present in 2 limbs
8. Sensory (pin prick to face, arm, trunk and legs; comparing side to side)	0: normal
	1: partial loss
	2: severe loss
9. Best language (name item, describe a picture, read sentences)	0: no aphasia
	1: mild to moderate aphasia
	2: severe aphasia
	3: mute
10. Dysarthria (evaluate speech clarity by patient repeating listed words)	0: normal articulation
	1: mild to moderate slurring of words
	2: near to unintelligible or worse
	X: untested (intubated or other physical barrier)
11. Extinction and inattention (use information from prior testing to identify neglect or double simultaneous stimuli testing)	0: no neglect
	1: partial neglect
	2: complete neglect

Note: NIHSS max score 42: no stroke (0), minor (1–4), moderate (5–15), moderate-severe (16–20), severe (21–42).

Table 16.22 Tissue plasminogen activator checklist for acute stroke

Inclusion	• Witnessed time of onset of symptoms or last known normal < 3 h (additional criteria if 3–4.5 h, see below) • Age ≥ 18 y
Exclusion	• Neurosurgery, significant head trauma or prior stroke in previous 3 mo • Clinical presentation suggests subarachnoid hemorrhage • Uncontrolled hypertension (> 185 mm Hg systolic or > 110 mm Hg diastolic) • Known intracranial arteriovenous malformation, neoplasm, or aneurysm • Active internal bleeding • Known coagulopathy: (1) platelet count < 100,000, (2) patient received heparin within 48 h and has elevated PTT greater than upper limit of normal for lab, (3) current use of oral anticoagulants (e.g., warfarin) and INR > 1.7, (4) current use of direct thrombin inhibitors or direct factor Xa inhibitors • Abnormal blood glucose (< 50 mg/dL)
Relative contraindications	• Only minor or rapidly improving stroke symptoms • Major surgery or serious non–head trauma in previous 14 d • History of gastrointestinal or urinary tract hemorrhage within 21 d • Seizure at stroke onset • Recent arterial puncture at noncompressible site • Recent lumbar puncture • Post-myocardial infarction pericarditis • Pregnancy
Additional warnings TPA 3–4.5 h)	• Age > 80 y • History of prior stroke and diabetes • Any active anticoagulant use (even with INR < 1.7) • NIH Stroke Scale (NIHSS) > 25 • CT showing multilobar infarction (hypodensity > 1/3 cerebral hemispheres)

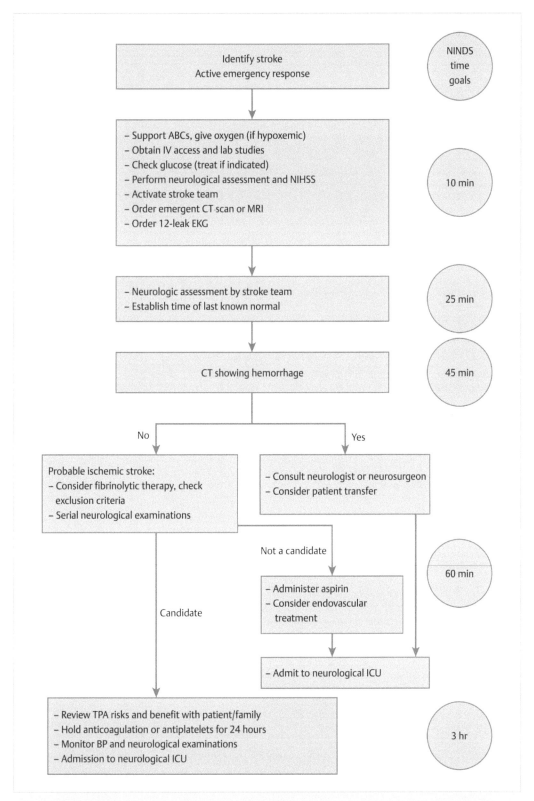

Fig. 16.5 Stroke protocol. See tissue plasminogen activator (TPA) checklist (▶ Table 16.20). ABC, airway, breathing, circulation; NINDS, National Institute of Neurological Disorders and Stroke.

References

[1] Chou R, Gordon DB, de Leon-Casasola OA, et al. Management of postoperative pain: a clinical practice guideline from the American Pain Society, the American Society of Regional Anesthesia and Pain Medicine, and the American Society of Anesthesiologists' Committee on Regional Anesthesia, Executive Committee, and Administrative Council. J Pain. 2016; 17(2):131–157

[2] Devlin JW, Skrobik Y, Gélinas C, et al. Clinical Practice Guidelines for the Prevention and Management of Pain, Agitation/Sedation, Delirium, Immobility, and Sleep Disruption in Adult Patients in the ICU. Crit Care Med. 2018; 46(9):e825–e873

[3] Lexicomp. Drug Information Handbook with International Trade Names Index. 25th ed. Hudson, OH: Lexi-Comp; 2016

[4] Becker DE, Reed KL. Local anesthetics: review of pharmacological considerations. Anesth Prog. 2012; 59(2):90–101, quiz 102–103

[5] Micromedex Solutions. Greenwood Village, CO: Truven Health Analytics 2019. Available at: https://www.micromedexsolutions.com/micromedex2. Accessed January 5, 2019

[6] Walsh K, Arya R. A simple formula for quick and accurate calculation of maximum allowable volume of local anaesthetic agents. Br J Dermatol. 2015; 172(3):825–826

[7] Stollings JL, Diedrich DA, Oyen LJ, Brown DR. Rapid-sequence intubation: a review of the process and considerations when choosing medications. Ann Pharmacother. 2014; 48(1):62–76

[8] Kowey PR. Pharmacological effects of antiarrhythmic drugs. Review and update. Arch Intern Med. 1998; 158(4):325–332

[9] Tsu LV. Antiarrhythmic therapy for Atrial Fibrillation. US Pharm. 2013; 38(2):20–23

[10] Evidence-based medicine consult. Available at: https://www.ebmconsult.com/. Reviewed 2018. Accessed January 9, 2019

[11] Frontera JA, Lewin JJ, III, Rabinstein AA, et al. Guideline for reversal of antithrombotics in intracranial hemorrhage: a statement for healthcare professionals from the Neurocritical Care Society and Society of Critical Care Medicine. Neurocrit Care. 2016; 24(1):6–46

[12] Rogers KC, Finks SW. A new option for reversing the anticoagulant effect of factor Xa inhibitors: andexanet alfa (ANDEXXA). Am J Med. 2019; 132(1):38–41

[13] Johnson W, Nguyen ML, Patel R. Hypertension crisis in the emergency department. Cardiol Clin. 2012; 30(4):533–543

[14] Aggarwal M, Khan IA. Hypertensive crisis: hypertensive emergencies and urgencies. Cardiol Clin. 2006; 24(1):135–146

[15] Muiesan ML, Salvetti M, Amadoro V, et al. Working Group on Hypertension, Prevention, Rehabilitation of the Italian Society of Cardiology, the Societa' Italiana dell'Ipertensione Arteriosa. An update on hypertensive emergencies and urgencies. J Cardiovasc Med (Hagerstown). 2015; 16(5):372–382

[16] 2018 GINA Report, Global Strategy for Asthma Management and Prevention. Available at: https://ginasthma.org/2018-gina-report-global-strategy-for-asthma-management-and-prevention/. Published 2018. Accessed January 2, 2019

[17] Müller-Lissner S, Bassotti G, Coffin B, et al. Opioid-induced constipation and bowel dysfunction: a clinical guideline. Pain Med. 2017; 18(10):1837–1863

[18] Paquette IM, Varma M, Ternent C, et al. The American Society of Colon and Rectal Surgeons' Clinical Practice Guideline for the evaluation and management of constipation. Dis Colon Rectum. 2016; 59(6):479–492

[19] See S, Ginzburg R. Choosing a skeletal muscle relaxant. Am Fam Physician. 2008; 78(3):365–370

[20] Schwenk ES, Viscusi ER, Buvanendran A, et al. consensus guidelines on the use of intravenous ketamine infusions for acute pain management from the American Society of Regional Anesthesia and Pain Medicine, the American Academy of Pain Medicine, and the American Society of Anesthesiologists. Reg Anesth Pain Med. 2018; 43(5):456–466

[21] Brophy GM, Bell R, Claassen J, et al. Neurocritical Care Society Status Epilepticus Guideline Writing Committee. Guidelines for the evaluation and management of status epilepticus. Neurocrit Care. 2012; 17(1):3–23

[22] Field JM, Hazinski MF, Sayre MR, et al. Part 1: executive summary: 2010 American Heart Association Guidelines for Cardiopulmonary Resuscitation and Emergency Cardiovascular Care. Circulation. 2010; 122:S640

[23] Powers WJ, Rabinstein AA, Ackerson T, et al. Guidelines for the early management of patients with acute ischemic stroke: 2019 update to the 2018 guidelines for the early management of acute ischemic stroke: A guideline for healthcare professionals from the American Heart Association/American Stroke Association. Stroke. 2010; 50:e344

Index

Note: Page numbers set **bold** or *italic* indicate headings or figures, respectively.